Difficult and Complicated Cases in Refractive Surgery

Jorge L. Alió • Dimitri T. Azar
Alessandro Abbouda • Amr El Aswad
Editors

Difficult and Complicated Cases in Refractive Surgery

Springer

Editors
Jorge L. Alió, MD, PhD
Department of Anterior Segment & Refractive Surgery
Vissum Corporation Instituto Oftalmológico
Alicante
Spain

Dimitri T. Azar, MD, MBA
Ophthalmology and Visual Sciences
Illinois Eye and Ear Infirmary
University of Illinois at Chicago
Chicago, IL
USA

Alessandro Abbouda, MD
R&D Department
Vissum Corporation Instituto Oftalmológico
Alicante
Spain

Amr El Aswad, MD
R&D Department
Vissum Corporation Instituto Oftalmológico
Alicante
Spain

Additional material to this book can be downloaded from http://extras.springer.com

ISBN 978-3-662-52130-4 ISBN 978-3-642-55238-0 (eBook)
DOI 10.1007/978-3-642-55238-0

Springer Heidelberg New York Dordrecht London

Softcover re-print of the Hardcover 1st edition 2015

Printed on acid-free paper

Springer is part of Springer Science+Business Media (www.springer.com)

To my Father,
All your help and support has allowed me to become a doctor. Thank you from the bottom of my heart.

Alessandro

Foreword

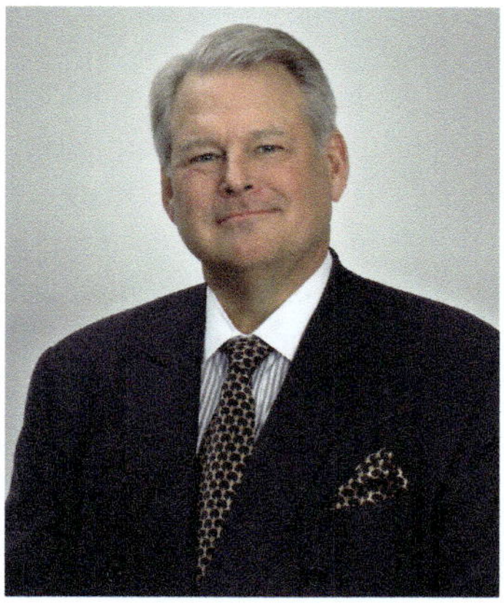

Refractive corneal surgery, including Lasik, PRK/Lasek, corneal inlays, collagen cross-linking, intracorneal ring segments, thermal keratoplasty, incisional refractive surgery including radial and astigmatic keratotomy/limbal relaxing incisions, and phakic intraocular lenses, together represent the second most common surgical procedure performed by the ophthalmic surgeon worldwide. While cataract surgery dominates at approximately 20,000,000 procedures per year globally, refractive corneal surgery including those procedures used in combination with cataract surgery together accounts for over 5,000,000 surgical interventions annually. In the modern era of ophthalmology, every ophthalmic surgeon must consider the refractive outcomes generated by every procedure, as a patient's daily visual function and quality of life are significantly impacted by their residual refractive error following surgery. Like every invasive procedure, refractive corneal surgery and phakic intraocular lenses are associated with complications. The proper prevention and timely management of intraoperative and postoperative complications is the hallmark of the master ophthalmic surgeon.

In their new book, *Complicated Cases in Refractive Surgery*, two master surgeons, Jorge Alio, M.D., and Dimitri Azar, M.D., along with a carefully selected group of highly experienced and respected colleagues present us with an extraordinary compilation of 101 select cases of both common and rarer complications, including their presentation, management, and clinical outcomes. This style of teaching using real-life cases is extremely effective and popular with surgeons, as it provides a learning experience that is impactful and more easily remembered than the typical didactic chapter referencing the published literature.

This new book, a follow-on publication to the same two editors' popular *Management of Complications in Refractive Surgery*, published in 2009 and translated into multiple languages, is a must read for every ophthalmic surgeon who performs refractive surgery along with those who help manage or encounter these patients in daily practice. The case presentation format is engaging and an easy read. The cases presented are well selected, are edited for maximum educational value, and provide the reader with one clinically useful pearl after another. Drs. Alio and Azar, thank you again for providing us with such a powerful and pleasant learning experience that is certain to benefit surgeons and patients worldwide for years to come.

Richard L. Lindstrom, MD
Department of Ophthalmology,
UC Irvine Gavin Herbert Eye Institute,
Minnesota Lions Eye Bank,
University of Minnesota,
Minneapolis, MN, USA

Preface

This is a unique book in which a clinical cases affected by complications of refractive surgery are presented as a series of cases to illustrate how, in practical terms, such complications can be managed.

In 2007, we published our book *Complicated Cases in Refractive Surgery*, which was well received and which has been translated into many different languages including Chinese. In that book, we offered state of the art pathogenesis and knowledge of management of complications in refractive surgery from classical techniques to the most recent innovations. In this book, we illustrate the practical knowledge and details that are necessary to achieve successful outcomes in many of these complex cases.

This book has been created based on the didactic technique known as "problem resolution." Problem resolution is a modern, innovative pedagological method of teaching medicine. We should not forget, however, that 2400 years ago, on the island of Kos, Hippocrates and the Hippocratic doctors were applying the hands on method to teach their students. The practice of medicine was basically empirical, and it was not until later that the volume of medical science enabled formal theoretical teachingto be incorporated into the curriculum.

In this book, the reader will find a series of interesting cases that illustrate the most frequent and complicated cases in refractive surgery and how different authors have accomplished their solutions successfully. While mostly-cases with successful outcomes have been included we have tried to illustrate in 101 cases how potential nightmares can have happy endings. We have simplified the process of analyzing the cases and extracting what is really the practical message that each case offers.

Our hope is that the reader will learn how difficult cases can be approached and solved, using the latest technology and medical knowledge available. Reproduction is a way to demonstrate, and demonstration is the basis of medical science. The art of being a doctor is using the scientific background that the doctor has jointly with his/her practice and experience that guides the medical judgment toward the best option for the patient. We hope that you will find the chosen cases of interest and be intrigued by the medical challenge they represent. Finally, the successful outcome that has been accomplished by the talented and innovative coauthors of this book.

We want to thank our talented coauthors for providing cases with innovative techniques and successful outcomes. We also would like to thank our associate editors for the many hours of work devoted to gathering together these cases, to simplify the process of editing, and to offer a unique format which can be easily comprehended and readily applied to your own patients. In editing this book, we have felt that we have been walking on the island of Kos and writing this book jointly with our Hippocratic colleagues.

Signed in Alicante and Chicago 2015

Alicante, Spain Jorge L. Alió, MD, PhD
Chicago, IL, USA Dimitri T. Azar, MD, MBA

Contents

How This Medical Book Was Inspired

Aesculapius: The Symbol of Medicine and Hippocratic Medicine
Our Aesculapius in Alicante
By Jorge L. Alió and Alessandro Abbouda

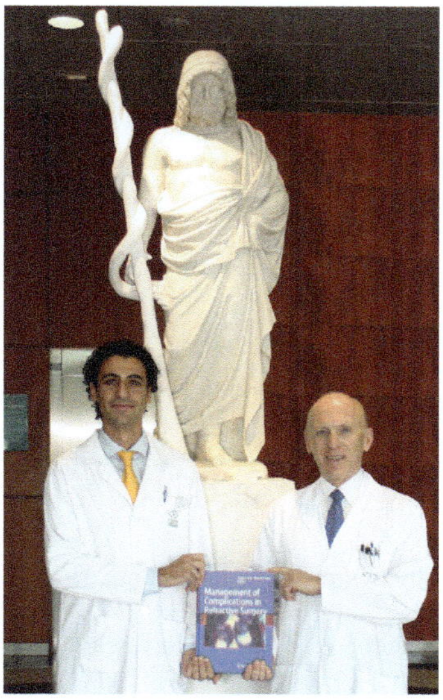

Vissum Corporation Instituto Oftalmologico of Alicante exhibits an original roman statue dating from the first century A.D. The statue was found near a temple in the south of Messina. Our Aesculapius travelled around the word from the Chicago collection to Seville, and in September 2011 this statue arrived in Alicante thanks to the patronage of Prof. Alio who donated the piece to the center as a sign of respect for all patients and the medical profession.

The ground floor of the clinic was built based on the distribution of the Epidaurus temple where the statue could be observed from above and meanwhile the sick could sleep overnight on the bare ground beside the statue.

The statue possesses all the typical elements of Aesculapius. A mature man with a calm expression, a tunic around his waist, then draped over one of his shoulders and wrapped around his lower torso and legs; curly beard; thick hair; one arm resting on the snake staff and the other on his hip. The right arm and the snake staff have both been restored.

According to the ancient Greek legends, Aesculapius was the son of Apollo and Coronis. Coronis was unfaithful to Apollo, and Artemis, Apollo's twin sister, killed her for her unfaithfulness. Apollo felt sorrow for his unborn son and snatched the child Asclepius from his mother's corpse, saving him from death. Apollo then handed Aesculapius over to the centaur Chiron who became his tutor and mentor.

Chiron taught Aesculapius the art of healing. According to Pindar (Pythian Odes), Aesculapius also acquired the knowledge of surgery, the use of drugs, love potions and incantations, and according to Apollodorus (the Library), Athena gave Aesculapius a magic potion made from the blood of the Gorgon. With these gifts Aesculapius transcended the bounds of human knowledge.

The main attribute of Aesculapius is a physician's staff with a snake wrapped around it; this is how he was distinguished in the art of healing, and his attribute still survives to this day as the symbol of the modern medical profession. The World Health Organization has used Aesculapius' symbols as its emblem since its foundation in 1947.

There were many centers and schools of medicine, from Trikkis in Thessaly to the island of Cos. It is believed that Hippocrates, a great doctor of antiquity, practiced his trade on the island of Cos. It is also said that Hippocrates was a descendant of Aesculapius. His disciples received the teaching of medicine, listening to the explanation walking with him while he was attending patients.

The format of our book is inspired by Hippocrates' style of teaching medicine based on the resolution of problems.

References

Christou P, Papastamatis K (eds) (2003) Gods and heroes in greek mythology. Bonechi (Bonechi), Sleaford, LINCS, UK

Adkins L, Adkins RA (1997) Ancient Greece a handbook. Oxford University Press, New York

Hallam E (1996) Gods and goddesses. MacMillan Publishing Company, Pembrokeshire, UK

Part I

Complications in Refractive Laser Treatment Plan

Dear reader,

This chapter includes cases related to the importance of preoperative planning before performing refractive surgery. Refractive surprise is not common today with excimer laser technology, but in cases such as elevated myopia and hyperopia and more in cases of astigmatism, an error in power or axis may be devastating for the patient and the surgeon. Furthermore, it is increasingly common to receive patients for cataract surgery who have previously undergone a corneal refractive procedure. The expectations of these patients are very high in terms of refractive outcomes and until the present we lacked an exact formula to determine the best IOL power.

The cases in this chapter describe situations such as management of refractive shifts, IOL calculations following refractive surgery, cataract surgery prior to refractive surgery, management of high astigmatism, and avoiding corneal grafts. After reading this chapter, we hope that the planning and management techniques from these cases will allow you to plan and select safe refractive treatments for your patient and to manage unexpected problems.

For a theoretical complement, we suggest the first book of this series: J. L. Alio', D. Azar *Management of Complications in Refractive Surgery*, Chapter 6: Refractive Miscalculation with Refractive Surprise (pp. 103–112) and Chapter 7: Optical Aberration (pp. 113–152).

Furthermore, in the appendix of this book, you will find a "step-by-step approach for planning refractive correction of highly aberrated eyes in excimer laser refractive corneal surgery." This will help to explain the application of customized treatment described in some of the cases in this chapter.

Specific topics covered by the cases include hyperopic shift following RK resolved by corneal wavefront PRK (Case 1) and how to manage high refractive defect choosing two procedures, IOL and LASIK/PRK (Cases 2 and 3). Other cases cover the challenge of IOL calculation and the optical quality of hyperopic or myopic patients previously treated by refractive surgery (Cases 4 and 5); intraoperative aberrometry, a new tool used for post-refractive surgery IOL power calculations (Case 6); high amount of refractive astigmatism solved by using a toric IOL and subsequent LASIK (Case 7); and the corneal epithelium's ability to alter in thickness profile and compensate for changes in stromal surface curvature (Case 8). Other cases cover sequential custom therapeutic keratectomy, a new tool for high irregular astigmatism (Case 9); how to manage high astigmatism after a penetrating keratoplasty (Case 10); how to solve corneal leukoma without a corneal transplant (Case 11); how to manage high astigmatism after a penetrating phaco wound burn (Case 12); and automated superficial lamellar keratectomy augmented with hyaluronic-assisted PTK as a new tool to avoid corneal graft (Case 13). We end with cases focused on the multifocal lens property and visual acuity (Case 14), an alternative treatment to amblyopia in consideration of difficult cases (Case 15), higher order of aberrations, the principal cause of poor scotopic vision after laser vision correction (Case 16), managing an unsatisfied patient after cataract surgery, a didactic case of monovision (Case 17), and errors in the excimer refractive program (Case 18).

Lesson to learn in these cases:

Case 1: Hyperopic result after corneal wavefront-guided PRK on an RK eye

A postradial keratotomy patient developed hyperopic shift and was treated by corneal wavefront PRK improving the refraction and the values of high order of aberrometry.

Case 2: Refractive laser treatment post phakic IOLs by LASIK

The complete correction of high refractive defect can find advantage from the joint effect of two different refractive procedures.

Case 3: Refractive laser treatment post ICL in high myopia by PRK

When a complete emmetropia is not achieved by ICL implantation and cornea is thick enough, a secondary PRK treatment could be a good solution.

Case 4: IOL calculation in a previous refractive hyperopic patient

How to solve the challenge of IOL power calculation and IOL selection in a hyperopic patient previously treated by corneal refractive surgery?

Case 5: Refractive surprise after cataract surgery solved in a patient that underwent corneal refractive surgery 12 years ago

The challenge of IOL calculation and the optical quality in a myopic patient previously treated by corneal refractive surgery. How to obtain a good result?

Case 6: Post-refractive surgery IOL power calculation, intraoperative aberrometry

The use of intraoperative wavefront aberrometry appears to increase the accuracy in post-refractive surgery IOL power calculation.

Case 7: Refractive lens exchange for high hyperopic astigmatism followed by LASIK

Different solutions to manage the high amount of refractive astigmatism remaining after the IOL implantation: to rotate the toric IOL, to explant the toric IOL, or to replace it with one with a different toricity?

Case 8: Transepithelial phototherapeutic keratectomy for irregularly irregular astigmatism

A transepithelial phototherapeutic keratectomy (PTK) procedure is a more appropriate and effective treatment than topography- or wavefront-guided

treatment due to the error introduced by significant topographic changes due to epithelial thickness remodeling.

Case 9: Sequential custom therapeutic keratectomy for irregular astigmatism

Sequential custom therapeutic keratectomy is a custom corneal topography-based excimer laser ablation, followed by a second intraoperative corneal topography to evaluate residual irregularities and to immediately plan on-site further custom-based ablation.

Case 10: Combined post-keratoplasty LASIK/AK to treat high astigmatism

When conservative method fails, the residual high astigmatism after penetrating keratoplasty can be treated by astigmatic keratotomy followed by LASIK.

Case 11: Avoiding a corneal graft: from corneal surgery to phakic IOL

A central corneal leukoma can be solved without corneal transplant using corneal excision followed by the correction of the residual refractive error by a phakic IOL.

Case 12: Excimer laser treatment of irregular astigmatism following phaco wound burn

A 93-year-old patient with dense nucleus cataract suffered a corneal phaco burn. PRK was an excellent solution to restore a good visual acuity.

Case 13: Femtosecond laser-assisted superficial lamellar keratectomy for the treatment of superficial corneal leukomas

An automated superficial lamellar keratectomy augmented with hyaluronic-assisted PTK is a reasonable treatment in a patient with central corneal leukoma after an infection to avoid a corneal graft.

Case 14: How to manage with LASIK hyperopic shift after multifocal lens?

How to manage the tricky problem of an unexpected refractive outcome following multifocal IOL implantation?

Case 15: LASIK and severe anisometropia in a child

An alternative treatment to reverse anisometropic amblyopia should take into account when the traditional methods are not suitable.

Case 16: Refractive laser treatment plan, night vision disturbance

A decreased contrast sensitivity, uncorrected lower-order aberrations, and induced higher-order aberration are the main causes of poor scotopic vision after laser vision correction. How to find a solution to the problem?

Case 17: Use of excimer laser surgery for monovision in cases of unsatisfactory outcome following cataract surgery

Pseudophakic monovision is an effective approach for managing loss of accommodation after cataract surgery, and it can be very useful in a patient who wants to be free from glasses.

Case 18: Error in the excimer refractive program. From a simple mistake to a major clinical problem

To remember the importance of a good refractive planning, we present a nightmare case for the surgeon and the patient but with the happy end.

Hyperopic Result After Corneal Wavefront-Guided PRK on an RK Eye

1

Jaime Aramberri Agesta

Contents

J.A. Agesta, MD
Department of Refractive Surgery, Begitek, San Sebastian, Spain

Okular, Vitoria, Spain
e-mail: jaimearamberri@telefonica.net

Why Is This Case Relevant for the Refractive Surgeon?

Refractive surgery on a cornea with a previous radial keratotomy can be challenging in terms of laser programming, as corneal response to PRK can differ significantly from a normal cornea.

Case Background

A 50-year-old man complains of low vision on his RE after radial keratotomy (RK) surgery which was performed 12 years before. RE BCVA was 20/63 with +2.25 sph −3.25 cyl × 135°, and LE BCVA, also operated by RK, was 20/32 with +0.50 sph −1.00 cyl × 80°. Slit lamp exploration revealed 12-cut radial keratotomy on both eyes. There was a slight nasal decentration on the RE with respect to the pupil center. Corneal topography displayed a small optical zone and asymmetric bow-tie pattern with flatter inferior hemicornea. Total aberrometry confirmed high optical irregularity with a higher-order aberration RMS of 4.43 μ for a 6 mm area of analysis. Most affected coefficients were fourth-order spherical aberration and third-order coma. Fundus exploration showed a mild myopic macular atrophy and tilted optic disc in both eyes.

J.L. Alió et al. (eds.), *Difficult and Complicated Cases in Refractive Surgery*,
DOI 10.1007/978-3-642-55238-0_1, © Springer-Verlag Berlin Heidelberg 2015

Main Problem to Solve

The objective of the treatment is to improve corneal optics, increasing and centering the optical zone and decreasing high-order aberrations.

Ancillary Tests

Ectasia risk can be determined by corneal tomography and Ocular Response Analyzer (ORA) studies. Corneal aberrometry is the key point to calculate the shotfile to eliminate the higher-order aberrations. Spherical aberration correction will induce some sphere change that needs compensation when the case is programmed. It is important that the user knows the sign of this refractive change as depending on how the software is programmed it can be myopic or hyperopic. In this case, Schwind ORK-W software was used and the induced myopia was compensated using a surgeon-developed nomogram.

Surgical/Medical Intervention

Epithelium removal prior to PRK was performed mechanically after 20 s of 20 % ethanol solution. First, the high-order correction pattern, as calculated by the Schwind ORK-W software from corneal topography aberrometry with the Schwind ESIRIS laser, was ablated, and second, the refractive pattern with the correspondent sphere and cylinder compensation for the depth of the ablated Z(4,0), Z(3,−1), and Z(3,1) coefficients. The ORK-W software version was used to undercorrect HOA treatments, so 20 % overcorrection of all coefficients was programmed. The target refraction was −0.50 sph. 0.02 % mitomycin C was applied for 30 s on the ablated surface at the end of surgery.

Outcome

Three months after surgery, BCVA was 20/50 with +1.00 sph −0.50 cyl × 180°. This meant a 1 D sphere equivalent refractive prediction error in the hyperopic side. Six months after surgery, a new PRK was performed and final refraction, 3 months later, was planned. Higher-order aberrations improved significantly, with a relevant decrease of most affected Zernike coefficients.

What to Learn from This Case

PRK sphere equivalent results are more variable than normal eyes, especially when higher-order corrections are added. Predictability can be even worse if subepithelial irregularity correction via transepithelial approach is aimed [1–5]. In our experience the variability is random and can be in both the myopic and hyperopic side. Therefore, programming has to be carefully designed and patients are informed about a higher rate of retreatment need. This case also illustrates the need for mitomycin application after PRK in patients with prior RK (Figs. 1.1, 1.2, 1.3, 1.4, and 1.5).

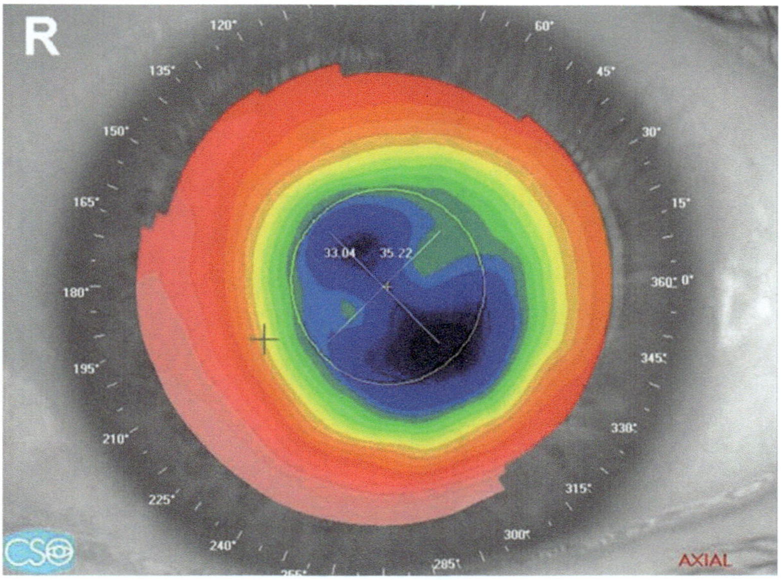

Fig. 1.1 RE corneal topography at first clinical visit: small optical zone with a slight nasal decentration. Irregular astigmatism with a flatter inferior component of the bow tie. Sim K astigmatism magnitude was −2.18 × 135°

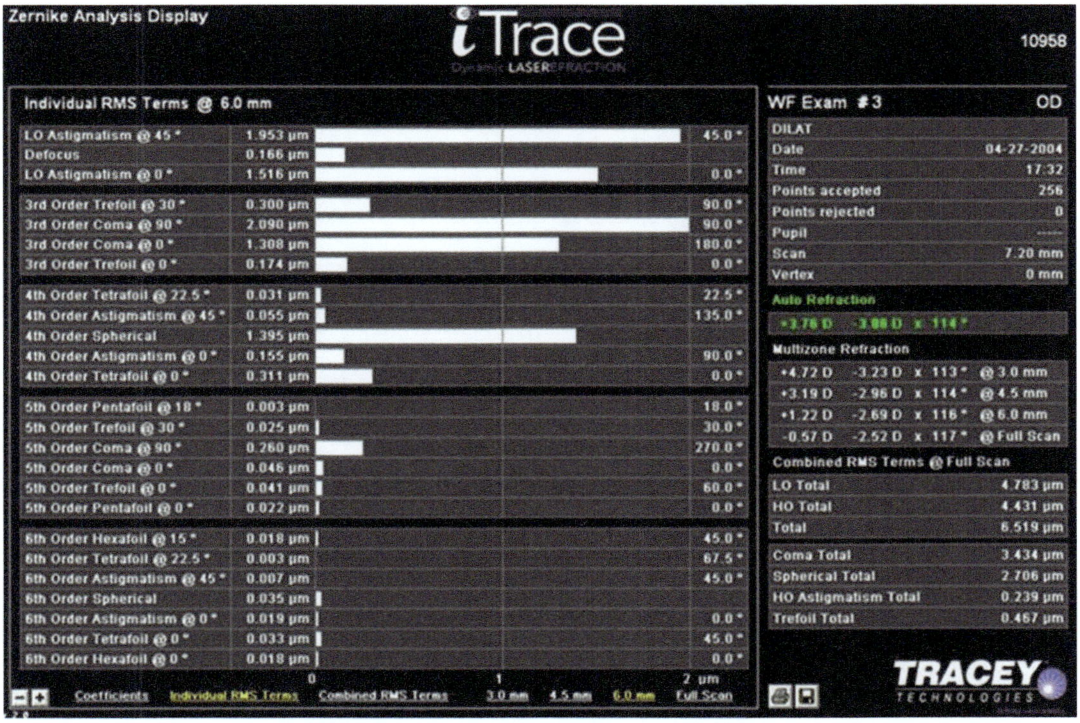

Fig. 1.2 Total aberrometry: high low-order astigmatism, third-order coma, and fourth-order spherical aberration. High-order aberration RMS is 4.43 µ (for a 6.00 mm area of analysis)

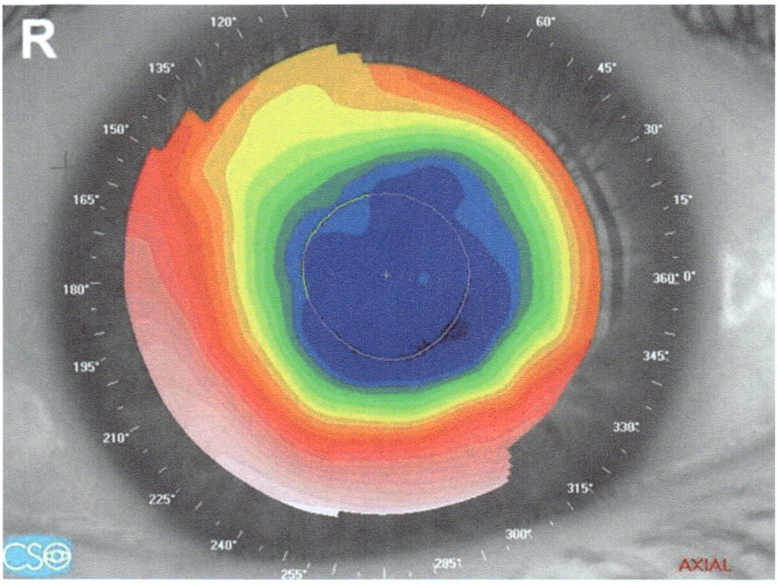

Fig. 1.3 Postoperative corneal topography: clear improvement of astigmatism and higher-order aberrations. Optical zone is wider, better centered, and more regular

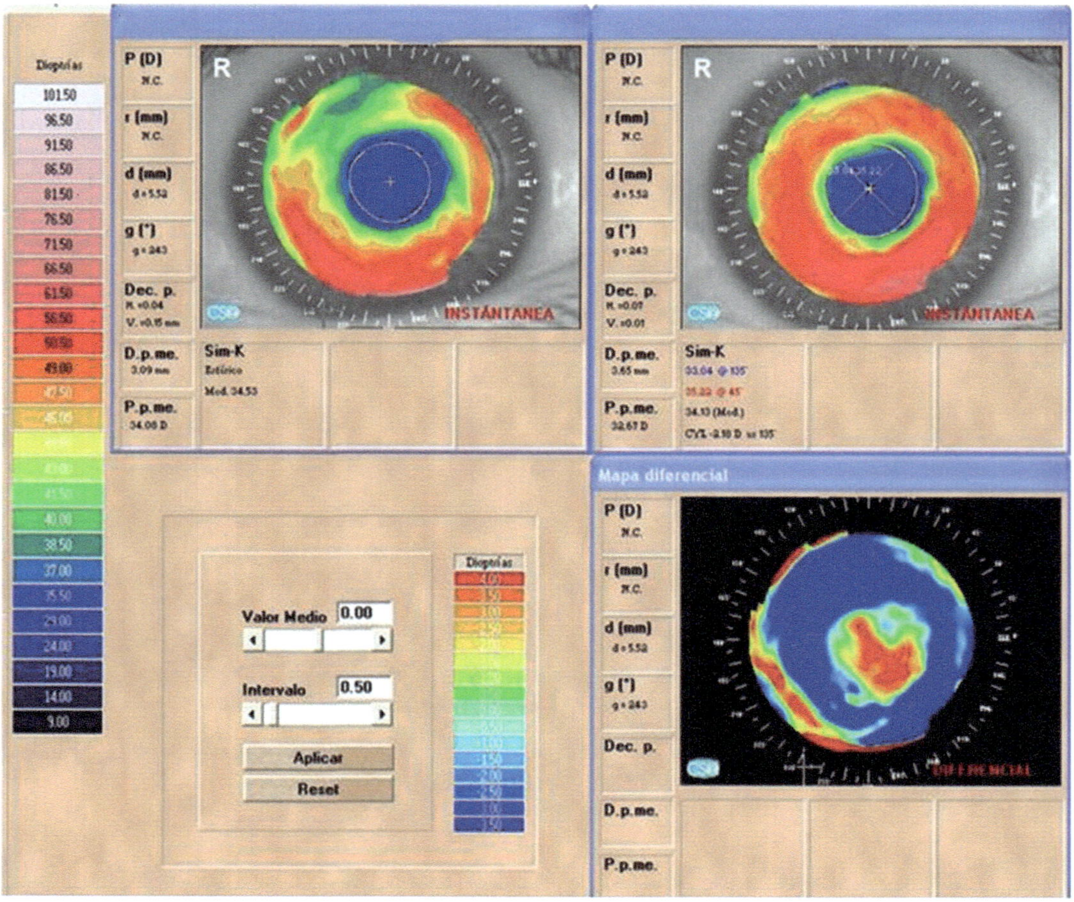

Fig. 1.4 The differential map helps in understanding the achieved correction in corneal curvature

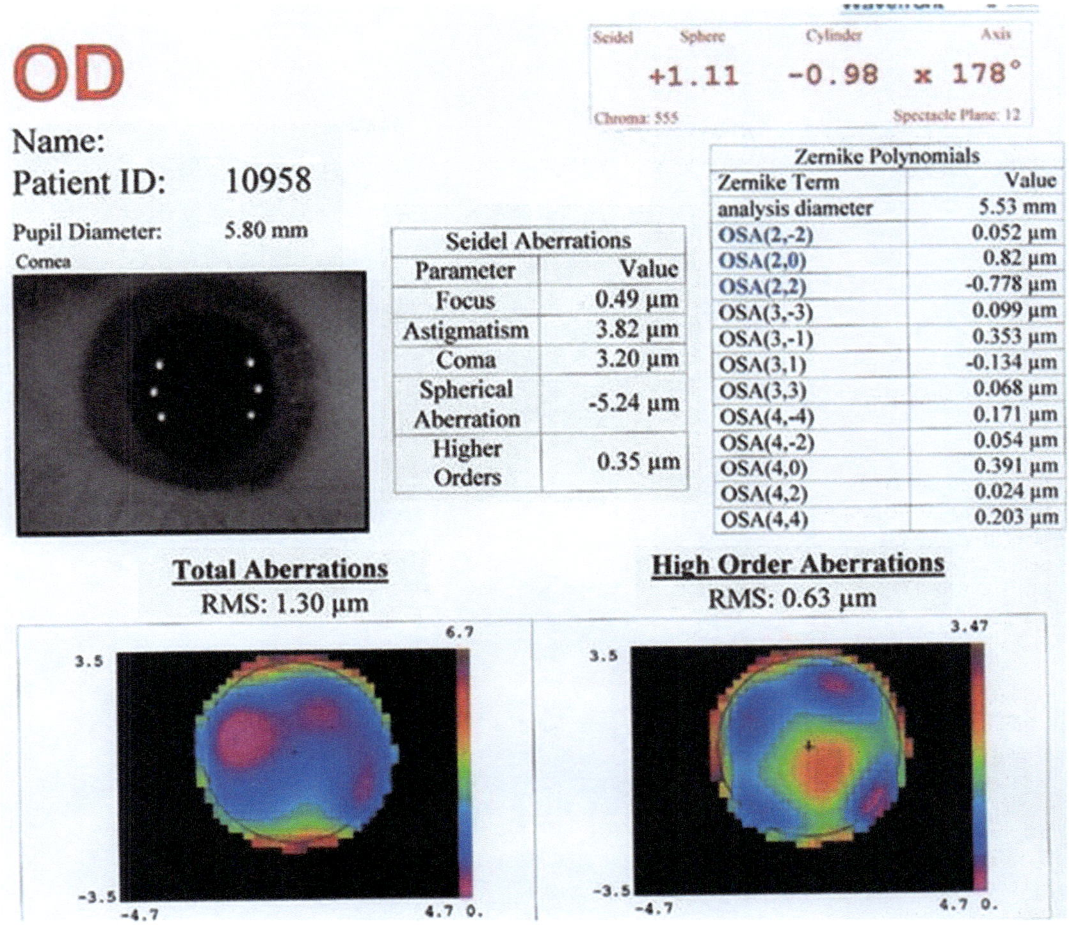

Fig. 1.5 Postoperative total aberrometry. Lower figures can be seen in the most affected Zernike coefficients. Higher-order aberrations RMS was 0.63 µ (for a 5.53 mm area of analysis)

References

1. Ghanem RC, Ghanem VC, Ghanem EA, Kara-Jose N (2012) Corneal wavefront-guided photorefractive keratectomy with mitomycin-C for hyperopia after radial keratotomy: two-year follow-up. J Cataract Refract Surg 38:595–606
2. Afshari NA, Schirra F, Rapoza PA, Talamo JH, Ludwig K, Adelman RA, Kenyon KR (2005) Laser in situ keratomileusis outcomes following radial keratotomy, astigmatic keratotomy, photorefractive keratectomy, and penetrating keratoplasty. J Cataract Refract Surg 31:2093–2100
3. Applegate RA, Howland HC, Sharp RP, Cottingham AJ, Yee RW (1998) Corneal aberrations and visual performance after radial keratotomy. J Refract Surg 14:397–407
4. Koch DD, Maloney R, Hardten DR, Dell S, Sweeney AD, Wang L (2009) Wavefront-guided photorefractive keratectomy in eyes with prior radial keratotomy; a multicenter study. Ophthalmology 116:1688–1696.e2
5. Azar DT, Tuli S, Benson RA, Hardten DR (1998) Photorefractive keratectomy for residual myopia after radial keratotomy; the PRK After RK Study Group. J Cataract Refract Surg 24:303–311

2 Refractive Laser Treatment Post Phakic IOLs by LASIK

Jorge L. Alió, Dominika Wróbel, and Alessandro Abbouda

Contents

J.L. Alió, MD, PhD (✉)
Department of Refractive Surgery, Vissum Corporación Oftalmológica, Alicante, Spain
e-mail: jlalio@vissum.com

D. Wróbel, MD
Glaucoma Diagnostic and Microsurgery Department, Medical University of Lublin, Lublin, Poland

R&D Department, Vissum Corporacion, Alicante, Spain
e-mail: ddudzinska@interia.pl

A. Abbouda, MD
Department of Refractive Surgery, Vissum Corporación Oftalmológica, Alicante, Spain

Department of Ophthalmology-Policlinico Umberto I of Rome, University of Rome "Sapienza", Viale del Policlinico, 155, 00186 Roma, Italy

R&D Department, Vissum Corporación Oftalmológica, 03016, Alicante, Spain
e-mail: a.abbouda@gmail.com

Why Is This Case Relevant for the Refractive Surgeon?

It is known that the complete correction of high myopia can be achieved by few surgical procedures. Bioptics (the term introduced by Roberto Zaldivar) is the combination of intraocular surgical techniques and corneal surgery [1–5]. In this technique, most of the refractive defects are corrected with the phakic intraocular lens and then LASIK is performed to correct any residual refraction errors. Bioptics offers several advantages, but we should keep in mind the possible endothelium complication related to the phakic IOL [6].

Case Background

A 37-year-old man, wearing contact lenses since the age of 15, presented for refractive surgery evaluation. His contact lens tolerance has deteriorated significantly over the last year. The patient's manifest refraction was −10.00 −0.75 70° in the right eye (RE) and −17.00 −0.75 110° in the left eye (LE). His best corrected visual acuity (BCVA) was 20/20 for distance and near in both eyes. Slit-lamp examination revealed papillary conjunctivitis; fundus examinations were normal. According to the topography, his cornea surface was regular. Keratometry value was 42.37/42.95 × 166 in the RE and 43.11/43.69 × 49 in the LE. The keratoconus

J.L. Alió et al. (eds.), *Difficult and Complicated Cases in Refractive Surgery*, DOI 10.1007/978-3-642-55238-0_2, © Springer-Verlag Berlin Heidelberg 2015

index was normal in both eyes (KPI 0 %). His RE pachymetry was 553 μm and his LE pachymetry was 562 μm. The endothelial cell count for the RE was 2,625 cells/mm² and the LE was 2,674 cells/mm².

The OCT Visante examination presented an anterior chamber depth (ACD) of 3.12 mm in the RE and 2.84 mm in the LE. The anterior chamber width (ACW) was 12.01 mm in both eyes.

Refractive surgical treatment was considered because the patient did not tolerate wearing contact lenses any longer. To avoid the risk of ectasia, we decided to perform a phakic intraocular lens implantation (IOL).

He underwent an uneventful surgery with the implantation of AcrySof Cachet lenses. The lens calculation software selected a lens power of −11.0 diopters (D) for the RE and of −16.0 D for the LE. Ciprofloxacin (Oftacilox) one drop three times a day for 7 days and dexamethasone (Maxidex) one drop three times a day for 10 days were prescribed. The postoperative evaluation was normal, the slit-lamp examination showed no anomalies, the lenses were centered, but the intraocular pressure (IOP) was 30 mmHg in both eyes. The patient started acetazolamide (Edemox) one tablet three times a day. His next appointment was after 3 days and the intraocular pressure was still 30 mmHg in the RE and 40 mmHg in the LE. He was then given antiglaucoma drops brinzolamide with timolol (Azarga) to be taken three times a day, and the steroid drops were stopped because there was a suspicion that he was corticoresponsive. After 4 days, the IOP was 17 mmHg in the RE and 19 mmHg in the LE.

After 1 month, the patient's manifest refraction was −0.50 −1.25 60° in the RE and −0.50 −1.00 135° in the LE. His BCVA was 20/20 for distance and near in both eyes. Slit-lamp and fundus examinations were normal, and the IOP was 13 mmHg in the RE and 15 mmHg in the LE. After 3 months, the uncorrected visual acuity (UCVA) was 20/32. The residual defect would be related to the difficulty to estimate the refraction in the high myopic patient. Moreover, the patient complained about reduced vision. The topography showed no risk for ectasia, pellucid marginal degeneration, or suspected keratoconus. Index of high order of aberration (HOA) was normal in both eyes with a value of RMS 0.067 in RE and 0.180 in LE. His right eye pachymetry was 562 μm and his left eye pachymetry was 563 μm. The endothelial cell count for the RE was 2,571 cells/mm² and 2,498 cells/mm² for the LE. LASIK treatment was performed, the flap was created using microkeratome Moria M2 in order not to cause an increase of intraocular pressure and not to shift the anterior chamber lenses. Corneal stromal ablation was performed by the AMARIS SCHWIND excimer laser (residual stromal in the RE was 391 and 405 μm in the LE).

The Main Problem to Solve

In case of high myopia, we need to consider the combination of different refractive procedures. The implantation of a phakic angle-supported IOL AcrySof Cachet does not correct the astigmatism defect, and the second step by LASIK can be very useful to achieve the best uncorrected visual acuity (UCVA) as far as variability in refraction, insufficient intraocular lens power, or astigmatism is concerned [2–5]. We should keep in mind the possible endothelium complication related to the phakic IOL [6].

Ancillary Tests

The following ancillary examinations were performed:

Best corrected visual acuity (BCVA), uncorrected visual acuity (UCVA), manifest and cycloplegic refraction, slit-lamp biomicroscopy, corneal topography, B-scan biometry, keratometry, central corneal and endothelial cell count with Nidek, and anterior segment measurements through OCT Visante.

Surgical/Medical Intervention

The patient underwent surgery with the implantation of AcrySof Cachet lenses in the anterior chamber. The residual refractive error (myopia and astigmatism) was corrected by LASIK after 3 months of the previous one. The flap was created using the microkeratome.

Outcome

After 3 months, postoperatively, the evaluation was normal, the slit-lamp examination showed no anomalies: no epithelial defects at the flap edge, a clear interface, and a well-positioned flap, well-centered anterior chamber lenses, no pupillary block, no pigment dispersion, and no iris atrophy (Fig. 2.1). His uncorrected visual acuity (UCVA) was 20/20 and his corrected distance visual acuity (CDVA) was 20/20.

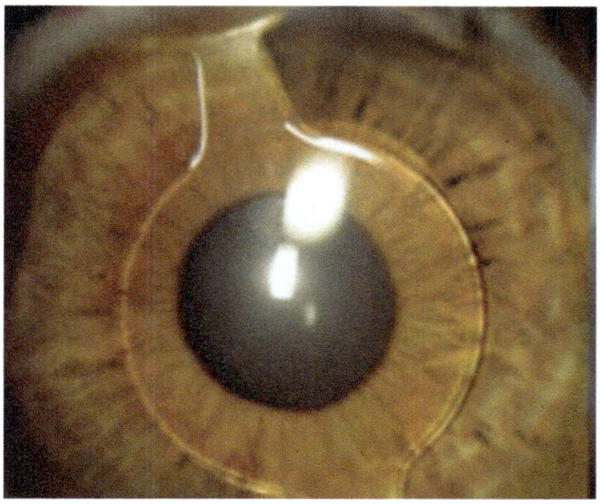

Fig. 2.1 Slit-lamp examination showed a well-positioned flap and well-centered anterior chamber lens

What to Learn from This Case

To achieve good results in the case of high myopia, the combination of corneal and intraocular surgical techniques (bioptics or adjustable refractive surgery) is beneficial. The phakic IOL (AcrySof Cachet) and LASIK is a safe, effective, and predictable method to correct high myopia. Bioptics play an important role in expanding the effectivity and success of phakic intraocular lenses for treating a wide range of refractive errors.

References

1. Zaldivar R, Davidorf JM, Oscherow S et al (1999) Combined posterior chamber phakic intraocular lens and laser in situ keratomileusis: bioptics for extreme myopia. J Refract Surg 15:299–308
2. Muñoz G, Alió JL (2005) Artisan iris-claw phakic intraocular lens followed by laser in situ keratomileusis for high hyperopia. J Cataract Refract Surg 31(2): 308–317
3. Malecaze FJ, Hulin H (2002) A randomized paired eye comparison of two techniques for treating moderately high myopia: LASIK and artisan phakic lens. Ophthalmology 109(9):1622–1630
4. Velarde JI, Anton PG, deValentin-Gamazo L (2001) Intraocular lens implantation and laser in situ keratomileusis (bioptics) to correct high myopia and hyperopia with astigmatism. J Refract Surg 17(2 Suppl):S234–S237
5. Meltendorf C, Cichocki M (2008) Laser in situ keratomileusis following the implantation of iris-fixated phakic intraocular lenses. Ophthalmologica 222:69–73
6. Alió JL, Abdelrahman AM, Javaloy J, Iradier MT, Ortuño V (2006) Angle-supported anterior chamber phakic intraocular lens explantation causes and outcome. Ophthalmology 113(12):2213–2220

Refractive Laser Treatment Post ICL in High Myopia by PRK

3

Jorge L. Alió, Alessandro Abbouda, and Angelo Rampone

Contents

J.L. Alió, MD, PhD (✉)
Department of Refractive Surgery, Vissum Corporación Oftalmológica, Alicante, Spain
e-mail: jlalio@vissum.com

A. Abbouda, MD
Department of Refractive Surgery, Vissum Corporación Oftalmológica, Alicante, Spain

Department of Ophthalmology-Policlinico Umberto I of Rome, University of Rome "Sapienza", Viale del Policlinico, 155, 00186 Roma, Italy

R&D Department, Vissum Corporación Oftalmológica, 03016, Alicante, Spain
e-mail: a.abbouda@gmail.com

A. Rampone, MD
Department of Ophthalmology, Seconda Università degli Studi di Napoli, Naples, Italy

R&D Department, Vissum Corporación, Alicante 03016, Alicante, Spain
e-mail: angelo.rampone@gmail.com

Why Is This Case Relevant for the Refractive Surgeon?

Corneal refractive surgeries are the preferred and safest surgical techniques for the correction of mild and moderate myopia [1]. In the case of high myopia and thick cornea, it is preferable to use phakic intraocular lenses (PIOLs). PIOLs induce very few ocular high-order aberrations and the contrast sensitivity is better than corneal refractive surgery.

We present a case that needed, after the implantation of an Implantable Collamer Lens (ICL; STAAR Surgical Co., Monrovia, Calif.), a corneal refractive treatment to achieve a good visual acuity.

Case Background

A 24-year-old woman with no ocular surgical history presented in our institute for refractive surgery evaluation. Her manifest refraction was −9.75, −1.00 × 95° in the right eye (RE) and −12.5, −1.0 × 50° in the left eye (LE). Keratometry reading were 43.08/43.56 × 13 in the RE and 42.84/43.56 × 143 in the LE. The topography showed a warpage aspect in both eyes (Fig. 3.1). Her best corrected visual acuity (BCVA) was 20/20. Both slit-lamp and fundus examinations were normal. The endothelial count was 2,589 in the RE and 2,318 in the

J.L. Alió et al. (eds.), *Difficult and Complicated Cases in Refractive Surgery*,
DOI 10.1007/978-3-642-55238-0_3, © Springer-Verlag Berlin Heidelberg 2015

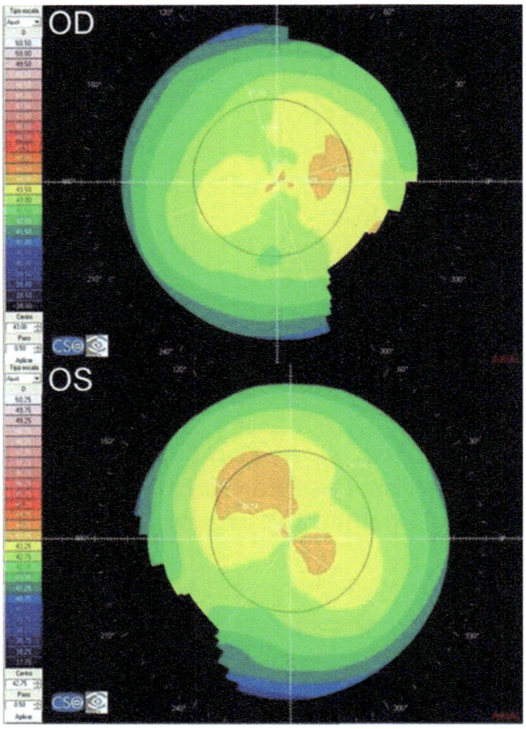

Fig. 3.1 Preoperative corneal topography

LE. AS-OCT showed an anterior chamber depth (ACD) of 3.15 mm and anterior chamber width (ACW) 12.05 mm in the RE and an ACD of 3.17 mm and an ACW of 12.07 mm in the LE. The pachymetry was 420 μm in the RE and 410 μm in the LE. The axial length was 28.34 mm in the RE and 28.9 mm in the LE. We decided to implant a posterior chamber phakic lens. The ICL calculation software selected a lens power for the RE of −13 sphere and in the LE −16 sphere. The ICLs were implanted in both eyes and the postoperative was uneventful. Three months after the surgery, her manifest refraction was −1.0, −0.50 × 105 in the RE and −1.0, −0.50 × 85 in the LE.

Main Problem to Solve

The final result deviated by 1 diopter of the refractive target. It is possible that it was related to an inaccurate refraction or a mistake in the ICL calculation. The axial length measurement did not show any changes with respect to the beginning. The patient was not satisfied with her refraction because she was hoping to be completely spectacle-free. According to the pachymetry value, we decided to perform a trans-epithelial PRK.

Ancillary Tests

Manifest refraction after ICL, visual acuity, corneal topography, aberrometry, ultrasound pachymetry, and pupil diameter were calculated.

Surgical/Medical Intervention

Trans-epithelial PRK procedure was applied. The standard ablation through SCHWIND AMARIS laser excimer was performed. The treatment planning was −1.0, −0.50 × 105 in the RE and −1.0, −0.50 × 85 in the LE. Mitomycin 0.02 % for 15 s and a bandage contact lens were applied. The patient followed the standard post-PRK treatment (ciprofloxacin five times a day for 1 week, dexamethasone 0.1 % three times a day for 1 week, and then fluorometholone three times a day tapering for a month and cyclopentolate three times for 48 h).

Outcome

Two months after the PRK procedure, her manifest refraction was 20/20 in both eyes. The slit-lamp examination was normal. The topography aspect showed a normal myopic profile ablation. Keratometric reading were 40.92/41.84X8 in the RE and 41.06/41.39X135 in the LE (Fig. 3.2). The slit-lamp examination revealed normal ICL vaulting.

What to Learn from This Case?

The higher the level of ametropia, the more difficult it is to obtain a reliable measurement [2]. The selection of ICL IOL size and power includes

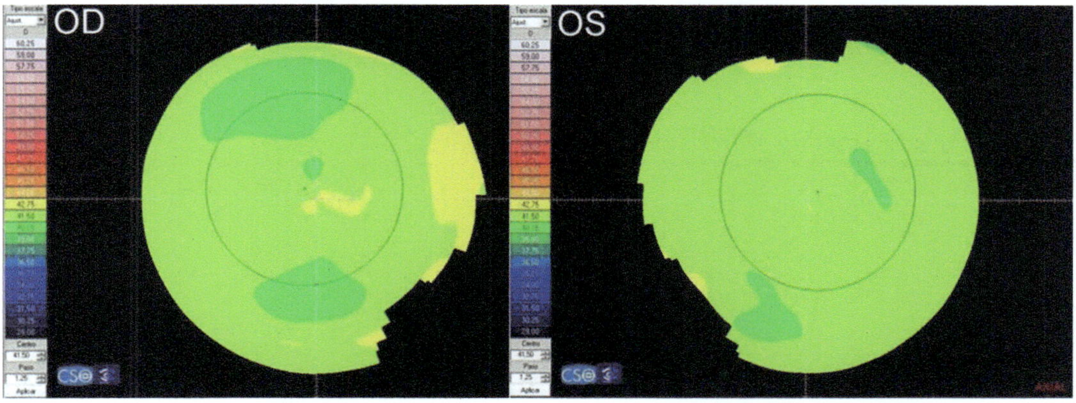

Fig. 3.2 Postoperative corneal topography

biometric analysis, pachymetry, endothelial cell count (ECC), and anterior chamber OCT.

ICL (STAAR Surgical Co., Monrovia, Calif.) and PRK is a safe, effective and predictable method to correct high myopia. The combination of corneal refractive surgery and phakic IOL can offer a good solution in case some refractive defects occur after phakic IOL implantation.

References

1. Comaish IF, Domniz YY, Lawless MA, Webber SK, Rogers CM, Sutton GL (2002) Laser in situ keratomileusis for residual myopia after photorefractive keratectomy. J Cataract Refract Surg 28(5):775–781
2. Petermeier K, Gekeler F, Messias A, Spitzer MS, Haigis W, Szurman P (2009) Intraocular lens power calculation and optimized constants for highly myopic eyes. J Cataract Refract Surg 35(9):1575–1581

IOL Calculation in a Previous Refractive Hyperopic Patient

4

Jorge L. Alió and Felipe A. Soria

Contents

J.L. Alió, MD, PhD (✉)
Department of Refractive Surgery, Vissum Corporación Oftalmológica, Alicante, Spain
e-mail: jlalio@vissum.com

F.A. Soria, MD
Department of Refractive Surgery, Instituto de la Visión, Universidad de Montemorelos, Montemorelos, Mexico
e-mail: soriafelipe.md@gmail.com

A 48-year-old female presented complaining of a decrease in her visual acuity for distance and near since 6 months ago. The patient had undergone uncomplicated bilateral simultaneous laser-assisted in situ keratomileusis (LASIK) for the correction of hyperopia 15 years prior.

Visual complaints were attributed to the regression of hyperopia and cataract, so cataract extraction was planned. Pre-LASIK refractive data was available.

Why Is This Case Relevant for the Refractive Surgeon?

The challenge of IOL calculation and the optical quality of an already treated cornea, which IOL to select.

We find two relevant aspects to analyze:

1. LASIK treatment in high hyperopes and the induced aberrations due to centration [1].

   In the following study [2], an acceptable predictability for the treatment of high levels of hyperopia (>4 D of spherical equivalent) with a laser platform with a 500 Hz repetition rate and 1,050 Hz eye tracker as well as the use of optimized aberration-free ablation profiles after a 6-month follow-up was found. This technique is still effective (index 0.85) and should be considered acceptable for correcting hyperopia up to +8.50 D. Regression in hyperopes is well documented; some studies have

J.L. Alió et al. (eds.), *Difficult and Complicated Cases in Refractive Surgery*,
DOI 10.1007/978-3-642-55238-0_4, © Springer-Verlag Berlin Heidelberg 2015

found an average increase in hyperopia of +0.54 D over a 5-year follow-up.

2. IOL calculation in a previous refractive hyperopic patient.

We are starting to perform cataract surgery in the first wave of patients with previous refractive surgery. The “tsunami” of these patients is near, and knowing all the previous history data of each patient will help us to offer them, for a second time, the possibility of emmetropia.

In the European Registry of Quality Outcomes for Cataract and Refractive Surgery (EUREQUO), the recommended refractive outcome should be an absolute mean biometry prediction error of 0.6 D or less. A biometry error with a correct sign should be centered on 0 D, and 87 % or more of the values should be within ±1.0 D of error [3].

These standards are based on virgin eyes and are the best markers of what we should expect for eyes that have had a corneal refractive surgery. Biometry is an essential step in these situations and it is difficult. Also, an important factor is that we are managing a patient that has previously achieved emmetropia in a refractive procedure, so the expectations are to be spectacle-free in most of the cases.

(a) Incorrect estimation of the effective lens position by third- or fourth-generation IOL power calculation formulas when the postoperative corneal power is used
(b) Improper determination of the true total corneal refractive power

In general, the accuracy of calculations after hyperopic LASIK is somewhat better than after myopic LASIK. Hyperopic patients typically receive smaller amounts of refractive correction, and the measurement error by small-zone autokeratometry is relatively small compared with myopic LASIK. Treatment regression combined with lens-induced myopia may render the historical method inaccurate. As with myopic LASIK, the Masket, modified Masket, and Haigis-L methods give good overall results; the Haigis-L is very useful when there are no prior refractive surgery data for review.

Case Background

At the time of consultation, she presented with the following data:

RE: +8.50 −1.25 × 15 20/40
LE: 8.50 −0.75 × 170 20/40
Keratometry measures:
RE: 46.80/47.20 at 20
LE: 47.21/47.54 at 178
Pre-LASIK information available:
RE: +8.00 −2.50 × 30
LE: +8.50 −2.00 × 180

On examination, the patient had clear corneas and normal LASIK flaps in both eyes. She had a NO2 (LOCS III) cataract in the right eye and a NO1 (LOCS III) in the left eye.

Using the ASCRS online calculator [4, 5], the power of the IOL was calculated for both eyes. The Haigis-L formula was used (Fig. 4.1).

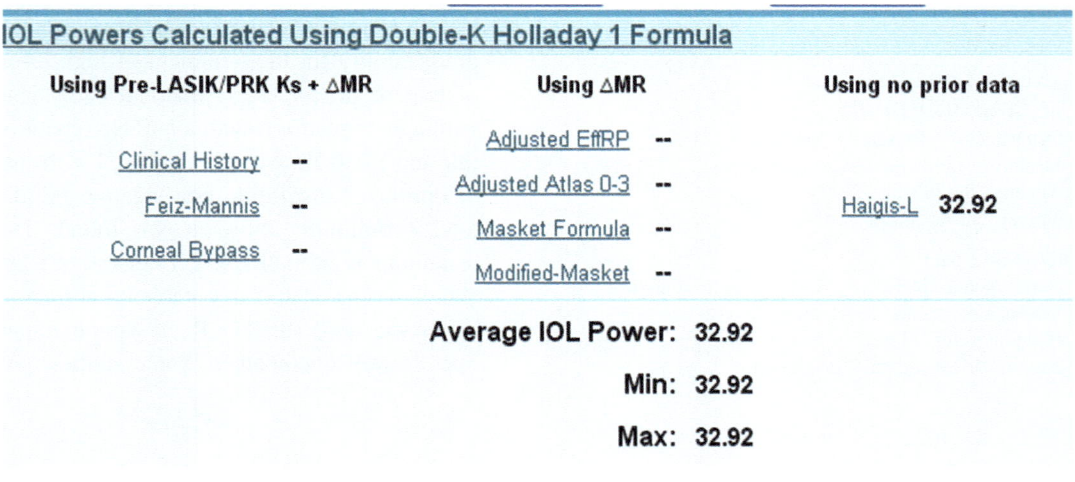

Fig. 4.1 ASCRS IOL power calculator result

The IOL power for the right eye determined to a target of 0.00 was 33.0 for a 118.74 A-Constant.

The IOL power for the left eye determined to a target of 0.00 was also 33.0 for a 118.74 A-Constant.

The patient underwent a noncomplicated bilateral cataract surgery with an implantation of an IOL.

Main Problem to Solve

The main problem to solve was to determine the exact power of the IOL in order to make this patient emmetropic.

Ancillary Tests

Topography
IOL Master
ASCRS online IOL power calculator

Surgical/Medical Intervention

Cataract Surgery

Outcome

One month after the surgery, the data obtained was as follows:

RE:		
UCDVA:		20/40
BCDVA:	−0.75	20/30
LE:		
UCDVA:		20/40
BCDVA:	+0.75	20/25

The patient was very satisfied with the procedure.

What to Learn from This Case

1. Regression in hyperopes is well documented.
2. Biometry must be exact.
3. The more that we use technology, a rational understanding in biometry values and the correct election of the IOL power is completely necessary. The optimal assessment of the optical quality of the cornea is also indispensable.
4. The overall satisfaction of the patient according to their needs is better than achieving emmetropia.
5. It is important that every patient that is operated with a refractive procedure must keep their refractive information to help with IOL power calculation when cataract surgery is needed.

References

1. Ibarrán-Diego C, Muñoz G, Montés-Micó R, Rodriguez A, Alió JL (2006) Corneal aberration changes after hyperopic LASIK: a comparison between the VISX Star S2 and the Asclepion-Meditec MEL 70 G Scan excimer lasers. J Refract Surg 22:34–42
2. Alió JL, El Aswad A, Vega-Estrada A, Javaloy J (2013) Laser in situ keratomileusis for high hyperopia (>5.0 diopters) using optimized aspheric profiles: Efficacy and safety. J Cataract Refract Surg 39(4):519–27
3. Lundström M, Barry P, Henry Y, Rosen P, Stenevi U (2012) Evidence-based guidelines for cataract surgery: guidelines based on data in the European Registry of Quality Outcomes for Cataract and Refractive Surgery database. J Cataract Refract Surg 38:1086–1093
4. Wang L, Hill WE, Koch DD (2010) Evaluation of intraocular lens power prediction methods using the American Society of Cataract and Refractive Surgeons Post-Keratorefractive Intraocular Lens Power Calculator. J Cataract Refract Surg 36:1466–1473
5. ASCRS online calculator. Available at: http://iolcalc.org/. Accessed Jan 2013

Refractive Surprise After Cataract Surgery Solved by Surface Ablation of a Patient That Underwent Corneal Refractive Surgery 12 Years Ago

5

Jorge L. Alió and Felipe A. Soria

Contents

J.L. Alió, MD, PhD (✉)
Department of Refractive Surgery, Vissum Corporación Oftalmológica, Alicante, Spain
e-mail: jlalio@vissum.com

F.A. Soria, MD
Department of Refractive Surgery, Instituto de la Visión, Universidad de Montemorelos, Montemorelos, Mexico
e-mail: soriafelipe.md@gmail.com

Why Is This Case Relevant for the Refractive Surgeon?

Nowadays, it is more and more common to receive patients that are seeking cataract surgery and have previously undergone a corneal refractive procedure. The expectations of these patients are very high in terms of refractive outcomes. We do not have an exact formula to determine the best IOL power.

Case Background

A 75-year-old male presented complaining of glare and trouble seeing at distance and near. The patient had undergone uncomplicated bilateral simultaneous laser-assisted in situ keratomileusis (LASIK) for the correction of myopia 12 years prior. Visual complaints were attributed to cataract so cataract extraction was planned. No pre-LASIK biometric or refractive data was available.

At the moment of consultation, he presented with the following data:

RE: −1.00 −3.00 × 110	20/30
LE: −1.50 −2.25 × 110	20/50
Keratometry measures:	
OS: 39.21/40.74 at 98	

On examination, the patient had clear corneas and normal LASIK flaps in both eyes. He had a

J.L. Alió et al. (eds.), *Difficult and Complicated Cases in Refractive Surgery*, DOI 10.1007/978-3-642-55238-0_5, © Springer-Verlag Berlin Heidelberg 2015

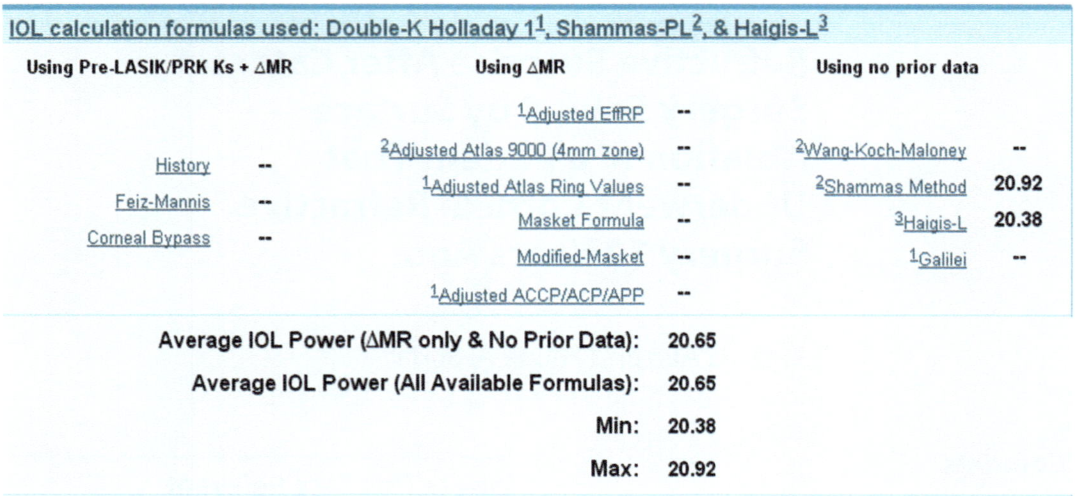
IOL calculation formulas used: Double-K Holladay 1[1], Shammas-PL[2], & Haigis-L[3]

Using Pre-LASIK/PRK Ks + ΔMR		Using ΔMR		Using no prior data	
		[1]Adjusted EffRP	--		
History	--	[2]Adjusted Atlas 9000 (4mm zone)	--	[2]Wang-Koch-Maloney	--
Feiz-Mannis	--	[1]Adjusted Atlas Ring Values	--	[2]Shammas Method	20.92
Corneal Bypass	--	Masket Formula	--	[3]Haigis-L	20.38
		Modified-Masket	--	[1]Galilei	--
		[1]Adjusted ACCP/ACP/APP	--		

Average IOL Power (ΔMR only & No Prior Data):	20.65
Average IOL Power (All Available Formulas):	20.65
Min:	20.38
Max:	20.92

Fig. 5.1 ASCRS IOL power calculator result

NOI (LOCS III) cataract in the right eye and a NOII (LOCS III) in the left eye.

Using the ASCRS online calculator, the power of the IOL was calculated (Fig. 5.1). The IOL power determined to a target of −1.00 was 20.6 for a 118.74 A-Constant.

The patient underwent a noncomplicated cataract surgery with an implantation of a Toric IOL.

One month after the surgery, the data obtained was as follows:

LE:		
UCDVA:		20/70
BCDVA:	−1.50	20/30

The patient was not satisfied with the vision in his left eye. He expected to have better vision in that eye.

A LASIK enhancement was performed in the left eye treating the residual myopia.

Main Problem to Solve

Determine the exact power of the IOL in order to achieve the target refraction and the correction of the astigmatism. After the cataract surgery and obtaining a −0.50 of difference from the estimated target refraction, the patient kept complaining about his distance vision. His expectations were high.

Ancillary Tests

Topography
IOL Master
ASCRS online IOL power calculator

Surgical/Medical Intervention

Cataract Surgery

Outcome

After the laser enhancement, the patient achieved a spontaneous visual acuity of 20/30.

What to Learn from This Case

1. IOL power calculation following refractive surgery is not accurate, and patients must be informed about this.
2. The biometry must be exact.

3. The more that we use technology, a rational understanding in biometry values and the correct election of the IOL power is completely necessary. It is important to compare the results of multiple IOL power calculations.
4. It is important that patients who undergo refractive procedures must keep their refractive information.

In a normal eye, the anterior corneal surface and the posterior corneal K readings in (D) are derived from the radius in mm measured using an effective refractive index (1.3375 in most instruments). This false value is considering a single refractive lens representing anterior and posterior surfaces. This effective refractive index is considered valid as long as radii of anterior and posterior surfaces of the cornea are proportionate and resemble that of the model eye.

After a myopic ablation (central), the radius of the anterior corneal surface is increased and the distance between both refractive surfaces is decreased. Therefore, calculating keratometric diopters from anterior radius of curvature is not accurate.

The two main errors following this condition are an incorrect estimation of the effective lens position by third- or fourth-generation IOL power calculation formulas when the postoperative corneal power is used and an improper determination of the total corneal refractive power.

The accuracy of calculations after myopic LASIK is somewhat worse than after hyperopic LASIK. Myopic patients typically receive larger amounts of refractive correction, and what is more significant is that the ablation is on the center, the place where all the instruments are going to measure the anterior corneal curvature. As with hyperopic LASIK, the Masket, modified Masket, and Haigis-L methods give good overall results; the Haigis-L is very useful when there are no prior refractive surgery data for review. The percentage of eyes achieving a postoperative spherical equivalent refraction within 0.5 and 1.0 D of the target and the total range of refractive error are the best markers of the quality of a biometry service.

References

1. Gale RP, Saldana M, Johnston RL, Zuberbuhler B, McKibbin M (2009) Benchmark standards for refractive outcomes after NHS cataract surgery. Eye (Lond) 23:149–152
2. Lundström M, Barry P, Henry Y, Rosen P, Stenevi U (2012) Evidence-based guidelines for cataract surgery: guidelines based on data in the European Registry of Quality Outcomes for Cataract and Refractive Surgery database. J Cataract Refract Surg 38:1086–1093
3. Wang L, Hill WE, Koch DD (2010) Evaluation of intraocular lens power prediction methods using the American Society of Cataract and Refractive Surgeons Post-Keratorefractive Intraocular Lens Power Calculator. J Cataract Refract Surg 36:1466–1473
4. Demill DL, Moshirfar M, Neuffer MC, Hsu M, Sikder S (2011) A comparison of the American Society of Cataract and Refractive Surgery post-myopic LASIK/PRK intraocular lens (IOL) calculator and the Ocular MD IOL calculator. Clin Ophthalmol 5:1409–1414
5. ASCRS online calculator. Available at: http://iolcalc.org/. Accessed Jan 2013

Post-refractive Surgery IOL Power Calculation, Intraoperative Aberrometry

6

Michael W. Raciti and Jonathan B. Rubenstein

Contents

M.W. Raciti, MD (✉) • J.B. Rubenstein, MD
Department of Ophthalmology,
Rush University Medical Center, Chicago, IL, USA
e-mail: racitim@gmail.com;
jonathan_rubenstein@rush.edu

Why Is This Case Relevant for the Refractive Surgeon?

Optical biometry, corneal power measurement, and simple intraocular lens (IOL) power calculations provide accurate intraocular lens power determination in most eyes. However, for eyes with altered corneal power after refractive surgery for the correction of myopia, hyperopia, or astigmatism, traditional IOL power calculations are inaccurate. Patients presenting for cataract surgery today have increasingly undergone previous refractive procedures. The refractive outcomes of cataract surgery are important and patient-centered healthcare is responding with new advancements [1]. Optimal postoperative outcomes with minimal refractive error are especially important for patients who have already made significant investments in refractive surgery to be spectacle-free, with high expectations to remain so after cataract surgery. The demand for accurate refractive outcomes has driven the development of new IOL power calculations and methods for determining IOL power in post-refractive surgery eyes. The development of intraoperative wavefront aberrometry appears to increase the accuracy in post-refractive surgery IOL power determination.

J.L. Alió et al. (eds.), *Difficult and Complicated Cases in Refractive Surgery*,
DOI 10.1007/978-3-642-55238-0_6, © Springer-Verlag Berlin Heidelberg 2015

Case Background

A 75-year-old male presented complaining of glare and with trouble seeing near and far distances. The patient underwent an uncomplicated bilateral simultaneous laser-assisted in situ keratomileusis (LASIK) for the correction of myopia 12 years prior. Visual complaints were attributed to the cataract so a cataract extraction was planned. No pre-LASIK biometric or refractive data was available.

Post-LASIK manifest refraction
OD: +0.25 +0.25 × 180 20/25
OS: −0.50 +1.75 × 170 20/30
Post-LASIK manual keratometry
OD: 41.10/41.25
OS: 41.00/41.50 @ 150

Upon examination, the patient had clear corneas and normal LASIK flaps in both eyes. He had a 2+ nuclear sclerotic cataract with 2+ cortical change in the right eye and a 3+ nuclear sclerotic cataract with 2+ cortical change in the left eye.

Main Problem to Solve

IOL power calculation is problematic in post-refractive surgery eyes because it is difficult to determine these eyes' true keratometric power. Corneal power is overestimated in eyes that have undergone previous refractive surgery for the correction of myopia, which leads to unexpected hyperopic outcomes after cataract surgery. There are multiple reasons for this overestimation [2]. First, correction of myopia results in a small effective central optical zone. Keratometers and Placido disc-based topography units measure outside this central area in the midperiphery where the cornea is steeper. Second, correction for myopia thins the central cornea, causing a larger disparity between the anterior and posterior curvatures and underestimating the divergence of the posterior curvature relative to the anterior. Because of this disparity, the value for the index of refraction, which is used to calculate corneal power from curvature measurements, overestimates the power. A third source of error results from third-generation formulas that use corneal power to predict pseudophakic anterior chamber depth, which is calculated to be artificially shallow in corrected myopic eyes [3]. This error leads to an underpowered IOL that sits more posteriorly than predicted and results in unplanned hyperopia.

Ancillary Tests

Various formulas and nomograms are available to correct for the prediction errors of traditional IOL power calculation methods post-LASIK. The "clinical history method" for IOL power calculation requires pre-refractive surgery refraction, keratometry, and post-refractive surgery refraction [4]. However, pre-refractive surgery data is often either unavailable or inaccurate. Therefore, several methods have been developed that do not rely on pre-refractive surgery biometric and refractive data. The American Society of Cataract and Refractive Surgery (ASCRS) website contains an online Post-Keratorefractive IOL Power Calculator developed by Hill et al. [5]. A recent study by Wang et al. with the online calculator showed that methods using no prior data had smaller IOL prediction errors than methods requiring only pre-LASIK/PRK K values and surgically induced changes in manifest refraction [6]. Fourier-domain optical coherence tomography (OCT)-based IOL power calculation is another new method developed by Tang et al. They found that this OCT-based method was equal to or better than current standards in post-laser vision correction [7].

Intraoperative wavefront aberrometry is a new technology that captures real-time refractive information during cataract surgery to help with IOL power calculation. The latest intraoperative aberrometry model is the ORA System™ (WaveTec® Vision, Aliso Viejo, CA, USA). The unit attaches to the operating room microscope and displays data on an external monitor. To determine the refractive state of the eye, a narrow beam of light is directed into the eye, reflects off the retina and produces an aberrated wavefront. Talbot-Moiré interferometry is used to capture the wavefront and analyzed to reveal the spherocylindrical error of the eye [8]. Proprietary technology allows the aberrometer to be compact and lightweight and also increases the dynamic range of capture from −20 to +20 diopters. The wavefront can be captured in the aphakic state for IOL power calculation or in the pseudophakic state to confirm IOL power, adjust toric IOLs, or guide the placement of peripheral corneal relaxing incisions. Intraoperative aberrometry is especially useful for IOL power determination in the post-refractive surgery patient because it relies on the reflected wavefront from the eye rather than corneal curvature. It eliminates many of the errors in standard IOL calculation post-refractive surgery.

Surgical/Medical Intervention

The case above portrays a post-myopic LASIK patient who presents for cataract surgery. As described, identifying the appropriate IOL power to insert during cataract surgery is difficult. IOL Master (Carl Zeiss Meditec, Inc., USA), corneal topography (ATLAS™ Carl Zeiss Meditec, Inc., USA), and Pentacam (Oculus USA, Lynnwood, WA) measurements were performed. The corneal data from these tests were consistent with prior LASIK for correction of myopia. There was no irregular astigmatism, ectasia, or abnormal posterior corneal curvature. Corneal thickness was ≥570 μm in both eyes. Using the above data, the average IOL power was calculated using the ASCRS online Post-Keratorefractive IOL Power Calculator <iolcal.org>. The online Post-Keratorefractive IOL Power Calculator provided an IOL power for the following formulas: Wang-Koch-Maloney, Shammas method, and Haigis-L. The IOL Master recommended lens was also calculated.

Outcome

The calculated IOL powers for the different methods are shown in Tables 6.1 and 6.2. Intraoperatively, the ORA System calculated an IOL power of 19.50 diopters for both eyes based on aphakic measurements. The ORA predicted a residual refractive error of −0.20 and −0.13 diopters in the right and left eye, respectively. There was considerable variation in calculated IOL power between the various preoperative calculations and the ORA System. Postoperatively, the patient had a favorable refractive outcome after implantation of the ORA system calculated IOL. Uncorrected distance visual acuity was 20/25 and 20/30 in the right and left eye, respectively. Corrected distance visual acuity was 20/20 in both eyes with the following manifest refraction:

OD: −0.25 +0.50 × 180	
OS: −0.50 sphere	

Table 6.1 IOL calculation method and IOL power (diopters) for the right eye

OD: method	IOL (D)
Wang-Koch-Maloney	18.65
Shammas	19.04
Haigis-L	18.92
IOL Master	18.50
ORA	**19.50**

Table 6.2 IOL calculation method and IOL power (diopters) for the left eye

OS: method	IOL (D)
Wang-Koch-Maloney	18.86
Shammas	19.13
Haigis-L	18.48
IOL Master	18.00
ORA	**19.50**

What to Learn from This Case

Post-refractive surgery IOL calculation is complicated and patients must be informed that IOL calculations are less accurate after refractive surgery. Comparing the results of multiple IOL power calculations is important. Intraoperative aberrometry is a new tool that is useful for post-refractive surgery IOL power calculations because it relies on principles other than corneal curvature. Intraoperative aberrometry is especially useful because it may improve the accuracy of refractive outcomes in a patient group who desires spectacle independence. We have also found intraoperative aberrometry useful for patients who cannot undergo standard measurements due to physical or mental cooperation limitations and in patients with extremely long and short eyes in which standard IOL calculations may be less accurate.

References

1. Talley-Rostov A (2008) Patient-centered care and refractive cataract surgery. Curr Opin Ophthalmol 19(1):5–9
2. Mimura T, Azar DT (2004) Current concepts, classification, and history of refractive surgery. In: Yanoff M, Duker JS (eds) Ophthalmology, 3rd edn. Mosby/Elsevier, St Louis
3. McCarthy M, Gavanski GM, Paton KE, Holland S (2011) Intraocular lens power calculations after myopic laser refractive surgery: a comparison of methods in 173 eyes. Ophthalmology 118(5): 940–944
4. Holladay JT (1989) Consultations in refractive surgery [comment]. Refract Corneal Surg 5:203
5. Hill W, Wang L, Koch DD (2012) IOL. Power calculation in eyes that have undergone LASIK/PRK/RK. Version 4.4. Available from http://iolcalc.org/. Cited 26 Dec 2012
6. Wang L, Hill WE, Koch DD (2010) Evaluation of intraocular lens power prediction methods using the American Society of Cataract and Refractive Surgeons Post-Keratorefractive Intraocular Lens Power Calculator. J Cataract Refract Surg 36(9): 1466–1473
7. Tang M, Wang L, Koch DD, Li Y, Huang D (2012) Intraocular lens power calculation after previous myopic laser vision correction based on corneal power measured by Fourier-domain optical coherence tomography. J Cataract Refract Surg 38(4):589–594
8. Wiley WF, Bafna S (2011) Intra-operative aberrometry guided cataract surgery. Int Ophthalmol Clin 51(2):119–129

Refractive Lens Exchange for High Hyperopic Astigmatism Followed by LASIK

7

Noel Alpins

Contents

N. Alpins, FRANZCO, FRC Ophth., FACS
NewVision Clinics, Melbourne, VIC, Australia

Department of Ophthalmology,
University of Melbourne, Melbourne, VIC, Australia
e-mail: alpins@newvisionclincis.com.au

Why Is This Case Relevant for the Refractive Surgeon?

This case highlights some of the interesting complications resulting from an unrecognised low correlation between corneal and refractive values in a refractive lens exchange. A refractive lens exchange with a toric IOL was called for in this case. Although one would have expected the toric implant to correct for corneal astigmatism, subsequent excimer laser surgery (LASIK) was necessary.

Case Background

A 47-year-old male underwent an excimer laser surgery assessment with the hope of achieving a level of unaided visual acuity suitable to enter the police force (which requires unaided 6/18 in better eye, 6/36 in other eye). He was found unsuitable for laser surgery due to a high amount of hypermetropia and astigmatism in his subjective refraction.

Unaided visual acuity	R 20/60	L 20/60
Subjective refraction	R +6.50/−5.75 × 95	L +6.00/−5.525 × 75
Cycloplegic refraction	R +7.25/−5.75 × 95	L +6.75/−5.25 × 75
Aided visual acuity	R 20/20 ++	L 20/20 ++
Topography (Sim K)	R 37.59/41.39 @ 7	L 37.44/41.46 @ 164
Keratometry	R 37.87/41.75 @ 13	L 37.75/41.62 @ 168

J.L. Alió et al. (eds.), *Difficult and Complicated Cases in Refractive Surgery*,
DOI 10.1007/978-3-642-55238-0_7, © Springer-Verlag Berlin Heidelberg 2015

Internal and external examinations were normal with no evidence of cataracts.

The patient was advised to receive a refractive lens exchange procedure for each eye and counselled regarding the risks, side effects, near spectacle prescription required with a monofocal lens implant and the possibility of part-time spectacles postoperatively.

Uncomplicated bilateral same-day IOL surgery was performed using a Tecnis Toric Aspheric IOL.

OD: 2.2 mm incision at 193°; Tecnis ZCT400 +26.0 D SE 4.00 D CYL

OS: 2.2 mm incision at 0°; Tecnis ZCT400 +26.0 D SE 4.00 D CYL

Figure 7.1 displays the Assort toric planning module demonstrating the effect of placing the phaco incision at the steepest corneal meridian, reducing the corneal astigmatism, which now requires targeting with the toric IOL.

Figure 7.2 shows the effect of implanting a toric IOL with 24.00 D sphere, 4.00 D cylinder at an axis of 13°. The expected subjective refraction is shown under 'toric target' as '0.04/−0.08 × 103', indicating that we expect to under-correct the corneal astigmatism by 0.08 D at a meridian of 13°.

It is interesting to note that the IOL toric power at the lens plane of 4.00 DC converts to 3.30 D @ 103 at the corneal plane; this is calculated using the effective lens position and the A-constant from the SRK/T formula.

Ocular residual astigmatism (ORA) [1, 2, 3] was not calculated preoperatively.

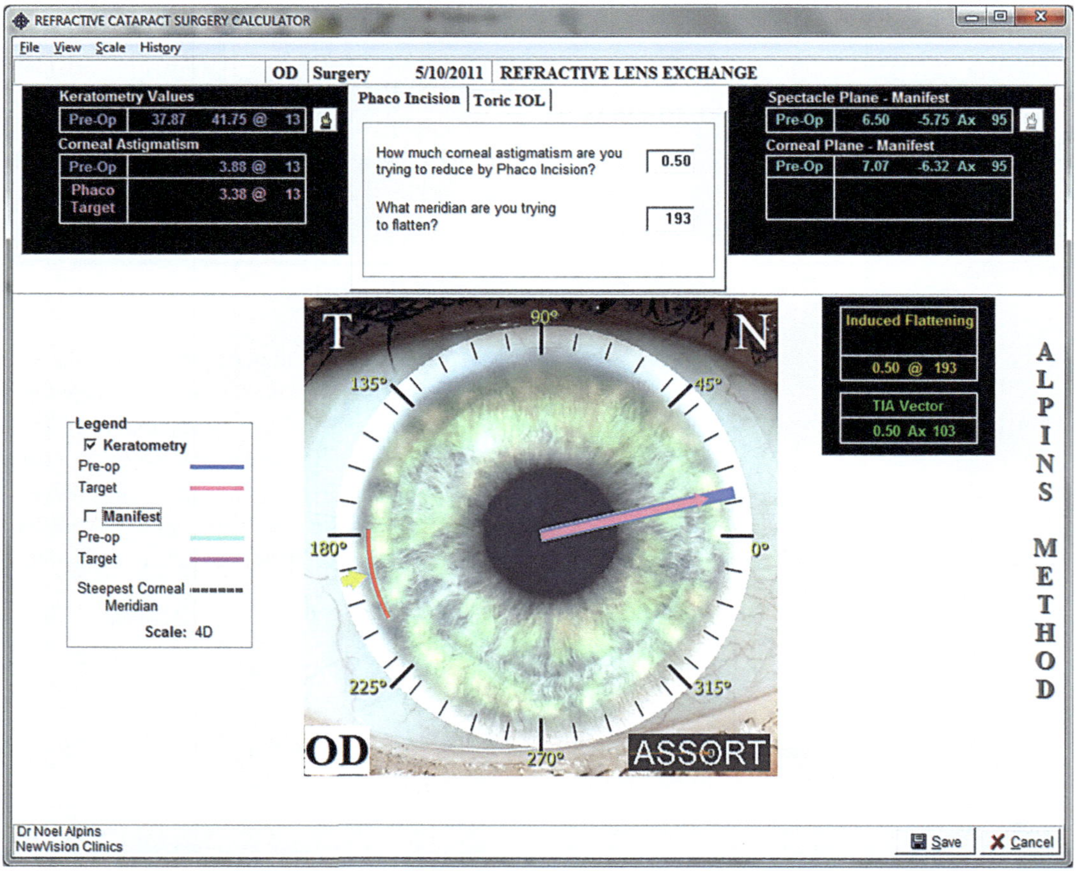

Fig. 7.1 Effect of the phaco incision on the preoperative corneal astigmatism of the right eye. Note that the flattening effect of the phaco incision of 0.50 D determined from previous cases reduces the preoperative astigmatism of 3.88–3.38 D

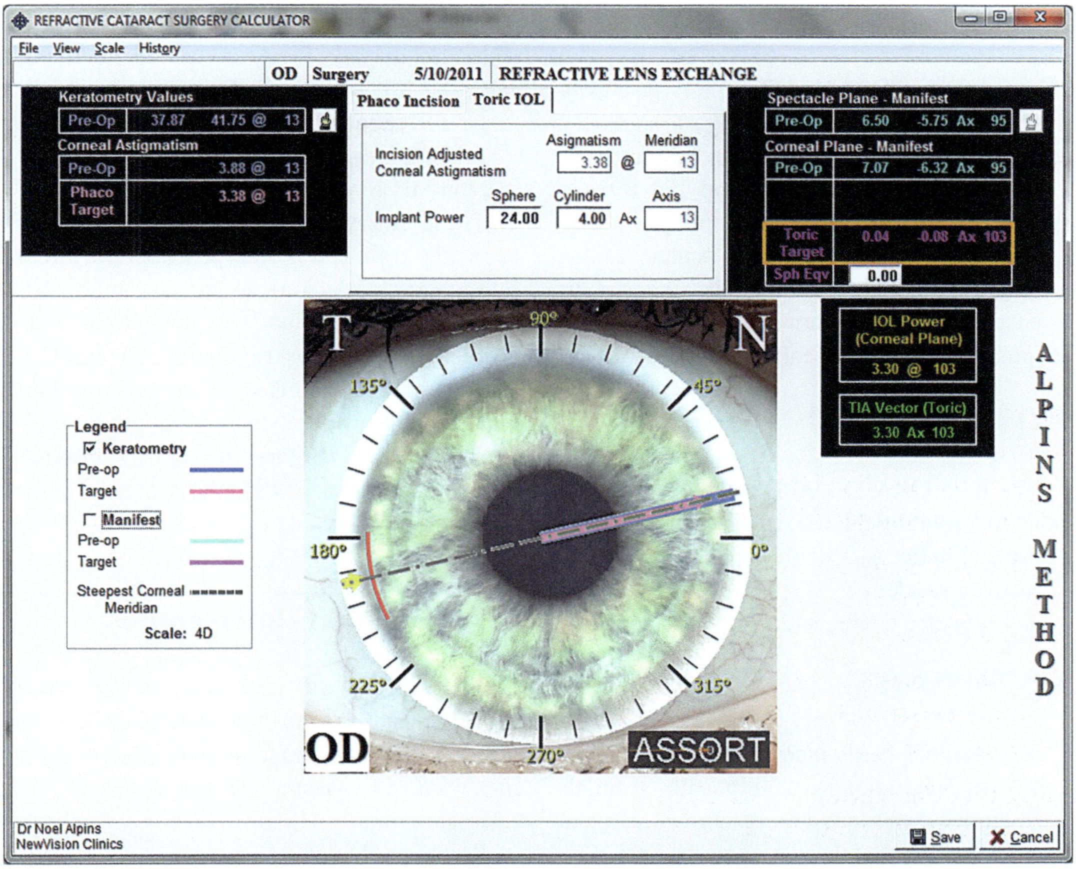

Fig. 7.2 Display of theoretical refractive astigmatism outcomes using a toric IOL of 24.00 D sphere and 4.00 D cylinder. The expected refractive cylinder is +0.08 D × 13

Main Problem to Solve

The high degree of astigmatism remaining postoperatively in the subjective refraction in both eyes was a refractive surprise.

One month postoperatively:

Unaided visual acuity	R 20/40 –	L 20/80 –
Subjective refraction	R +0.25/−2.00 × 70	L +0.25/−2.25 × 50
Aided visual acuity	R 20/25 +	L 20/30 ++
Keratometry	R 38.25/41.60 @ 14	L 37.75/41.60 @ 170
Slit lamp	R IOL markings @ 13/193° as intended	L IOL markings @ 0/180° instead of 168/348°

Options

(a) Rotate the toric IOL to reduce the postoperative subjective cylinder.
(b) Explant the toric IOL and replace with a different toricity.
(c) Perform excimer laser surgery on the existing toric IOL to correct for the refractive astigmatism.

The toric IOL in the right eye was inconsistent in lining up exactly where it should have been (at 193°), resulting in a refractive cylinder of 2.00 D postoperatively. The toric IOL in the left eye was sitting 18° clockwise from its intended position of 168°, resulting in a 2.25 D refractive cylinder postoperatively.

Ancillary Tests

The patient was reviewed 2 months postoperatively to reassure refractive stability. No significant change in the subjective refraction was noted.

Slit-lamp examination showed the IOLs at exactly the same position as 1 month previously.

Calculation of preoperative ocular residual astigmatism (ORA), defined as the vectorial difference between the corneal and the refractive astigmatism (at the corneal plane), was:

ORA	R 2.27 D×116	L 2.66 D×91

The high ORA (>1.00 D) in both eyes indicated that rotating the IOL towards the refractive positive cylinder axis could reduce the manifest refractive cylinder.

Keratometry readings (2 months postop):

R 38.10/41.60 @ 14	L 37.75/41.75 @ 177

The manual keratometry parameters do not appear to have changed significantly from the preoperative measurements of corneal astigmatism, indicating that there was no unusual effect of the incision procedure on the cornea.

In analysing the outcome of a toric IOL procedure, it is important to compare the postoperative subjective cylinder (at the corneal plane) to the preoperative corneal astigmatism adjusted for any effect in magnitude and steep meridian by the phaco incision. Two overriding parameters must be calculated:

1. The Angle of Error (AE) [1, 2, 4, 5]: The angle between the intended astigmatic treatment vector (target-induced astigmatism vector – TIA) and the surgically induced astigmatism vector (SIA). This shows the degree that the IOL needs to be rotated for the minimum amount of spectacle cylinder to remain postoperatively.
2. The Magnitude of Error (ME) [1, 2, 4, 5]: The arithmetic difference between the magnitudes of the SIA and the TIA. This indicates whether the IOL implanted has over- or under-corrected the corneal astigmatism.

In this case, the toric IOL astigmatism analysis using the preoperative manual keratometry parameters adjusted for the phaco incision (Fig. 7.3), displays the AE to be +18° in the right eye. The ME was −0.49 D, indicating a minor under-correction of astigmatism in the right eye.

In the left eye, the AE was calculated as +20° and the ME as −0.67 D.

These analyses demonstrate an angle of error; the right eye is well positioned while the left eye is not. Considering the high ORA, rotation of the implant was not guaranteed to correct the cylinder remaining. Because the two eyes were inconsistent in IOL alignment and calculations, we decided to proceed with excimer laser surgery to most effectively reduce the refractive cylinder without rotating the implant.

Surgical/Medical Intervention

LASIK surgery was performed in the left eye 6 weeks post IOL toric implantation and 16 weeks post IOL toric implantation in the right eye using the ViSX S4 system and the Amadeus (*SiS*) microkeratome.

Right eye: Mixed astigmatism

Treatment parameters: −2.07 DS +2.37 DC×165°

This was converted to cross-cylinders to minimise the amount of corneal tissue removal:

Plano/+0.78×165 was treated at the cornea in the 5.0–9.0 mm zone.

Plano/−1.59×75 was treated at the cornea using an ellipse of 6.0×5.5 mm.

Left eye: Mixed astigmatism (with spherical shifts of astigmatism treatment included)

Treatment parameters (corneal plane): −2.26 DS +2.11 DC×140°

This was converted to cross-cylinders to minimise the amount of corneal tissue removal:

Plano/+0.34×140 was treated at the cornea in the 5.0–9.0 mm zone.

Plano/−1.77×50 was treated at the cornea using an ellipse of 6.0×5.5 mm.

Excimer laser treatments were based on 100 % refractive parameters. Vector planning, which incorporates both corneal and refractive parameters into the treatment plan, was not used as the corneal values were not relevant.

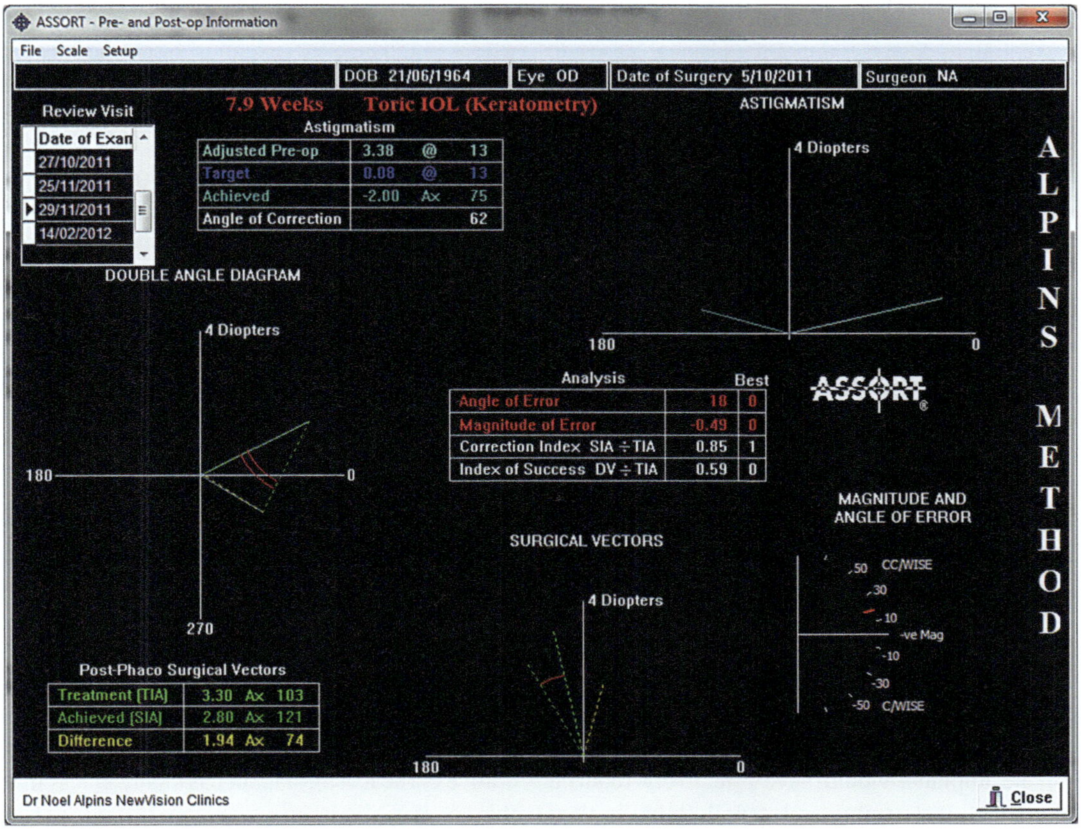

Fig. 7.3 Toric IOL astigmatism analysis displays an 'angle of error' of 18°, meaning that the IOL could be rotated clockwise 18° to reduce the postoperative refractive cylinder. The 'magnitude of error' is –0.49 D, indicating a minor under-correction of astigmatism with the toric IOL selected

Outcome

Three months after LASIK surgery in the right eye and 5 months after LASIK in the left eye (8 months after bilateral toric IOL implantation):

Unaided visual acuity	R 20/20–	L 20/25–
Subjective refraction	R +0.25/–0.25 × 75	L +0.75/–0.75 × 55
Aided visual acuity	R 20/20	L 20/20
Slit lamp (cornea)	R clear and quiet	L clear and quiet

The patient was extremely pleased with the outcome!

What to Learn from This Case

It is important to calculate the ORA presurgery (using the iAssort software: www.assort.com) to determine treatment possibilities, particularly LASIK or lenticular surgery which can remove the crystalline lens and lenticular astigmatism.

Given the excellent astigmatic outcomes of this case, we conclude that the ORA calculated preoperatively was likely due to lenticular astigmatism.

When planning for toric IOL surgery, it is important to factor into the lens choice any effect of the phaco incision on the preoperative corneal astigmatism. The magnitude of the toricity of the IOL may be more or less than that measured preoperatively, and the steepest corneal meridian may also have shifted as a result of the phaco incision not being placed on axis. Hence, it is essential to analyse previous surgical cases to establish the flattening effect, if any, of your phaco incisions [2].

When assessing outcomes of toric IOL implants, the markings on the lens (which indicate the least power of the IOL) may be at the intended steepest corneal meridian, but mathematically this may not be the optimum axis of the IOL.

If there is a refractive surprise as indicated by a significant amount of cylinder remaining in the subjective refraction postoperatively, a toric astigmatic analysis must be performed, which compares the postoperative refractive cylinder (corneal plane) to the preoperative corneal astigmatism, adjusted for any effect of the phaco incision. The treatment in these cases is the IOL toricity at the corneal plane allowing for the effective lens position and the spherical component of the IOL. These calculations can be done using the ASSORT(R) toric IOL calculator (www.assort.com).

Perhaps early intervention and early rotation of the implants would have effectively reduced the functional (right) and actual (left) implant misalignment. However, there was concern that either one could have independently caused the remaining refractive cylinder.

There are essentially three options available to the surgeon:

1. Rotate the existing toric IOL to reduce the refractive cylinder to a minimum.

   Consider rotating the toric IOL when the AE is greater than 10°.
2. Exchange the IOL as the toric power selected is too strong or too weak.

   In cases where the ME is greater than 1.00 D, consider changing the toric IOL to a more suitable cylinder power selection.
3. Perform excimer laser surgery to correct for any unexpected cylinder in the subjective refraction.

It is important to note that if there is a coexisting spherical component postoperatively, this may influence a surgeon's decision between a lens exchange or excimer laser surgery. In cases where the preoperative ORA is greater than 1.25 D and the AE and ME are not significant, excimer laser surgery to correct the postoperative refractive cylinder may be indicated.

Importantly, before considering any of the above suggestions, it is necessary to establish that the phaco incision has performed as expected by measuring the corneal astigmatism postoperatively (topography or manual keratometry). This should be very similar to what you allowed for when determining the amount of astigmatism the toric IOL would neutralise and the steepest meridian that the toric IOL was aligned to. If the corneal astigmatism or the steepest meridian is now significantly different, with an unexpectedly large SIA, then all three options above should be reconsidered.

The significance of postoperative corneal and/or refractive astigmatism can be determined by the indicated steps of a toric IOL. If the toric IOL comes in 0.75 steps of cylinder and the postoperative corneal astigmatism has changed less than this, or the ME is less than this, it may not be beneficial to change to toric IOL.

References

1. Alpins NA (1997) New method of targeting vectors to treat astigmatism. J Cataract Refract Surg 23: 65–75
2. Alpins NA (1997) Vector analysis of astigmatism changes by flattening, steepening, and torque. J Cataract Refract Surg 23:1503–1514
3. Kugler L, Cohen I, Haddad W, Wang MX (2010) Efficacy of laser in situ keratomileusis in correcting anterior and non-anterior corneal astigmatism: comparative study. J Cataract Refract Surg 36:1745–1752
4. Alpins NA (1993) A new method of analyzing vectors for changes in astigmatism. J Cataract Refract Surg 19:524–533
5. Alió JL, Piñero DP, Tomás J (2011) Vector analysis of astigmatic changes after cataract surgery with implantation of a new toric multifocal intraocular lens. J Cataract Refract Surg 37:1217–1229

Trans-epithelial Phototherapeutic Keratectomy for Irregularly Irregular Astigmatism

8

Dan Z. Reinstein, Timothy J. Archer, and Marine Gobbe

Contents

D.Z. Reinstein, MA(Cantab), FRCSC, FRCOphth (✉)
London Vision Clinic, London, UK

Department of Ophthalmology, Columbia University Medical Center, New York, NY, USA

Centre Hospitalier National d'Ophtalmologie, Paris, France
e-mail: dzr@londonvisionclinic.com

T.J. Archer, MA (Oxon) DipCompSci(Cantab)
M. Gobbe, MST(Optom) PhD
London Vision Clinic, London, UK
e-mail: tim@londonvisionclinic.com; marine@londonvisionclinic.com

Why Is This Case Relevant for the Refractive Surgeon?

The corneal epithelium has the ability to alter its thickness profile, which compensates for changes in stromal surface curvature and re-establishes a smooth, symmetrical optical surface. Such compensatory epithelial thickness changes have been noted after myopic excimer laser ablation, hyperopic excimer laser ablation, radial keratotomy, orthokeratology, and in keratoconus and ectasia. In cases of irregular astigmatism, the compensatory mechanism of the epithelium has a significant effect, as epithelial thickness changes mask the true curvature of the irregular stromal surface [1–4].

Surface topography and aberrometry, primary sources of diagnostic testing in the repair of post refractive surgery complications, have greatly enhanced quantitative understanding of how irregular astigmatism and other shape irregularities produce subjective visual complaints. However, topography and wavefront cannot provide a diagnosis for the exact anatomy of the pathology that needs correcting (i.e. the irregular stromal surface) due to the masking effect of the epithelium. Therefore,

Electronic supplementary material The online version of this chapter (10.1007/978-3-642-55238-0_8) contains supplementary material, which is available to authorized users.

J.L. Alió et al. (eds.), *Difficult and Complicated Cases in Refractive Surgery*,
DOI 10.1007/978-3-642-55238-0_8, © Springer-Verlag Berlin Heidelberg 2015

topography-guided or wavefront-guided treatments may lead to a sub-optimal treatment because of epithelial compensation mechanisms inherent to the cornea [1–4].

Here we describe an example case that demonstrates why a trans-epithelial phototherapeutic keratectomy (PTK) procedure can be a more appropriate and effective treatment than topography- or wavefront-guided treatment due to the error introduced by significant epithelial thickness remodeling.

Case Background

A 50 year-old male was referred to our clinic (London Vision Clinic, London, UK) with complaints of severe visual disturbances after LASIK including diplopia, halos and starbursts. He had undergone a primary LASIK procedure in October 2009 for low hyperopia using the Technolas 217z and Moria 130 disposable microkeratome with a nasal hinge in the left eye. The surgeon notes say that a large, well-centered flap was created on the visual axis. A decentration was diagnosed, so the surgeon lifted the flap and performed a topography-guided retreatment a few months later, which improved the refraction but left the patient with visual symptoms of ghosting. Because the topography-guided treatment was unsuccessful, there was the possibility that whole-eye aberrations had gone uncorrected. A wavefront-guided retreatment was then performed which left the patient much worse than before. On presentation at the London Vision Clinic, the topography showed a nasally truncated ablation zone and had some similarities to those seen in a decentration.

Main Problem to Solve

The primary problem was understanding why both a topography-guided and a wavefront-guided retreatment had not improved the topography or the subjective symptoms.

Ancillary Tests

An Artemis very high-frequency digital ultrasound exam measured the individual layers of the cornea including the epithelial thickness profile and revealed the true diagnosis (Fig. 8.1). The flap was found to have a short nasal hinge and the stromal surface was indented near the hinge. At this nasal location, the epithelial thickness profile showed a localized step with a region of thin epithelium (41 μm) immediately nasal to a region of thick epithelium (77 μm); the epithelium had compensated by 36 μm within 1-mm for the stromal irregularity by thinning over the ridge and thickening to fill in the crevice. The diagnosis was that a short flap had been created with laser ablation performed on the underside of the flap near the hinge, resulting in a region of double ablation adjacent to a region of no ablation.

Surgical/Medical Intervention

The epithelial thickness compensation masked the true stromal surface irregularity from front surface topography, which explains the failure of topography- and wavefront-guided treatments. A better treatment plan was trans-epithelial PTK. Trans-epithelial PTK requires an ablation of constant depth over a large zone with an equal amount of tissue removed throughout the treatment zone. It uses the epithelium as a natural masking agent to target the ablation onto the peaks of the irregular stromal surface.

Prior to surgery, we generated a topography-guided ablation profile based on Atlas topography and compared this to the stromal ablation map predicted for a trans-epithelial PTK (Fig. 8.2). In order to correct the stromal irregularity, the logical approach was to remove tissue from the nasal ridge where no ablation was performed in the primary procedure due to the short flap. A trans-epithelial PTK procedure would concentrate the stromal ablation in this location because the epithelium was thinnest here. Conversely, the area of maximum ablation was not matched in the topography-guided ablation and therefore the procedure would not address the main irregularity on the stromal surface.

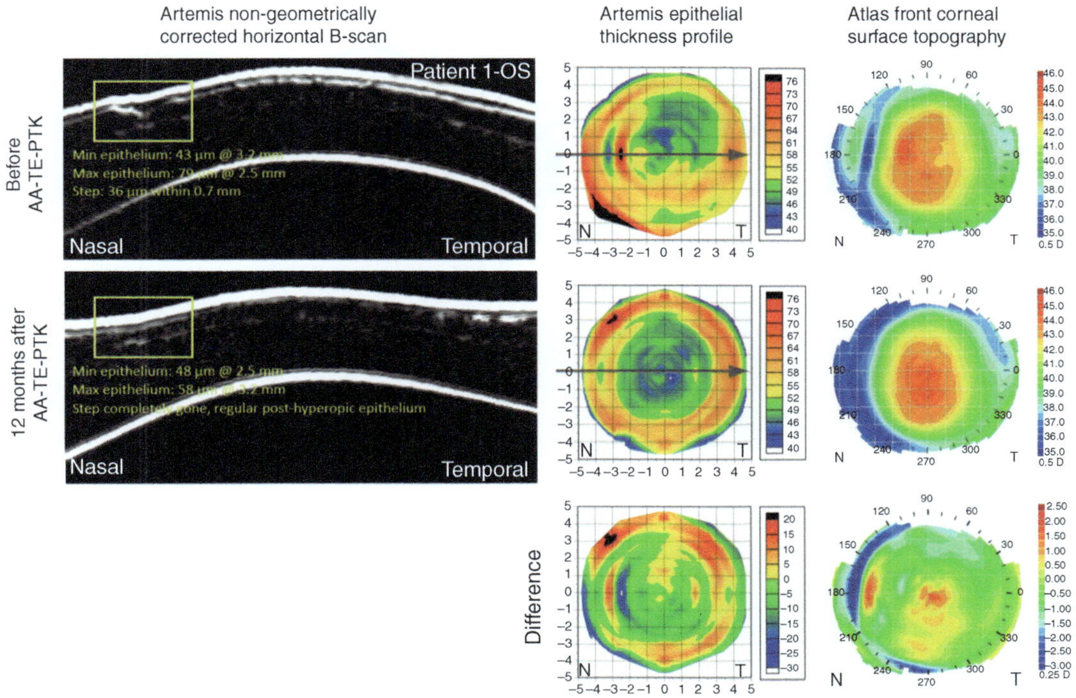

Fig. 8.1 *Left column*: Artemis non-geometrically corrected horizontal B-scans before and after the AA-TE-PTK procedure. The *yellow box* highlights the nasal region where the flap interface stops abruptly. In this area, there is a crevice on the stromal surface over which the epithelium has thickened with thin epithelium overlying the adjacent ridge. *Middle column*: Artemis epithelial thickness maps before and after the AA-TE-PTK procedure plotted on the same scale. These show the nasal step in epithelial thickness which has been completely smoothed after the procedure. The difference map is plotted underneath, which shows the significant epithelial remodeling in the nasal region after the procedure. *Right column*: Atlas corneal front surface topography before and after the AA-TE-PTK procedure plotted on the same scale. The difference map is plotted underneath, which demonstrates a significant improvement in topographic irregularity after the procedure (Reprinted with permission from Reinstein et al. [3])

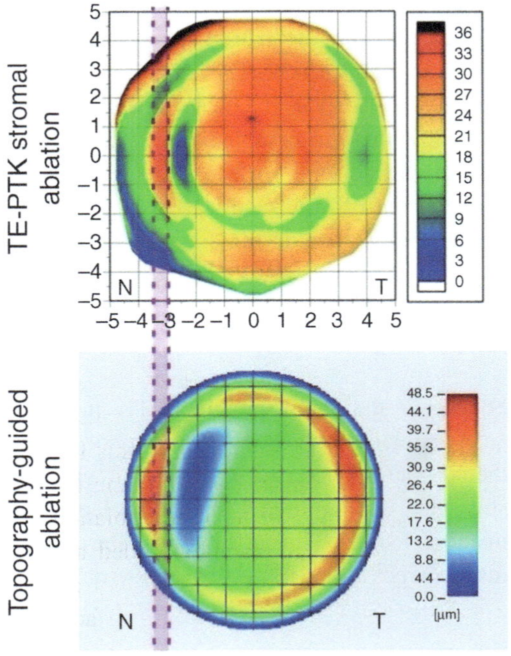

Fig. 8.2 Stromal ablation predicted for a trans-epithelial PTK (*top*) calculated from the Artemis epithelial thickness data and topography-guided custom ablation profile (*bottom*) generated from the Atlas front corneal surface topography using the CRS-Master software. The maximum ablation of the topography-guided profile was too far nasal and would have resulted in creating a second crevice nasal of the ridge. This highlights a benefit of the trans-epithelial PTK approach, in which errors associated with centration are eliminated as the natural epithelial masking effect locates peaks in the stromal surface (Reprinted with permission from Reinstein et al. [3])

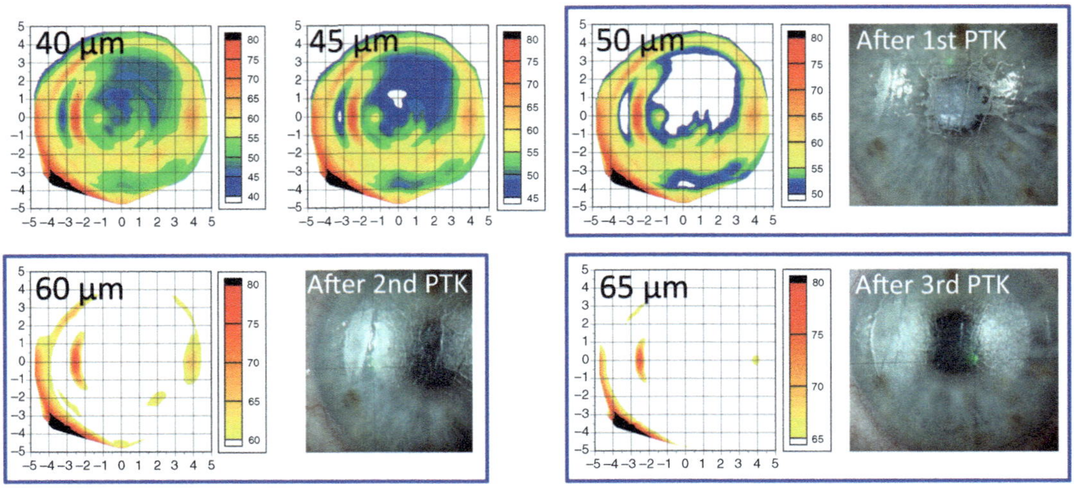

Fig. 8.3 Artemis digital subtraction pachymetry simulation of the pattern of remaining epithelium that would be expected after increasing trans-epithelial PTK ablations from 40 to 65 µm in 5 µm steps. The *white* represents the regions where all of the epithelium would have been ablated after the labeled trans-epithelial PTK ablation, and hence the regions where ablation of stromal tissue would occur. Due to epithelial masking, the stromal ablation was concentrated onto the nasal ridge immediately adjacent to the crevice on the stromal surface. During the procedure, the trans-epithelial PTK ablation was performed in three steps, with a planned 50 µm ablation as the first step. After the first ablation, the cornea was examined (as shown in the intraoperative photograph) and the pattern of remaining epithelium closely matches the predicted pattern with a strip of isolated epithelium overlying the crevice in the stroma, confirming that the first ablation was close to 50 µm. The second and third trans-epithelial PTK ablations were then planned to reach the intended end point of 65 µm accurately. The intraoperative photographs show that the pattern of remaining epithelium was similar to the predicted pattern with only a small line of epithelium remaining overlying the stromal crevice. This stepwise method provides a means to accurately reach the intended end point and to reserve stromal tissue, which is often at a premium in repair cases (Reprinted with permission from Reinstein et al. [3])

We then used our Artemis-assisted trans-epithelial PTK technique which employs Digital Subtraction Pachymetry (DSP) [1, 2] software to display maps showing the breakthrough pattern and remaining epithelium at regular lamellar depths of PTK ablation. The details of the stepwise trans-epithelial PTK ablations are described in Fig. 8.3. Trans-epithelial PTK can also have a refractive impact, which can be predicted based on the epithelial thickness map. In this case, the epithelium was thinner centrally, so a trans-epithelial PTK ablation would act as a myopic ablation. Therefore, a +1.00 D hyperopic ablation in a 7-mm zone was performed to account for this.

There were a few small microfolds remaining on the stromal surface, so a 'wet' PTK ablation was performed to polish the surface of these sharp-edge irregularities. This involved flooding the cornea with balanced salt solution (BSS) followed immediately by a PTK ablation of 8 s' duration (after 8 s, the BSS surface tension begins to break-up) in an 8-mm zone. The BSS acts as a masking agent and naturally spreads across the surface, leaving the ridges of any microfolds closer to the surface. The shockwaves of the excimer laser expose the peaks of the microfolds and allow them to be ablated in isolation of the rest of the stromal surface. This process was repeated until the surface was visibly smoothed of microfolds upon drying.

Outcome

Following the trans-epithelial PTK procedure, an Artemis scan showed that the nasal ridge on the stromal surface had been almost completely smoothed. The epithelial thickness map showed that the localized nasal 36 µm difference had disappeared and the postop epithelium had a regular thickness profile (Fig. 8.1). The truncation of the optical zone of the hyperopic ablation on topography was also restored, with the difference map showing the significant change in the nasal region. Finally, the nasal ridge was no longer visible with fluorescein negative staining. Subjectively, the patient reported virtual disappearance of his preoperative best spectacle corrected image ghosting.

What to Learn from This Case

This case demonstrates how compensatory epithelial thickness mechanisms can detrimentally affect wavefront- or topography-guided custom ablation, as the true stromal irregularity is partially masked by the epithelium. In fact, a topography-guided treatment might have made the irregularity worse in this case: the maximum ablation of the topography-guided profile was further nasal than the ridge, which would have created a second crevice on the opposite side of the ridge.

Ideally, an epithelial thickness measurement is required in cases of irregular astigmatism in order to diagnose the cause of the irregularity and to determine the most appropriate treatment plan. In the absence of an epithelial thickness measurement, the likely epithelial remodeling can be estimated according to a few basic rules.

1. The more irregular the topography, the more epithelial remodeling has occurred.
2. The amount of epithelial remodeling is defined by the rate of change of curvature of the irregularity; more epithelial remodeling occurs in more localized irregularities [1–4].
3. The epithelium thickens in areas where tissue has been removed or the curvature has flattened.
4. The epithelium is thinner over elevated regions such as in the center of a hyperopic ablation.

An advantage of the trans-epithelial PTK approach is that careful centration is not required, as stromal ablation is guided by epithelial thickness and the epithelium is thin over relative peaks on the stromal surface. However, trans-epithelial PTK may only treat the proportion of the stromal irregularity compensated for by the epithelium, thus multiple procedures are usually required. In exceptional cases such as the one presented here, the irregularity is localized to a small region, indicating that the rate of change of curvature was high and the epithelium could compensate almost 100 %. In this case, the stromal irregularity was almost completely smoothed by a single procedure. In contrast, most cases require a second procedure to further treat the stromal surface irregularity after allowing the epithelium to compensate for the irregularity remaining after the first procedure [4]. This stepwise approach means that the patient may only experience a limited improvement after the first procedure since the irregularity has only been partially corrected [3].

We have found that a topography-guided treatment works very well for large-scale global "regular" irregularities such as small optical zone and decentration because the rate of change of curvature is relatively low and hence there is less epithelial remodeling [5, 6]. Following the guidelines above, if the topography is "irregularly" irregular, a trans-epithelial procedure is almost always the best first option because a large proportion of the irregularity will have been compensated for by the epithelium and hence masked from topography. The epithelium contains more irregularities than the topography and these irregularities need to be addressed first. Also, given the nature of the compensatory epithelial remodeling mechanism, a trans-epithelial PTK must smooth the stromal surface to some degree, so it is virtually impossible to make the symptoms worse although it can induce a change in refraction. Following a trans-epithelial procedure, if the topography only has "regular" irregularities remaining, a topography-guided treatment can correct these irregularities which the epithelium compensates for the least [2].

The trans-epithelial PTK procedure itself can be performed relatively easily without an epithelial thickness measurement. The mean central epithelial thickness in a normal eye is 53 μm [7], so the thinnest epithelium in an irregularly irregular cornea will be less than this (as there must be compensatory thinning for an irregularity). Therefore, the first ablation of a stepwise trans-epithelial PTK can be programmed as 53 μm, which should guarantee a breakthrough in the epithelium, exposing the stromal surface somewhere. From this point, trans-epithelial PTK ablations can be performed sequentially in 10 μm steps. The amount of remaining epithelium can be reviewed after each ablation so that the procedure can be stopped once only a small patch of epithelium is left in order to avoid unnecessary stromal tissue removal (since there will be no smoothing effect once all of the epithelium has been ablated).

References

1. Reinstein DZ, Archer T (2006) Combined Artemis very high-frequency digital ultrasound-assisted transepithelial phototherapeutic keratectomy and wavefront-guided treatment following multiple corneal refractive procedures. J Cataract Refract Surg 32:1870–1876
2. Reinstein DZ, Archer TJ, Gobbe M (2012) Refractive and topographic errors in topography-guided ablation produced by epithelial compensation predicted by three-dimensional Artemis very high-frequency digital ultrasound stromal and epithelial thickness mapping. J Refract Surg 28:657–663
3. Reinstein DZ, Archer TJ, Gobbe M (2013) Improved effectiveness of transepithelial PTK versus topography-guided ablation for stromal irregularities masked by epithelial compensation. J Refract Surg 29(8):526–533
4. Reinstein DZ, Archer TJ, Dickeson ZI, Gobbe M (2014) Transepithelial phototherapeutic keratectomy protocol for treating irregular astigmatism based on population epithelial thickness measurements by artemis very high-frequency digital ultrasound. J Refract Surg 30(6):380–387
5. Reinstein DZ, Archer TJ, Gobbe M (2009) Combined corneal topography and corneal wavefront data in the treatment of corneal irregularity and refractive error in LASIK or PRK using the Carl Zeiss Meditec MEL80 and CRS Master. J Refract Surg 25:503–515
6. Reinstein DZ, Archer TJ, Gobbe M (2012) Is topography-guided ablation profile centered on the corneal vertex better than wavefront-guided ablation profile centered on the entrance pupil? J Refract Surg 28:139–143
7. Reinstein DZ, Archer TJ, Gobbe M, Silverman RH, Coleman DJ (2008) Epithelial thickness in the normal cornea: three-dimensional display with Artemis very high-frequency digital ultrasound. J Refract Surg 24:571–581

Sequential Custom Therapeutic Keratectomy for Irregular Astigmatism

9

Paolo Vinciguerra and Fabrizio I. Camesasca

Contents

P. Vinciguerra, MD (✉) • F.I. Camesasca, MD
Department of Ophthalmology,
Istituto Clinico Humanitas, Rozzano, MI, Italy
e-mail: paolo.vinciguerra@humanitas.it

Why Is This Case Relevant for the Refractive Surgeon?

A highly irregular and astigmatic cornea following refractive surgery or infective keratitis is a therapeutic challenge. Phototherapeutic keratectomy (PTK) is an effective tool for partial or total corneal transplantation, preventing more invasive surgery. Here we present two cases of irregular astigmatism, one after refractive surgery and the other after acanthamoeba keratitis, both treated with transepithelial sequential custom therapeutic keratectomy (SCTK).

Background

Case 1

A 36-year-old male underwent PRK in his right eye for −8.00 sph −1.00 cyl (180). Due to the onset of haze and regression, he underwent retreatment with PRK and mitomycin application 8 months later. His final vision was 0.1 with −7.00 sph −2.00 cyl (125), and his cornea had a 4+ haze with irregular subepithelial scar down to 180 μ in depth (Fig. 9.1). Vision in the other eye was 0.4 with −4.00 sph −1.50 cyl (135). Corneal pachymetry in the thinnest point was 507 μ. DALK was suggested as a possible treatment.

J.L. Alió et al. (eds.), *Difficult and Complicated Cases in Refractive Surgery*,
DOI 10.1007/978-3-642-55238-0_9, © Springer-Verlag Berlin Heidelberg 2015

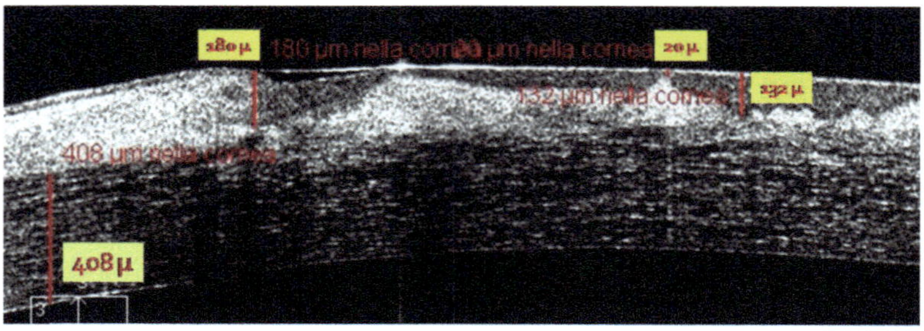

Fig. 9.1 Case 1, right eye. OCT of cornea showing stromal opacities extending in depth down to 180 μ, with 408 of residual clear stroma

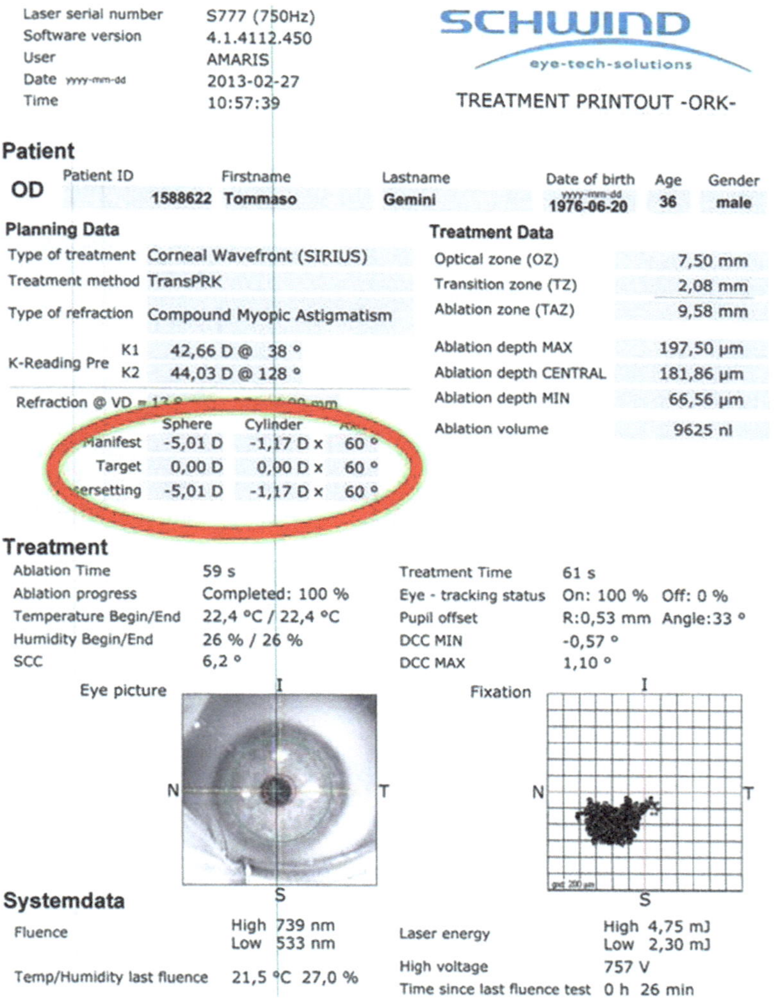

Fig. 9.2 Case 1, right eye. Schwind Amaris shotfile of first ablation phase

We treated the right eye with transepithelial SCTK. Given the patient's opacities of significant depth, a first ablation phase aimed at resolving the bulk of corneal high-order aberrations (HOA) and the refractive error (Fig. 9.2). However, excimer laser ablation, especially of high-volume, induces biomechanical changes that influence corneal shape, creating HOA and refractive error. A second custom-based ablation phase was aimed at partially reducing myopia, avoiding anisometropia, and treating residual high-order aberrations. Refraction and visual

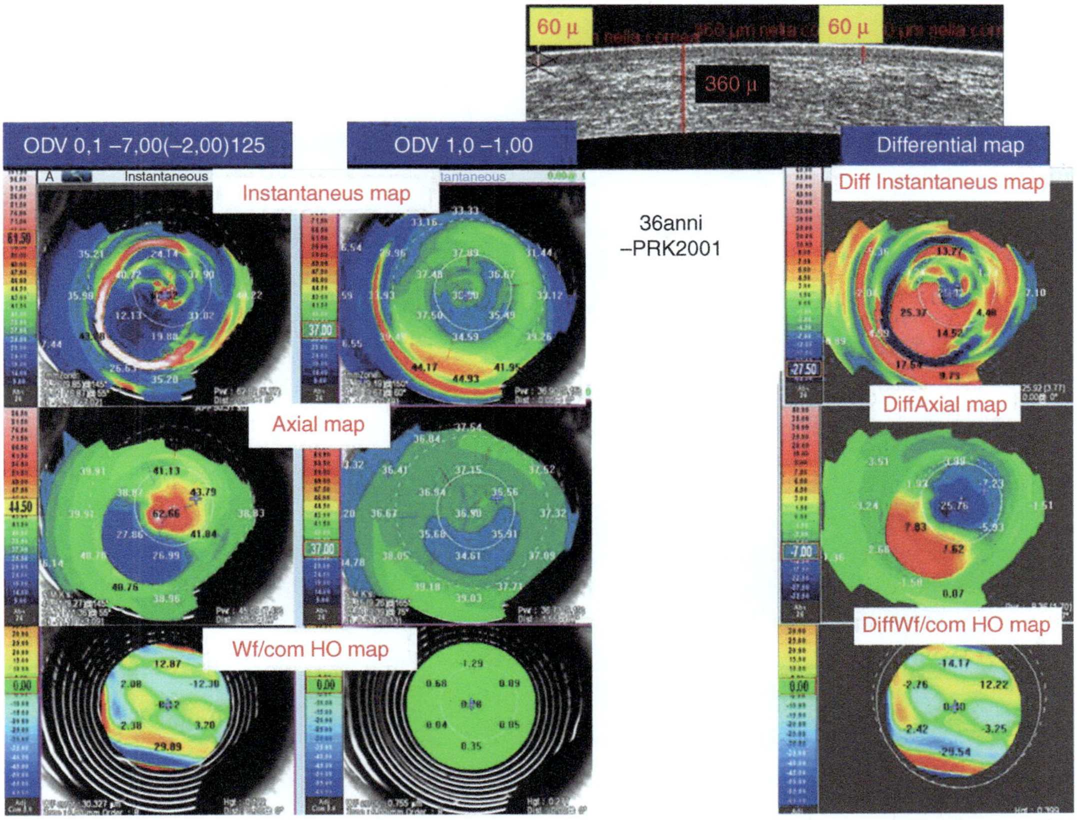

Fig. 9.3 Case 1, right eye. Pre- and postoperative corneal topography, axial and instantaneous algorithm, corneal wave front map. Note at the differential maps, on the *right*, the almost complete disappearance for the peripheral high-curvature ring generated by previous treatments. Above, *right*, postoperative OCT featuring a regular epithelium as well as a regular stroma without opacities

acuity improved after each phase. Figure 9.3 shows pre- and postoperative corneal topography with differential maps.

Case 2

A 26-year-old female contact lens wearer incurred an Acanthamoeba infection in her right eye. Her preoperative vision was 0.1 +1.00 sph −7.00 cyl (65) and vision in her left eye was 0.9 −4.00 sph. Anterior segment examination of the right eye showed a vascularized, central-paracentral corneal leukoma, with stromal thinning. The preoperative OCT showed a mild stromal opacity extending down to 184 µ in the stroma (Fig. 9.4). Total corneal pachymetry in the thinnest point was 444 µ, with an epithelial thickness of 104 µ, thus a residual stroma of 340 µ (Fig. 9.4). Preoperative topography (Fig. 9.5) revealed a wide superotemporal area of corneal flattening, corresponding to the leukomatous cornea with stromal thinning. Transepithelial SCTK was applied. The first custom ablation phase targeted regularizing the optical zone by flattening only the steep inferonasal cornea as well as sparing the thinned cornea. In fact, steepening a flattened portion of the cornea can be achieved by flattening the surrounding steep cornea. Such an asymmetrical ablation may induce corneal relaxation and changes in both HOA and refraction. Thus, a second phase was necessary. Figure 9.6 shows the Schwind Amaris shotfile for the second phase highlighting a residual myopia

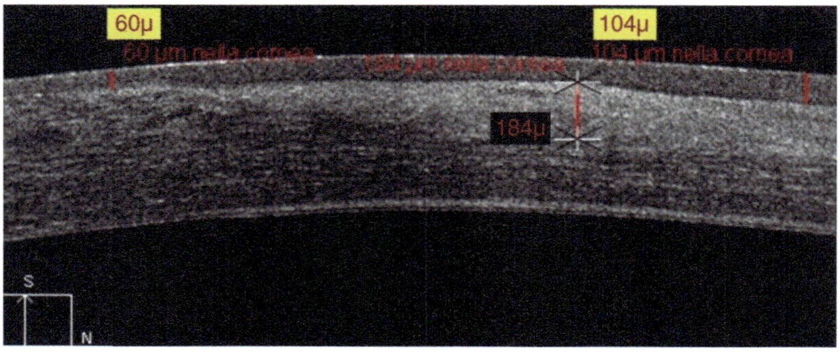

Fig. 9.4 Case 2, right eye. Preoperative OCT shows a mild stromal opacity extending for 184 µ

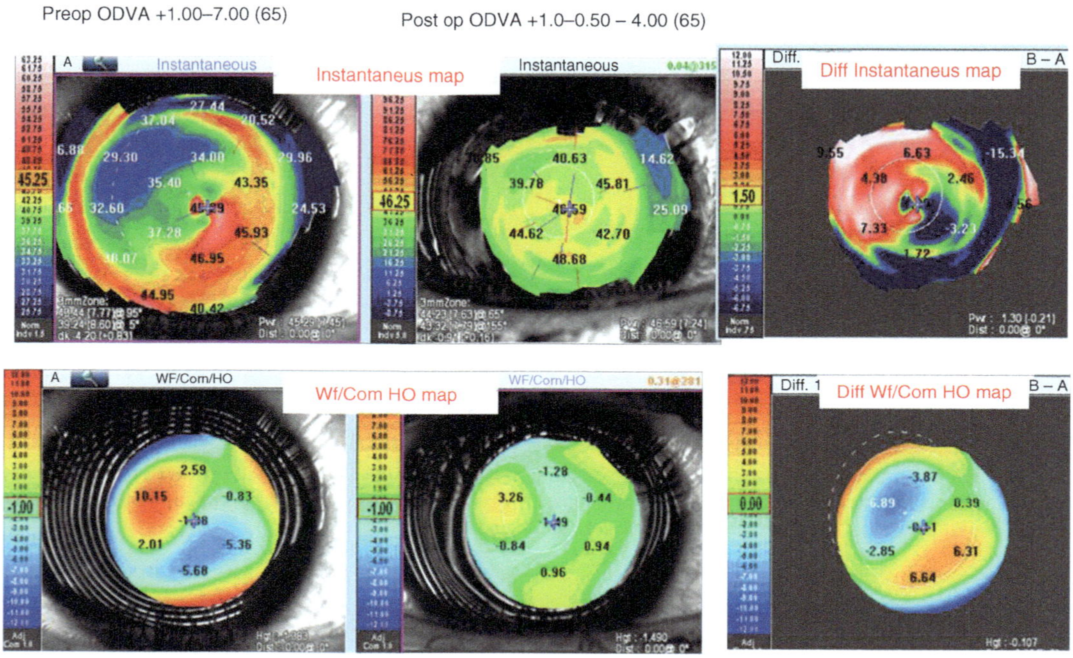

Fig. 9.5 Case 2, right eye. Preoperative topography shows a wide superotemporal area of corneal flattening, corresponding to the leukomatous cornea with stromal thinning. Postoperative maps (*center*) show regularization of central corneal and decrease of high-order aberrations

planned (target: −2.50 SE) to avoid anisometropia. Vision improved after each phase.

The Problem

Case 1: The main problems were irregular astigmatism due to a highly irregular cornea, stromal haze with a deeply irregular subepithelial scar, and a peripheral high-curvature ring generated by previous treatments.

Case 2: The main problems were high astigmatism due to the eccentrical area of corneal flattening and a vascularized corneal leukoma with stromal thinning.

Ancillary Tests

Corneal topography, aberrometry, corneal spectral domain OCT, Pentacam.

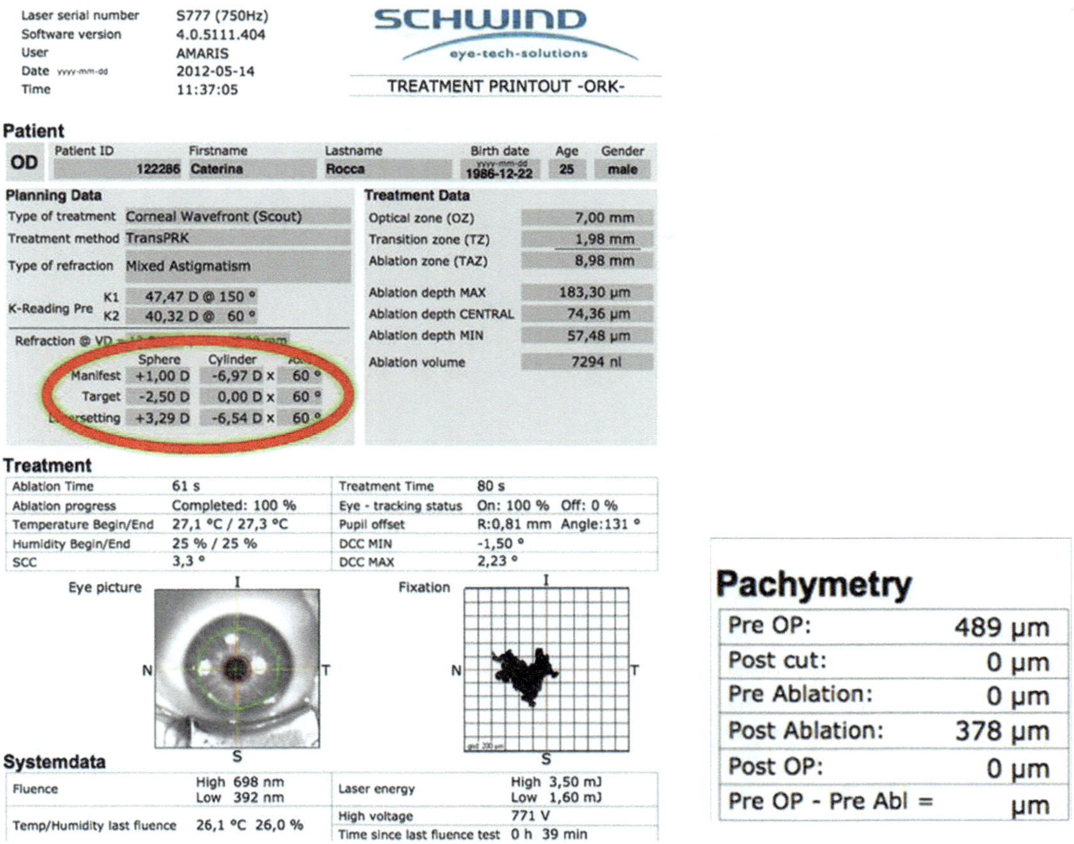

Laser serial number	S777 (750Hz)
Software version	4.0.5111.404
User	AMARIS
Date yyyy-mm-dd	2012-05-14
Time	11:37:05

SCHWIND eye-tech-solutions

TREATMENT PRINTOUT -ORK-

Patient

	Patient ID	Firstname	Lastname	Birth date yyyy-mm-dd	Age	Gender
OD	122286	Caterina	Rocca	1986-12-22	25	male

Planning Data

Type of treatment	Corneal Wavefront (Scout)
Treatment method	TransPRK
Type of refraction	Mixed Astigmatism
K-Reading Pre K1	47,47 D @ 150 °
K-Reading Pre K2	40,32 D @ 60 °

Refraction @ VD

	Sphere	Cylinder	Axis
Manifest	+1,00 D	-6,97 D x	60 °
Target	-2,50 D	0,00 D x	60 °
…rsetting	+3,29 D	-6,54 D x	60 °

Treatment Data

Optical zone (OZ)	7,00 mm
Transition zone (TZ)	1,98 mm
Ablation zone (TAZ)	8,98 mm
Ablation depth MAX	183,30 µm
Ablation depth CENTRAL	74,36 µm
Ablation depth MIN	57,48 µm
Ablation volume	7294 nl

Treatment

Ablation Time	61 s	Treatment Time	80 s
Ablation progress	Completed: 100 %	Eye - tracking status	On: 100 % Off: 0 %
Temperature Begin/End	27,1 °C / 27,3 °C	Pupil offset	R:0,81 mm Angle:131 °
Humidity Begin/End	25 % / 25 %	DCC MIN	-1,50 °
SCC	3,3 °	DCC MAX	2,23 °

Systemdata

Fluence	High 698 nm Low 392 nm	Laser energy	High 3,50 mJ Low 1,60 mJ
Temp/Humidity last fluence	26,1 °C 26,0 %	High voltage	771 V
		Time since last fluence test	0 h 39 min

Pachymetry

Pre OP:	489 µm
Post cut:	0 µm
Pre Ablation:	0 µm
Post Ablation:	378 µm
Post OP:	0 µm
Pre OP - Pre Abl =	µm

Fig. 9.6 Case 2, right eye. Schwind Amaris shotfile highlighting planning of residual myopia (target: –2.50 sph), in order to avoid anisometropia. Pachymetry is inclusive of corneal epithelium

Surgical/Medical Intervention

Transepithelial SCTK consists of a custom corneal topography-based excimer laser ablation, followed by a second corneal topography to evaluate residual irregularities and plan a further custom-based ablation [1–4]. This sequence may be repeated until a regular cornea is achieved or residual stromal thickness approaches safety limits. Custom ablation was performed with the Schwind Amaris excimer laser linked to the ORK-CAM platform (Schwind GMBH & Co., Kleinostheim, Germany). Corneal topography was performed with Sirius or Keratron Scout topographers (CSO, Florence, Italy; Optikon 2000, Rome, Italy), directly linked to the custom ablation platform. Finally, a corneal smoothing phase was performed applying a sodium hyaluronate 0.25 % solution (Laservis, TRB Chemedica, AG, Haar/Munchen, Germany) featuring the same ablation rate of the cornea. This solution acts as a masking fluid: a Castroviejo spatula was used to diffuse the fluid over the cornea and allow irregularities to emerge while a 10-mm wide ablation was performed for a theoretical depth of 20 µ. The irregularities were ablated, producing a very smooth corneal surface.

In the first phase of case 2, we used a special feature of the Schwind ORK-CAM platform that treats only corneal irregularities generating HOA. Our clinic collaborated with Schwind to develop this special feature. Figure 9.5 shows the final instantaneous map (center, above), featuring a much more regular cornea. Postoperative HOA map (Fig. 9.5, center, below) demonstrates significant reduction of preoperative coma.

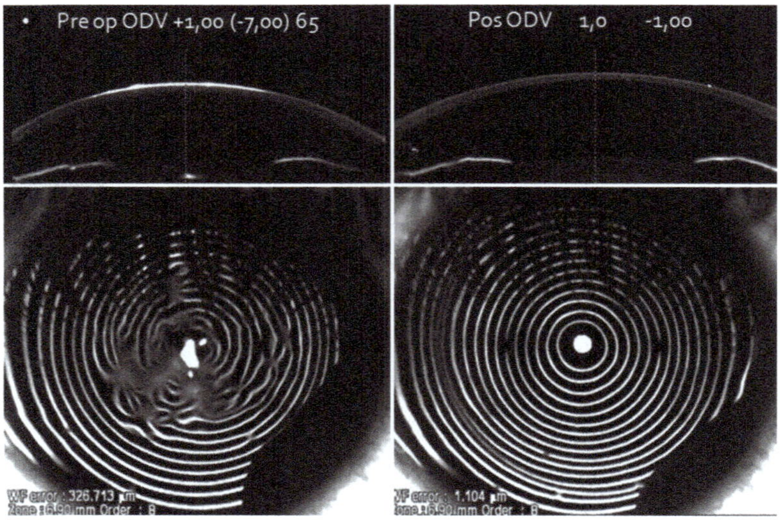

Fig. 9.7 Case 1, right eye. Pre- and postoperative keratoscopy, note nice regularization of the rings

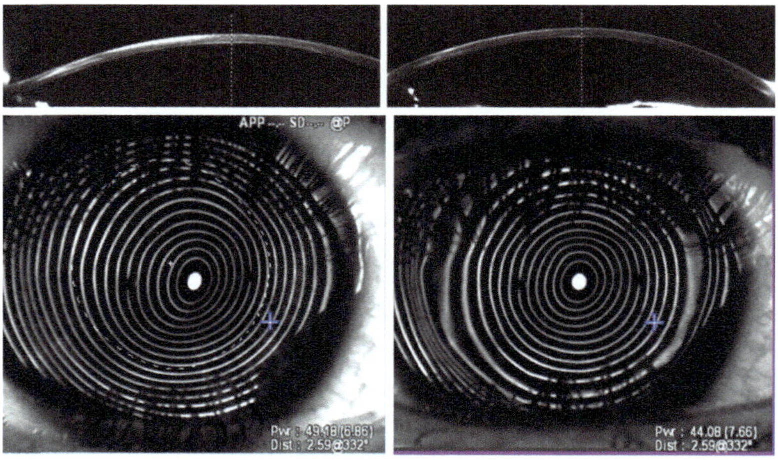

Fig. 9.8 Case 2, right eye. Pre- and postoperative keratoscopy, with significant regularization of ovalized rings. Pentacam shows decrease in stromal opacities

Outcome

Case 1: Two months after surgery, vision in the right eye was 1.0 with −1.00 sph, and the cornea was transparent without residual haze. Figure 9.3 shows regularization of the optical zone, with near-complete disappearance of the peripheral spherical aberration and the high-curvature ring generated by previous treatments. Furthermore, Fig. 9.3 shows the postoperative OCT featuring a regular 60 μ thick epithelium and a stroma without opacities. Figure 9.7 shows the pre- and postoperative keratoscopy featuring regularization of the rings.

Case 2: Two weeks after surgery, vision was 0.8 with –0.50 sph and –4.00 cyl (65). Planned SE was attained, but complete correction of astigmatism was prevented by the scarce residual stromal thickness that discouraged further ablation. Figure 9.8 shows pre- and postoperative keratoscopy, with significant regularization of ovalized rings, as well as a decrease in stromal opacities at Pentacam. Corneal new vessels appear regressed.

What We Learned

Both cases revealed that a well-conducted SCTK may provide excellent results and spare the patient complications including a long postoperative period and high final refractive error related to partial or total corneal transplantation.

Concentrating SCTK ablation on the thickest corneal portions spares thinned portions and provides corneal regularization even in the case of highly irregular astigmatism. In case 2, we spared the patient a partial or total keratoplasty with increased possibilities of rejection due to the presence of a vascularized leukoma.

Finally, as demonstrated in case 1, it is interesting to notice how a single-phase PTK may not lead to reliable results, even when mitomycin is added.

References

1. Roberts C (2002) Biomechanics of the cornea and wavefront-guided laser refractive surgery. J Refract Surg 18:S589–S592
2. Vinciguerra P, Camesasca FI (2004) Custom phototherapeutic keratectomy with intraoperative topography. J Refract Surg 20:S555–S563
3. Vinciguerra P, Camesasca FI (2004) One-year follow-up of custom phototherapeutic keratectomy. J Refract Surg 20(5 Suppl):705–710
4. Vinciguerra P, Camesasca FI (eds) (2007) Refractive surface ablation: PRK, LASEK, Epi-LASIK, PTK and retreatment. Slack Inc., Thorofare

10 Combined Post-keratoplasty LASIK/AK to Treat High Astigmatism

Joann J. Kang and Dimitri T. Azar

Contents

J.J. Kang, MD (✉)
Department of Ophthalmology,
University of Illinois at Chicago, Chicago, IL, USA
e-mail: kang.joann@gmail.com

D.T. Azar, MD, MBA
Department of Ophthalmology and Visual Sciences
Illinois Eye and Ear Infirmary,
University of Illinois at Chicago, Chicago, IL, USA
e-mail: dazar@uic.edu

Why Is This Case Relevant for the Refractive Surgeon?

Refractive unpredictability and postoperative astigmatism are common complications following penetrating keratoplasty [1–5]. High astigmatism may result in decreased visual acuity, anisometropia, image distortion, and monocular diplopia, thus challenging the visual rehabilitation of patients [1]. Spectacle correction or soft contact lenses are used to manage small amounts of cylinder, while rigid gas permeable lenses are effective for higher levels of regular astigmatism or in the presence of irregular astigmatism [1]. However, contact lenses may not be successful for all patients due to a variety of factors including corneal abnormalities, dry eye, lid abnormalities, or contact lens intolerance. Therefore, when conservative methods fail, other refractive treatments for post-keratoplasty astigmatism are needed.

Case Background

An 83-year-old retired high school teacher was referred for a "corneal problem." He had a past medical history of mild asthma, arthritis, and migraine headaches and also underwent removal of a gastrointestinal tumor and prostate surgery. His medications included aspirin, Asmanex, and Cafergot. The patient's past ocular history included bilateral cataract extraction 9 years prior to presentation and subsequent penetrating

J.L. Alió et al. (eds.), *Difficult and Complicated Cases in Refractive Surgery*,
DOI 10.1007/978-3-642-55238-0_10, © Springer-Verlag Berlin Heidelberg 2015

keratoplasty in the right eye 1 year later and in the left eye seven years later for presumed pseudophakic bullous keratopathy. He also reported a history of corrective surgery one year prior for astigmatism of the left eye. Using his current spectacles, his vision in the right eye was 20/100 with a −5.00 +4.25×015 correction and 20/200 with −6.25 +5.50×022 correction. Manifest refraction improved his vision to 20/25 in the right eye with a −5.00 +4.25×032 correction and $20/25^{-3}$ in the left eye with −12.75 +12.00×180 correction. His corneal pachymetry was 612 and 616 µm in the right and left eye, respectively. Slit-lamp biomicroscopy showed clear corneal grafts without any signs of rejection or wound override and all sutures were removed. Posterior intraocular lens implants were present for both eyes. Fundus examination was notable for peripapillary atrophy and showed some peripheral pigmentary change. Keratometry and corneal topography were performed and showed high against the rule astigmatism in the left eye greater than the right.

Main Problem to Solve

This patient presented with high post-keratoplasty astigmatism greater in the left eye. Although spectacle correction was satisfactory for his right eye, his left eye had a higher amount of cylinder, resulting in significant anisometropia and image distortion. He was unable to be corrected adequately with spectacles and was contact lens intolerant. The corneal transplant in his left eye was performed 2 years prior to presentation and all sutures were removed postoperatively; thus, selective suture removal or adjustment of a running suture was not possible at the time of presentation. Alternative surgical options for correction of this patient's post-keratoplasty astigmatism were needed.

Ancillary Tests

Post-keratoplasty astigmatism should be evaluated using a combination of manifest refraction, keratometry, corneal topography, and wave front analysis (Fig. 10.1). Slit-lamp examination is also important for evaluating graft centration, size, clarity, as well as the graft-host interface for wound apposition. Corneal thickness is another important parameter to measure when considering refractive surgery.

Surgical/Medical Intervention

In this case, a combined astigmatic keratotomy (AK) and laser assisted in situ keratomileusis (LASIK) was performed in two steps:

- First, femtosecond laser (IntraLase) was used to make symmetric paired arcuate incisions (laser settings of 90 % of graft thickness, 7 mm diameter, 90° arc length, anterior side cut energy 3 µJ) centered at the steep meridian and inside the graft-host interface.
- Next, a nasal flap was created with a thickness set at 150 µm and directly measured to be 115 µm, avoiding the incision at the graft-host interface.
- The flap was then lifted, the arcuate incisions opened, and the flap replaced. Afterward, keratoscopy mires were checked and significant residual astigmatism was noted.
- Finally, VISX laser treatment was performed to correct an additional 8D of cylinder (using two −4.00 treatments) with a residual stromal bed noted of 526 µm. The procedure was uneventful with no intraoperative complications.

Outcome

The patient did well postoperatively. At 1 month after the procedure, his vision was 20/25 in the left eye with a refraction of −3.00 +3.50×45 (Fig. 10.2). Slit-lamp examination revealed a clear graft, a nasal hinged LASIK flap, and the two arcuate incisions under the LASIK flap. His refraction (−4.00 +3.25×017) and topography remained stable at 6 months postoperatively (Fig. 10.3). At his last documented follow-up, 3 years later, his best-corrected spectacle vision was 20/20 in the right eye (−5.50 +5.50×010) and 20/20 in the left eye (−5.25 +4.75×018) (Fig. 10.4). There was a total decrease in

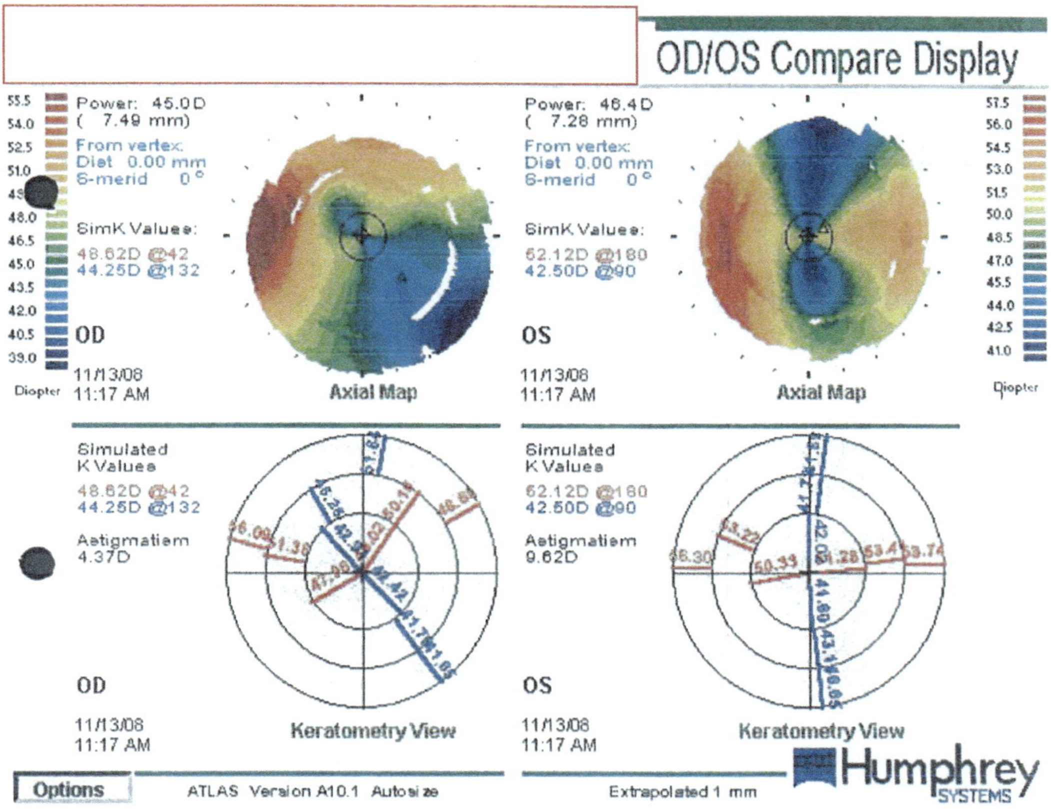

Fig. 10.1 Preoperative Humphrey corneal topography of both eyes, demonstrating higher corneal astigmatism in the left eye. The simulated keratometry OS showing 42.50 D; 52.12 D at 180°

astigmatic correction by 7.25D in the left eye as measured by manifest refraction. The patient was satisfied with his excellent vision with spectacle correction and without anisometropia.

What to Learn from This Case

High astigmatism after penetrating keratoplasty presents a challenge for visual rehabilitation despite an optically clear corneal graft. There are several refractive options for the correction of post-keratoplasty astigmatism including astigmatic keratotomy, refractive surgery such as LASIK and photorefractive keratectomy (PRK), compression sutures, and wedge resections [1–4]. Other surgical procedures include cataract extraction and intraocular lens (IOL) implantation for phakic patients or placement of a piggyback IOL for pseudophakic patients [3]. One-step LASIK (lamellar cut and ablation in one procedure) or two-step LASIK (lamellar cut then ablation in two successive procedures) has also been investigated in treating post-keratoplasty astigmatism [5]. A two-step procedure with LASIK flap creation before ablation leads to a more precise and better refractive outcome in PKP eyes [5]. It is important to note that prior to any surgical intervention, we should ensure that the graft-host junction is well healed and all sutures have been removed to ensure a stable refraction and topography.

In this particular case, AK was combined with LASIK for optimal astigmatic correction as our patient had high myopic astigmatism. AK is a well-established technique that reduces high

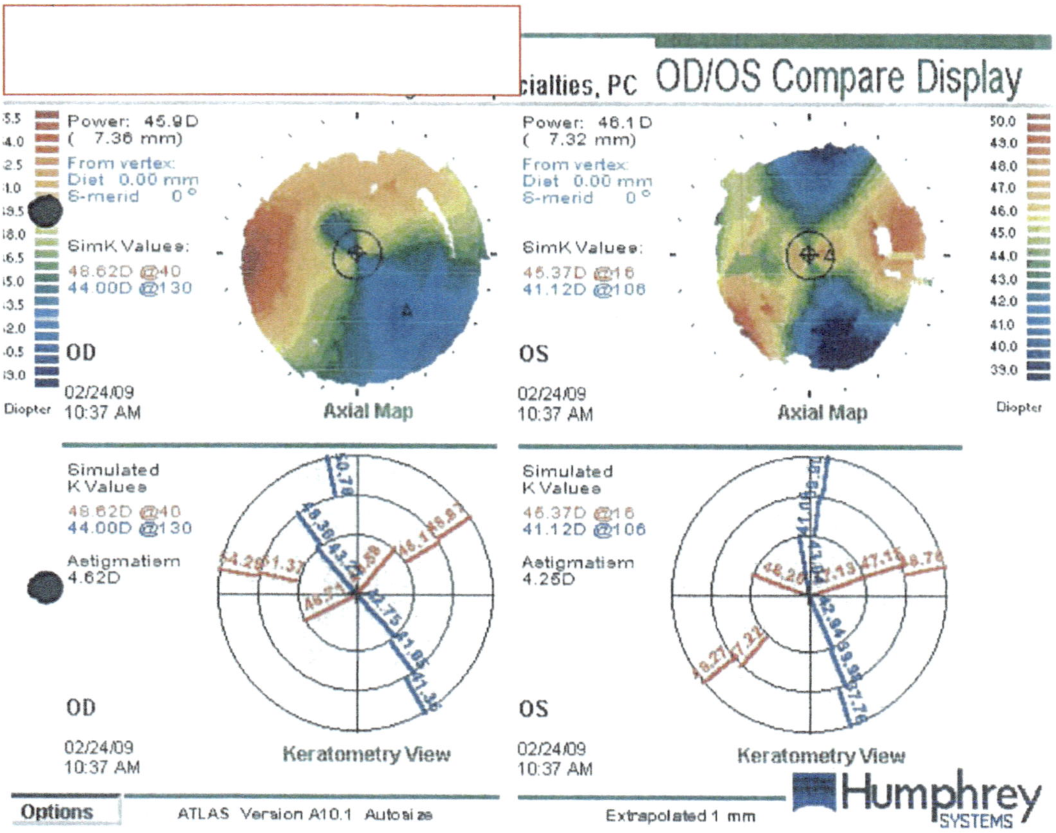

Fig. 10.2 Humphrey corneal topography of both eyes at 1 month post AK and LASIK procedure of the left eye

astigmatism by flattening the steep corneal meridian with the placement of one or two incisions perpendicular to the steep axis. Outcomes may vary based on the number of incisions, incision length and depth, as well as the use of freehand, mechanical, or femtosecond laser techniques. In our case, we placed the arcuate incisions central to the graft-host junction at the 7.0 mm optical zone and used 90 % depth for maximal effect. We also used femtosecond laser to improve the precision of AK as the accuracy of depth and length of the incisions made by the laser may result in better final outcomes.

A stepped approach was planned with AK performed first, followed by refractive surgery to address the residual astigmatic and spherical component as our patient had a very high preoperative astigmatism of 12D. Refractive surgery options, including PRK and LASIK, show effectiveness in treating post-keratoplasty astigmatism as they correct not only astigmatism but also myopia and hyperopia. LASIK has the advantage of correcting a wider range of refractive disorders and offering more effective and predictable outcomes, faster visual rehabilitation, and less stromal scarring than PRK. Femtosecond laser may also be used to create the LASIK flap and has more uniform and thinner flaps than mechanical microkeratomes. However, the accuracy of these procedures is less predictable after penetrating keratoplasty, as wound healing may differ from the normal healing response of a patient's cornea. In addition, although minimized with the

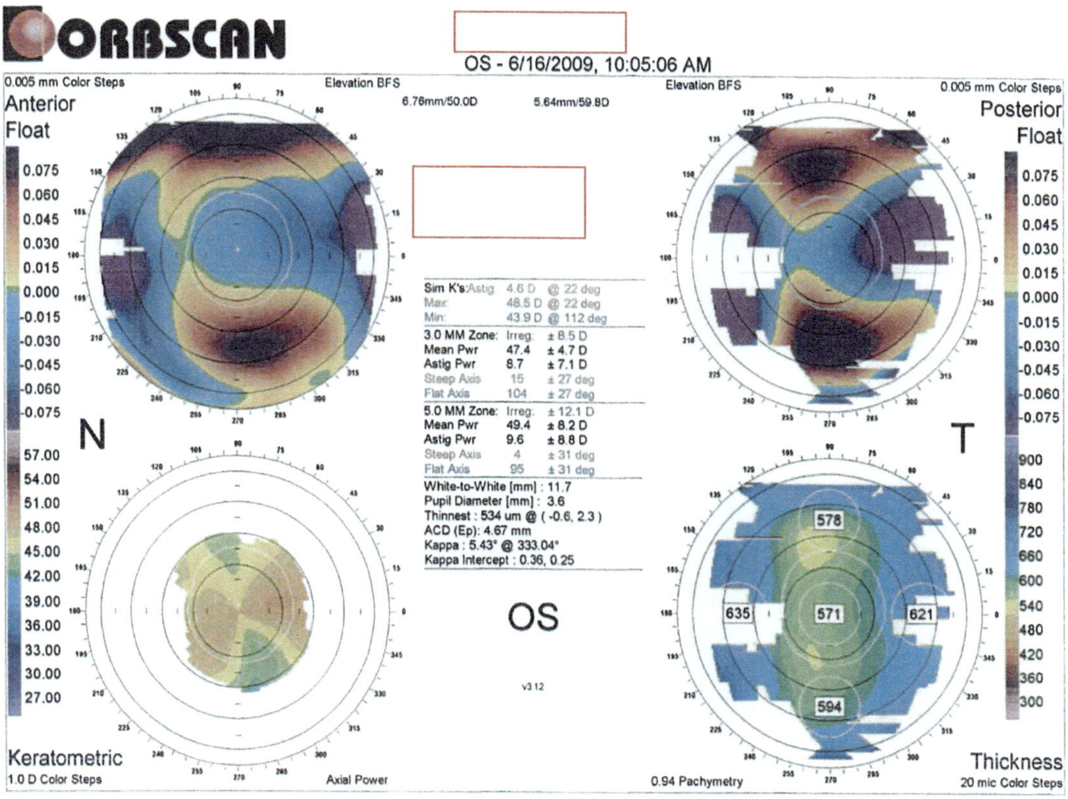

Fig. 10.3 Orbscan corneal topography of the left eye 6 months post AK and LASIK procedure

use of prophylactic mitomycin C, there is a risk of late-onset haze formation in PRK and graft-host destabilization during the creation of the LASIK flap. However, most studies have found that refractive surgery following penetrating keratoplasty is safe, effective, and predictable and results in satisfactory refractive outcomes.

In conclusion, post-keratoplasty astigmatism is very common and may limit visual recovery in otherwise successful grafts. Multiple options exist for treating post-keratoplasty astigmatism, including a combination of incisional techniques and refractive surgery for high astigmatism, with the ultimate goal of spectacle-corrected binocularity.

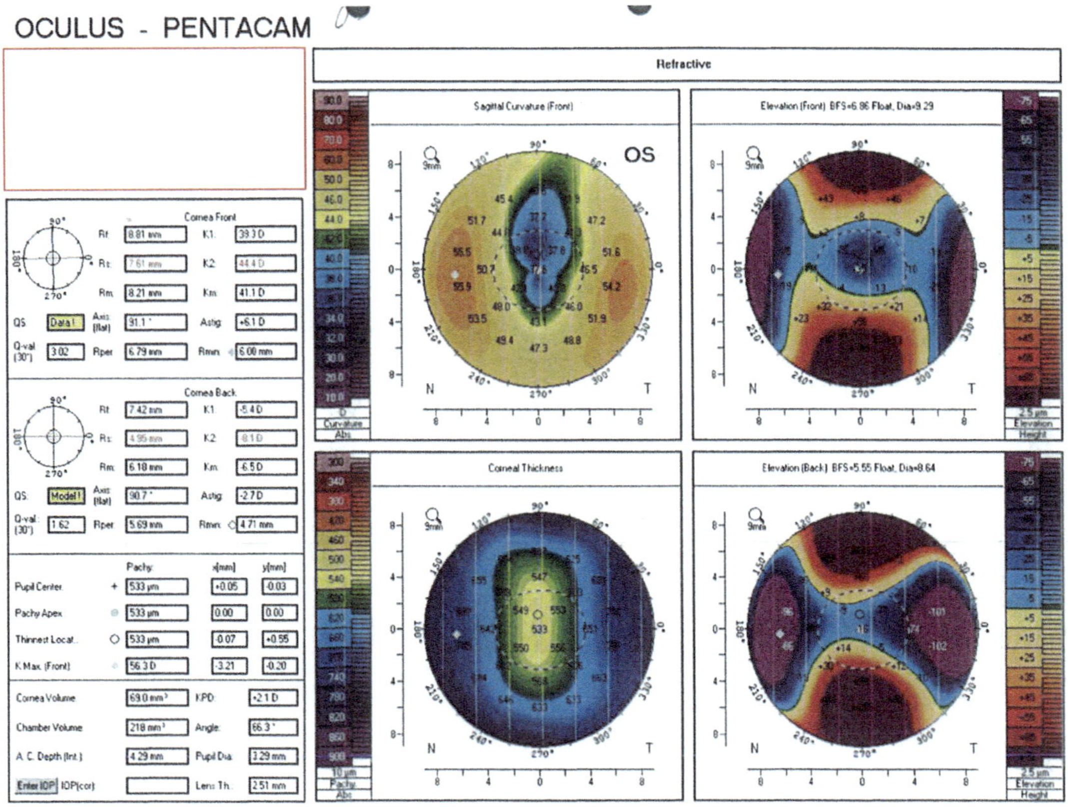

Fig. 10.4 Pentacam topography of the left eye, 3 years postoperatively, demonstrating stable corneal curvature and astigmatism consistent with minimal progressive increase in refractive astigmatism

References

1. Butrus SI, Ashraf F, Azar DT (2007) Postkeratoplasty astigmatism: etiology, management and femtosecond laser applications. In: Azar DT (ed), Gatinel D, Hoang-Xuan T (associate editors) Refractive surgery, 2nd edn. Elsevier-Mosby, St. Louis. pp 549–559
2. Buzard K, Febbraro JL, Fundingsland BR (2004) Laser in situ keratomileusis for the correction of residual ametropia after penetrating keratoplasty. J Cataract Refract Surg 30:1006–1013
3. Ghanem RC, Azar DT (2006) Femtosecond-laser arcuate wedge-shaped resection to correct high residual astigmatism after penetrating keratoplasty. J Cataract Refract Surg 32:1415–1419
4. Fares U, Sarhan AR, Dua HS (2012) Management of post-keratoplasty astigmatism. J Cataract Refract Surg 38:2029–2039
5. Alio JL, Javaloy J, Osman AA, Galvis V, Tello A, Haroun HE (2004) Laser in situ keratomileusis to correct post-keratoplasty astigmatism: 1-step versus 2-step procedure. J Cataract Refract Surg 30: 2303–2310

Avoiding Corneal Graft: From Corneal Surgery to Phakic IOL

11

Jorge L. Alió and Alessandro Abbouda

Contents

J.L. Alió, MD, PhD (✉)
Department of Refractive Surgery, Vissum Corporación Oftalmológica, Alicante, Spain
e-mail: jlalio@vissum.com

A. Abbouda, MD
Department of Refractive Surgery, Vissum Corporación Oftalmológica, Alicante, Spain

Department of Ophthalmology-Policlinico Umberto I of Rome, University of Rome "Sapienza", Viale del Policlinico, 155, 00186 Roma, Italy

R&D Department, Vissum Corporación Oftalmológica, 03016, Alicante, Spain
e-mail: a.abbouda@gmail.com

Why Is This Case Relevant for the Refractive Surgeon?

Irregular astigmatism, one of the worst sequelae of corneal injuries, is a frequent complication of corneal refractive surgery. Options for the correction of irregular astigmatism are scarce, with limited results. Discovering new surgical methods to improve corneal regularity for the correction of astigmatism is of primary importance, especially as corneal refractive surgery techniques including laser in situ keratomileusis.

Case Background

A 43-year-old woman was evaluated for low vision in the right eye after infectious keratitis related to contact lens use. Best corrected visual acuity (BCVA) was 20/40 with a manifest refraction of -1×170. She presented with a central leukoma (Fig. 11.1a). Preoperative central thickness was 430 μm. The keratometry reading was $43.49/46.17 \times 70$. The corneal topography showed a flat area in correspondence to the leukoma (Fig. 11.1b). Corneal aberrometry showed RMS of 6.51 μm (Fig. 11.1c). On November 2011, the patient underwent superficial lamellar keratectomy with FM laser, assisted by a viscous masking solution of 0.25 % sodium hyaluronate (ELASHY's technique) [1, 2].

J.L. Alió et al. (eds.), *Difficult and Complicated Cases in Refractive Surgery*,
DOI 10.1007/978-3-642-55238-0_11, © Springer-Verlag Berlin Heidelberg 2015

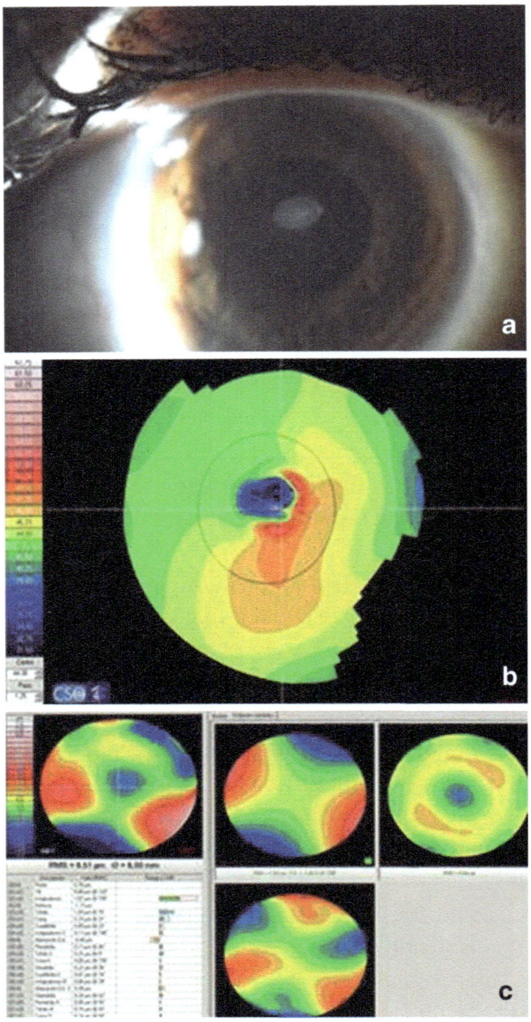

Fig. 11.1 (**a**) Slit lamp showed a central leukoma. (**b**, **c**) Preoperative topography and aberrometry pattern. Topography showed a flat area in the same area of leukoma, and corneal aberrometry showed the presence of highest value of trifolio, trifolio II, spherical aberration II, trifolio III, and coma IV

The ablation was 30 μm. The postoperative period was uneventful. The slit-lamp examination showed a persistence of leukoma in the temporal area. After 3 months, the corrected distance visual acuity (CDVA) was 20/50 with a manifest refraction of +4 in the right eye. The keratometry reading was 29.65/31.39 × 136 in the right. The aspect of the images showed a diffuse inferior flattening area (Fig. 11.2a). The corneal aberrometry showed RMS of 13.24 (Fig. 11.2b).

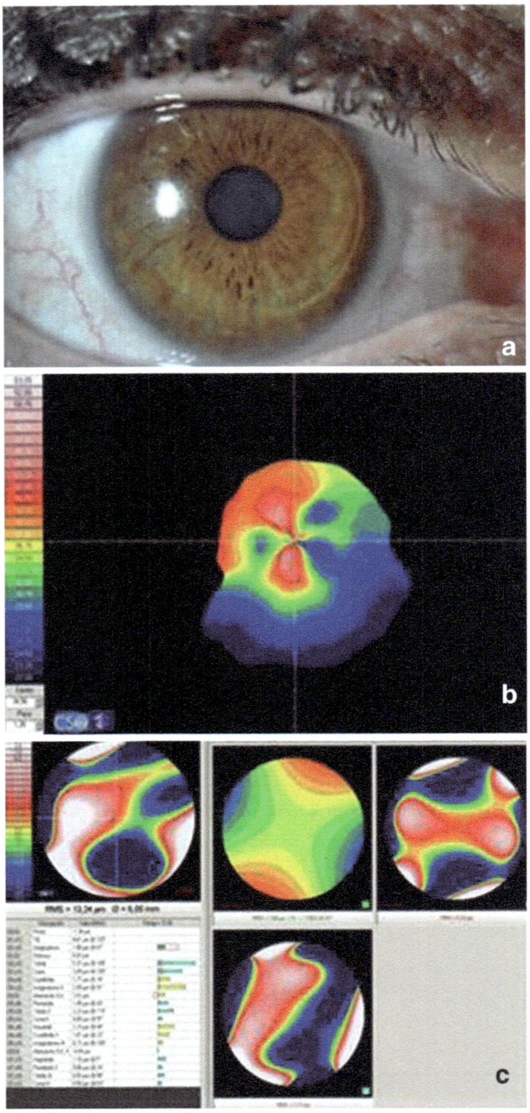

Fig. 11.2 (**a**) Slit lamp showed a clear cornea. (**b**, **c**) Postoperative topography and aberrometry pattern. Topography showed a large inferior flat area, and corneal aberrometry showed the presence of the highest value for each aberration

We decided on PTK treatment. The ablation was 80 μm. On January 2011, the CDVA was 20/25 with a manifest refraction of +5 −2 × 180 in the right eye. The slit-lamp examination revealed a resolution of leukoma (Fig. 11.3a). The keratometry reading was 37.83/39.95 × 90, showing a central flat area (Fig. 11.3b). The corneal aberrometry showed RMS of 8.92 (Fig. 11.3c).

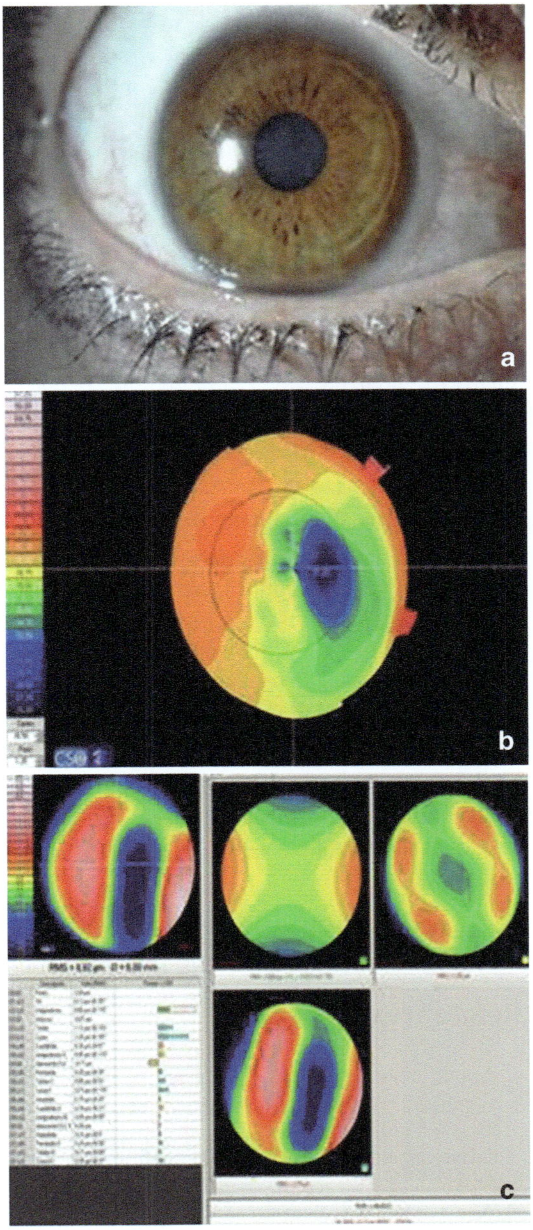

Fig. 11.3 (**a**, **b**) Post-PTK topography and aberrometry pattern. Topography showed a reduction of the flat area, and corneal aberrometry showed the presence of the highest value in astigmatism, trifolio, coma, and spherical aberration, (**b**) Post-operative Topography showed a large inferior flat area, (**c**) Post operative corneal aberrometry pattern showed the presence of highest value for each aberration

Her vision was getting worse. In February, the CDVA was 20/25 with a manifest refraction of +10 −4 × 10 in the right.

Main Problem to Solve

ELASHY's technique can induce corneal thinning and requires a prolonged follow-up to determine its biomechanical effects and stability. However, in this case, the procedure allowed removal of the corneal scar without the biological problems and long follow-up required with a corneal graft.

Ancillary Tests

Modern corneal topography shows certain patterns and numerical indexes of corneal irregularity that can be useful for follow-up. However, today the most useful clinical examination technique is corneal aberrometry. Based on this patient's clinical information, auxiliary clinical examination techniques were options. The most relevant for this case were anterior segment optical coherence tomography (OCT), very high-frequency (VHF) ultrasound bioimaging of the anterior segment of the eye, and corneal confocal microscopy. Corneal confocal microscopy allows a precise estimation of the corneal depth at which to remove the leukoma.

Surgical/Medical Intervention

The first treatment was superficial corneal excision with FM laser assisted by a viscous masking solution of 0.25 % sodium hyaluronate (ELASHY). The procedure intended to produce a uniform corneal surface while improving best corrected visual acuity. A viscous masking agent increased the procedure's efficiency by protecting the valley between the irregular corneal peaks while leaving the peaks exposed to laser treatment. Then, we performed PTK to obtain a resolution of leukoma and a better corneal surface. Finally, we decide to implant an iris supported phakic IOL (Artisan) of power +12 −5.5 axis 0. We defined the axis of implantation by marking the limbus with a surgical pen.

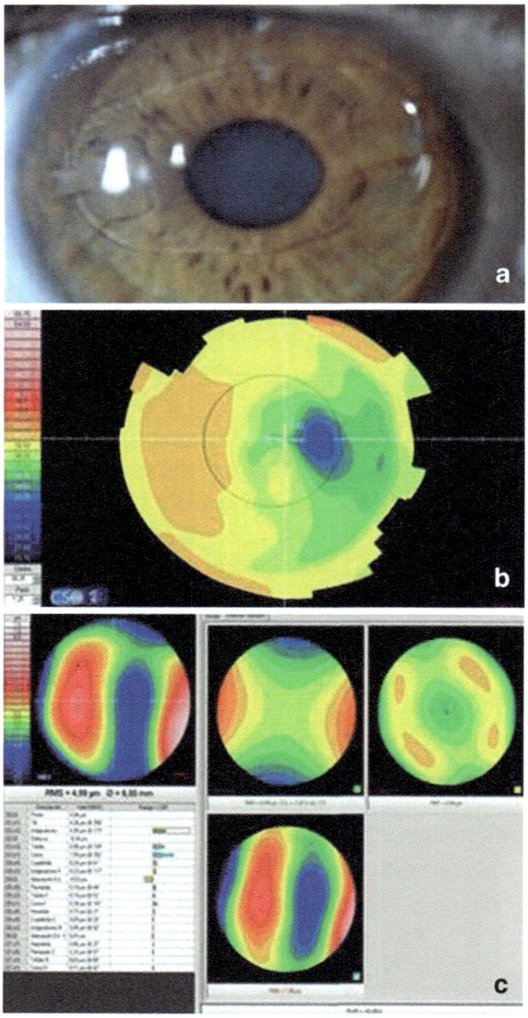

Fig. 11.4 (**a**) Slit-lamp examination showed clear cornea and a well-centered phakic IOL. (**b**, **c**) Topography and aberrometry pattern at the end of follow-up. Topography showed a further reduction of flat area, and corneal aberrometry showed the persistence of the highest value in astigmatism and coma

Outcome

Three months post phakic IOL implantation, the patient's refraction was 20/20 with a manifest refraction of −1 −1×120 in the right eye. The slit lamp showed a clear cornea and the anterior chamber lens was well centered (Fig. 11.4a). The keratometry reading was 39.86/39.62×82 (Fig. 11.4b). The corneal aberrometry showed RMS of 4.99 μm (Fig. 11.4c).

What to Learn from This Case

Irregular astigmatism is very common after corneal surgery, trauma, dystrophies, and infections. Visual disability characterized by a steep or flattened area of the cornea extending larger than 2 mm is classified as macro-irregular, while a disperse irregularity of the cornea that does not create a well-defined elevated or flattened area is described as micro-irregular. Mixed patterns showing aspects of both macro- and micro-irregularity are common, as occurred in this case. This initial classification obtained from the corneal topography map has important clinical implications [3]. As described in the literature, various treatments for irregular astigmatism exist, including contact lens adaptation, wavefront-guided excimer laser surgery, internal corneal ring segment (ICRS) implantation, deep anterior lamellar keratoplasty (DALK), and penetrating keratoplasty (PK) [4, 5].

As an alternative to corneal grafting, automated superficial corneal excision with sodium hyaluronate 0.25 % may be used to manage severe superficial corneal opacities. Phakic IOL can be used to obtain a refractive target after this procedure,

References

1. Alió JL, Javaloy J, Merayo J, Galal A (2004) Automated superficial lamellar keratectomy augmented by excimer laser masked PTK in the management of severe superficial corneal opacities. Br J Ophthalmol 88:1289–1294
2. Alio JL, Belda JI, Shalaby AM (2001) Correction of irregular astigmatism with excimer laser assisted by sodium hyaluronate. Ophthalmology 108:1246–1260
3. Alió JL, Belda JI, Patel S (2004) Treating irregular astigmatism and keratoconus. Highlights of Ophthalmology International, Miami, pp 1–14
4. Alió JL (2008) Chapter 7.4 Corneal irregularity. In: Alio JL, Azar D (eds) Management of complications in refractive surgery. Springer, Berlin/Heidelberg, pp 141–152
5. Alió JL, Belda JI (2004) Practical guidelines for the correction of irregular astigmatism and keratoconus. In: Alió JL, Belda JI, Patel S (eds) Treating irregular astigmatism and keratoconus. Highlights of Ophthalmology International, Miami, p 335, 342

12 Excimer Laser Treatment of Irregular Astigmatism Following Phaco Wound Burn

Scott Kelly and Dimitri T. Azar

Contents

S. Kelly (✉) • D.T. Azar, MD, MBA
Department of Ophthalmology and Visual Sciences
Illinois Eye and Ear Infirmary, University of Illinois at Chicago, Chicago, IL, USA
e-mail: scottkellyy@gmail.com; dazar@uic.edu

Why Is This Case Relevant for the Refractive Surgeon?

Thermal burn from phacoemulsification is much less prevalent today than it was even 10 or 20 years ago. However, when it occurs it causes irregular astigmatism of varying degrees [1]. In severe cases such as the one presented here, exposure to treatment options and maintaining uncorrected visual acuity are critical to patient satisfaction.

Case Background

Our patient is a 93-year-old Caucasian hyperopic patient who underwent cataract extraction in his left eye 1 year prior to referral for treatment. His cataract extraction was complicated by a dense nucleus, posterior capsular tear, and thermal phacoemulsification burn of the main 2.4 mm temporal corneal wound. An anterior vitrectomy was performed, and an intraocular lens was placed in the sulcus. Initial postoperative management included closure of the gaping wound with multiple 10-0 nylon sutures, which were removed prior to presentation.

He currently has a cataract in his right eye, but no other ocular history.

He has a past medical history of early dementia, hearing loss, and hypertension, for which he takes lisinopril, metoprolol, and tamsulosin. He has no allergies.

J.L. Alió et al. (eds.), *Difficult and Complicated Cases in Refractive Surgery*,
DOI 10.1007/978-3-642-55238-0_12, © Springer-Verlag Berlin Heidelberg 2015

His vision with presurgical glasses in the right eye was 20/60 with +4.75 +1.50 × 180. His uncorrected vision in the left eye was 20/60. Manifest refraction improved his right eye vision to 20/30 with +3.50 +1.75 × 180, and his left eye improved to 20/25 with −5.00 +2.75 × 165. The patient was unable to tolerate the anisometropia caused by his new refraction and favored wearing his presurgical glasses for both eyes.

Ocular motility and confrontational fields were full in both eyes, and pachymetry was 595 right and 626 left. Intraocular pressures were 13 right and 19 left. Pupillary exam showed 5 mm brisk pupils OD, with an irregular and minimally reactive pupil in the left eye.

Slit-lamp examination showed a 3+ nuclear sclerotic cataract OD. The left cornea had an area of corneal scarring and edema temporally with underlying IK touch. A three-piece lens was in the sulcus. Fundoscopic exam revealed healthy nerves in both eyes and normal macula, veins, and periphery in both eyes.

Given the outcome of his first surgery, the patient was hesitant to undergo intraocular surgery OD. He chose to observe and wanted to attempt spectacle correction. He returned 6 months later with complaints of aniseikonia secondary to his anisometropia and a similar exam. His refraction upon return visit was +3.25 +2.50 × 175 = 20/40 in the right eye and −4.75 +4.25 × 160 = 20/20 in the left eye.

Main Problem to Solve

What are the patient's best surgical options OU given his reluctance to undergo further intraocular surgery OD? Cataract extraction of the right eye is a viable option to reduce the anisometropia, with associated spectacle correction. Intraocular lens exchange for a Toric IOL is inadvisable given the sulcus intraocular lens and incomplete posterior capsule OS. Arcuate incisions are less reliable and would likely not neutralize the amount of astigmatism present. Contact lenses would also be a viable option, except for the patient's age and dexterity issues handling the lenses.

Myopic astigmatic LASIK and PRK are viable options in this case.

Ancillary Tests

Wavefront analysis and corneal topography are vital to the diagnosis and treatment of this condition [1–3]. However, wavefront aberrometry could not be performed to guide the laser treatment, given the extent of astigmatism in the patient.

Outcome

The patient chose to undergo PRK with MMC in the left eye prior to seeking cataract extraction in the right eye. Non-custom treatment of −5.00 +4.00 × 165 was chosen, with a total ablation depth of 39 μm. Non-custom treatment in plus-cylinder format was used to preserve more tissue [1]. Preferably, PRK patients will have myopia less than −6.0 D and less than 6.0 D of astigmatism. However, we will treat myopia greater than −6.0 D with the addition of prophylactic mitomycin C 0.2 mg/ml application for 10–20 s. Our threshold is less for astigmatism, and mitomycin C application is generally used for astigmatism of 4.0 diopters or greater.

At the 1-week postoperative visit, the patient had uncorrected visual acuity of $20/40^{-2}$, which improved to $20/25^{+2}$ with a −0.50 sphere. At the postoperative 1 month visit, his uncorrected vision was $20/70^{-1}$ OS and improved to 20/40 with 0.25 +2.25 × 040. He had significant central corneal dryness and punctate epithelial erosions. Later follow-up confirmed stability of the refractive correction. The patient reported symptomatic benefit from the artificial tears. He was instructed to continue using them on an as-needed basis.

What to Learn from This Case

LASIK and PRK are excellent options to tweak postoperative refractive error in patients who are unable or unwilling to tolerate spectacles or contact lenses [2, 3].

Phaco wound burn causes steepening of the central and mid peripheral cornea (Figs. 12.1 and 12.2). The burn itself causes flattening of the involved cornea, often exaggerated by the

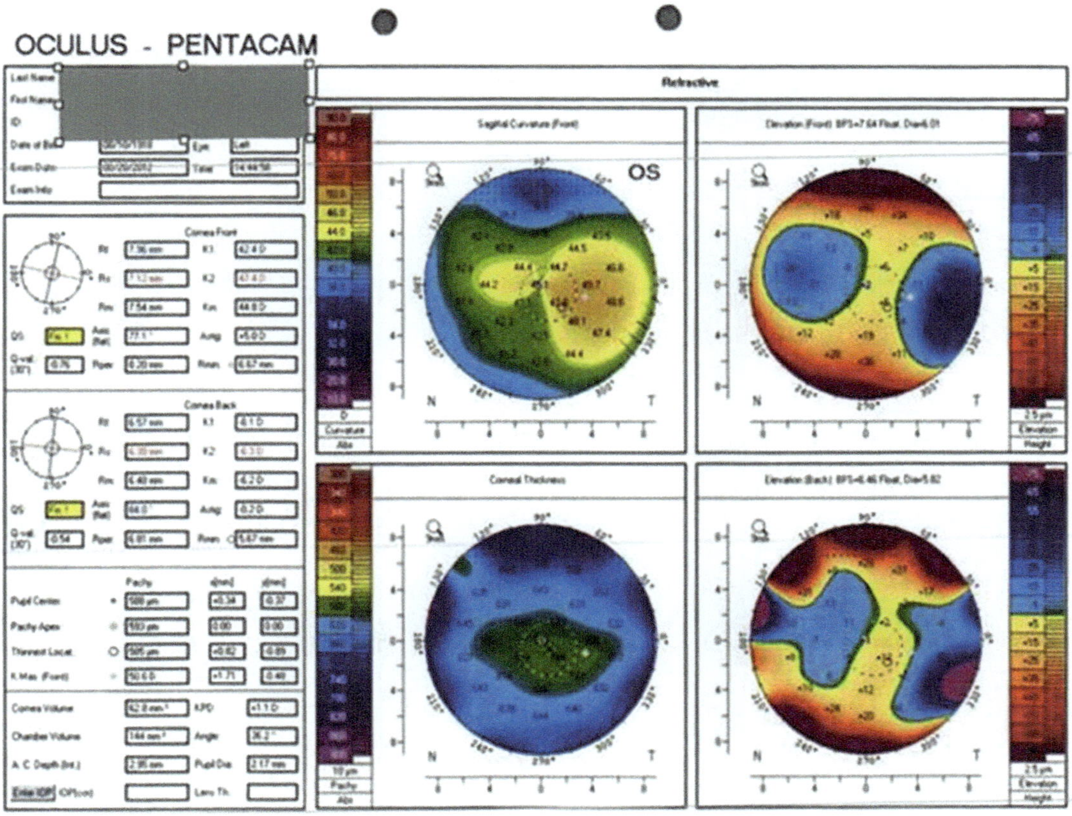

Fig. 12.1 Left eye topography, showing compensatory steepening

tightness from sutures used to close the gaping corneal incision. Thermal damage to the corneal stroma causes collagen shrinkage and retraction of the wound wall, thus flattening the vault of the peripheral cornea in the affected area. The cornea must then vault at a much greater degree to maintain the same position at the corneal center as the remainder of the cornea.

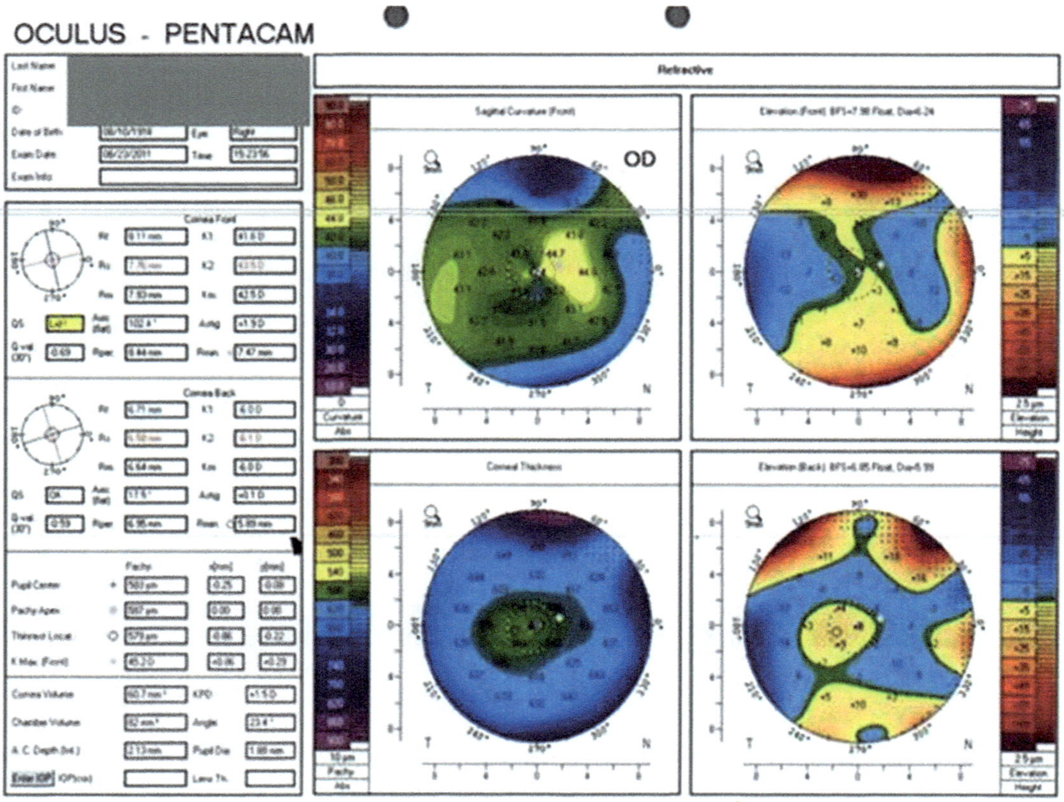

Fig. 12.2 Right eye for comparison

References

1. Bradley MJ, Olson RJ (2006) A survey about phacoemulsification incision thermal contraction incidence and causal relationships. Am J Ophthalmol 141: 222–224
2. Gatinel D, Hoang-Xuan T, Azar DA (2002) Three-dimensional representation and qualitative comparisons of the amount of tissue ablation to treat mixed and compound astigmatism. J Cataract Refract Surg 28:2026–2034
3. D'Arcy F (2012) Prospective contralateral eye study to compare conventional and wavefront-guided laser in situ keratomileusis. Acta Ophthalmol 90:76–80

13 Femtosecond Laser-Assisted Superficial Lamellar Keratectomy for the Treatment of Superficial Corneal Leukomas

Jorge L. Alió, Alessandro Abbouda, and Felipe Soria

Contents

J.L. Alió, MD, PhD (✉)
Department of Refractive Surgery, Vissum Corporación Oftalmológica, Alicante, Spain
e-mail: jlalio@vissum.com

A. Abbouda, MD
Department of Refractive Surgery, Vissum Corporación Oftalmológica, Alicante, Spain

Department of Ophthalmology-Policlinico Umberto I of Rome, University of Rome "Sapienza", Viale del Policlinico, 155, 00186 Roma, Italy

R&D Department, Vissum Corporación Oftalmológica, 03016, Alicante, Spain
e-mail: a.abbouda@gmail.com

F.A. Soria, MD
Department of Refractive Surgery, Instituto de la Visión, Universidad de Montemorelos, Montemorelos, Mexico
e-mail: soriafelipe.md@gmail.com

Why Is This Case Relevant for the Refractive Surgeon?

Superficial corneal opacities following infections are a frequent cause of visual loss [1]. In 2011, the authors published the results of femtosecond laser-assisted superficial lamellar keratectomy for the treatment of corneal leukomas [2]. They showed that superficial corneal excision with femtosecond laser augmented with PTK laser smoothening assisted with 0.25 % sodium hyaluronate improved visual acuity. This allows an alternative to more invasive procedures in patients with severe opacities.

Case Background

A 40-year-old man referred to our clinic presented complaining of pain and blurred vision in his left eye (LE). He reported contact lens use. His best corrected visual acuity (BCVA) was finger count. Slit-lamp examination revealed conjunctival injection and circumscribed focus of infiltration in the pupil area. Infectious keratitis was diagnosed and vancomycin and ceftazidime drops were applied every hour. After 1 week, BCVA improved to 20/63 and the epithelial defect appeared closed. Ofloxacin, one drop two times per day, and dexamethasone, one drop four times per day tapering to one drop each week, were prescribed. After 6 months, BCVA was 20/25

J.L. Alió et al. (eds.), *Difficult and Complicated Cases in Refractive Surgery*,
DOI 10.1007/978-3-642-55238-0_13, © Springer-Verlag Berlin Heidelberg 2015

with −3.75 −1 × 175°. The slit-lamp examination revealed central leukoma (Fig. 13.1a). The OCT Visante showed the depth of the lesion (Fig. 13.1b). The pachymetry was 509 μm. The keratometry reading was 45.6/48.6 × 163°. The corneal topography showed a flat area in correspondence with the leukoma (Fig. 13.2). The patient underwent superficial lamellar keratectomy with FM laser assisted by a viscous masking solution of 0.25 % sodium hyaluronate (ELASHY's technique) [3].

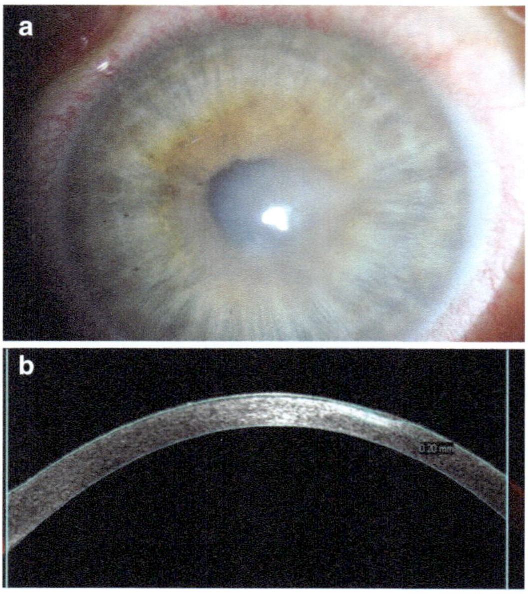

Fig. 13.1 (**a**) Slit-lamp examination revealed central leukoma. (**b**) OCT Visante depth and localization of leukoma

The Main Problem to Solve

Preserving the cornea of the patient is of tremendous importance. Avoiding corneal grafting is necessary when facing a superficial corneal leukoma.

Ancillary Tests

Anterior optical coherence tomography (OCT) is a mandatory preoperative study. Measuring the depth and longitude of the corneal scarring allows us to determine the parameters for surgical planning.

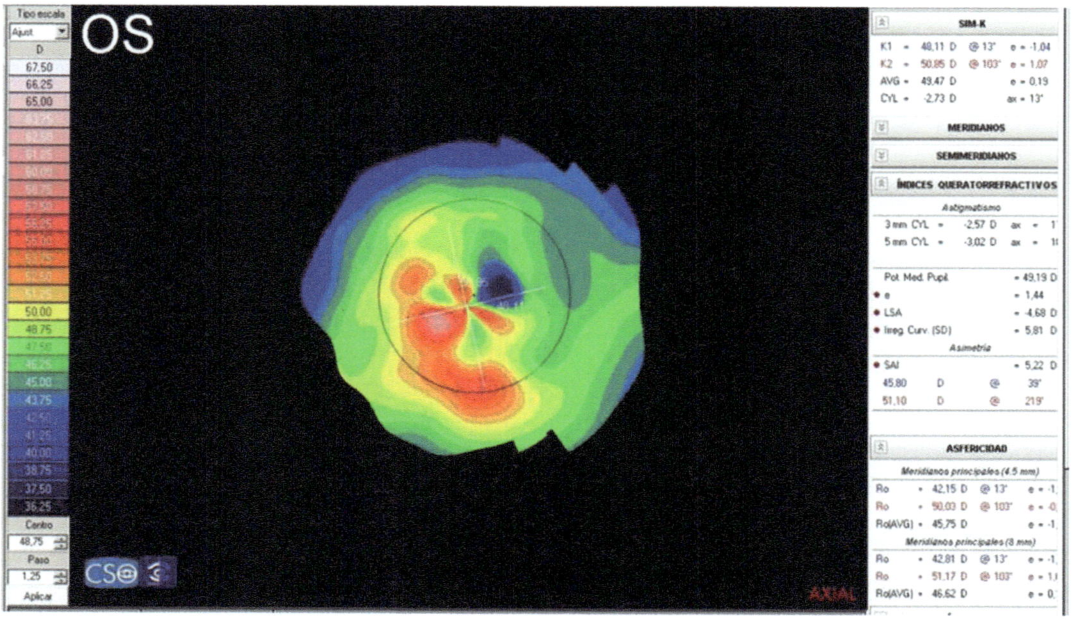

Fig. 13.2 Preoperative topography

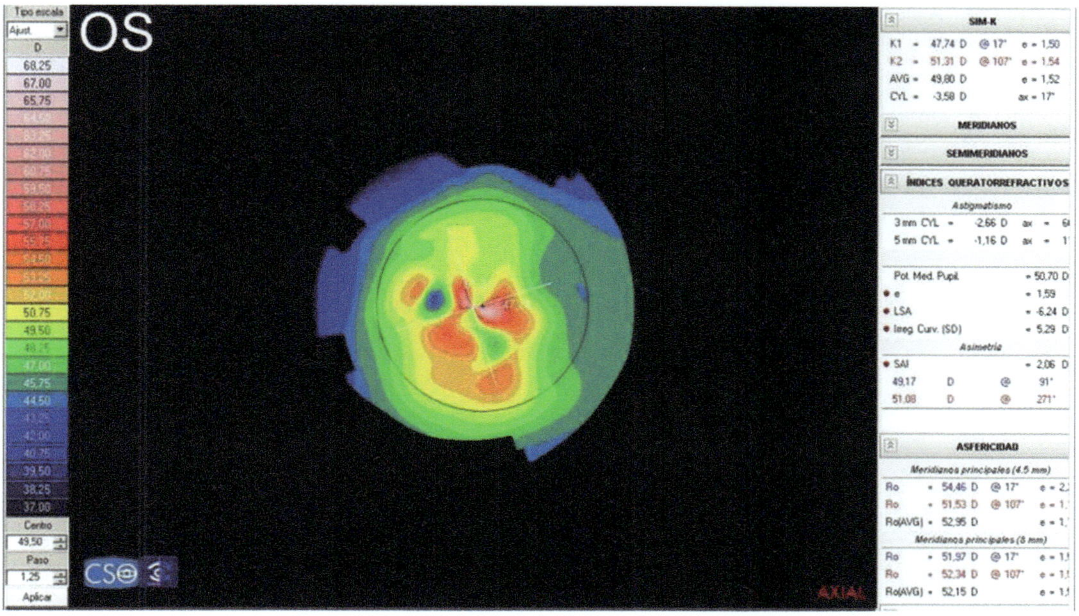

Fig. 13.3 Postoperative topography

Surgical/Medical Intervention

The first step consisted of creating a free corneal cap using the femtosecond laser. As a rule of thumb, the energy used in this procedure must double the amount of corneal refractive procedures, as we are aiming to guarantee corneal dissection in the presence of opacities. The corneal cap thickness is selected according to the depth measured by the OCT and a superior 4 mm hinge is created. The second step consisted in the excimer laser ablation. Before activating the laser, a free cap is created removing it with a crescent blade, and a drop of 0.25 % of sodium hyaluronate is instilled. As soon as the ablation is finished, mitomycin C 0.02 % is applied for 1 min following an intense washing with a balanced salt solution. Finally, a bandage contact lens is placed.

Outcome

After 1 month, the corrected distance visual acuity (CDVA) was 20/50 with a manifest refraction of −1.5=−1 −5×15°. The keratometry reading was 48.11/50.85×103°. The aspect of the image showed a diffuse irregular area (Fig. 13.3). A gas-permeable contact lens was applied. After 8 months, the slit-lamp examination revealed a resolution of leukoma and the vision had improved to 20/25.

What to Learn from This Case

Automated superficial lamellar keratectomy augmented with hyaluronic-assisted PTK has proven a viable alternative to corneal grafting for the management of severe superficial corneal opacity. Femtosecond technology has allowed ophthalmic surgeons to perform a variety of corneal refractive procedures with high precision, offering numerous advantages over mechanical microkeratome devices in terms of visual quality, reproducibility, and safety [3–5]. This procedure can improve visual acuity and optical quality vision of patients with superficial corneal opacities.

References

1. Whitcher JP, Srinivasan M, Upadhyay MP (2001) Corneal blindness: a global perspective. Bull World Health Organ 79:214–221

2. Alió JL, Agdeppa MC, Uceda-Montanes A (2011) Femtosecond laser assisted superficial lamellar keratectomy for the treatment of superficial corneal leukomas. Cornea 30:301–307
3. Alio JL (2013) Femtosecond laser assisted keratoplasty, 1st edn. Jaypee, Philadelphia
4. Soong HK, Malta JB (2009) Femtosecond lasers in ophthalmology. Am J Ophthalmol 147:189–197
5. Durrie DS, Kezirian GM (2005) Femtosecond laser versus mechanical keratome flaps in wavefront-guided laser in situ keratomileusis: prospective contralateral eye study. J Cataract Refract Surg 31:120–126

Managing LASIK Hyperopic Shift with a Multifocal Lens

14

Jorge L. Alió and Alessandro Abbouda

Contents

J.L. Alió, MD, PhD (✉)
Department of Refractive Surgery, Vissum Corporación Oftalmológica, Alicante, Spain
e-mail: jlalio@vissum.com

A. Abbouda, MD
Department of Refractive Surgery, Vissum Corporación Oftalmológica, Alicante, Spain

Department of Ophthalmology-Policlinico Umberto I of Rome, University of Rome "Sapienza", Viale del Policlinico, 155, 00186 Roma, Italy

R&D Department, Vissum Corporación Oftalmológica, 03016, Alicante, Spain
e-mail: a.abbouda@gmail.com

Why Is This Case Relevant for the Refractive Surgeon?

Multifocal intraocular lenses (MIOLs) are designed to reduce dependence on spectacles for all vision ranges after cataract surgery or clear lens extraction. The Lentis Mplus IOL (Oculentis GmbH, Berlin) is a sectorial piece refractive multifocal lens made of hydrosmart with an aspheric posterior surface. The multifocality is achieved by implementing a distance piece and a distinct near sector of +3.0 D in the lower IOL segment, comparable to a multifocal spectacle lens. Here we report the case of a patient who developed a hyperopic shift following MIOL implantation and needed additive excimer laser treatment to achieve an adequate visual result [1].

Case Background

A 63-year-old man presented complaining of both near and far distance visual problems in both eyes that had been present for many years. The patient had a strong motivation to be independent from spectacles for all his daily activities. His manifest refraction was +1 −0.5 × 90 in the right eye (RE) and +1.5 −0.5 × 110 in the left eye (LE). His best corrected visual acuity (BCVA) was 20/20 for far and near distance in both eyes (adding a lens of +2 sphere). Both slit lamp and fundus examinations were normal. According to

J.L. Alió et al. (eds.), *Difficult and Complicated Cases in Refractive Surgery*, DOI 10.1007/978-3-642-55238-0_14, © Springer-Verlag Berlin Heidelberg 2015

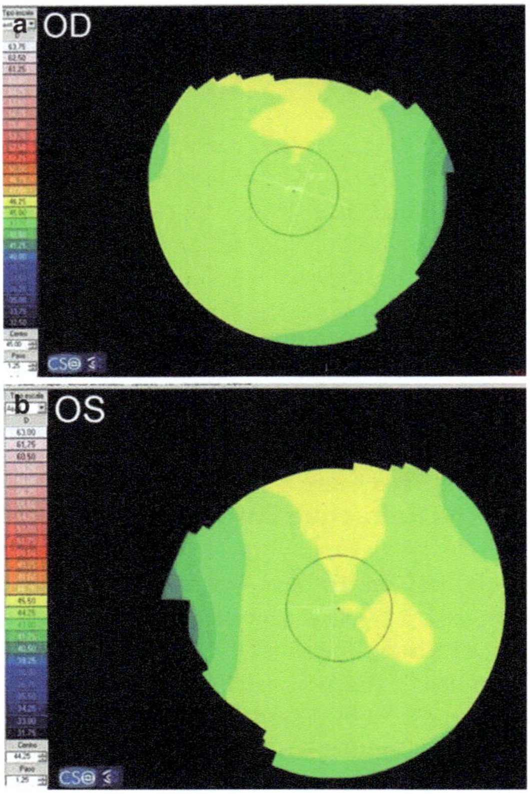

Fig. 14.1 (a, b) Corneal topography before the LASIK procedure

the topography, his cornea surface was regular. According to LOCS III classification [2], a nuclear sclerosis cataract N01 was diagnosed. Cataract surgery was performed with implantation of Lentis Mplus, +19 diopter (Δ) in the RE and +18.5Δ in the LE. The postoperative was uneventful. After 4 months, the patient was not satisfied with his near vision. His manifest refraction was +2.5 −0.5 × 75 in the right eye (RE) and +1.25 −0.5 × 70 in the left eye (LE). His uncorrected visual acuity was 20/20 for far distance and 20/50 for near in both eyes. The topography showed a regular surface. Keratometric value was 44.57/45.35 × 70 in the RE and 44.5/44.5 × 90 in the LE (Fig. 14.1a, b). High order of aberrometry was analyzed through KR-1W|Topcon. The values of RMS at 4 mm were 0.4 in both eyes. Pachymetry was 553 μm in the RE and 559 μm in the LE.

Main Problem to Solve

It must be kept in mind that in the presence of a multifocal IOL, far vision can be corrected by using the two principal foci of the IOL, but only if the far focus is adjusted for far vision will the near focus be useful for near vision. A near focus focused for far vision is not useful for near vision. The subjective refraction value when using the near focus for far vision is equal to the real refractive error minus the addition of the IOL for near vision. For a patient with a real hyperopia after refractive multifocal IOL implantation, BCVA can be achieved using an addition of a positive lens. On the contrary, when the near focus is used for far vision, the patient needs a negative lens to achieve a BCVA. This patient's defocus curve (Fig. 14.2) showed a BCVA with an addition of −1.0 Δ. The patient was able to read 20/20. Near vision was insufficient to properly perform his near vision daily activities, as he read 20/40. We decided to perform hyperopic LASIK to improve his BCVA.

Ancillary Tests

BCVA for near and far distance, defocus curve, corneal topography, and corneal and internal aberrometry were indicated.

Surgical/Medical Intervention

Hyperopic LASIK treatment was performed. The flap was created using microkeratome and corneal stromal ablation by the AMARIS SCHWIND excimer laser. The residual stroma after the procedure was 461 and 472 μm.

Outcome

Six months post LASIK procedure, the patient's manifest refraction was +0.5 in both eyes. The distance and near uncorrected visual acuity in the RE was 20/20 and 20/32 in the LE. The topography showed an irregular aspect in the RE.

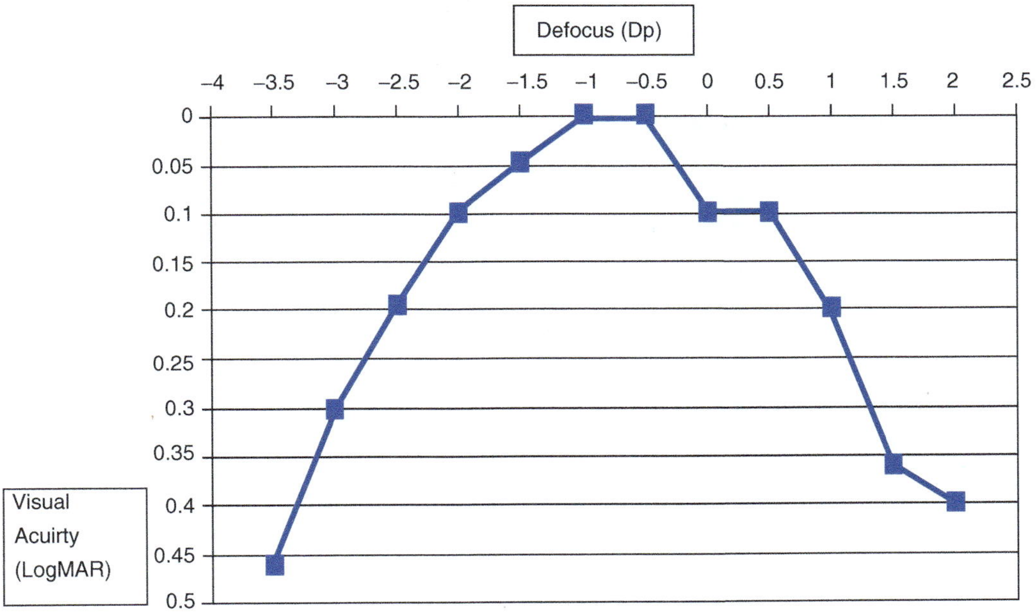

Fig. 14.2 Defocus curve

The hyperopic ablation profile appeared evident in both eyes (Fig. 14.3a, b). The corneal aberrometry was normal in both eyes (Fig. 14.3c, d).

What to Learn from This Case

If visual acuity is not within the expected values for the IOL, one possibility is the patient's use of the near or intermediate focus of the IOL for distance vision correction. However, in patients implanted with refractive MIOLs, vision improves over time by a neuroadaptation process in which the brain reduces the noise-to-signal ratio produced by multifocality [3]. Optimal refractive outcomes with multifocal IOLs are achieved when used appropriately with patients. Also, precise measurements performed by keratometry/topography and axometer ensure the correct sizing of the anterior segment and the accurate prediction of the effective lens position [4]. A final consideration is that an inappropriate preoperative refraction can be the source of a refractive surprise.

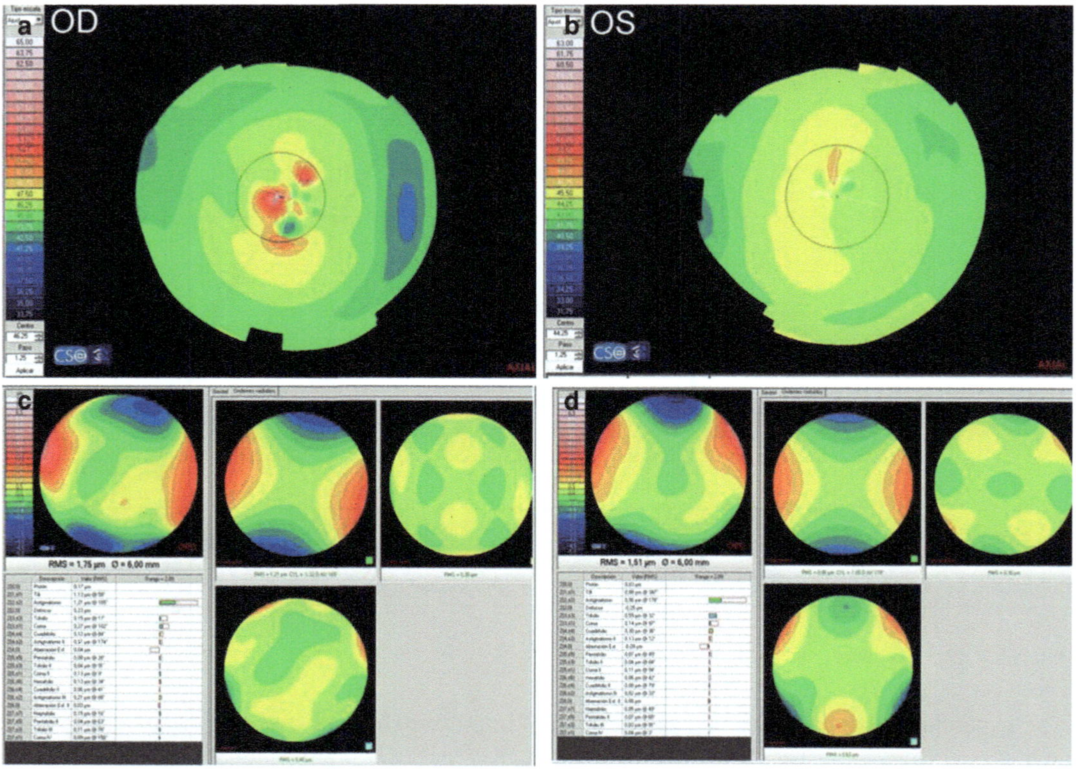

Fig. 14.3 Corneal topography and aberrometry 6 months post LASIK procedure. (**a**, **b**) Anterior corneal topography of both eyes showing hyperopic ablation profile. (**c**, **d**) The corneal aberrometry was normal in both eyes

References

1. Ayala MJ, Pérez-Santonja JJ, Artola A, Claramonte P, Alió JL (2001) Laser in situ keratomileusis to correct residual myopia after cataract surgery. J Refract Surg 17(1):12–16
2. Chylack LT Jr, Wolfe JK, Friend J, Tung W, Singer DM, Brown NP, Hurst MA, Köpcke W, Schalch W (1995) Validation of methods for the assessment of cataract progression in the Roche European-American Anticataract Trial (REACT). Ophthalmic Epidemiol 2:59–75
3. Montés-Micó R, Alió JL (2003) Distance and near contrast sensitivity function after multifocal intraocular lens implantation. J Cataract Refract Surg 29:703–711
4. Holladay JT. IOL power calculations for multifocal lenses research has identified seven key measurements for success. http://www.crstoday.com/PDF%20 Articles/0807/CRST0807_11.php

LASIK and Severe Anisometropia in a Child

15

Jorge L. Alió and Alessandro Abbouda

Contents

J.L. Alió, MD, PhD (✉)
Department of Refractive Surgery, Vissum Corporación Oftalmológica, Alicante, Spain
e-mail: jlalio@vissum.com

A. Abbouda, MD
Department of Refractive Surgery, Vissum Corporación Oftalmológica, Alicante, Spain

Department of Ophthalmology-Policlinico Umberto I of Rome, University of Rome "Sapienza", Viale del Policlinico, 155, 00186 Roma, Italy

R&D Department, Vissum Corporación Oftalmológica, 03016, Alicante, Spain
e-mail: a.abbouda@gmail.com

Why Is This Case Relevant for the Refractive Surgeon?

Pediatric laser refractive surgery was first reported in 1995 [1]. Two types of pediatric refractive surgery are intraocular refractive surgery with the implantation of intraocular lenses (IOL) and corneal refractive surgery (PRK and LASIK). Either option may help reverse refractive amblyopia, especially in cases in which either severe anisometropia does not improve with spectacles or when contact lens adaptation is impossible. In such cases, surgery can eliminate or reduce aniseikonia and correct for high myopia and astigmatism.

Case Background

A 5-year-old child came to our department with a diagnosis of severe anisometropia. His manifest refraction was −12 −3 × 70 in the right eye and 0.75 −1.5 × 100 in the left eye. His best corrected visual acuity (BCVA) was 20/20 in the RE and 20/25 in the LE. The preoperative central thickness was evaluated through OCT Visante. The value in the RE was 660 μm (Fig. 15.1). The keratometry reading of the RE was 40.61/42.16 × 13.

J.L. Alió et al. (eds.), *Difficult and Complicated Cases in Refractive Surgery*, DOI 10.1007/978-3-642-55238-0_15, © Springer-Verlag Berlin Heidelberg 2015

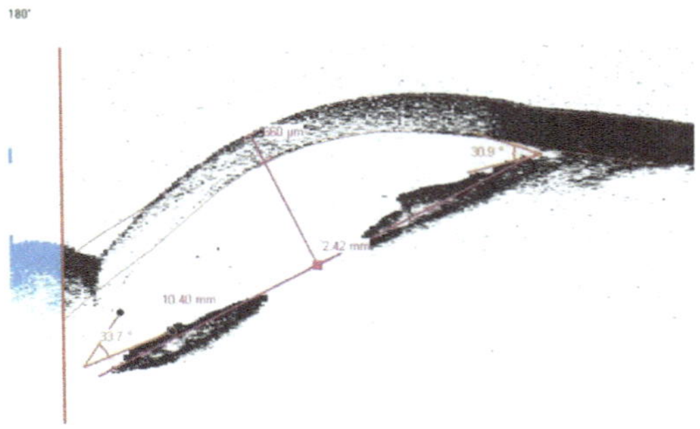

Fig. 15.1 Preoperative OCT Visante

The Main Problem to Solve

Corneal refractive surgery in pediatric patients has unique risks, including an uncertain preoperative examination. A child's lack of cooperation may affect preoperative tests and reduce final visual acuity. Treatment performed under anesthesia theoretically has a higher risk of decentration because fixation is very difficult in children, especially in very young children. Sometimes the pupil center does not correspond with the visual axis, resulting in minimal decentration [2].

Ancillary Tests

The first option proposed to the parents was a contact lens in the RE and occlusion of the LE. However, the child did not tolerate the contact lens. Therefore, refractive treatment was proposed.

Surgical/Medical Intervention

The child underwent an uneventful LASIK procedure targeted for distance in the RE. Flap creation was performed using the Alcon Wavelight® FS200 femtosecond laser and corneal stromal ablation by the Alcon Allegretto® excimer laser. One hour postoperatively, the slit-lamp examination showed no anomalies, no epithelial defects at the flap edge, a clear interface, and a well-positioned flap. One week postoperatively, the slit-lamp examination showed a normal flap.

Outcome

After 3 months, the manifest refraction was −1.75. The child's BCVA was 20/80. The topography showed an ablation profile (Fig. 15.2). The parents reported that the child did not steadily follow the occlusion therapy. At 1 year, the BCVA was 20/60.

What to Learn from This Case

The goal of surgical treatment is to reduce or eliminate refractive errors, facilitating the treatment of amblyopia and promoting functional binocular vision. However, controversy surrounds pediatric refractive surgery [3]. LASIK surgery of short duration with minimal postoperative pain and rapid visual recovery make it a suitable option for children. On the other hand, the greatest advantages of surface ablation techniques for children are no risks of rubbing the eye; reepithelialization also appears to occur more rapidly in children than in adults [4].

We believe that refractive surgery is a viable option to reverse refractive amblyopia, especially in cases of severe anisometropia that do not improve with spectacles or for patients unable to withstand contact lens adaptation.

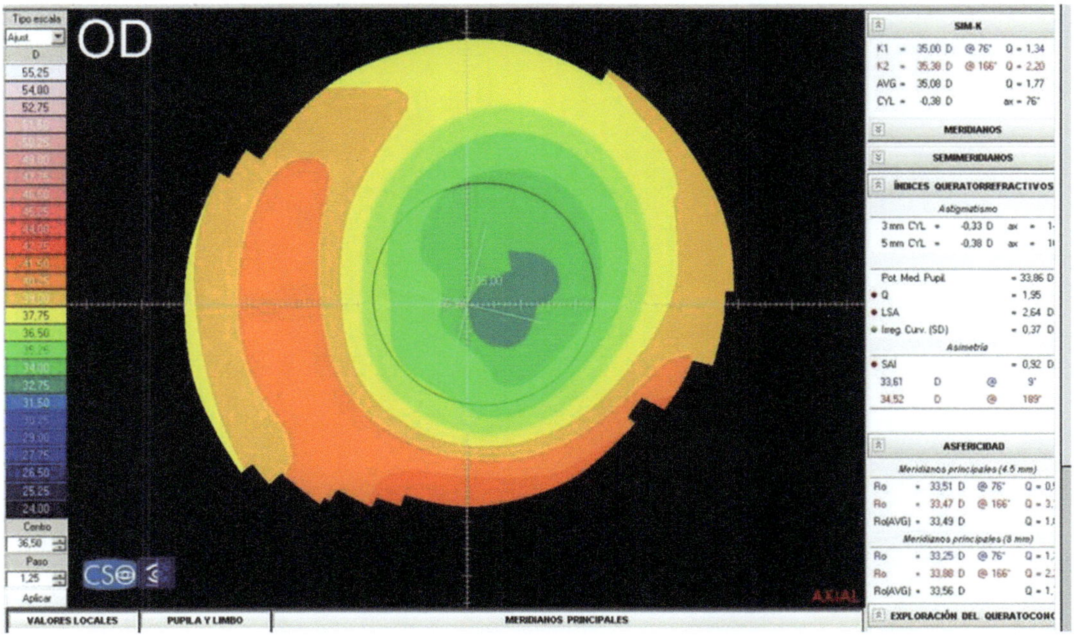

Fig. 15.2 Topography at 1-year post-refractive treatment

References

1. Singh D (1995) Photorefractive keratectomy in pediatric patients. J Cataract Refract Surg 21:630–632
2. Moore AT (1985) Refraction in childhood. Trans Ophthalmol Soc UK 104:648–652
3. Alió JL, Wolter NV, Piñero DP, Amparo F, Sari ES, Cankaya C, Laria C (2011) Pediatric refractive surgery and its role in the treatment of amblyopia: meta-analysis of the peer-reviewed literature. J Refract Surg 27:364–74
4. Pediatric Eye Disease Investigator Group (2004) A randomized trial of atropine regimens for treatment of moderate amblyopia in children. Ophthalmology 111:2076–2085

Refractive Laser Treatment Plan, Night Vision Disturbance

16

Roberto Pineda and Jnanankar Medhi

Contents

R. Pineda, MD (✉)
Department of Refractive Surgery, Massachusetts Eye and Ear Infirmary, Harvard Medical School, Boston, MA, USA
e-mail: roberto_pineda@meei.harvard.edu

J. Medhi, MD
Department of Refractive Surgery, Massachusetts Eye and Ear Infirmary, Boston, MA, USA
e-mail: jmedhimail@gmail.com

Why Is This Case Relevant for the Refractive Surgeon?

Night-related complaints are not uncommon after laser vision correction. Causes include decreased contrast sensitivity [1], uncorrected lower-order aberrations, or induced higher-order aberration (HOA), i.e., spherical aberration [2]. Understanding how to address night-related complaints will result in higher postoperative patient satisfaction.

Case Background

A 30-year-old female presented with complaints of hazy vision and difficulty while driving at night. Her symptoms included poor distance vision, glare, and haloes. Her history was significant for laser vision correction (moderate myopic femtosecond wavefront-optimized LASIK) in both eyes 6 months previously for a refraction of −6.50 −0.50 at 175 and −7.00 −0.25 at 035 with a 6 mm OZ. She had trialed topical brimonidine, artificial tears, and cyclosporine 0.05 % without symptomatic improvement.

Current exam:

UCVA	OD 20/20	OS $20/20^{-2}$
MRx	OD: +0.25/−0.25@ 45	20/20
	OS: −0.50	20/20

J.L. Alió et al. (eds.), *Difficult and Complicated Cases in Refractive Surgery*,
DOI 10.1007/978-3-642-55238-0_16, © Springer-Verlag Berlin Heidelberg 2015

Scotopic pupil size: 6.0 mm (OU)
SLE: no striae, folds, or haze. Other findings unremarkable
IOP: 12 mmHg OU
Fundoscopy: normal

Post-LASIK wavefront aberrometry prior to re-treatment

	OD	OS
tHOA	0.74	0.90
Coma	0.550 @ 201	0.510 @ 7
Spherical aberration	0.433	0.672

Diagnosis: symptomatic HOAs (spherical aberration, coma) after femtosecond LASIK in both eyes

Main Problem to Solve

Improvement of visual acuity, glare, and haloes at night

Ancillary Tests

We conducted wavefront aberrometry and analysis.

Surgical/Medical Intervention

VisX WaveScan was performed and lower-order and higher-order aberrations were evaluated (see table below). Once the WaveScan was confirmed as stable, wavefront-guided ablation in both eyes using VisX Customvue IR (Software version 5.22) technology was performed.

Outcome

The patient underwent the procedure first in the right eye, followed 4 weeks later by the left eye. The immediate postoperative period was unremarkable. She reported improved night visual acuity after the procedure but felt haloes at night had not improved. Repeat wavefront aberrometry following the re-treatment shows reduction in HOA, comas, and spherical aberration values (Figs. 16.1 and 16.2; Table 16.1 below).

What to Learn from This Case

Spherical aberration is the principal cause of poor scotopic vision following laser vision

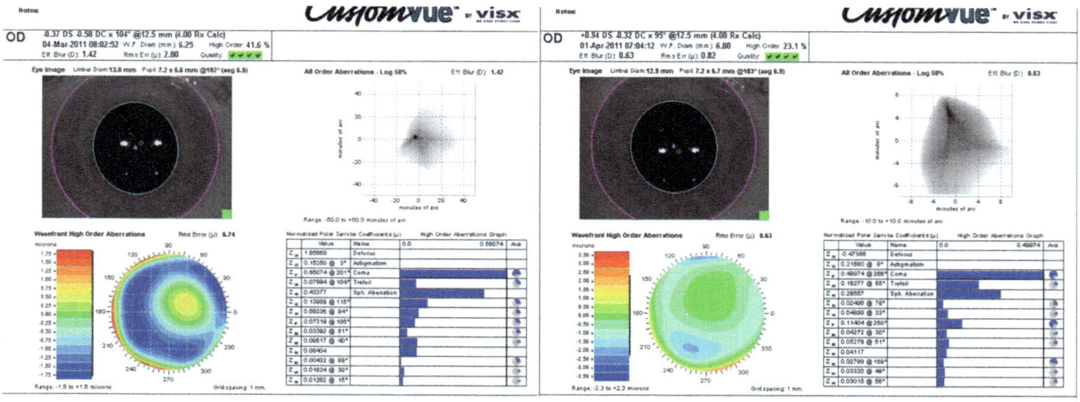

Fig. 16.1 Pre- and posttreatment wavefront picture (OD) showing reduction of HOA, coma, and aberration values

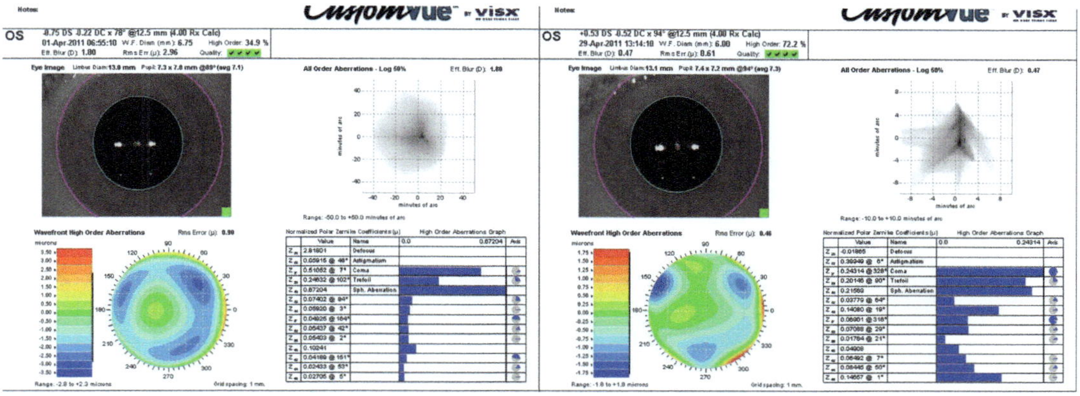

Fig. 16.2 Pre- and posttreatment wavefront picture (OD) showing the reduction of HOA, coma, and aberration values posttreatment wavefront picture (OD and OS)

Table 16.1 Pre and 1 month Post treatment Wavefront values showing reduction of HOA, Coma and Spherical aberration values

	OD		OS	
	Preop	Postop[a]	Preop	Postop[a]
tHOA	0.74	0.63 (Δ−0.11)	0.90	0.46 (Δ−0.44)
Coma	0.550 @ 201	0.499 @256	0.510 @ 7	0.243 @ 328
Sph. aberration	0.433	0.295(Δ−0.138)	0.672	0.215 (Δ−0.457)

[a]Fourth week postoperative visit

correction in higher-order aberrations. Other vision problems are caused by untreated lower-order aberrations or other residual HOAs. These may be visually debilitating in low light and result in scotopic glare and haloes. Wavefront-guided excimer laser enhancement or topography-guided laser vision correction can also reduce lower- and higher-order aberrations [2].

References

1. Tuan KM, Liang J (2006) Improved contrast sensitivity and visual acuity after wavefront guided laser in situ keratomileusis: In-depth statistical analysis. J Cataract Refract Surg 32:215–220
2. Alio JL, Pinero DP, Plaza Puche AB (2008) Corneal wavefront guided enhancement for high levels of corneal coma aberration after laser in situ keratomileusis. J Cataract Refract Surg 34:222–231

Use of Excimer Laser Surgery for Monovision in Cases of Unsatisfactory Outcome Following Cataract Surgery

17

Jaime Javaloy and Alessandro Abbouda

Contents

Why Is This Case Relevant for the Refractive Surgeon?

Monovision is the adjustment of one eye for near vision and the other for distance vision. Pseudophakic monovision is a type of monovision used in lens surgery to correct postoperative presbyopia by programmed refractive error from biometry calculations [1].

In this case we decided to correct the patient for far distance, but after 1 year the patient decided to try monovision.

Case Background

A 48-year-old woman came to our department interested in refractive surgery and complaining about the refractive change in her RE. Her manifest refraction was −7 in the right eye (RE) and −5.75 −0.75×70 in the left eye (LE). Her best corrected visual acuity (BCVA) was 20/20 for distance and near vision in both eyes (adding a lens of +2). Both slit lamp and fundus examinations were normal. According to the topography, her cornea surface was regular. According to LOCS III classification [2], a nuclear (N01) and cortical (C1) cataract was diagnosed. The patient used to drive during the night, so we avoided implantation of a multifocal IOL. Cataract surgery was performed with implantation of Alcon Acrysof MA60 +17 Diopter (Δ) in the RE and +16.5Δ in the LE. The postoperative was

J. Javaloy, MD, PhD (✉)
Department of Anterior Segment and Refractive Surgery, Vissum Corporacion Oftalmológica, Alicante, Spain
e-mail: javaloy@coma.es

A. Abbouda, MD
Department of Refractive Surgery, Vissum Corporación Oftalmológica, Alicante, Spain

Department of Ophthalmology-Policlinico Umberto I of Rome, University of Rome "Sapienza", Viale del Policlinico, 155, 00186 Roma, Italy

R&D Department, Vissum Corporación Oftalmológica, 03016, Alicante, Spain
e-mail: a.abbouda@gmail.com

J.L. Alió et al. (eds.), *Difficult and Complicated Cases in Refractive Surgery*, DOI 10.1007/978-3-642-55238-0_17, © Springer-Verlag Berlin Heidelberg 2015

uneventful. After 6 months, her manifest refraction was −1.5 −0.75 × 145 in the right eye (RE) and −1 in the left eye (LE). Her uncorrected visual acuity for distance was 20/50 in the RE and 20/25 in the LE and for near vision was 20/40 in the RE and 20/32 in the LE. The topography showed a regular surface. The pachymetry was 482 μm in the RE and 489 μm in the LE. Keratometric index was 44.59/44.87 × 101° in the RE and 43.99/44.85 × 86° in the LE. The axial eye length measurement using the Zeiss IOL Master was 25.13 in the RE and 24.84 in the LE.

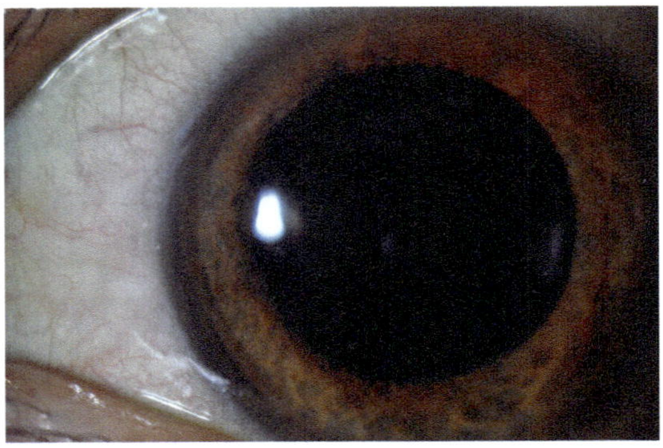

Fig. 17.1 Slit-lamp examination showed pseudophakic eye with a previous flap

Main Problem to Solve

The patient presents a thin cornea. The amount of ablation was 20.34 μm. The cutting of the flap was set at 90 μm.

Ancillary Tests

It is important to define the dominant eye and the posttest tolerance and adaptation of monovision with a contact lens [3]. In this case, the right eye was dominant.

Surgical/Medical Intervention

LASIK treatment was performed. Flap creation was performed using the Alcon Wavelight® FS200 femtosecond laser and corneal stromal ablation by the Alcon Allegretto® excimer laser.

Outcome

After 6 months, the patient's manifest refraction was −1.5 −0.75 × 145 in the right eye (RE) and plano in the left eye (LE). Her uncorrected visual acuity was 20/50 (RE) and 20/20 (LE) for distance and 20/20 (RE) and 20/30 (LE) for near vision (Fig. 17.1).

What to Learn from This Case

Pseudophakic monovision is an effective approach to manage loss of accommodation following cataract surgery, especially for a patient who wants to be free from glasses while the implantation of a MFIOL it is not possible. The preoperative refractive status of the patient should not determine which eye should be corrected. Rather, a full exam determining the sensorial and motor dominance is necessary to avoid mistaking the effect that an incipient cataract or even a different refractive status of the patient during his infancy might provoke. In our case, both eyes had similar features of axial length and keratometry, but had a different refraction (more myopic in the dominant RE before cataract surgery). A bilateral refractive treatment after cataract surgery can promote good near and distance vision, but only with correction of the dominant eye.

References

1. Chylack LT Jr, Wolfe JK, Friend J, Tung W, Singer DM, Brown NP, Hurst MA, Köpcke W, Schalch W (1995) Validation of methods for the assessment of cataract progression in the Roche European-American Anticataract Trial (REACT). Ophthalmic Epidemiol 2:59–75
2. Fernandes PR, Neves HI, Lopes-Ferreira DP, Jorge JM, González-Meijome JM (2013) Adaptation to multifocal and monovision contact lens correction. Optom Vis Sci 90:228–235
3. Ito M, Shimizu K, Iida Y, Amano R (2012) Five-year clinical study of patients with pseudophakic monovision. J Cataract Refract Surg 38:1440–1445

Error in the Excimer Refractive Program: From a Simple Mistake to a Major Clinical Problem

18

Jaime Javaloy, Alessandro Abbouda, and Jorge L. Alió

Contents

J. Javaloy, MD, PhD (✉)
Department of Anterior Segment and Refractive Surgery, Vissum Corporacion Oftalmológica, Alicante, Spain
e-mail: jjavaloy@coma.es

A. Abbouda, MD
Department of Refractive Surgery, Vissum Corporación Oftalmológica, Alicante, Spain

Department of Ophthalmology-Policlinico Umberto I of Rome, University of Rome "Sapienza", Viale del Policlinico, 155, 00186 Roma, Italy

R&D Department, Vissum Corporación Oftalmológica, 03016, Alicante, Spain
e-mail: a.abbouda@gmail.com

J.L. Alió, MD, PhD
Department of Refractive Surgery, Vissum Corporación Oftalmológica, Alicante, Spain
e-mail: jlalio@vissum.com

Why Is This Case Relevant for the Refractive Surgeon?

Every refractive surgeon should be very careful when typing or writing the refractive plan before surgery. Preventable human errors are one of the most common sources of sphere error after surgery [1]. Here we describe a case in which the transposed cylinder form was incorrect.

Case Background

A 36-year-old male was referred for refractive surgery. Cycloplegic refraction was +2.25 = −2 × 5° in the right eye (RE) and +4.5 = −5.25 × 170° in the left eye (LE), with the best spectacle-corrected visual acuity (BSCVA) of 20/20 in both eyes. The ultrasound pachymetry was 530 μm in both eyes. Keratometry indices were 41.36/43.15 × 98° in the RE and 39.7/44.34 × 78° in the LE. The topography showed a vertical bow tie according to astigmatism with rule in both eyes (Fig. 18.1). The flap creation was performed using Hansatome microkeratome and corneal stromal ablation by the Technolas 217z B&L® excimer laser. Three weeks post surgery, the patient was very worried. He complained of very bad vision in the LE. His visual acuity was 20/20 in the RE and finger count in the LE. The refraction of the patient was (RE) plano, and the LE improved to 20/40 with the refraction of +7 = −10 × 170°.

J.L. Alió et al. (eds.), *Difficult and Complicated Cases in Refractive Surgery*, DOI 10.1007/978-3-642-55238-0_18, © Springer-Verlag Berlin Heidelberg 2015

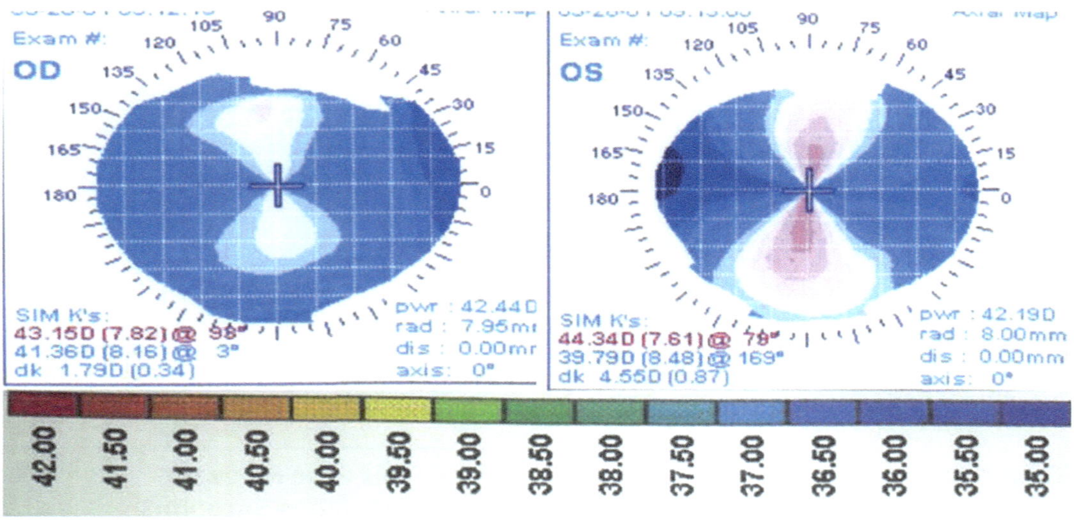

Fig. 18.1 Preoperative topography showed a vertical bow tie in both eyes according to astigmatism with rule

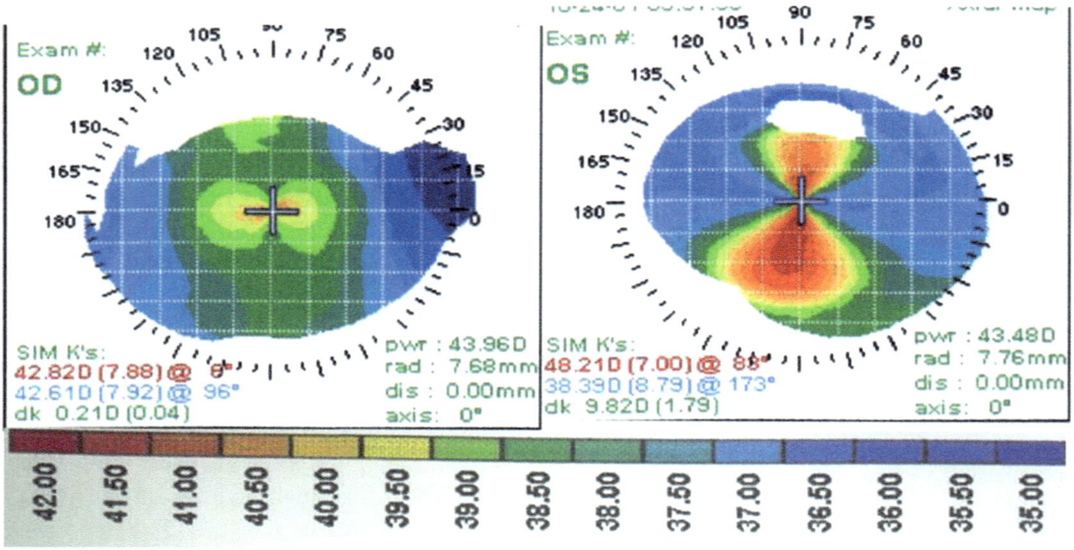

Fig. 18.2 Topography after the first treatment showed a horizontal bow tie in the RE and an increase of the vertical bow tie profile in the LE

The ultrasound central pachymetry was 514 μm in the RE and 480 μm in the LE. Keratometry indices were 42.6/42.8 × 6° in the RE and 38.3/48.2 × 88° in the LE. The topography showed a horizontal bow tie in the RE and an increase of the vertical bow tie profile in the LE (Fig. 18.2).

Main Problem to Solve

It was evident that some mistake had occurred. Upon analyzing the history, we realized that the transposed cylinder form was wrong. The refraction in the LE at the first visit was +4.5 = −5.25 × 170°, and in the surgery planning

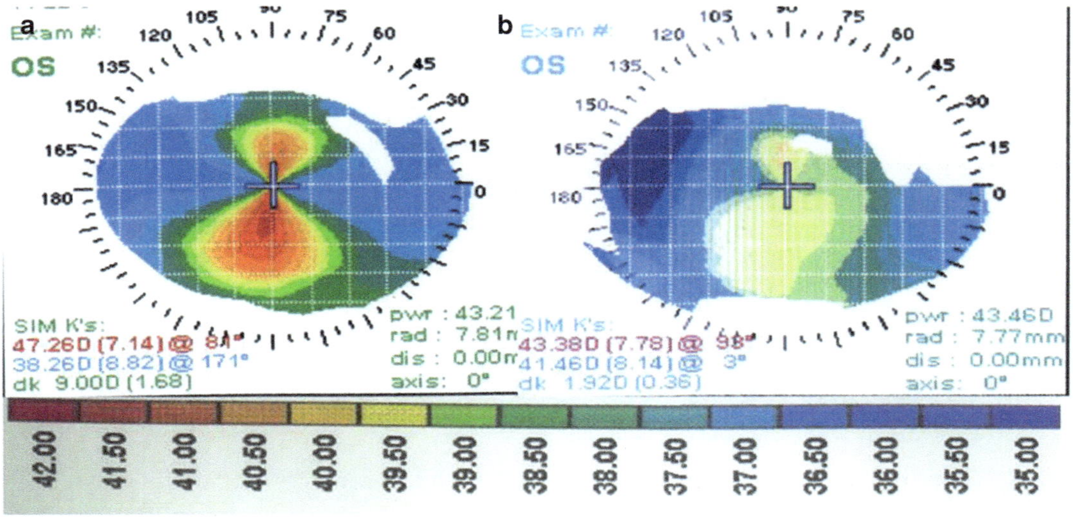

Fig. 18.3 (**a**) Left eye. Topography after 3 months of KTA showed astigmatism with rule. (**b**) Left eye. Topography after 3 months of LASIK re-treatment showed an irregular astigmatism with rule

it was −0.75 = +5.25 × 170°. The correct planning should have been −0.75 = +5.25 × 80°. The resultant refraction from this clinical mistake was finger count.

Ancillary Tests

Pachymetry was fundamental in this case. The previous laser did not waste a substantial amount of central corneal stroma because the profile applied was hypermetromic. This situation allowed us to follow a new laser ablation.

Surgical/Medical Intervention

The first approach was to reduce the high astigmatism. We chose to perform an arcuate relaxing incision (KTA). Two 80° opposite incisions were performed at 90 % depth at 7 mm of the center of the pupil on the LE. Both incisions of the arc were centered over the steeped axis at 80°. The second step, according to the residual refractive defect, was to perform a LASIK re-treatment over the remaining refractive defect after the incisional surgery.

Outcome

At 3 months post-KTA, the visual acuity in the LE was 20/25 with a manifest correction of 3 = −5 × 180°. The topography consistently showed a vertical bow tie. The keratometry index was 38.26/47.2 × 80° (Fig. 18.3a). On this refractive defect, the LASIK treatment was performed planning a crossed cylinder treatment. Three months after LASIK, the visual acuity in the LE was 20/25 without correction. The ultrasound central pachymetry was 430 μm in the LE. Keratometry indices in the LE were 41.46/43.38 × 98°. The topography showed an irregular vertical bow tie (Fig. 18.3b).

What to Learn from This Case

This case emphasizes the importance of carefully reviewing the refractive plan before surgery. The magnitude of this iatrogenic error was significant, and such a refractive surprise due to preventable transcription mistakes is possible for every surgeon. KTA was a good choice to reduce the astigmatism in this case, and the LASIK re-treatment resulted in a positive visual outcome.

Reference

1. Chayet AS, Torres LF, Alpins N, Walsh G (2008) Chapter 6: Refractive miscalculation with refractive surprise. In: Alio JL, Azar D (eds) Management of complications in refractive surgery. Springer, Berlin/Heidelberg, pp 103–112

Part II

LASIK Intraoperative Complications

Dear reader,

Our goal is to provide you with some of the most common clinical intraoperative complications of the LASIK procedure in order to provide you with the confidence and knowledge needed to confront some of these issues. The intraoperative complication rate of 0.7–6.6 % is most commonly microkeratome related, either mechanical or femtosecond laser. This chapter is divided in two sections: the first part analyzes intraoperative complications related to mechanical microkeratome and the second part addresses those related to the femtosecond laser.

We present cases related to microkeratome such as incomplete or dislocated flaps, as well as issues pertaining to femtosecond involving flap loss, a decentered flap, and suction break. Our hope is to provide you with case examples to help clinical involvement with LASIK intraoperative complications. Patient collaboration is also an important consideration when dealing with these issues.

For a theoretical complement, we suggest the first book of this series: J.L. Alio', D. Azar *Management of Complications in Refractive Surgery*, Chapter 3: LASIK Intraoperative Complications (pp. 16–31).

Specific topics covered by the cases include complication of microkeratome, the risk of subepithelial stromal scars, irregular astigmatism (Case 19), incomplete flap after mirokeratome solved by lamellar keratectomy and PTK (Case 20), how to manage a dislocated flap (Case 21), and how to manage vertical gas breakthrough (Case 22). Other cases cover what is important to know and do about thin flaps (Case 23), predisposing factors and methods for avoiding a gas bubble breakthrough (Case 24), how to manage free flap after LASIK (Case 25), proper orientation and management of a free cap during flap creation (Case 26), and flap loss (Case 27). We end with cases focused on hyperopic intra-LASIK: the importance of a centered flap (Case 28), how to manage suction loss before a side cut, an incomplete flap, or a complete raster pattern (Cases 29, 30, and 31).

Lesson to Learn

Case 19: Buttonhole flaps

Different stages or types of buttonhole flap complication are addressed and solved by different approaches: a delayed alcohol-assisted-PRK, a delayed laser PTK-PRK procedure, and an immediate PTK-PRK approach.

Case 20: Incomplete LASIK flap
A patient with previously aborted LASIK surgery due to an incomplete flap created with a microkeratome treated by lamellar keratectomy and PTK
Case 21: Dislocated flaps
A case of flap dislocation and epithelial ingrowth after microkeratome LASIK is treated and solved by hydration of the stroma and flap with hypotonic solution
Case 22: Perforated femtosecond laser-created flap
Vertical gas breakthrough is a unique complication of femtosecond LASIK. How to identify the risk factors?
Case 23: Thin flap complications
A case of flap divided into two parts during the femtosecond laser cutting. Risk factor and management
Case 24: Vertical gas breakthrough complicated a case of femtosecond LASIK in an eye with previous microkeratome flap.
What is better, to use femtosecond or mechanical microkeratome to create the flap in patient with previous LASIK procedure? What should be the safe distance between the new flap and the previous one?
Case 25: Intraoperative complications – free cap in femtosecond LASIK
A free flap with femtosecond LASIK can occur during flap manipulation rather than during flap creation. How to manage it?
Case 26: Limitations of reorientation of a LASIK free cap
The importance of the proper orientation and management of a free cap during a complicated LASIK case
Case 27: Flap loss
A conservative way to treat a patient with a flap lost after LASIK
Case 28: Decentered flap in hyperopic intra-LASIK: how to delay is to succeed
An appropriate flap centration is crucial for the success of hyperopic LASIK procedure to achieve a highest quality vision. What to do when the flap is decentered?
Case 29: Suction break during raster pattern and before side cut
Suction loss during the raster pattern can be treated immediately applying the same suction ring; use the same cone and the same femtosecond laser settings.
Case 30: Suction break after complete raster pattern and incomplete side cut
Suction loss during the side cut can be managed reapplying the suction and cone, decreasing the diameter of the ablation by 0.5 mm, and increasing the depth by 20 μm.
Case 31: Suction loss after complete raster pattern and no side cut, no flap lift, and rainbow glare
Rainbow glare is a rare complication which occurs after an incomplete flap that could not be lifted at the time of surgery. An attempt at lifting the original flap might be a better way to treat the complication than performing a PRK.

Buttonhole Flaps 19

Rosario Soriano and Fernando Llovet

Contents

R. Soriano, MD, PhD (✉)
CLINICA BAVIERA GROUP, Head of Ophthalmology Service of Henares University Hospital, Refractive Surgeon at Clínica Baviera Madrid, Madrid, Spain

Associate Professor of Francisco de Vitoria University, Madrid, Spain
e-mail: rcobo@clinicabaviera.com

F. Llovet, MD, PhD
Clínica Baviera,
Clínica-Baviera Medical Director, Madrid, Spain
e-mail: fllovet@clinicabaviera.com

Why Are These Cases Relevant for the Refractive Surgeon?

Among intraoperative LASIK complications, the buttonhole flap is perhaps the most challenging. The buttonhole flap affects the visual axis and compromises visual, anatomical, and functional recovery, as well as has significant psychological and medicolegal repercussions. While free caps and incomplete flaps do not usually cause long-term loss of vision, the buttonhole formation is the most likely complication to result in glare and substantial loss of best corrected visual acuity (BSCVA). Management also poses therapeutic risks, including the formation of subepithelial stromal scars in the visual axis and the induction of irregular astigmatism.

In this section, we present three cases representing different stages or types of buttonhole flap complication, treatment approaches, and outcomes. In the first case, the complication is treated with delayed alcohol-assisted PRK, in the second case with a delayed laser-PTK-PRK procedure with an optimal anatomical result but a refractive hypercorrection, and in the third with an immediate PTK-PRK approach, which involves a long and slow evolution but has relatively positive results.

J.L. Alió et al. (eds.), *Difficult and Complicated Cases in Refractive Surgery*,
DOI 10.1007/978-3-642-55238-0_19, © Springer-Verlag Berlin Heidelberg 2015

Background

Case report 1: A 32-year-old white female with a manifest refraction of −2.5, −0.5 115° in the right eye (BSCVA 20/20, mean $K=44.25$, central pachymetry of 548 μm) and −3.25, −0.75 × 15° in the left eye (BSCVA 20/20, $K=44.25$, central pachymetry of 555 μm), and normal elevation topography was programmed for LASIK surgery. The surgeon used a manual microkeratome (Moria-LSK-ONE 100 μm footplate and −1 suction ring). LASIK in the right eye was uneventful, resulting in a nasal-hinged 80 μm flap. However, a complicated surgery in the left eye resulted in a buttonholed central triangular-shaped lesion with a small dot of epithelial ingrowth (Fig. 19.1). The flap was repositioned without laser treatment and a bandage contact lens was applied.

Case report 2: A 34-year-old white male with a manifest refraction of −5, −0.5 × 15° in the right eye (BSCVA 20/20, mean $K=43.25$, central pachymetry of 545 μm) and − 4.5, −0.25 × 145° in the left eye (BSCVA20/20, $K=43.25$, central pachymetry of 546 μm), and normal elevation topography was programmed for LASIK surgery.

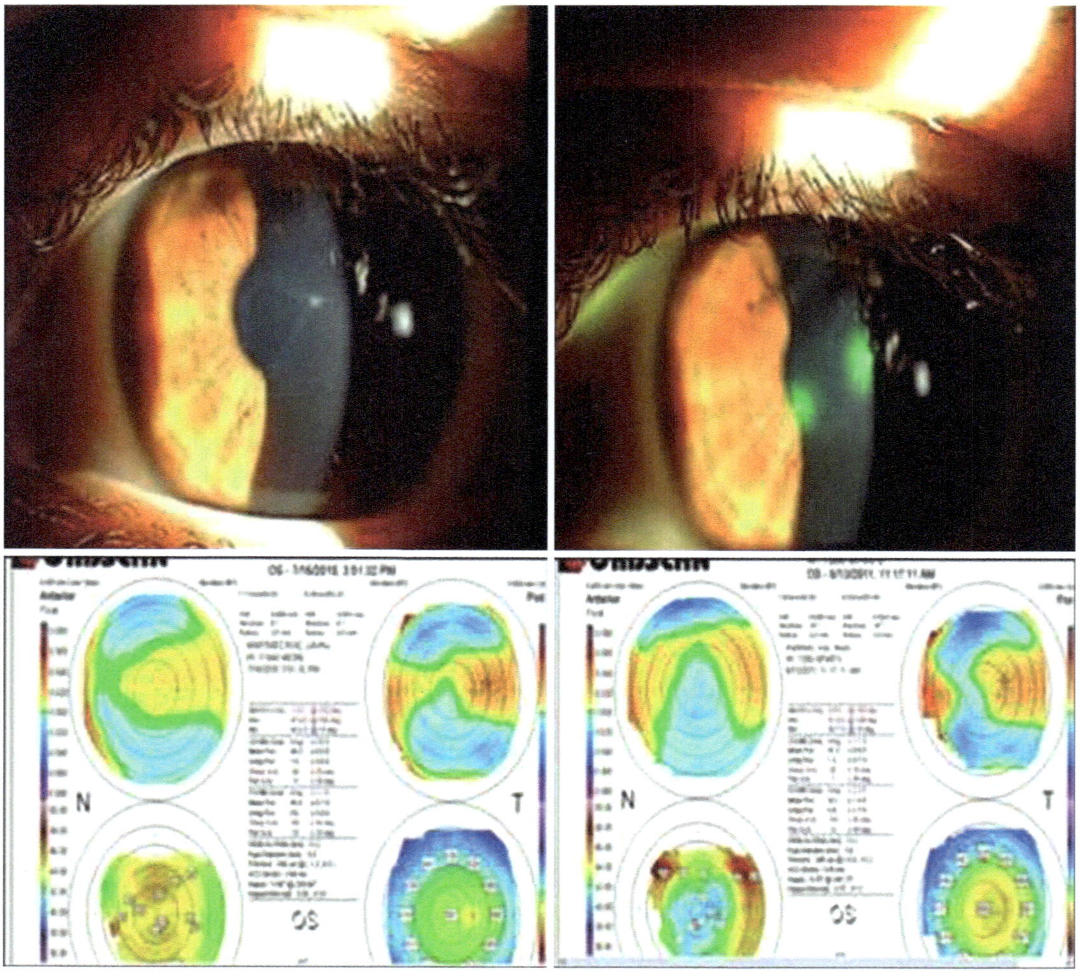

Fig. 19.1 Case 1. Buttonholed central triangular-shaped lesion with a small dot of epithelial ingrowing and natural evolution to a faint scar. Preoperative and postoperative topographies show a perfect recovery of the corneal surface and an optimal refractive outcome: UCVA = 20/20

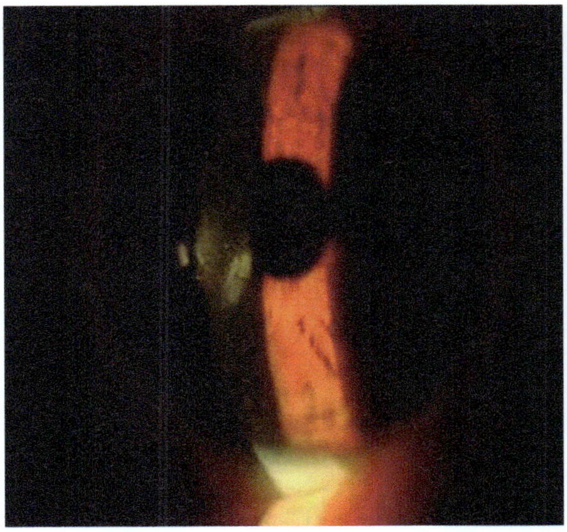

Fig. 19.2 Case 2. Paracentral inferior scar secondary to a buttonhole flap

The surgeon used a manual microkeratome (Moria-LSK-ONE, 100 μm footplate and −1 suction ring).

The microkeratome pass was apparently uneventful (OS), but a central buttonhole was noted once the flap was reflected. The flap was repositioned without laser treatment and a bandage contact lens was applied; the right eye was not operated on to prevent an anisometropia status (Fig. 19.2).

Case report 3: A 26-year-old male with no significant medical or ocular history elected to have LASIK for emmetropia. The preoperative refraction was −3.25, −0.5 × 15° in the right eye and −2.75, −0.5 × 185° in the left eye. In both eyes, the BSCVA was 20/20. Mean keratometry were 44.5 and 44.75 diopters (D) in OD and OS, respectively. Central ultrasonic pachymetry were 545 and 550 μm, respectively.

A corneal flap was attempted in the left eye using a Moria-LSK-ONE microkeratome with a 100 μm footplate and −1 suction ring. A buttonhole was noted centrally in the left eye when the flap was reflected, and a normal flap was created in the contralateral eye of 101 μm thickness. As the buttonhole was not manipulated and there was good apposition of the lesion edges, the surgeon decided to apply laser ablation in both eyes: standard LASIK in OD and in the left eye a PTK (50 μm, OZ = 7)/PRK/MMC. The OS in the immediate postoperative period progressed with a significant delay of reepithelialization lasting nearly 3 weeks, with redness and pain (Figs. 19.3 and 19.4).

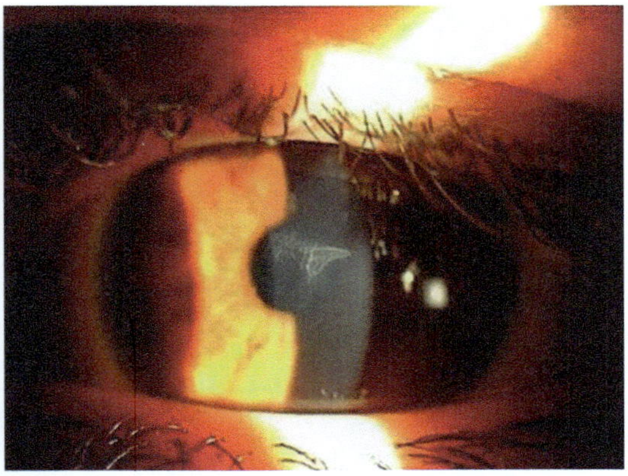

Fig. 19.3 Case 3. Central buttonhole scar with haze, epithelial ingrowth, and corneal irregularity

Main Problems to Solve

The buttonhole is an intraoperative LASIK complication resulting from an uncut portion of the corneal flap which usually occurs at the central corneal apex. The formation may result in vision loss due to an irregular astigmatism and central scarring and/or epithelial ingrowth. Buttonholes occur during surgery when the blade misses an area in the cornea, leaving an uncut hole (Fig. 19.5); an island of tissue left remaining on the corneal bed fits like a puzzle piece into the hole. The microkeratome blade exits the epithelium prematurely as it travels across the stroma and quickly reenters to follow the original path.

The incidence of LASIK buttonholes (BH) varies from 0.20 and 0.56 % [1], with several theories accounting for their occurrence. Traditionally, steep corneas were reported to be at greater risk for this complication; however, Albelda-Valles et al. [2] found no relationship between steep keratometry and buttonhole occurrence in a study of 34,099 eyes. Other proposed explanations include malfunctioning of the microkeratome motor, inadequate suction

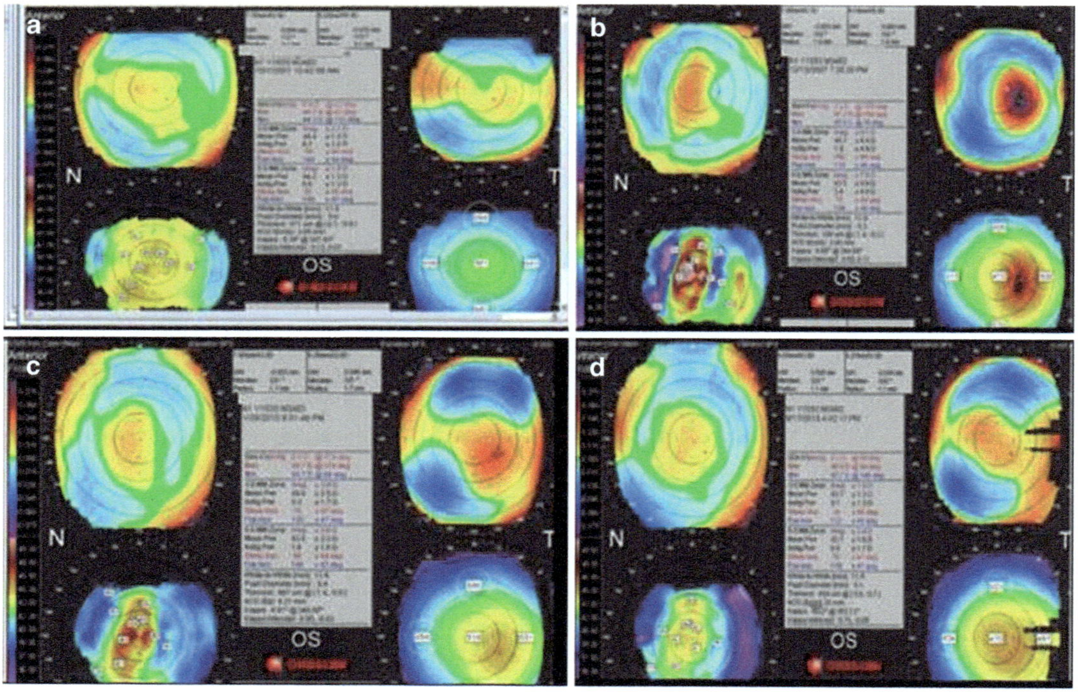

Fig. 19.4 Case 3. Topographic sequence: (**a**) preoperatively, (**b**) after first PRK/PTK, (**c**) after 1 year natural evolution, (**d**) after second treatment (PRK/PTK topo-guided)

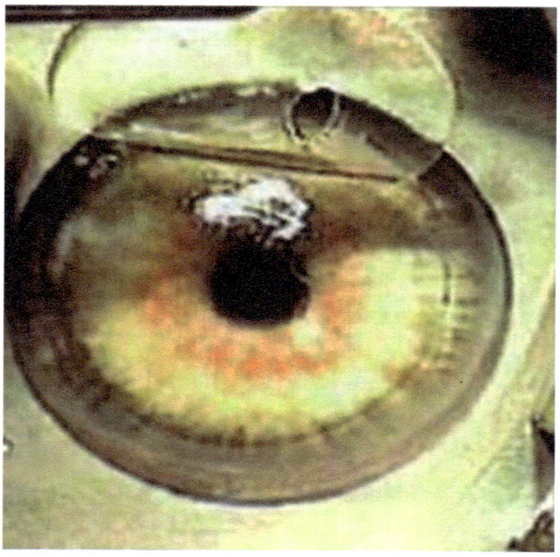

Fig. 19.5 Central buttonhole flap following the microkeratome pass (Taken from Randleman et al. [6]. Online course, American Academy of Ophthalmology)

(malfunctioning of vacuum unit or other etiologies that compromise the adherence of the suction ring to the cornea such as high astigmatism, conjunctival incarceration, etc.), and even poor quality of the blade [3].

Once a buttonhole occurs, we propose the following steps:

1. Ensure the best anatomical reposition.
2. Decide whether to cancel the procedure or perform an immediate laser treatment.
3. Avoid associated inflammatory complications.
4. Decide timing of re-treatment.
5. Decide on another re-treatment technique.
6. Treat severe anatomical complications.

Ancillary Tests

Harissi-Dagher [1] and coauthors reported a useful classification of buttonholes in three stages based on the development of epithelial ingrowth which determined a practical management approach: stage 1 (a full- or partial-thickness buttonhole without epithelial ingrowth), stage 2 (a full- or partial-thickness buttonhole with epithelial ingrowth), and stage 3 (a full- or partial-thickness buttonhole

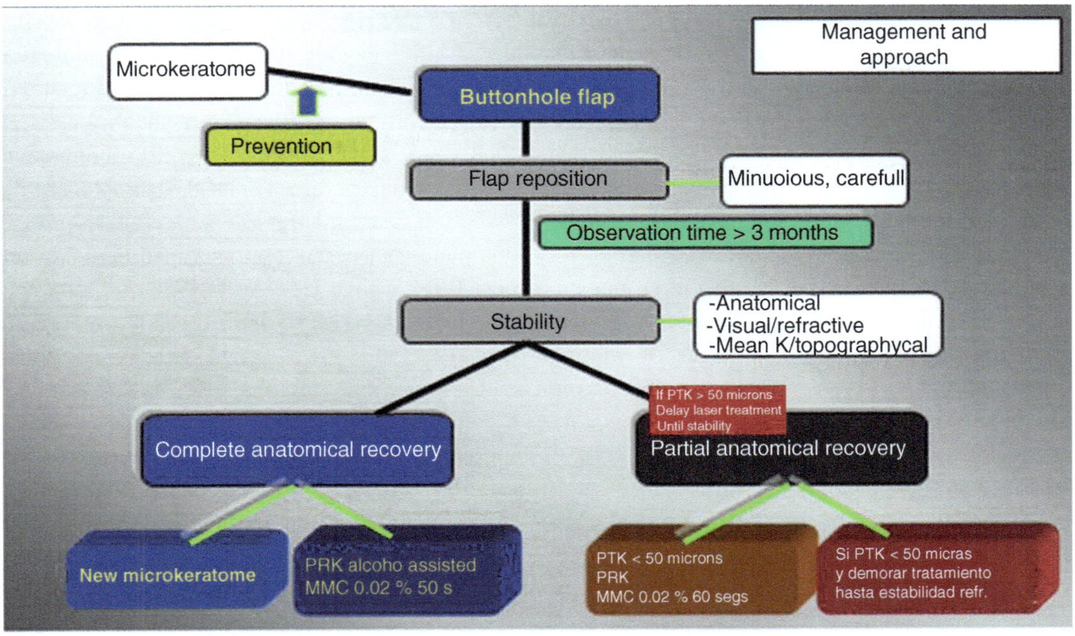

Llovet et al. Button Hole treatment algorithm oresented at the 26th SECOIR Congress. Valensia. Spain. 2011

Fig. 19.6 Algorithm decision in a buttonhole flap complication (Llovet et al. [7])

with epithelial ingrowth and resultant stromal melt/scarring or flap elevation).

Creation of a new LASIK flap beneath the buttonhole flap by means of a new microkeratome pass is another option in cases of good anatomical recovery without significant leukoma in the visual axis. Figure 19.6 shows our own decision-making algorithm regarding management and surgical approaches according to various levels of severity and complication.

Surgical/Medical Intervention

1. Ensure the best anatomical reposition. A meticulous intraoperative repositioning of the flap is extremely important to ensure good apposition of the buttonhole margins and to avoid irregular astigmatism and infiltration of the epithelial cells through the buttonhole edges, which would cause epithelial ingrowth. Although it is not always easy to reposition these flaps, it is important to be careful during this step and to take as long as necessary to align the edges of the disk correctly to achieve a correct reattachment.
2. Cancel the procedure. The most accepted response to buttonholes is to cancel the procedure and bypass treatment with laser, which can induce an irreversible irregular astigmatism. Although immediate (same day) surface ablation (PTK/PRK) has been reported [4] with initial success, the series was limited by a short-term follow-up. Concern regarding immediate treatment includes the possibility of activated stromal keratocytes creating scar tissue or a delay of reepithelialization and a corneal ulcer complicating the situation. Although prophylactic MMC may limit the development of scar tissue after immediate treatment, the rationale for delaying treatment by several weeks pertains to the surface epithelium as well as significant medicolegal issues of informed consent.
3. To avoid associated inflammatory complications, maintaining a postoperative steroid treatment for several months is important to avoid further complications such as DLK and to minimize further corneal scarring.

4. Decide on the timing of re-treatment. Usually the surgeon and patient are motivated to address the complication early in the postoperative period. However, a postoperative waiting period of at least 3 months is recommended in order to allow the cornea to heal and restore to its original refraction. Patients usually become anxious and demand an earlier re-treatment, especially if an anisometropia status has been created. Therefore, proper counseling as to the advantages of waiting (e.g., less haze, better surface regularity from epithelial remodeling) and postponing re-treatment lead to better results.
5. Re-treatment technique: Although a new, deeper flap can be created by repeating a microkeratome pass below the original flap, the safest way to manage buttonholes is to treat them with surface PRK assisted with mitomycin C 0.02 % for 60 s [5].
   Deciding between alcohol-PRK and laser-PTK-PRK, epithelial removal techniques depend on the epithelium conditions and topographic abnormalities. The most accepted transepithelial PTK ablation is 50 μm and for PRK should be readjusted to 80 % of subjective refraction. In the series reported by Harissi-Dagher, overcorrection occurred in 33 % of the PTK-PRK cases [1].
6. Treatment of severe anatomical complications. In cases of progressive epithelial ingrowth, a two-stage treatment is recommended. First, PTK applied therapeutically obliterates infiltrated epithelial cells and recovers as much transparency as possible. Second, a PRK procedure of residual refraction is called for, which can be modified by the PTK procedure.
   Cases of irregular astigmatism or significant scarring should also be treated in two stages, PTK followed by topographically guided ablations (Fig. 19.6).

Outcomes

Case 1: One month after initial surgery, there was a very faint line scar (Fig. 19.1). Three months later, BCVA recovered to 20/20 with sph −3.25 cyl −0.5 axis 15° (K=43.75, keratometric cylinder of −0.75 D, axis 30°), and the buttonhole was no longer visible at the slit lamp. Re-treatment was performed by means of alcohol-assisted PRK (20 % alcohol during 40 s plus mitomycin C and a bandage contact lens 8.8). Postoperative evolution was favorable, achieving a prompt complete transparent epithelialization at 1 week post-PRK, a final UCVA of 20/20, an emmetropia status (K=41.25), and a normal topography (Fig. 19.1).

Case 2: Two months after initial surgery, there was still a central scar with epithelial ingrowth, significant haze, and loss of BCVA (20/40) with sph − 5.0 D (K=43 keratometric cylinder of −1.75 D, axis 68°) (Fig. 19.2). Finally, 6 months after initial surgery and stabilization of refraction and topographies, we decided to perform the treatment in both eyes: PRK in OD and a PTK/PRK/MMC procedure (70 μm), optical zone of 7 plus a PRK (−5.0 D) in OS. Postoperative evolution showed a favorable anatomical outcome, achieving complete transparency of the cornea and resolution of the haze and the scar in OS. Unfortunately, however, the functional result was suboptimal, developing an overcorrection with a final refraction of +1.5 D. Refraction at 10 months postoperatively was OD (UCVA=20/20, +0.25 sph, mean K of 39 D) and OS (UCVA=20/30, BCVA with +1.5 sph=20/20, mean K of 38 D). As the patient did not tolerate the postoperative anisometropia, we recommended a hyperopic PRK re-treatment; however, the patient decided against it, and we lost follow-up contact.

Case 3: Over the 4 months following the procedure, the follow-up showed a corneal central scar with haze and epithelial ingrowth OS (Fig. 19.3) that derived in a myopic shift with irregular astigmatism and significant loss of BCVA. One month postoperatively, refraction in OD was emmetropia with UCVA of 20/20. In OS, UCVA was 20/200, refraction was −3.25, −4.5×57° (K=47.75), and BCVA=20/60.

Intensive steroid treatment applied over several months resulted in gradual restoration of the corneal surface and more regularity within the refraction and topographies. (Fig. 19.4 shows topographic sequence.) Eight months postoperatively the patient was very uncomfortable with the anisometropia, and a rigid contact lens had to be applied achieving a BCVA = 20/30.

One year post-op, the patient consented to a new PTK/MMC topographically guided by the Allegretto excimer laser system. PTK was 50 μm depth and OZ = 7 mm followed by a PRK programed with −1.0 D (28.9 μm of maximum depth). Finally, after the second re-treatment, the cornea achieved a transparency, a very light residual haze, a regular topographic appearance (Fig. 19.4) with a refraction of −2, −0.5 75°, and a BCVA of 20/20. A phakic intraocular lens (ICL) was recommended but the patient refused it at the moment.

What to Learn from These Cases

These cases demonstrate that the best approach to buttonhole flap formation is to cancel the laser treatment and proceed when the best spectacle-corrected visual acuity approaches the preoperative level or has stabilized. Secondly, if the flap allows an alcohol-assisted PRK, the laser refractive treatment will be more predictable. If choosing a PTK-PRK technique, it is very important to calculate both ablations in order not to induce hypercorrection. In Case 1, we obtained a better result with alcohol de-epithelialization, as the posterior refraction treatment by PRK is reliable and easily reproducible. However, in Case 2 we miscalculated the PRK/PTK ablation, leading to overcorrection and a hyperopic shift. In severe cases such as Case 3, more than one procedure separated by months may be required to eliminate the central cut or doughnut-shaped flap scar.

Although buttonhole flap formations are a potentially serious complication of LASIK, a planned, delayed reoperation after sufficient corneal healing that employs the proper technique can allow satisfactory recovery of UCVA and BCVA.

References

1. Harissi-Dagher M, Todani A, Melki SA (2008) Laser in situ keratomileusis buttonhole: classification and management algorithm. J Cataract Refract Surg 34:1892–1899
2. Albelda-Valles JC, Martin-Reyes C, Ramos F, Beltran J, Llovet F, Baviera J (2007) Effect of preoperative keratometric power on intraoperative complications in LASIK in 34,099 eyes. J Refract Surg 23:592–597
3. Leung ATS, Rao SK, Cheng ACK (2000) Pathogenesis and management of laser in situ keratomileusis flap buttonhole. J Cataract Refract Surg 26:358–362
4. Jain VK, Abell TG, Bond WI, Stevens G Jr (2002) Immediate transepithelial photorefractive keratectomy for treatment of laser in situ keratomileusis flap complications. J Refract Surg 18:109–112
5. Muller LT, Candal EM, Epstein RJ, Dennis RF, Majmudar PA (2005) Transepithelial phototherapeutic keratectomy/photorefractive keratectomy with adjunctive mitomycin-C for complicated LASIK flaps. J Cataract Refract Surg 31:291–296
6. Randleman JB, Azar D, Wachler BB. "LASIK and PRK: Managing Complications". Online course, ONE® Network.American Academy of Ophthalmology. http://one.aao.org/lms/courses/managing_lasik_complications/index.htm
7. Llovet F et al (2011) Button hole treatment algorithm presented at the 26th SECOIR Congress, Valencia, Spain

Incomplete LASIK Flap

20

Michael T. Andreoli and Dimitri T. Azar

Contents

M.T. Andreoli, MD • D.T. Azar, MD, MBA (✉)
Department of Ophthalmology and Visual Sciences
Illinois Eye and Ear Infirmary,
University of Illinois at Chicago, Chicago, IL, USA
e-mail: michaelandreoli@gmail.com; dazar@uic.edu

Why Is This Case Relevant for the Refractive Surgeon?

Large-scale studies have reported numerous intraoperative and postoperative laser in situ keratomileusis (LASIK) flap complications with use of a mechanical microkeratome [1]. Frequently, detection of an intraoperative flap complication causes the surgeon to abort the laser ablation process. These eyes then present a management dilemma, as a repeat attempt at refractive surgery is associated with higher risks of intraoperative and postoperative complications [2].

Case Background

A 32-year-old female with myopia presented for a second opinion regarding a failed attempt at LASIK surgery at an outside academic institution 2 months earlier. LASIK was performed on the right eye, but during the procedure, an incomplete flap was identified after passage of the microkeratome. The flap was lifted and found to have an irregular configuration. The surgeon repositioned the LASIK flap and aborted the laser ablation. The flap had irregular edges and a ridged bed, and it was not repositioned appropriately. The surgeon applied a bandage contact lens to it and did not continue with surgery on the contralateral eye. On the clinical exam 1 day postoperatively, the patient was noted to have

J.L. Alió et al. (eds.), *Difficult and Complicated Cases in Refractive Surgery*,
DOI 10.1007/978-3-642-55238-0_20,

formed corneal striae and a ridge adjacent to the microkeratome incision, limiting best visual acuity to 20/100. During follow-up with conservative management, the patient developed blurred vision and photosensitivity soon after the procedure. By postoperative week 1, early diffuse lamellar keratitis was suspected, which responded appropriately to topical steroids over the next 2 weeks. Two weeks postoperative, the patient's uncorrected visual acuity decreased to count fingers, with pinhole improvement to 20/80. At 3 postoperative weeks, the patient developed mild double vision, which prompted the patient to seek a second opinion. The corneal specialist at the second institution recommended contact lenses to improve vision, but the patient declined. At 2 months postoperative, the patient sought the opinion of a third corneal specialist. The patient complained of severe monocular glare and diplopia and was noted to have 10 D of oblique irregular astigmatism, corneal fixed folds, and interface haze, all potentially contributing to her severe loss of best spectacle-corrected visual acuity (20/80) OD.

Main Problem to Solve

This case represents the uncommon management predicament of a patient with previously aborted LASIK surgery due to an incomplete flap created with a microkeratome. Due to the intraoperative identification of this complication, laser ablation was not performed. A case series of such patients has suggested that patients with incomplete flaps that are repositioned without ablation tend to return to within one diopter of their preoperative spherical and astigmatic refraction [3]. However, this particular patient persisted with monocular diplopia and significantly diminished uncorrected and best corrected visual acuity due to corneal irregularity and high irregular astigmatism. The fixed folds, the history of DLK, and the irregularly cut flap present difficult management problems 2 months after surgery.

Ancillary Tests

The patient's manifest refraction at postoperative month 2 was −7.50 + 10.00 × 150, resulting in the best spectacle-corrected visual acuity of 20/80. The refractive error OS was −3.25 + 1.75 × 160 with visual acuity of 20/20^{+}. In a patient with previous LASIK flap creation OD, corneal pachymetry and topography offer a better understanding of the current architecture of the cornea. Central pachymetry OD was 651 μm, contrasting with 580 μm in the fellow eye. OCULUS Pentacam topography of the right eye at postoperative month 2 is depicted in Fig. 20.1. It confirms the presence of high irregular astigmatism as well as severe variability of pachymetry in the central cornea. The thinnest pachymetry, localized 2.76 mm temporal to the corneal apex, measured 495 μm. This was associated with 12.5 D of against-the-rule (ATR) astigmatism OD.

Surgical/Medical Intervention

The patient demonstrated significant irregular astigmatism on imaging with high astigmatism on manifest refraction, which was able to improve visual acuity to 20/80. Due to the corneal abnormalities, the options of lamellar keratectomy, deep anterior lamellar keratoplasty, penetrating keratoplasty, and phototherapeutic keratectomy were discussed with the patient. The patient elected to undergo lamellar keratectomy, 4 months after the incomplete LASIK flap was created. The rationale for surgery was to identify a surgical plane posterior to the irregular (thickened) flap, followed by PTK to provide a more regular optical surface, and to eliminate the irregularities, folds, and opacities caused by the LASIK flap. The lamellar keratectomy was followed 2 days later by phototherapeutic keratectomy with mitomycin C application. The plan was to establish a baseline refractive error measurement upon which subsequent PRK would be based. Prior to PTK treatment, we obtained direct ultrasonic pachymetry, the paracentral area showing 480 μm temporally,

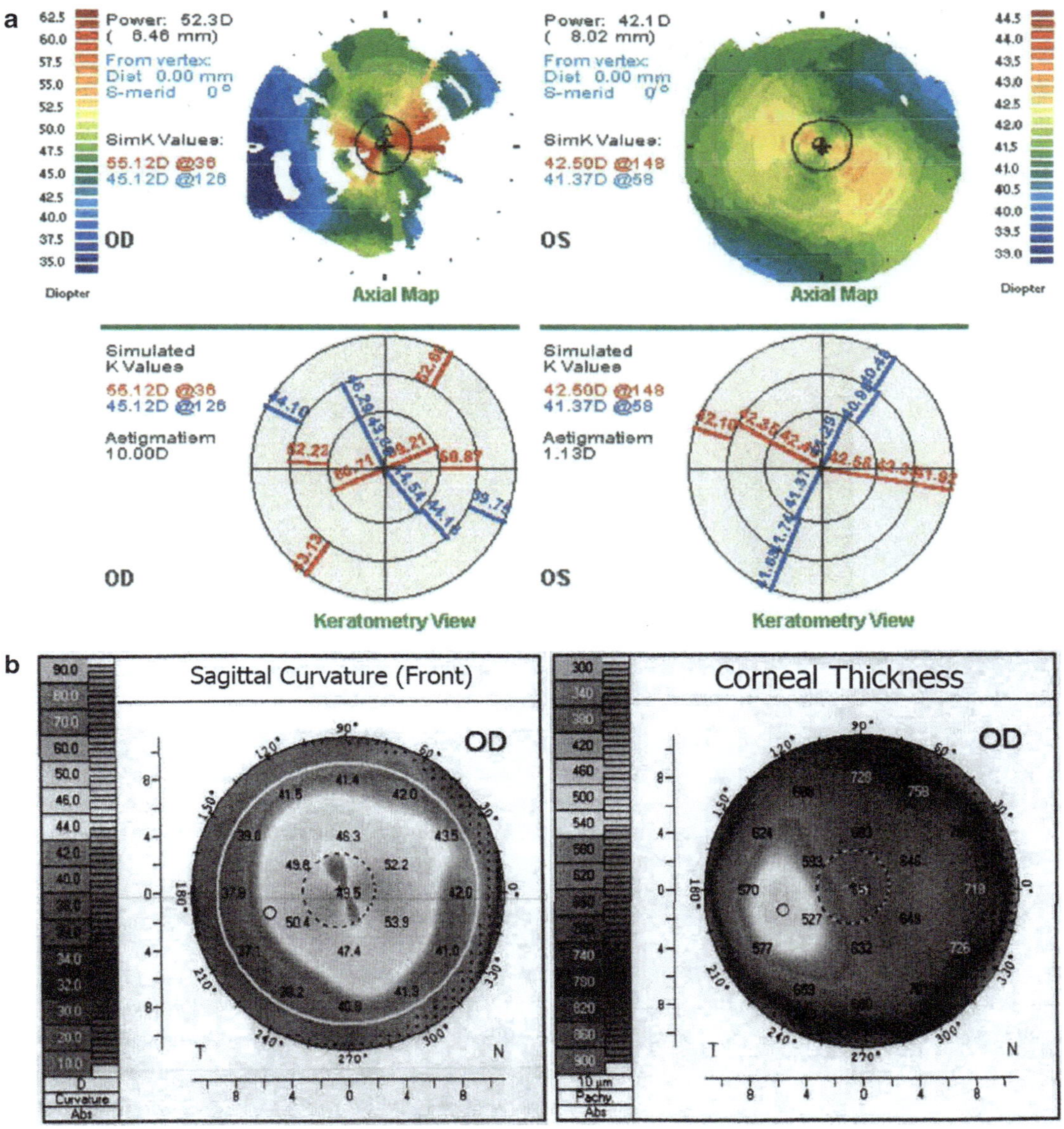

Fig. 20.1 Humphrey Orbscan corneal topography OU (**a**) and OCULUS Pentacam corneal topography of the right eye on 1/21/09, 7 weeks after an incomplete flap was created (**b**). Note the high astigmatism and corneal irregularities

500 μm nasally, and 455 μm inferiorly. Direct ultrasonic central pachymetry measured 515 μm. The procedure involved repeated application of a modulating agent prior to approximately every 10 μm of PTK laser applications (for a total of 57 μm PTK depth). Postoperative pachymetry measured 458 μm OD.

Outcome

Within 1 week of the lamellar keratectomy, the diplopia resolved with the improvement of best corrected visual acuity to 20/40. By 11 weeks after lamellar keratectomy, the patient's uncorrected visual acuity improved to 20/40, with a

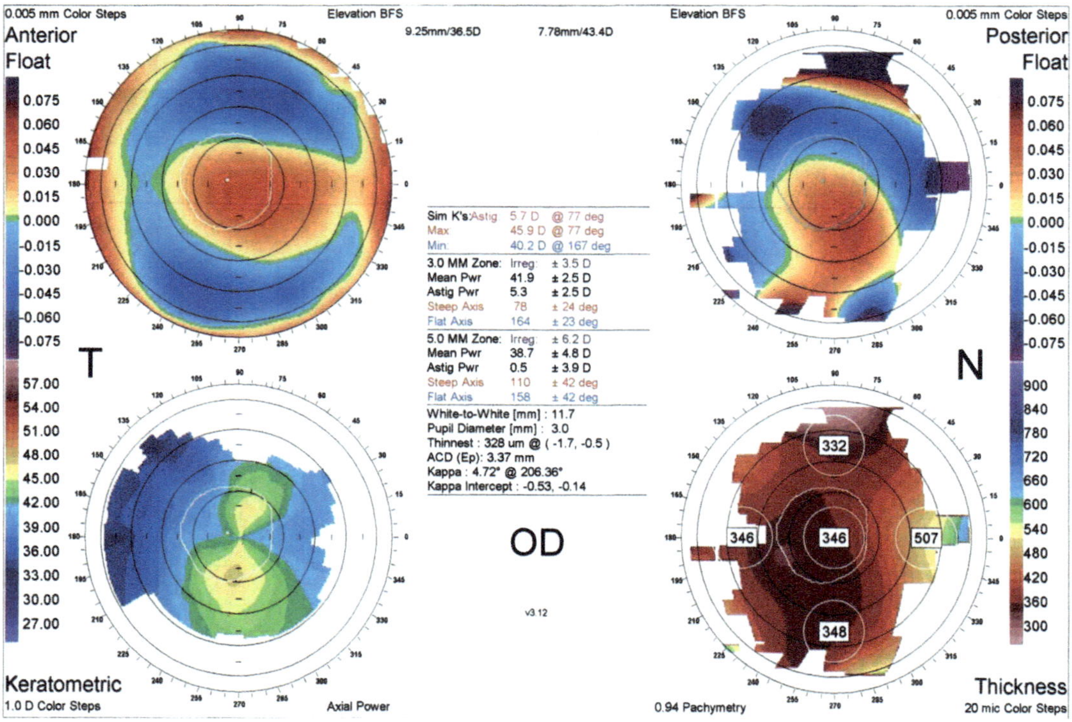

Fig. 20.2 Bausch & Lomb Orbscan corneal topography of the right eye on 6/30/09, 11 weeks after lamellar keratectomy and phototherapeutic keratectomy with mitomycin C. Note the improvement in corneal astigmatism

manifest refraction of −4.00+3.00×78 yielding the best corrected visual acuity of 20/20. The postoperative Orbscan topography is shown in Fig. 20.2. PRK surface treatment was offered to correct the residual/induced refractive error, but the patient was cautioned about the risks of postoperative ectasia (given the low postoperative pachymetry). The patient was content with the resolution of her symptoms and preferred to avoid additional surgical or laser interventions OD.

What to Learn from This Case

While intraoperative flap complications are a dreaded reality of LASIK surgery [4, 5], visual outcomes are often acceptable with close follow-up and continued management. Planned refractive interventions can often improve vision above pre-complication acuity. Management options for an incomplete flap include spectacles, contact lenses, lamellar keratectomy, deep anterior lamellar keratoplasty, penetrating keratoplasty, and phototherapeutic keratectomy. The particular treatment depends on the corneal dimensions, degree of irregularity, manifest refraction, subjective visual complaints, and patient expectations. With the advent of femtosecond laser flap creation, there has been a shift in the intraoperative and postoperative risks of LASIK surgery. However, studies have demonstrated a similar number of total flap complications between mechanical microkeratome and femtosecond laser flaps, with a greater number of epithelial defects with a microkeratome and a higher rate of diffuse lamellar keratitis with the femtosecond laser [1].

References

1. Moshirfar M, Gardiner JP, Schliesser JA, Espandar L, Feiz V, Mifflin MD, Chang JC (2010) Laser in situ keratomileusis flap complications using mechanical microkeratome versus femtosecond laser: retrospective comparison. J Cataract Refract Surg 36:1925–1933
2. Sharma N, Ghate D, Agarwal T, Vajpayee RB (2005) Refractive outcomes of laser in situ keratomileusis after flap complications. J Cataract Refract Surg 31:1334–1337
3. Tham VM, Maloney RK (2000) Microkeratome complications of laser in situ keratomileusis. Ophthalmology 107:920–924
4. Jacobs JM, Taravella MJ (2002) Incidence of intraoperative flap complications in laser in situ keratomileusis. J Cataract Refract Surg 28:23–28
5. Jabbur NS, Myrowitz E, Wexler JL, O'Brien TP (2004) Outcome of second surgery in LASIK cases aborted due to flap complications. J Cataract Refract Surg 30:993–999

Dislocated Flaps

21

Rosario Soriano and Julio Baviera-Sabater

Contents

R. Soriano, MD, PhD (✉)
Refractive surgery, CLINICA BAVIERA GROUP, Head of Ophthalmology Service of Henares University Hospital, Refractive Surgeon at Clínica Baviera Madrid, Madrid, Spain

Associate Professor of Francisco de Vitoria University, Madrid, Spain
e-mail: rcobo@clinicabaviera.com

J. Baviera-Sabater, MD
Baviera Group Chairman and Medical Director, Clinica Baviera, Madrid, Spain
e-mail: jbaviera@clinicabaviera.com

Why Is This Case Relevant for the Refractive Surgeon?

A dislocated flap is a mild complication of LASIK, ordinarily detected promptly (in less than 24 h) and managed easily, resulting in a favorable anatomic and functional outcome. The precise cause of flap dislocation is unclear, but wrinkling or dislodgment may result from poor adherence of the corneal flap to the stromal bed because of overhydration of the stromal bed or the flap, eye rubbing, excessive blinking, and eye squeezing from pain, photophobia, or other discomfort in the postoperative period. Although flap dislocation is a relatively rare complication of LASIK (incidences range from 0.012 to 5.8 %) when a flap remains wrinkled for several hours or overnight, visual recovery is delayed because of apposition and incongruous fitting between the edematous folded flap and the bed, despite prompt surgical repositioning. In these situations, refractive regression is often indicated, which requires an enhancement treatment and mild persistent microstriae that can affect quality of vision. In addition, severe cases of permanent wrinkles or an irregularly shaped corneal surface can lead to diminished UCVA and BCVA, additional surgical maneuvers, or even flap amputation.

Included in this chapter are the results of a descriptive study of dislocated flaps we have encountered in our practice. We highlight a case of prompt diagnosis and successful intervention with a favorable response and outcome.

J.L. Alió et al. (eds.), *Difficult and Complicated Cases in Refractive Surgery*,
DOI 10.1007/978-3-642-55238-0_21, © Springer-Verlag Berlin Heidelberg 2015

Case Background

A 50-year-old white female with a manifest refraction of −8, −0.5 × 10° in the right eye (BSCVA, 20/25) and −5, −0.5 × 174° in the left eye (BSCVA, 20/20) underwent uneventful bilateral simultaneous LASIK for the correction of myopia and astigmatism. Mean keratometry was 42.25, −1 × 176° OD and 42.5, −0.75 × 174° OS; preoperative pachymetry 568- and 565-µm OD/OS, respectively; normal topographies and Orbscan white-to-white distance 11.8-mm OU; biomicroscopic clear lenses; and myopic fundus without peripheral rhegmatogenous retinal lesions.

LASIK surgery was performed using a manual microkeratome (Moria LSK-ONE), 9-mm H-suction ring diameter and a 10-µm-thickness footplate without complications, creating nasal-hinged flaps of 125- and 80-µm thickness in OD and OS, respectively. The excimer laser (Technolas Zyoptix) performed ablation depths of 115 µm (optical zone OZ=6.0) and 80 µm (OZ=6.2) in OD and OS, respectively, aiming at monovision OD. An Alphagan® drop was instilled postoperatively in both eyes in order to minimize hyperemia and discomfort, and no eye shield was recommended. Twenty-four hours after surgery, the patient came to the office complaining of moderate discomfort, redness, and worse vision in the right eye. Apparently there was no history of eye rubbing, but the patient admitted that application of lubricant tear drops was not asymptomatic and painless (despite printed instructions).

Slit lamp examination revealed an edematous partially inferior dislodged corneal flap in OD with flap folds across the visual axis and an exposed area of temporal stroma (Fig. 21.1). The patient's flap was immediately stabilized in the slit lamp at the office, a bandage contact lens was applied, and the patient was sent to the surgery room to complete the flap-folding treatment.

In the surgery room, the flap was repositioned with the following technique:

- Hydration of the stroma and flap with hypotonic solution (destillate water) and physiologic 0.9 % saline.
- Lifting, repositioning, and flap stretching and drying of the flap cornea ring junction.
- Central epithelial removal was performed due to persistent deep striae beside de hinge despite a correct flap edge alignment.
- Placing of a bandage contact lens and cycloplegic plus dexamethasone-tobramycin drops.

Postoperatively, the eye developed a central area of small white dots of epithelial ingrowth (Fig. 21.2) after reepithelialization healing. A mild diffuse lamellar keratitis resolved with intensive topical dexamethasone-tobramycin drops in 6 weeks, leaving a clear, wrinkle-free cornea. Three months later, the BSDCVA was 20/20 (−1.25, −0.5 × 180°) and the UCNVA was J3.

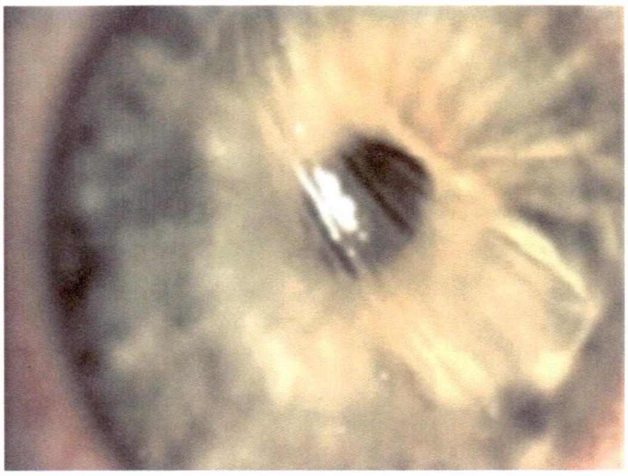

Fig. 21.1 Flap inferonasal dislocation with deep folds affecting visual axis of the RE

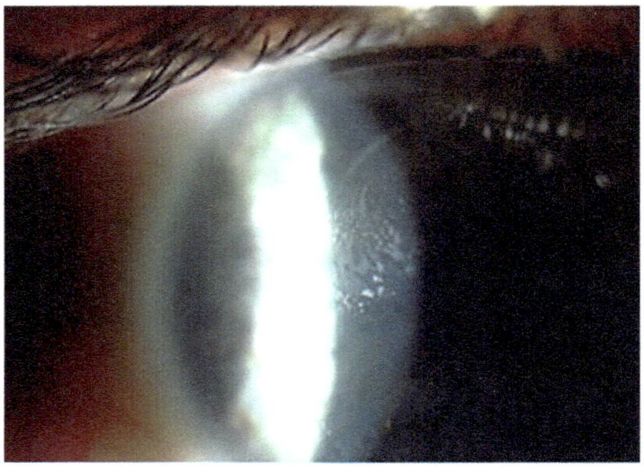

Fig. 21.2 Postoperative white-dot patches of epithelial ingrowth after flap reposition technique with epithelial removal

Main Problem to Solve

The primary problem is avoiding corneal fixed folds at the visual axis that produce an incongruent fitting of the flap and bed surfaces and which cause visual loss, haze, and refractive regression. Less frequent complications include epithelial ingrowth, stromal interface inflammation (DLK), infection, and recurrent shifting, which in severe cases can lead to lysis and necrosis of the flap, even requiring amputation to recover media transparency.

Ancillary Tests

Although this case has a clear surgical indication, sometimes the flap displacement can be mild with light striae out of the visual axis, requiring repositioning with the slit lamp. Some additional challenges for the refractive surgeon may include interpretation of the severity of striae, determination of its visual repercussion, deciding to work under the microscope in the surgery room (with the subsequent increase of patient anxiety), or cases requiring surgical stretching. Table 21.1 offers a decision algorithm for use in encountering some challenges.

Surgical/Medical Intervention

The repositioning described techniques are as follows:

- Lifting, hydration (refloating) of the flap with hyposmotic solutions, stretching it with blunt forceps and/or microsponges, and meticulous dryness of flap edge. This is the most extended technique, and it often takes a long time to obtain a good reposition.
- If folds persist after flap reposition and a correct alignment of the border (Fig. 21.3), central de-epithelialization can release mechanical tension and facilitate corneal stretching.
- Other fold-treatment techniques described are:
  - Llovet's rolling technique: ironing and pressing the folds using a heavy syringe filled with saline solution and performing a perpendicular movement to the folds direction (presented at the 82nd Congress of Spanish Society of Ophthalmology, Sept. 2006) (Fig. 21.4)

Table 21.1 Techniques for repositioning the LASIK flap

Slit lamp	Operating/laser room
Debridement; small amount	Debridement; large amount
Striae	Striae with sutures
Displaced flap	Epithelial ingrowth
	Infection; need for culture
	Irrigation of diffuse lamellar keratitis

Taken from Lichter et al. [1]

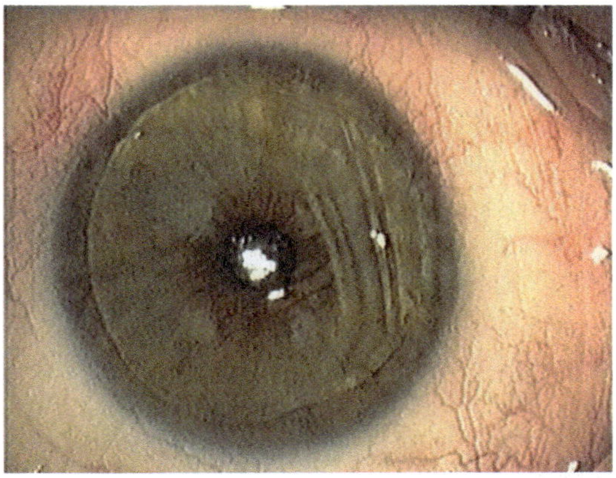

Fig. 21.3 Persistent deep flap striae beside the nasal hinge despite a correct flap edge alignment

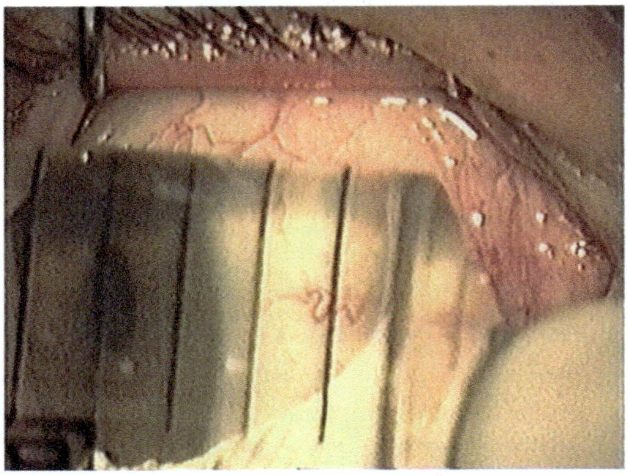

Fig. 21.4 Llovet's rolling technique fold treatment: ironing and pressing the folds using a heavy syringe filled with saline solution performed at a perpendicular movement to the striae direction

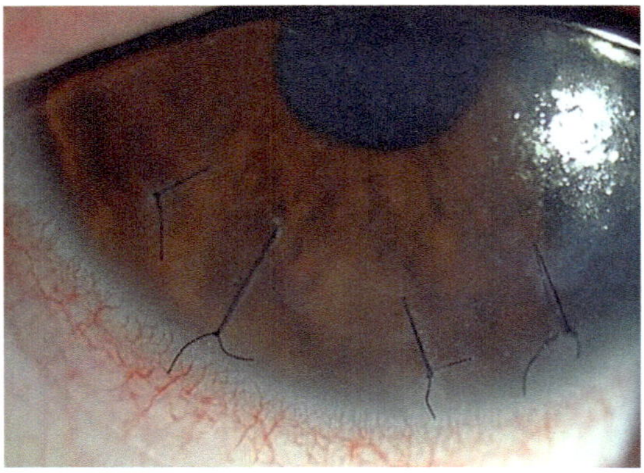

Fig. 21.5 Flap suturing (four 10-0 nylon stitches) in a refractory case (a 28-year-old male) with recurrent dislocations (three times), peripheral haze, and stromal edema

  - Donnenfeld hyperthermic treatment of the flap with a hot spatula (JCRS 2004)
  - Sandwich technique (Hernandez-Matamoros and Iradier, JCRS 2001)
- Sutures: Usually there is no need to suture the flap, but in cases of deep persistent folds after previously mentioned surgical maneuvers or repeated dislocations, flap suture with 10-0 nylon is sometimes necessary to maintain equal tension by pulling at opposite sides of the wrinkles (continuous or separated stitches) (Fig. 21.5).
- In cases of long-lasting flap dislocation with the suspicion of growing epithelium over bare stroma, removal and scraping of the epithelial cells with a knife, spatula, or both over the posterior surface of the flap and the bed are recommended.
- Finally, placing a bandage contact lens can stabilize the flap and reduce the risk of epithelial ingrowth.
- Prophylactic antibiotics, corticosteroids, intensive lubricant artificial drops, and in some cases cycloplegics are the treatments of choice to prevent further infectious and inflammatory complications.

Immediately following the repositioning procedure, the appearance of the flap worsens due to edema of the epithelium and stroma, with the folds initially becoming more evident and opaque. Twelve to 24 h later, the striae tend to diminish, and the cornea becomes flatter and clearer.

Outcome of Dislocated Flaps

This case had a favorable outcome despite an immediate postoperative epithelial inflammation. Topical corticoid therapy was used to achieve positive anatomic and functional results.

Reports of follow-up of patients with subluxated flaps are scarce. Recep et al. [2] reported the outcomes at 6 months in 19 cases, which were compared with the contralateral uneventful eye. These cases showed slightly worsening visual and refractive results, although results were not statistically significant. Another more recent study by Clare et al. [3] evaluated the risks factors for early flap displacements (less than 48 h) using a logistic regression model of ten eyes over 12 months. The study showed an extremely low incidence of flap displacement (0.012 %) and a higher risk for mechanical microkeratome compared with IntraLase femtosecond flaps. It showed a statistically significant higher risk for hyperopic eyes (eight cases) than myopic eye (two cases), reporting an OR of 19.29 for hyperopia and 10.53 for mechanical microkeratomes.

We are conducting a retrospective analysis of our own series of dislocated flaps through the Clinica Baviera Group data base from 2002 till present. Our purpose is firstly to investigate the outcomes of these complicated eyes and secondly to ascertain if particular preoperative and/or intraoperative conditions influence flap dislocation. Out of 300,000 cases, 429 (or 0.1 %) involved this flap dislocation. We compared the functional postoperative results of the study with a control LASIK group to determine whether outcomes were significantly different. Publication is pending. Most cases we found showed early dislocations; 77 % of cases were detected in less than 24 h. One hundred and twenty-one clients experienced dislocation within the same day of surgery and 209 the day after surgery (Clinica Baviera has a 24-h emergency service). Only 13 cases involved traumatic dislocation 3 months post-surgery, with a single case 2.5 years post-surgery. Table 21.2 identifies myopia as the main refractive defect, present in 78 % of cases; of these, 19 % were cases of high myopia (SE<−6D). Hyperopia comprised only 22 % of dislocated

Table 21.2 Preoperative data of the series

N (6 eyes with dislocation after enhancement procedures)	*429*
Spherical equivalent (SE) (mean, SD)	−2.81 (3)
Cylinder (mean, SD)	−1.24 (1.2)
Myopia (%) (spherical myopia, simple and compound myopic astigmatism)	78 %
Hyperopia (%) (spherical hyperopia, simple, compound and mixed astigmatism)	22 %
Significant astigmatism (≥2D) (%) Keratometric cylinder	23.3 %
Mean K	43.7 (1.8)
BSCVA	0.9 (0.13)

Table 21.3 Functional postoperative data

	Cases $N=429$ (%)	Control $N=165$ (%)	P
Efficacy[a]	72.7	73.9	>0.05
Safety[b]	9.1	2.4	<0.01
Predictability[c] (+/− 0.5D)	73.6	88.2	<0.01
% Enhancement	9.3	3.9	<0.05

[a]Percentage of eyes with difference between postoperative uncorrected visual acuity and preoperative best-corrected visual acuity (BVCA) ≥ 0 Snellen lines
[b]Percentage of eyes with loss of ≥1 lines between preoperative and postoperative BCVAs
[c]Percentage of eyes with postoperative spherical equivalent of ±0.5 D

flap cases, and significant astigmatism (>2D) comprised 23 %. The distribution of refractive error is similar to that found in standard LASIK surgery, indicating no influence of specific refraction in the flap dislocation.

Our series had poorer postoperative outcomes compared with uneventful LASIK procedures, showing a statistically significant worse predictability, percentage of enhancement, and safety parameters despite early detection and prompt treatment (Table 21.3). The most frequent anatomic complications were epithelial ingrowth (principally peripheral and stable), different grades of haze, recurrent keratitis, dryness, and persistent striae.

What to Learn from This Case

Post-LASIK flap dislocation is an infrequent complication (0.1 % in our series). Although severe further complications can occur, they are exceptional and typically result in good anatomic and functional outcomes (77 % in our series) when promptly and appropriately managed. However, flap dislocation cases typically have a slow recovery when they involve poor flap-bed surfaces fitting and persistent microstriae, causing loss of BSCVA and poorer quality of vision.

References

1. Lichter H, Russell GE, Waring GO III (2004) Repositioning the laser in situ keratomileusis flap at the slit lamp. J Refract Surg 20(2):166–169
2. Recep OF, Cagil N, Hasipiri H (2000) Outcome of flap subluxation after laser in situ keratomileusis: results of 6 month follow-up. J Cataract Refract Surg 26(8): 1158–1162
3. Clare G, Moore TC, Grills C, Leccisotti A, Moore JE, Schallhorn S (2011) Early flap displacement after LASIK. Ophthalmology 118:1760–1765

Perforated Femtosecond Laser-Created Flap

22

David R. Hardten, and Sumitra S. Khandelwal

Contents

D.R. Hardten, MD
Department of Ophthalmology, Minnesota Eye Consultants, Minneapolis, MN, USA

Department of Ophthalmology, University of Minnesota, Minneapolis, MN, USA
e-mail: drhardten@mneye.com

S.S. Khandelwal, MD
Assistant Professor, Department of Ophthalmology, Baylor College of Medicine, Houston, TX, USA

Why Is This Case Relevant for the Refractive Surgeon?

The incidence of flap-related complications with a mechanical keratome is about 5 % and includes flap tears, buttonholes, free flaps, and decentered flaps [1]. The creation of a buttonhole does not specifically occur with the femtosecond laser; instead the laser can create a unique type of flap complication: vertical gas breakthrough. With early recognition, patients can do well despite this complication. However, if this complication is not recognized and the flap is lifted, the femtosecond flap vertical gas breakthrough may be converted into a buttonhole.

Case Background

A patient with myopia, wearing contacts approximately 12 h a day, sought refractive surgery. Due to his/her busy schedule, she desired LASIK. An eye examination revealed clear corneas except for one scratch in his/her right cornea from several years ago. The surgeon did not notice a small faint scar in his/her right eye and found his/her topography normal (Figs. 22.1 and 22.2). The patient proceeded with femtosecond-assisted LASIK. During flap creation, there was good suction. The femtosecond made its normal flap, when suddenly a small white area appeared, followed by a black area.

J.L. Alió et al. (eds.), *Difficult and Complicated Cases in Refractive Surgery*,
DOI 10.1007/978-3-642-55238-0_22, © Springer-Verlag Berlin Heidelberg 2015

The surgeon immediately took his/her foot off the pedal, confirmed vertical gas breakthrough (VGB), and did not continue with the procedure.

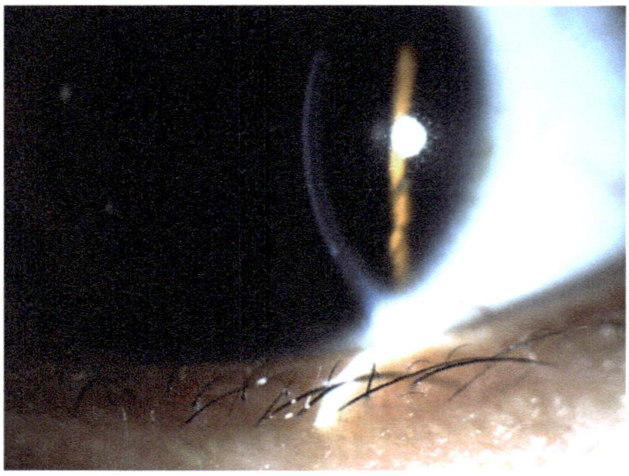

Fig. 22.1 Slit lamp photo of patient with contact lens corneal scar. Though this scar is very apparent, some patients will have very light scarring from prior erosions or subclinical breaks in Bowman's membrane. Careful history and imaging are necessary

Main Problem to Solve

Managing vertical gas breakthrough.

Ancillary Tests

If the surgeon had not noticed the VGB, he would have continued to cut the flap. Upon attempting to lift the flap, the surgeon may have noticed some resistance in that area. If he continued to lift the flap, he would likely have torn it, creating a buttonhole.

Surgical/Medical Intervention

Early recognition: If the surgeon suspects VGB, he should take his/her foot off the pedal and assess the suspicious area. Although some experts advocate lifting the new flap and recutting a flap

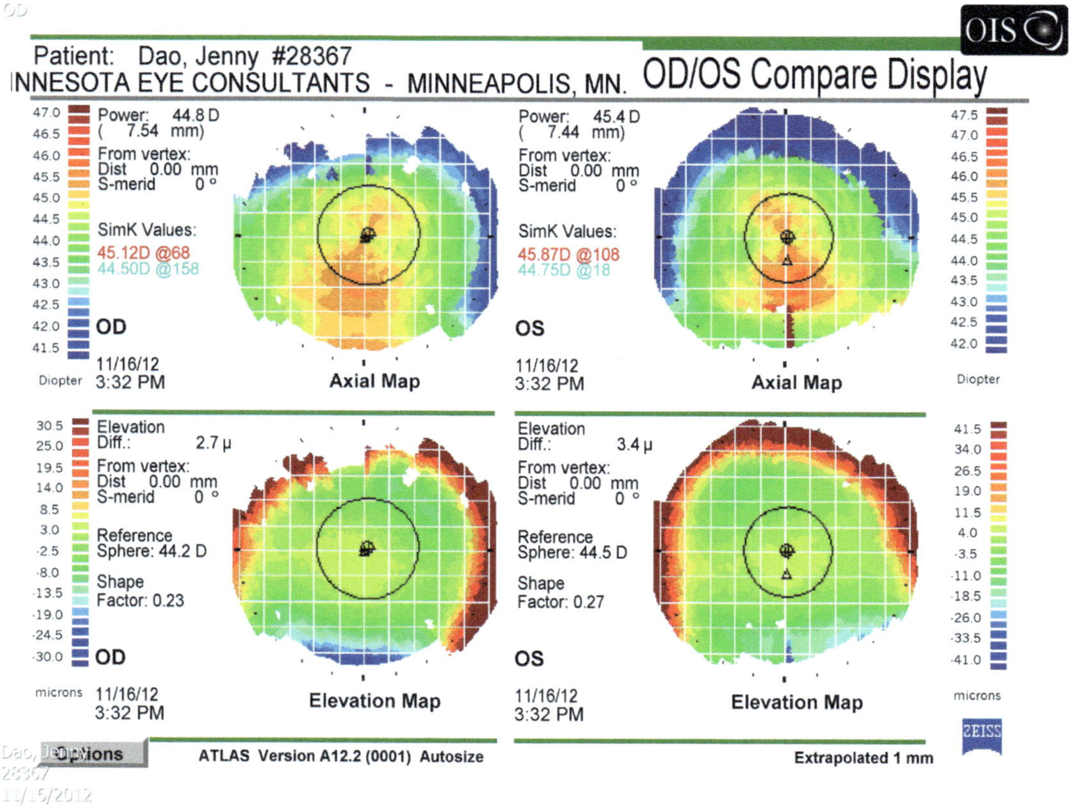

Fig. 22.2 Topography shows mild irregular astigmatism in this patient with mid-peripheral corneal scars

40–50 μm below the current attempted depth with care, our preferred approach is to change to PRK while being careful not to dislodge the edge of the vertical gas breakthrough during epithelial removal. We typically use mitomycin C with PRK in this situation. We do not attempt to lift the flap if we recognize VGB, as this would risk tearing the flap [2] (Fig. 22.3).

Late recognition: If the surgeon lifts the flap and sees the mini-buttonhole, it is best to lay down the flap and perform surface ablation at a later date. Of concern is epithelial ingrowth under the flap. In addition, MMC is typically utilized (Fig. 22.4).

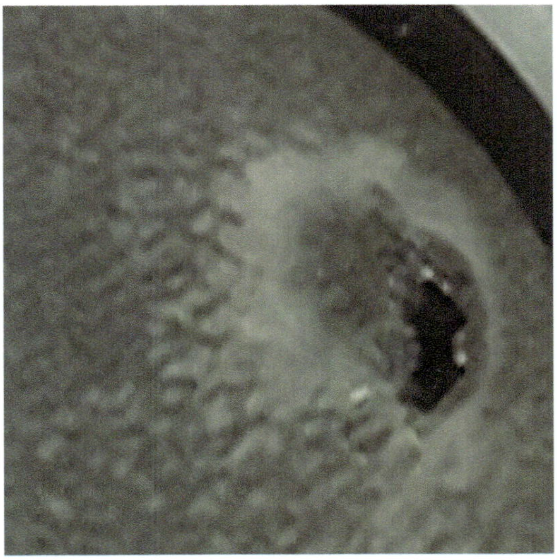

Fig. 22.3 An example of vertical gas breakthrough

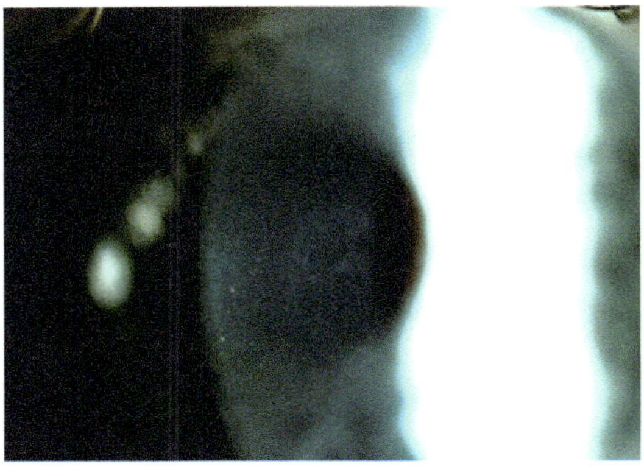

Fig. 22.4 Buttonhole flap

When performing surface ablation after a prior femtosecond flap that hasn't been lifted, surgeons have reported good success with timing that subsequent treatment immediately after the problem is noted in the flap as long as the surface is regular in the area of the ablation. Some surgeons prefer to wait 1 day to 3 months to allow the patient to adapt to the idea of a surface treatment instead of a lamellar treatment, and surgeon judgment on the timing should be exercised.

Outcome

The surgeon stopped the procedure prior to completing the flap or lifting the flap. The patient was told about the vertical gas breakthrough in the recovery area, given drops, and told to return the following day. The following day, surface ablation was performed in both eyes without complication. The patient did very well and accepted the change in surgical treatment. In this case, direct communication with the patient about the course of action and preoperative counseling were helpful in managing the patient's expectations.

What to Learn from This Case

Vertical gas breakthrough is unique to laser flap creation. Risk factors include loss of suction, a thin flap, and focal breaks in Bowman's membrane such as a scar or past trauma [3]. At times these scars can be difficult to see, so careful examination and a thorough history should be performed. A patient with a history of possible erosions in the eyes despite a normal exam may also benefit from thicker flap creation or PRK. When the surgical procedure cannot be completed in one eye, it is typically best to delay surgery in the second eye. If a minor issue occurs in the first eye which allows completion of the procedure with a good expected outcome, many surgeons will proceed with the second eye. In this case, the patient chose surface ablation in both eyes.

References

1. Gimbel HV, Penno EE, van Westenbrugge JA (1998) Incidence and management of intraoperative and early postoperative complications in 1000 consecutive laser in situ keratomileusis cases. Ophthalmology 105(10): 1839–1847
2. Srinivasan S, Herzig S (2007) Sup-epithelial gas breakthrough during the femtosecond laser flap creation for LASIK. Br J Ophthalmol 91(10):1373
3. Seider MI, Ide T, Kymionis GD, Culbertson WW, O'Brien TP, Yoo SH (2008) Epithelial breakthrough during IntraLase flap creation for laser in situ keratomileusis. J Cataract Refract Surg 34(5):859–863

Thin Flap Complications

23

Jorge L. Alió, Dominika Wróbel, and Alessandro Abbouda

Contents

J.L. Alió, MD, PhD (✉)
Department of Refractive Surgery,
Vissum Corporación Oftalmológica, Alicante, Spain
e-mail: jlalio@vissum.com

D. Wróbel, MD
Glaucoma Diagnostic and Microsurgery Department,
Medical University of Lublin, Lublin, Poland

R&D Department, Vissum Corporacion,
Alicante, Spain
e-mail: ddudzinska@interia.pl

A. Abbouda, MD
Department of Refractive Surgery,
Vissum Corporación Oftalmológica, Alicante, Spain

Department of Ophthalmology-Policlinico Umberto I
of Rome, University of Rome "Sapienza",
Viale del Policlinico, 155, 00186 Roma, Italy

R&D Department, Vissum Corporación
Oftalmológica, 03016, Alicante, Spain
e-mail: a.abbouda@gmail.com

Why Is This Case Relevant for the Refractive Surgeon?

The poor-quality flaps like thin, irregular, or buttonhole flaps occur in 0.3–2.6 % of mechanical microkeratomes LASIK procedures. The incidence with the femtosecond laser seems lower. During the creation of the corneal flap using the femtosecond IntraLASIK procedure, the flap may be cut leaving a hole in the center or mid-periphery of the flap. It is important to use caution when lifting such a flap. Clinical concerns when dealing with poor-quality flaps include the potential for epithelial cells to infiltrate the stroma, causing epithelial ingrowth in the central axis. This may result in corneal scarring in the visual field, affecting visual acuity. In addition, invasive epithelial ingrowth can lead to more severe complications such as stromal melting [1–4].

Case Background

A 37-year-old woman, who has worn contact lenses since age 16, presented for refractive surgical evaluation. Her contact lens tolerance had deteriorated over the last few months. The patient's manifest refraction was +3.75 diopters (D) in the right eye (RE) and +3.25 = −0.50×180° in the left eye (LE). Her best corrected visual acuity was 20/20 in the RE and 20/16 in the LE. The slit

J.L. Alió et al. (eds.), *Difficult and Complicated Cases in Refractive Surgery*,
DOI 10.1007/978-3-642-55238-0_23, © Springer-Verlag Berlin Heidelberg 2015

lamp and fundus examination were normal. Intraocular pressure (IOP) was 13 mmHg in the RE and 15 mmHg in the LE. The keratometry value was 42.35/43.66×69° in the RE and 42.40/43.49×79° in the LE. The keratoconus index was normal in both eyes (KPI 0 %). Her right eye pachymetry was 554 μm, and her left eye pachymetry was 557 μm.

She underwent refractive surgery, and the flap thickness was set at 100 μm for both eyes. Uneventful LASIK treatment was performed in the left eye with a temporal hinge. In the right eye, the thin flap was divided into two parts; the tear did not affect the pupil area. The flap was lifted, and corneal stromal ablation was performed. A bandage contact lens was placed. After 1 day, her uncorrected visual acuity (UCVA) was 20/50 in the RE and 20/25 in the LE. Slit lamp examination showed epithelial defect on inferior-nasal border of flap in the RE (Fig. 23.1). After 15 days, her UCVA was 20/32 in the RE and 20/20 in the LE. The slit lamp examination showed no anomalies, no epithelial defects at the flap edge, a clear interface, and a well-positioned flap on the LE. On the RE, the area of epithelial defect disappeared, but a line from the 5 h position direct to the pupil was observed, without affecting it (Fig. 23.2).

Main Problem to Solve

Usually, to prevent loss of BCVA, it is recommended to avoid the ablation procedure when the corneal flap is of poor quality. In this case we decided to proceed with the treatment because the affected zone was outside the ablation zone. Some surgeons would advise PRK laser ablation; however, this procedure may not be good for a hyperopic patient.

Ancillary Tests to Make a Decision

UCVA, BCVA, IOP, topography, and pachymetry.

Surgical/Medical Intervention

Femto-LASIK treatment was performed in both eyes. Flap creation was performed using the IntraLase FS™ CORP femtosecond laser system

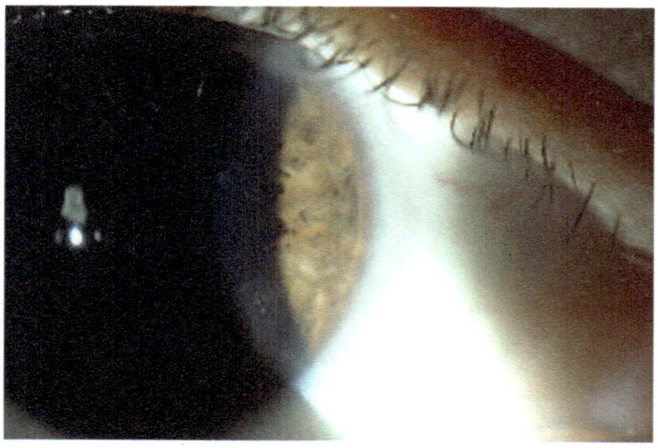

Fig. 23.1 Slit lamp examination showed: epithelial defect on inferior-nasal border of flap

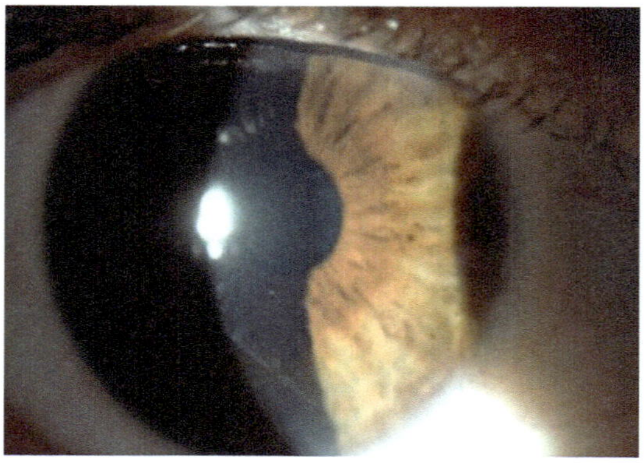

Fig. 23.2 Slit lamp examination revealed: The area of epithelial defect disappeared, but a line from the 5 h position direct to the pupil was observed, without affecting it

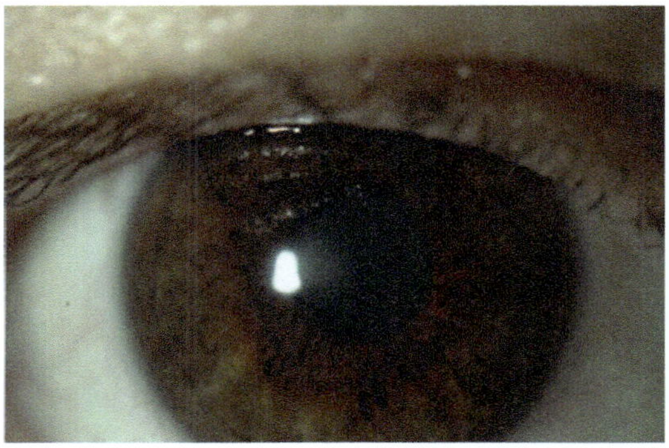

Fig. 23.3 Slit lamp examination revealed a transparent, clear cornea in both eyes, no epithelial defects at the flap edge, a clear interface, and a well-positioned flap

and corneal stromal ablation by the AMARIS SCHWIND excimer laser.

Outcome

After 6 months, UCVA was 20/20 in both eyes. Slit lamp examination revealed a transparent, clear cornea in both eyes, no epithelial defects at the flap edge, a clear interface, and a well-positioned flap (Fig. 23.3).

What to Learn from This Case

A poor-quality flap can occur with all keratomes, including the new femtosecond devices. The causes are often unclear and can be multifactorial. They may include low pressure, poor corneal lubrication, poor blade quality, preexisting corneal pathology, or a keratome malfunction. Those complications may cause delayed recovery of visual acuity as we observed in our case. Similar cases are presented in the literature with long-term loss of vision, postoperative irregular astigmatism, and epithelial defects.

References

1. Leung ATS, Rao SK, Cheng ACK (2000) Pathogenesis and management of laser in situ keratomileusis flap buttonhole. J Cataract Refract Surg 26(3):358–362
2. Sharma N, Ghate D, Agarwal T, Vajpayee RB (2005) Refractive outcomes of laser in situ keratomileusis after flap complications. J Cataract Refract Surg 31(7): 1334–1337
3. Jacobs JM, Taravella MJ (2002) Incidence of intraoperative flap complications in laser in situ keratomileusis. J Cataract Refract Surg 28(1):23–28
4. Cobo-Soriano R (2005) Thin flap laser in situ keratomileusis: analysis of contrast sensitivity, visual, and refractive outcomes. J Cataract Refract Surg 31(7):1357–1365

24 Vertical Gas Breakthrough During Femtosecond Laser Flap Creation for Laser In Situ Keratomileusis in an Eye with Previous Microkeratome Flap

Jorge L. Alió, Dominika Wróbel, and Alessandro Abbouda

Contents

Electronic supplementary material The online version of this chapter (10.1007/978-3-642-55238-0_24) contains supplementary material, which is available to authorized users.

J.L. Alió, MD, PhD (✉)
Department of Refractive Surgery, Vissum Corporación Oftalmológica, Alicante, Spain
e-mail: jlalio@vissum.com

D. Wróbel, MD
Glaucoma Diagnostic and Microsurgery Department, Medical University of Lublin, Lublin, Poland

R&D Department, Vissum Corporacion, Alicante, Spain
e-mail: ddudzinska@interia.pl

A. Abbouda, MD
Department of Refractive Surgery, Vissum Corporación Oftalmológica, Alicante, Spain

Department of Ophthalmology-Policlinico Umberto I of Rome, University of Rome "Sapienza", Viale del Policlinico, 155, 00186 Roma, Italy

R&D Department, Vissum Corporación Oftalmológica, 03016, Alicante, Spain
e-mail: a.abbouda@gmail.com

Why Is This Case Relevant for the Refractive Surgeon?

Using the femtosecond laser to create the corneal flap during laser in situ keratomileusis (LASIK) has many advantages in predictability and reliability over the microkeratome. However, each surgical procedure may have complications. One of them is vertical gas breakthrough as a result of escaping gas bubbles from the dissection plane into the subepithelial space. In this case, the cause would be related to a previous thin flap or a focal break in the Bowman's layer. The refractive surgeon should be aware that this complication can be associated with epithelial down growth, corneal scar, and microstriae. A decrease of best corrected visual acuity (BCVA) may occur if the pupillary area is involved [1–4].

Case Background

A 29-year-old man had a LASIK procedure 8 years ago. An unsatisfied patient, with the result of previous refractive surgery, appeared in our clinic to correct a residual refractive error. The manifest refraction (MR) was +3.25 −3.25 × 10° in the right eye (RE) and +2.75 −1.75 × 160° in the left eye (LE). The uncorrected visual acuity (UCVA) was 20/63 in the RE and 20/40 in the LE. The best corrected visual acuity (BCVA) was 20/20 in both eyes. The corneal pachymetry was 518 μm in RE and 527 μm in the LE. The corneal

J.L. Alió et al. (eds.), *Difficult and Complicated Cases in Refractive Surgery*, DOI 10.1007/978-3-642-55238-0_24, © Springer-Verlag Berlin Heidelberg 2015

topography values were 41.93/44.83 × 101° in the RE and 42.21/44.69 × 73° in the LE. An IntraLase treatment was performed. Tobramycin/dexamethasone (Tobradex® Alcon) six times a day for both eyes was prescribed.

Main Problem to Solve

In this case, it is important to consider two important questions: (1) What is better to use femtosecond laser or mechanical microkeratome to create the flap in patient with previous LASIK procedure? (2) What should be the safe distance between the new flap and previous one? What to do in case of vertical gas breakthrough?

Ancillary Tests to Make a Decision

UCVA, BCVA, IOP, pupillometry, topography, and pachymetry.

Surgical/Medical Intervention

The flap creation was performed using the IntraLase FS™ CORP femtosecond laser system, and the corneal stromal ablation was performed with the AMARIS SCHWIND excimer laser.

The IntraLase flap thickness parameter was set at 150 μm for both eyes because of the previous LASIK procedure. The residual stroma was 359 μm in the RE and 345 μm in the LE. In both eyes, during the flap creation, the vertical bubbles breakthrough was observed between the previous flaps and new ones. Nevertheless, the flap creation step was completed; the bubbles did not perforate the previous flaps. The flaps were then lifted gently without creating a buttonhole. The excimer ablation procedure was performed (Video 24.1).

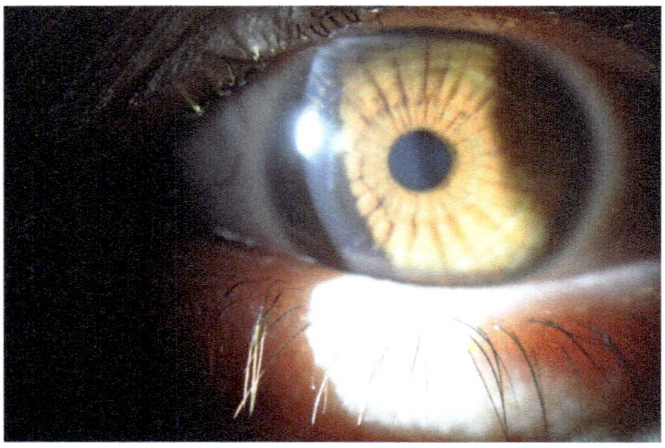

Fig. 24.1 Slit lamp examination after 10 days of procedure showed a vertical epithelial line in the nasal side

Outcome

After 15 days of surgery, the uncorrected visual acuity (UCVA) was 20/20 in the RE and 20/25 in the LE. The corneal topography values were 44.42/45.79 × 107° in the RE and 43.94/45.24 × 73° in the LE. The slit lamp examination showed small epithelial linear opacities in the area of the vertical gas breakthrough (Fig. 24.1). The OCT Visante was performed. The examination showed a two list flap lines in both eyes (Fig. 24.2a, b).

What to Learn from This Case

Predisposing factors and methods for avoiding a gas bubble breakthrough remain unknown. Even though we came across the complication during the flap creation, the gas bubble breakthrough in this case was possible to follow the ablation procedure. It is very important to lift the flap very cautiously and not make a buttonhole. A long follow-up is needed to examine the long-term effect of this phenomenon during femtosecond IntraLASIK.

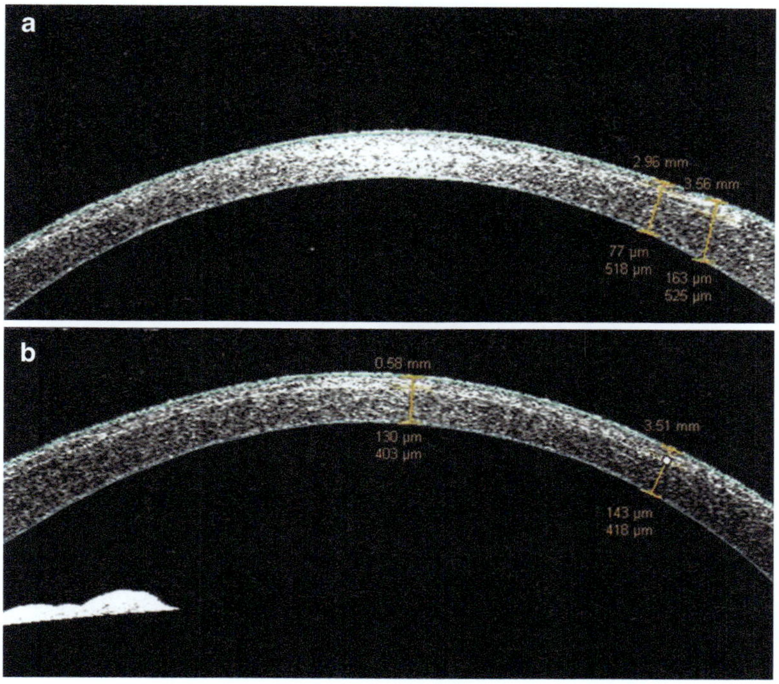

Fig. 24.2 OCT Visante in both eyes (**a**, **b**) showed two hyper reflective lines of the previous flap

References

1. Durrie DS, Kezirian GM (2005) Femtosecond laser versus mechanical keratome flaps in wavefront-guided laser in situ keratomileusis; prospective contralateral eye study. J Cataract Refract Surg 31(1):120–126
2. Kezirian GM, Stonecipher KG (2004) Comparison of the IntraLase femtosecond laser and mechanical keratomes for laser in situ keratomileusis. J Cataract Refract Surg 30:804–811
3. Srinivasan S, Herzig S (2007) Sub-epithelial gas breakthrough during femtosecond laser flap creation for LASIK. Br J Ophthalmol 91:1373
4. Seider MI (2008) Epithelial breakthrough during IntraLase flap creation for laser in situ keratomileusis. J Cataract Refract Surg 34:8 59–863

Intraoperative Complications: Free Cap in Femtosecond LASIK

25

Samir Melki

Contents

Why This Case Is Relevant for the Refractive Surgeon?

A free flap or a cap is a rare but significant complication that can occur with femtosecond LASIK [1]. This can happen during flap manipulation rather than during flap creation as seen with the microkeratome. Following the creation of the corneal flap, the flap can be inadvertently severed from the hinge in the process of lifting, positioning, and refloating. Some of the potential complications include irregular astigmatism, recurrent flap dislodgement, and complete flap loss.

Background of the Case

A 45-year-old woman with no prior ocular history presented for LASIK evaluation. All appropriate testing revealed that she would be an adequate candidate for LASIK for the treatment of myopia and astigmatism.

Corneal flaps were created using the standard protocol at a requested thickness of 90 μm. Radial gentian violet marks were applied using an optical zone marker at the intersection of the flap edge and corneal bed.

S. Melki, MD, PhD
Department of Refractive Surgery, Massachusetts Eye and Ear Infirmary, Harvard Medical School, Boston, MA, USA
e-mail: samir_melki@meei.harvard.edu

Electronic supplementary material The online version of this chapter (10.1007/978-3-642-55238-0_25) contains supplementary material, which is available to authorized users.

J.L. Alió et al. (eds.), *Difficult and Complicated Cases in Refractive Surgery*, DOI 10.1007/978-3-642-55238-0_25, © Springer-Verlag Berlin Heidelberg 2015

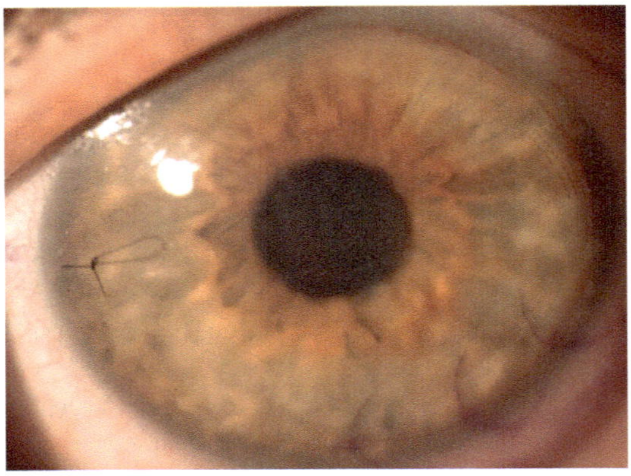

Fig. 25.1 Slit lamp photo of the right eye: free flap secured in place with a single anchoring 10-0 nylon suture. Fiduciary markings are visible confirming adequate alignment. Bandage contact lens (BCL) is in place

The flap was carefully lifted, and excimer laser ablation was applied. In the process of repositioning the flap back onto the ablated corneal bed, its tight adherence to the lid speculum resulted in a full-thickness detachment of the flap from its superior hinge.

Main Problem to Solve

A free flap detached from its superior hinge, which needs to be repositioned in proper orientation and secured in place.

Ancillary Tests to Make a Decision

None.

Surgical/Medical Intervention

The free flap was repositioned using the fiduciary markings. A single 10-0 nylon suture was placed at 9 o'clock position with an air knot to minimize any torque, irregular astigmatism, or decentration tension. A bandage contact lens was placed (Fig. 25.1).

Outcome

On the first postoperative day, the free flap was in good position. The 10-0 nylon suture was removed at the slit lamp without any complications. The flap remained clear and in position throughout the remainder of the postoperative course. Final refraction of −2.50 sphere was achieved, consistent with desired monovision aim in the involved eye.

What to Learn from This Case

The free flap in this case resulted from tight adherence of the flap to the lid speculum. This was thought to be a result of relatively longer excimer laser treatment time from anterior chamber bubbles hindering the tracker's ability to recognize the pupillary contour. Pre-placed fiduciary markings were crucial in allowing for proper positioning with significant visual aberrations. Free flap was secured with a single loose anchoring suture, which had not been reported previously. Traditional methods for securing free flaps include air drying, patching, bandage contact lens, and running or interrupted sutures. A loose anchoring suture avoids the possible complications of the traditional methods such as flap loss or asymmetric torque with irregular astigmatism while providing a fail-safe method for managing a free flap.

Reference

1. Choi CJ, Melki SA (2012) Loose anchoring suture to secure a free flap after laser in situ keratomileusis. J Cataract Refract Surg 38:1127–1129

Limitations of Reorientation of a LASIK Free Cap

26

Samuel H. Lee and Dimitri T. Azar

Contents

S.H. Lee, MD (✉) • D.T. Azar, MD, MBA
Department of Ophthalmology and Visual Sciences
Illinois Eye and Ear Infirmary, University of Illinois at Chicago, Chicago, IL, USA
e-mail: samuel.lee.md@gmail.com; dazar@uic.edu

Why Is This Case Relevant for the Refractive Surgeon?

Refractive surgeons performing LASIK should be aware of the importance of the proper orientation and management of a free cap during flap creation. Although increased use of the femtosecond laser has decreased the incidence of free cap formation, knowledge of its management is important.

Case Background

A 38-year-old female was referred to our institution for possible management of a free cap, which occurred during LASIK surgery. She underwent bilateral LASIK 12 years ago with her local surgeon. Her left eye surgery was uneventful, but her right eye had a free cap during flap creation with a mechanical microkeratome. The cap was placed aside, and the procedure was completed. There were no marks to help align and position the cap. The surgeon replaced the cap and placed a bandage lens placed over it. The next day, the cap was found to be displaced nasally and was refloated and repositioned without the ability to determine the correct orientation of the cap. The patient was referred to another surgeon, who recommended refloating the flap and stretching it, as there were significant striae. After refloating and stretching of the flap, the patient had persistent striae, and her best corrected visual acuity was in

J.L. Alió et al. (eds.), *Difficult and Complicated Cases in Refractive Surgery*,
DOI 10.1007/978-3-642-55238-0_26, © Springer-Verlag Berlin Heidelberg 2015

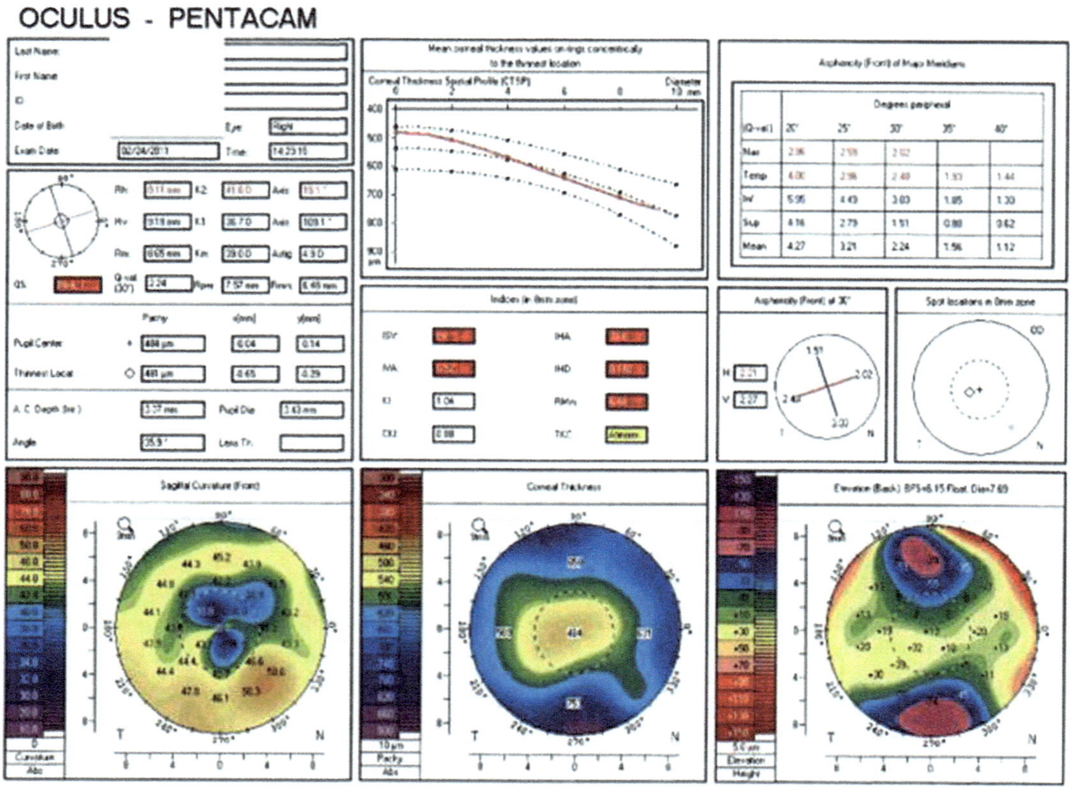

Fig. 26.1 Pentacam image of right eye

the 20/60 range. The patient was referred to another surgeon, who confirmed that the orientation of the cap was incorrect. He recommended refloating the cap, rotating the cap by 90° and suturing the cap in place. This helped with her flap striae, but did not improve her vision. There were still questions regarding the correct orientation of her cap and the potential benefits of reorientation of the cap.

Main Problem to Solve

There are a number of issues that are relevant to this case. The first problem is that no markings were used prior to flap creation. The second problem is that the surgeon went ahead with the treatment under the free cap. It would have been better not to remove the cap in the first place to avoid problems as the cap was perfectly circular, but its thickness was not uniform. The third problem that the surgeon operated on the right eye first had a complication and proceeded with the left eye. Fortunately the patient did not have a complication in the left eye. The question of whether or not to treat the eye under a free cap must be addressed, as a free cap is not uniform in width or thickness. An irregularly shaped flap would be easier to reposition than an oval or a round free cap [1–3].

Ancillary Tests

We wanted to use the depth of the stromal bed and compare it to the thickness of the flap at various medians. This would theoretically help us determine the best reorientation of the cap. However, 12 years had passed since the surgery, so we had very low expectations of success. Topography was obtained using a Pentacam, and anterior segment OCT was obtained using an Optovue FD-OCT anterior segment module (Figs. 26.1, 26.2, and 26.3).

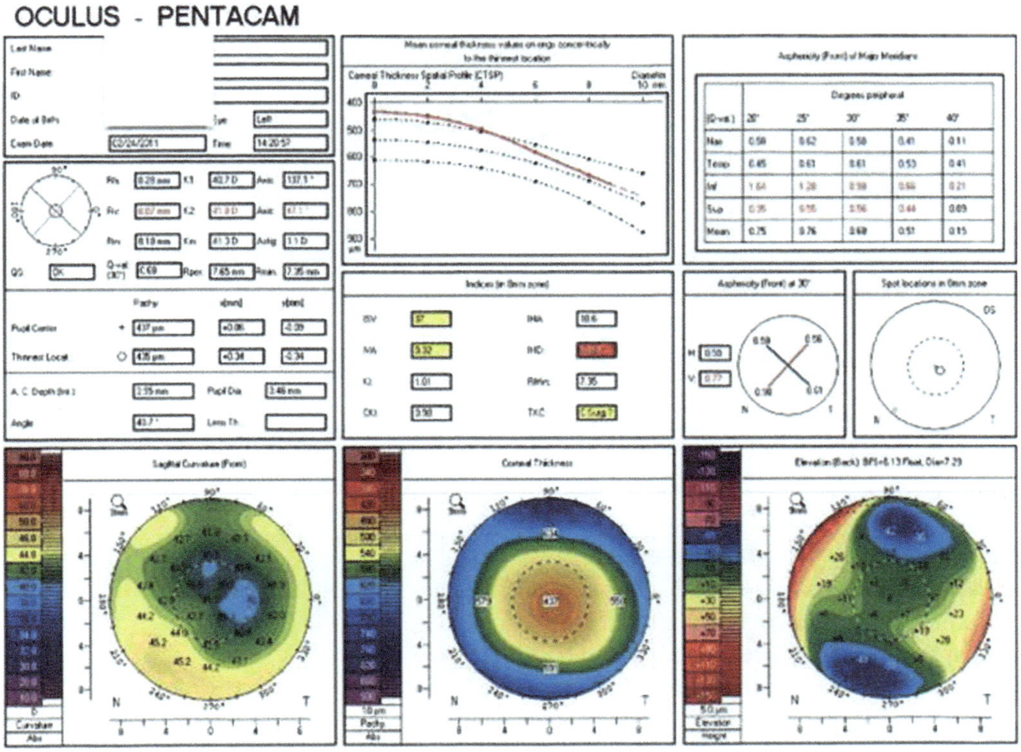

Fig. 26.2 Pentacam image of left eye

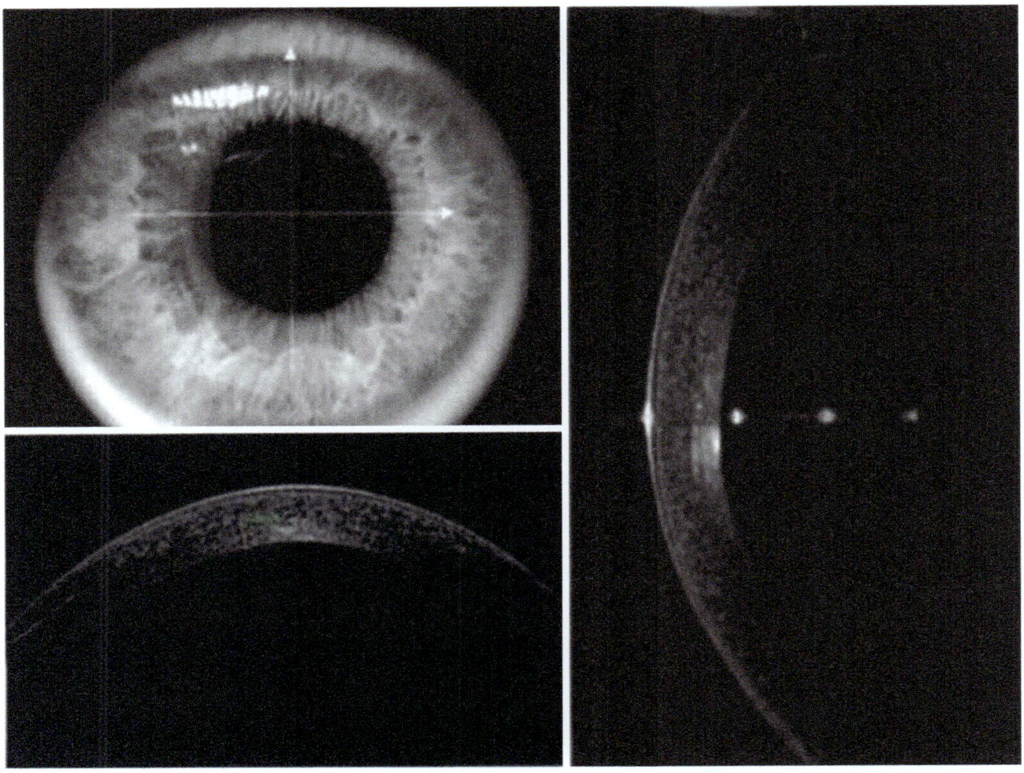

Fig. 26.3 Anterior segment OCT of right eye demonstrating a treated free cap 12 years after original surgery

Surgical/Medical Intervention

Anterior segment OCT was obtained at 16 meridians, and measurements were taken of the cap and underlying stroma at all meridians to see if there were any patterns for realignment. Treatment was discussed with the patient, with the option to use the femtosecond laser to create the inner side cut with rotation of the free cap for proper orientation versus wavefront-guided surface ablation. After risks, benefits, and alternatives were discussed with the patient, she decided to continue in her rigid gas permeable contact lens, as she had been for the last 11 years.

What to Learn from This Case

Key learning points from this case are to mark the flap each time, no matter how routine refractive surgery may become. The second point is to avoid treating the underlying stroma if there are intraoperative flap complications. A third point is that even though a free cap can be treated properly, proper alignment is imperative, making a circular free cap more difficult to treat than an irregularly shaped free cap.

References

1. Azar DT, Koch DD (2003) LASIK: fundamentals, surgical techniques, and complications. Marcel Dekker, Inc., New York/Basel
2. Utz VM, Krueger RR (2008) Management of irregular astigmatism following rotationally disoriented free cap after LASIK. J Refract Surg 24:383–391
3. Hovanesian JA, Maloney RK (2005) Treating astigmatism after a free laser in situ keratomileusis cap by rotating the cap. J Cataract Refract Surg 31: 1870–1876

Flap Lost

27

Jorge L. Alió and Alessandro Abbouda

Contents

J.L. Alió, MD, PhD (✉)
Department of Refractive Surgery,
Vissum Corporación Oftalmológica,
Alicante, Spain
e-mail: jlalio@vissum.com

A. Abbouda, MD
Department of Refractive Surgery,
Vissum Corporación Oftalmológica, Alicante, Spain

Department of Ophthalmology-Policlinico Umberto I of Rome, University of Rome "Sapienza",
Viale del Policlinico, 155, 00186 Roma, Italy

R&D Department, Vissum Corporación Oftalmológica, 03016, Alicante, Spain
e-mail: a.abbouda@gmail.com

Why Is This Case Relevant for the Refractive Surgeon?

Refractive surgeons should be able to manage flap loss and restore visual acuity with an adequate refractive outcome. Considering less aggressive treatment is important.

Case Background

The patient came to our center 3 days after refractive surgery with the diagnosis of flap loss. The patient had undergone FM laser treatment in his/her right eye (RE), and during surgery, a free flap occurred. The preoperative refraction was $-0.75 = -0.25 \times 5$. A bandage contact lens was applied and removed the day after surgery. The flap was lost the day after surgery. The patient was treated with a soft bandage contact lens for the abrasion, moxifloxacin hydrochloride ophthalmic solution (Vigamox; Alcon Laboratories Inc., Ft Worth, Texas) three times daily, and cyclopegic ophthalmic solution four times daily. The first visit to our clinic, the patient's visual acuity in the RE was finger counting. Slit lamp examination revealed diffused corneal edema. The ultrasound pachymetry was 730 μm. The topography showed an irregular profile (Fig. 27.1a), and the OCT Visante showed a high stromal thickness (Fig. 27.2).

J.L. Alió et al. (eds.), *Difficult and Complicated Cases in Refractive Surgery*,
DOI 10.1007/978-3-642-55238-0_27, © Springer-Verlag Berlin Heidelberg 2015

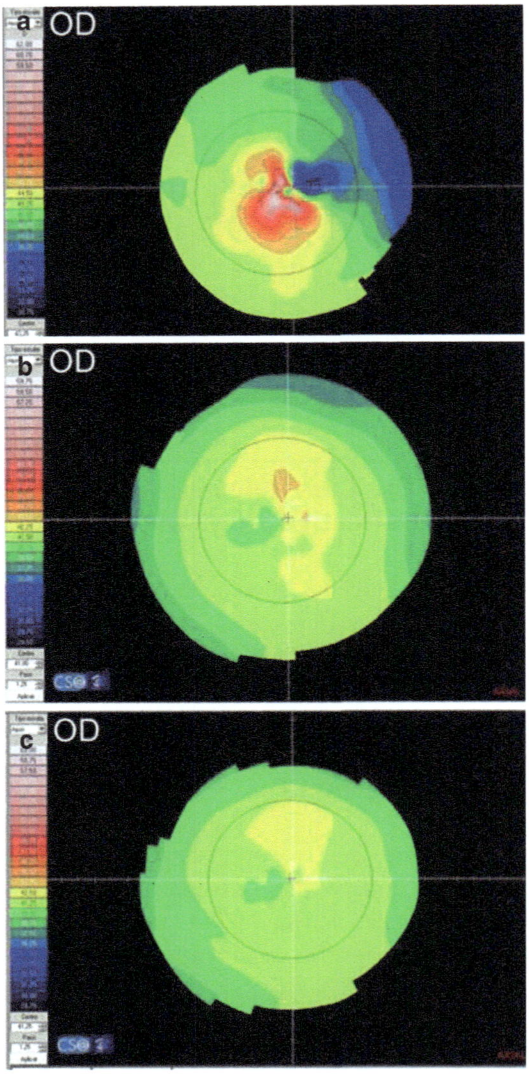

Fig. 27.1 Anterior corneal topography (**a**) at first visit, (**b**)1.5 month after treatment, (**c**) 1 year after treatment

Main Problem to Solve

Flap loss and resultant inflammation put the patient at risk for significant haze. Some authors [1] are proponents of performing anterior lamellar keratoplasty in cases of flap loss or flap removal. However, these procedures create risks of suturing and induced refractive error [2].

Ancillary Tests

What is the best way to improve the patient's significantly without further refractive surgery? Refraction, BCVA, topography, corneal aberrometry, pachymetry, and long follow-up are fundamental in this case. Also important are good communication and coaching with the patient. The flap was set to 110 μm, the epithelium about 50 more or less, and the stromal loss to 70. Even with significant stromal loss, this case demonstrated the epithelium's ability to regenerate itself and restore a good surface.

Surgical/Medical Intervention

The patient was treated with dexamethasone, one drop four times per day for 1 week, tapering to one drop each week, and cyclopentolate, one drop three times per day for 1 week. After the first month, the patient started fluorometholone 2 % (FML Forte Allergan) one drop three times per day tapering to one drop each week. At

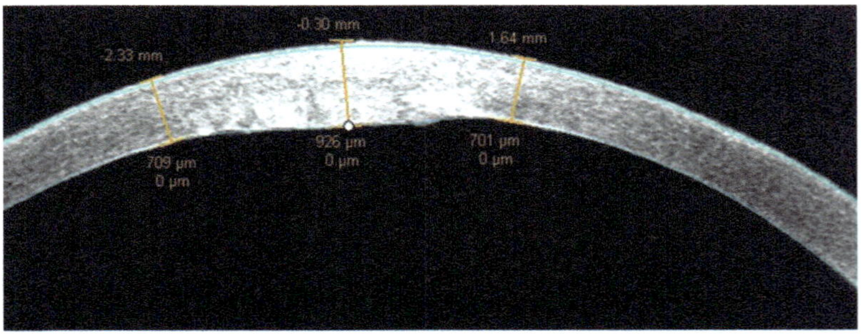

Fig. 27.2 OCT Visante at the first visit showed diffuse corneal edema

2 months, we decided to apply a SynergEyes® contact lens (contact lens characteristics: base curve 7.9; superior curvature 8.9; power −1.5; diameter 14.5). This lens combines two types of contact lens materials, a rigid gas permeable center and a soft hydrophilic outer skirt, into one unique "hybrid" lens.

Outcome

After 1.5 months, the patient's visual acuity was 20/50 with a refraction of +0.75 = −1 × 180. The slit lamp examination showed tender haze. The topography showed an irregular profile (Fig. 27.1b). The patient started to wear the contact lens, with a visual acuity of 20/20 after 1 year. The slit lamp showed a clear cornea (Fig. 27.3). The topography evidenced a superior steeping according to the use of the contact lens.

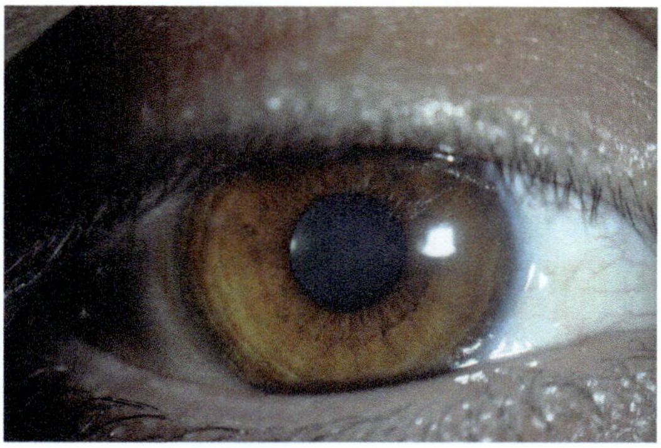

Fig. 27.3 Slit lamp examination at the end of follow-up showed a clear cornea

What to Learn from This Case

This case shows that excellent visual results can be obtained following flop loss without further procedures. The long-term outlook for this patient appears favorable, as he/she shows a stable 20/20 uncorrected vision in the RE with good topography and minimal aberrations. The most important thing is to follow the healing time to prevent haze formation. We advised the patient to wait for the follow-up before pursuing a more aggressive treatment.

References

1. Eggink FA, Eggink CA, Beekhuis WH (2002) Postoperative management and follow-up after corneal flap loss following laser in situ keratomileusis. J Cataract Refract Surg 28:175–179
2. Motwani M, Lizano GJ, Yam K, English C (2011) Photorefractive keratectomy after late traumatic LASIK flap loss. J Refract Surg 27:542–544

28 Decentered Flap in Hyperopic IntraLASIK: Sometimes to Delay Is to Succeed

Jorge L. Alió, Alessandro Abbouda, and Angelo Rampone

Contents

Why Is This Case Relevant for the Refractive Surgeon?

A decentered flap is a complication that occurs during the LASIK procedure which can affect the visual and refractive outcome, causing the loss of best corrected visual acuity (BCVA).

Prompt management of this situation is necessary to achieve the best visual outcome.

Case Background

A 33-year-old man with no previous ocular history presented for refractive surgery evaluation. His manifest refraction was +4.0, −1.25 × 90° in the right eye (RE) and +3.50, −0.75 × 65° in the left eye (LE). Keratometry readings were 42.76/43.21 × 169° in the RE and 42.78/42.48 × 90° in the LE. His BCVA was 20/20 in both eyes. Both slit lamp and fundus examinations were normal. According to the topography, his cornea surface was regular. RE pachymetry was 499 μm, and his LE pachymetry was 498 μm.

LASIK procedure was chosen. On the day of the surgery, the patient appeared troubled. During

Electronic supplementary material The online version of this chapter (10.1007/978-3-642-55238-0_28) contains supplementary material, which is available to authorized users.

J.L. Alió, MD, PhD (✉)
Department of Refractive Surgery, Vissum Corporación Oftalmológica, Alicante, Spain
e-mail: jlalio@vissum.com

A. Abbouda, MD
Department of Refractive Surgery, Vissum Corporación Oftalmológica, Alicante, Spain

Department of Ophthalmology-Policlinico Umberto I of Rome, University of Rome “Sapienza”, Viale del Policlinico, 155, 00186, Roma, Italy

R&D Department, Vissum Corporación Oftalmológica, 03016, Alicante, Spain
e-mail: a.abbouda@gmail.com

A. Rampone, MD
Department of Ophthalmology, Seconda Università degli Studi di Napoli, Naples, Italy

R&D Department, Vissum Corporacion, Alicante 03016, Alicante, Spain
e-mail: angelo.rampone@gmail.com

J.L. Alió et al. (eds.), *Difficult and Complicated Cases in Refractive Surgery*, DOI 10.1007/978-3-642-55238-0_28, © Springer-Verlag Berlin Heidelberg 2015

the femtosecond procedure, the patient was uncooperative, and a decentered flap was created in the RE.

Main Problem to Solve

In hyperopic IntraLASIK, a centered flap is very important because the excimer laser treatment must be applied in a peripheral area. In the case of a decentered flap, the refractive surgeon has two choices: (a) abort the procedure and repeat after 1 week creating a deeper flap or (b), if the ablation zone is near the flap edge, continue the procedure and apply a contact lens.

We chose the first option in this case.

Ancillary Test

The planning treatment predicted an ablation zone of 8.23 mm and a transition zone of 1.53 mm. The flap parameters were set to 9.2 mm diameter, but it was decentered on the nasal side. Based on this consideration, we decided to put off the treatment, and pachymetry was repeated to confirm the value.

Surgical/Medical Intervention

The patient was premedicated with a benzodiazepine. The planning of the second procedure provided a flap depth of 180 μm. The femtosecond procedure was uneventful.

Outcome

One week after LASIK, the patient's manifest refraction was −0.75, −0.50 × 180° in the RE. His BCVA was 20/22, and the slit lamp examination was normal.

What to Learn from This Case

Appropriate flap centration is crucial for the success of LASIK. Creating a flap with the largest possible diameter is necessary to create a bed sufficient for excimer laser treatment [1].

Patient and surgeon factors can also influence flap creation. Head position, ring position, and applanation can all influence the procedure. The femtolaser computer can make small adjustments in flap centration when suction is used to permit small realignment [2]. An important caution with hyperopic patients is avoiding performing an ablation if the flap is not well centered.

References

1. Salomão MQ, Wilson SE (2010) Femtosecond laser in laser in situ keratomileusis. J Cataract Refract Surg 36:1024–1032
2. Ertan A, Karacal H (2008) Factors influencing flap and INTACS decentration after femtosecond laser application in normal and keratoconic eyes. J Refract Surg 24:797–801

Suction Break During Raster Pattern and Before Side Cut

29

James J. Salz

Contents

J.J. Salz, MD
Department of Ophthalmology,
Keck School of Medicine,
University of Southern California,
Los Angeles, CA, USA

Laser Vision Medical Group, Los Angeles, CA, USA
e-mail: drjjsalz@gmail.com

Why Is This Case Important?

In a large study by Haft et al. of 4,772 eyes, only 3 (0.06 %) eyes had incomplete flaps due to suction loss [1]. By far the most common type of suction loss during femtosecond flap creation occurs during the raster pattern, either early (Fig. 29.1) or late but before the side cut is initiated. When suction loss occurs during a mechanical microkeratome LASIK procedure, the procedure should be terminated if the instrument actually started to cut the flap. Attempting to perform a recutting of the flap is not advisable since the same plane of dissection will not be attained.

Case Background

This case was the initial femtosecond flap for an experienced microkeratome surgeon who had performed over 1,000 LASIK procedures. The patient was a 34-year-old, cooperative male patient with normal-sized corneas and normal eyelid and orbital anatomy. I was acting as the proctor for this case. The surgeon had completed the AMO IntraLase training and had properly prepared the patient for the procedure. The intended flap parameters were 120 μm depth with a 9.0 mm optical zone diameter side cut angle of 70° and superior hinge angle of 55°. We were using the AMO iFS laser, and suction was obtained with a full applanation as evidenced by the meniscus to the periphery of the lens. The

J.L. Alió et al. (eds.), *Difficult and Complicated Cases in Refractive Surgery*,
DOI 10.1007/978-3-642-55238-0_29, © Springer-Verlag Berlin Heidelberg 2015

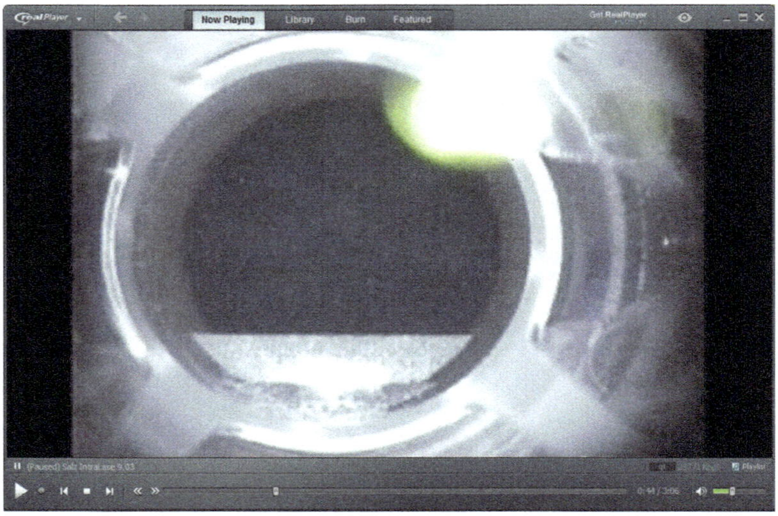

Fig. 29.1 Partial raster pattern with superior hinge and pocket

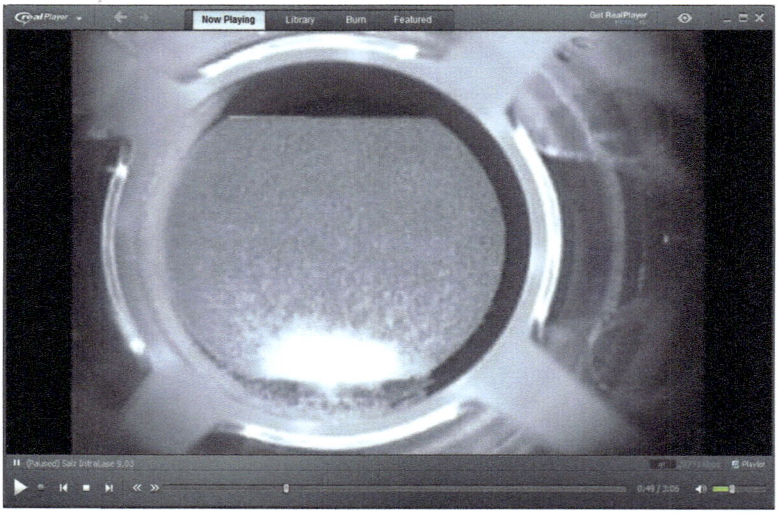

Fig. 29.2 Almost complete raster pattern with superior hinge (simulated not actual case)

suction loss occurred when the patient appeared to squeeze the lids near the completion of the raster pattern. (Figure 29.2 simulated photo since we did not have video of the actual procedure).

Main Problem to Solve

The problem to solve was to safely complete the flap while the raster pattern was still visible on the cornea. The situation was quickly explained to the patient who was told that this happens at times and is not a cause for concern in an effort to relax him before reapplying the suction ring.

Ancillary Tests

My normal technique for lifting a flap is to identify and open the side cut for about 1 clock hour on each side near the superior hinge with the small tip of a Seibel flap lifter (Fig. 29.3), then introduce the full Seibel rounded spatula across the flap near the hinge (Fig. 29.4), and pass it first toward the hinge and then inferiorly to the periphery in one sweep if there is little resistance and in two or three sweeps if the flap seems to be adherent. I change this technique in a case like this where there is a chance that the original raster pattern and the second raster pattern may not be

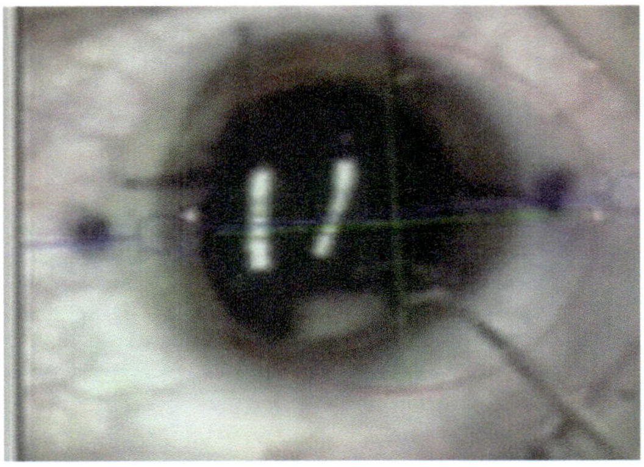

Fig. 29.3 Seibel flap lifter, short end, entering side cut near superior hinge

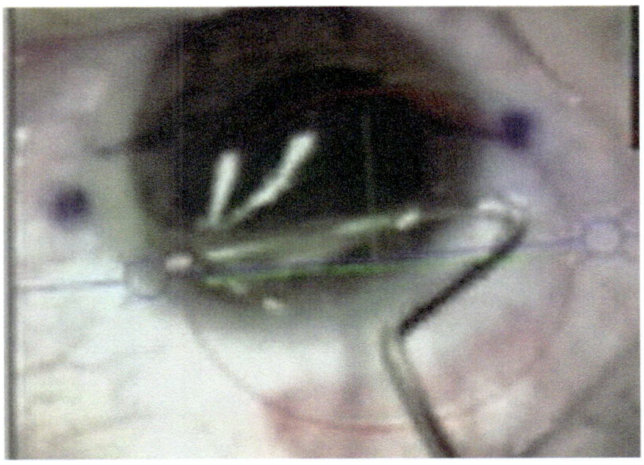

Fig. 29.4 Seibel flap lifter, long spatula end, lifting flap near superior hinge

at exactly the same level. In this case, the lower portion of the flap is elevated first by introducing the small tip of the Seibel flap lifter near the inferior edge of the side cut and opening it for one clock hour on each side. Since the lower edge of the flap has only had one pass of the raster pattern, entering and lifting from this point and then moving the spatula edge of the Seibel from inferior toward the superior hinge assures that you are lifting the flap in the correct plane and results in a smooth bed.

Surgical/Medical Intervention

We applied another drop of anesthetic and reminded the patient to try to keep his other eye open without squeezing during the 15 s it would take to complete the flap. The same suction ring and cone was applied, suction was obtained with good applanation, and the exact same settings for depth and diameter were used. The technician centered the flap outline on the screen to overlap the edge of the bubbles which were still clearly visible. Figure 29.5 is from the AMO teaching library and shows the application of the suction ring and the appearance of the bubbles on an eye with a nasally hinged flap. The raster pattern and side cut were accomplished without difficulty. The flap on the second eye was performed without incident.

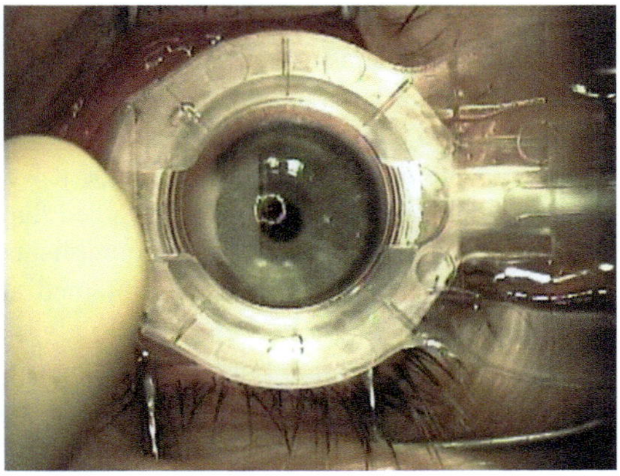

Fig. 29.5 Reapplication of suction ring, bubbles visible in case with nasal hinge and pocket (Courtesy of AMO from teaching library)

Outcome

Inspection of the flap at the slit lamp revealed a normal appearance with a complete raster pattern and what appeared to be a complete side cut.

What to Learn from This Case

What we have learned from this case is that suction loss during the raster pattern can be effectively treated immediately. When this happens before the raster pattern is completed, quickly apply the same suction ring, use the same cone, use the same femtosecond laser settings, align the template of the hinge pattern with the visible bubbles representing the raster pattern, and repeat a full raster pattern. Modify your flap-lifting technique to first lift the portion of the flap which was created with only one portion of the raster pattern. In this case it was the inferior edge of this superiorly hinged flap. The flap lift in this case was accomplished without difficulty and the patient obtained an excellent result in both eyes. In a study by Tomita et al. they found: "In patients requiring a second or third lamellar flap cut immediately after suction loss, 97.2 % of eyes achieved uncorrected distance visual acuity of 0.00 logMAR (20/20) or better and 100 % of eyes achieved corrected distance visual acuity of 0.00 logMAR (20/20) or better at most recent follow-up" [1]. In cases where suction cannot be obtained, PRK at a later date can usually be performed with good results [2].

References

1. Haft P, Yoo SH, Kymionis GD, Ide T, O'Brien TP, Culbertson WW (2009) Complications of LASIK flaps made by the IntraLase 15- and 30-kHz femtosecond lasers. J Refract Surg 25:979–984
2. Tomita M, Watabe M, Nakamura T, Nakamura N, Tsuru T, Waring GO IV (2012) Management and outcomes of suction loss during LASIK flap creation with a femtosecond laser. J Refract Surg 28:32–36

Suction Break After Complete Raster Pattern and Incomplete Side Cut

30

James J. Salz

Contents

J.J. Salz, MD
Department of Ophthalmology, Keck School of Medicine, University of Southern California, Los Angeles, CA, USA

Laser Vision Medical Group, Los Angeles, CA, USA
e-mail: drjjsalz@gmail.com

Why Is This Case Relevant for the Refractive Surgeon?

It can be difficult to determine if the side cut is complete when suction is lost before the complete side cut. It is also important to be certain you are lifting the flap at the correct interface. This chapter addresses both of these issues.

Case Background

This was my patient, a 32-year-old female patient's right eye, −.8.50 −0.75 × 165 = 20/20. She had successful IntraLASIK (IntraLase) and Allegretto WaveLight in her left with uncorrected vision of 20/20 several months ago and deferred surgery in the right eye for financial reasons. She is an Asian patient but had normal eyelid anatomy, corneal diameter, and pachymetry of 610 μm and was not apprehensive since this was her second eye. The settings for the iFS Laser were 120 μm depth, 8.85 mm diameter, side cut angle 70°, and hinge angle 55° with pocket on. Suction was obtained without difficulty with full applanation to the periphery. After a complete raster pattern and about 3 s of the side cut, suction was lost and the procedure terminated. The view through the video monitor of the iFS showed the outline

J.L. Alió et al. (eds.), *Difficult and Complicated Cases in Refractive Surgery*,
DOI 10.1007/978-3-642-55238-0_30, © Springer-Verlag Berlin Heidelberg 2015

of a compete side cut, but we were uncertain of the depth. The bubbles were still clearly visible.

Main Problem to Solve

The surgeon must be sure the side cut is completely through the epithelium and that the flap is lifted at the correct interface.

Ancillary Tests to Make a Decision

I elected to quickly perform a slit lamp examination. It was clear that the depth of the side cut was incomplete. This can be confirmed by looking at the glass applanation lens which would show either no etching of the glass or only partial etching. If the side cut is compete, the glass will show a complete side cut indicating that the laser has cut through the epithelium into the glass (Fig. 30.1).

Surgical/Medical Intervention

The patient was immediately positioned beneath the iFS laser which was programmed for side cut only with a diameter of 8.35 mm, depth of 130 μm. Suction was obtained, centration of the side cut was accomplished with the reticule aligned with the still visible bubbles, and the side cut was completed inside the incomplete side cut. The flap lift was initiated by inserting the Seibel short end into the inside side cut near the hinge and opening it for about 2'clock hours. The long end of the Seibel was then inserted, and the flap lifted easily with only one inferior sweep. The bed looked smooth, and the procedure was completed without difficulty.

Outcome

The patient obtained 20/20 uncorrected visual acuity. Slit lamp exam looks normal, and it is difficult to visualize the outer incomplete side cut (Fig. 30.2).

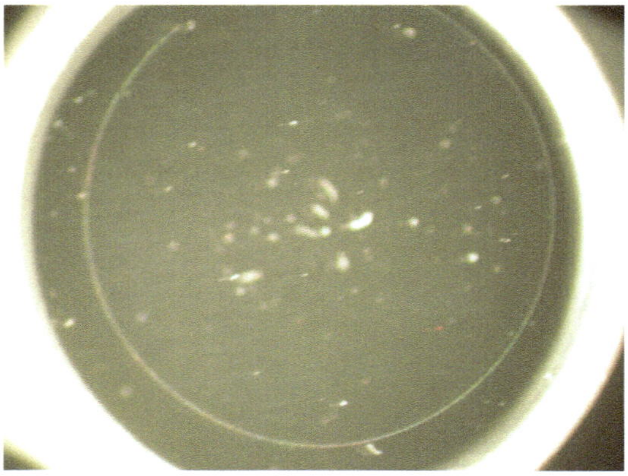

Fig. 30.1 Glass applanation lens showing a complete side cut pattern

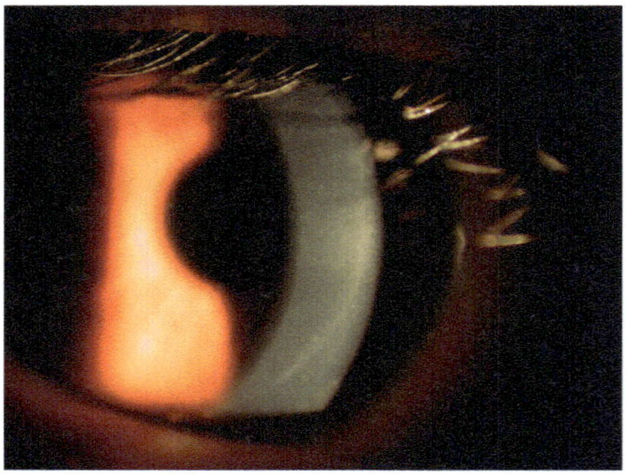

Fig. 30.2 Slit lamp photograph of Case 2 showing edge of second side cut

What to Learn from This Case

We learned from this case that suction loss during the side cut can be managed successfully by reapplying the suction and cone, decreasing the diameter of the ablation by 0.5 mm and increasing the depth by 20 μm, centering the reticule at the outer edge of the raster pattern bubble, and performing a side cut only.

Suction Loss After Complete Raster Pattern and No Side Cut, No Flap Lift, and Rainbow Glare

31

James J. Salz

Contents

J.J. Salz, MD
Department of Ophthalmology,
Keck School of Medicine,
University of Southern California,
Los Angeles, CA, USA

Laser Vision Medical Group, Los Angeles, CA, USA
e-mail: drjjsalz@gmail.com

Why Is This Case Relevant for the Refractive Surgeon?

It is rare to have a complete raster pattern and not be able to obtain suction to complete the side cut. The presence of the raster pattern in the cornea is invisible on slit-lamp examination, but this spectral pattern of disruption of the stroma can be a cause of troublesome "rainbow glare." This does not always resolve and a PRK on the surface would be above the original raster pattern and would not eliminate the "rainbow glare." Finding the same interface and performing a side cut only can be challenging.

Case Background

The patient was a 35-year-old male, optical engineer (naturally it would happen to him), refraction OD −7.00 −0.75 × 90 = 20/20. The IntraLase was one of the original models operating at 60 KHz. The left eye (−6.25 −0.75 × 85 = 20/20) had an uncomplicated IntraLase flap, 9.0 mm diameter and 110 μm depth with Visx Custom Wavefront-guided ablation. Suction was obtained without difficulty; a full raster pattern with good centration was completed when suction was lost without any side cut pulses. Despite three attempts to reapply the suction ring, the procedure was terminated without lifting the flap or performing the excimer treatment. Postoperatively the patient obtained an uncorrected vision of 20/20 in the left

J.L. Alió et al. (eds.), *Difficult and Complicated Cases in Refractive Surgery*,
DOI 10.1007/978-3-642-55238-0_31, © Springer-Verlag Berlin Heidelberg 2015

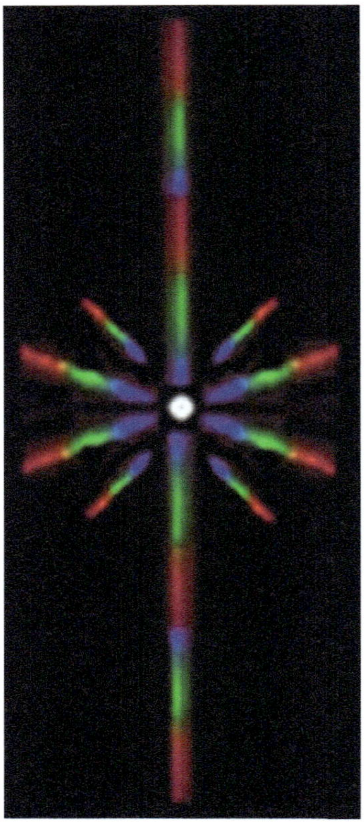

Fig. 31.1 Patient's simulation of the rainbow glare after first procedure

eye and was wearing a contact lens in the left eye. He had no complaints about the quality of vision in the left eye but was complaining of rainbow glare around lights at night in the right eye which also had 20/20 vision with his soft contact lens. As an optical engineer, he described the glare in great detail as follows: "Description of the streaks: Normal light source all streaks had the spectrum. Spectrum streaks before 2nd LASIK: 1 vertical up(repeated the spectrum two times);1 vertical down(repeated the spectrum two times); 4 on the left and 4 on the right (single spectrum on each)." Figure 31.1 is an attempt by the patient to portray the rainbow glare.

The original surgeon was planning on doing a PRK in the right eye after a few weeks, expecting the rainbow glare complaint to resolve. When the rainbow glare persisted, he asked me to see the patient for a second opinion. On examination, the right eye refraction was – 8.5 D=20/20, topography was normal, slit-lamp exam looked completely normal, the IntraLASIK raster pattern was not visible, and of course there was no side cut. When looking at a point of light in a darkened lane, the patient saw normal slight white streaks and no rainbow effect in the left eye but described rainbow glare around the light in the right eye as described previously. He stated that this rainbow glare was very bothersome at night, especially when driving.

Main Problem to Solve

The main problem to solve was decreasing or eliminating the rainbow glare while also correcting the refractive error in the right eye. I remembered reading an article by my friend Ron Krueger about rainbow glare following IntraLASIK [1].

Ancillary Tests

So I called Ron to discuss his thoughts in managing this patient. In their article, they reported on 37 patients with significant rainbow glare around lights, following IntraLASIK with an early model of the IntraLase with raster pattern which had a greater separation of spot size operating at 30 KHz. Their conclusion was as follows: "Light scattering from the back surface of the IntraLASIK flap creates a spectral pattern whose visual impact is clinically inconsequential in the majority of patients. The spectral pattern and visual angle correspond to a grating size that matches the raster spot separation of IntrLase pulsing. Eyes treated with newer focusing optics of higher numerical aperture reduced the rainbow symptom. Variance in optical quality and numerical aperture can impact the spot size and uniformity of IntrLase flap creation." Ron felt that because this patient did not receive the smoothing effect of the excimer on the bed side of the flap, he was more likely to be bothered by rainbow glare. Thus, a PRK, which would not reach the level of the raster pattern, was not likely to eliminate the rainbow glare. The best option would be to create a side cut only and lift the original flap and treat with the excimer which

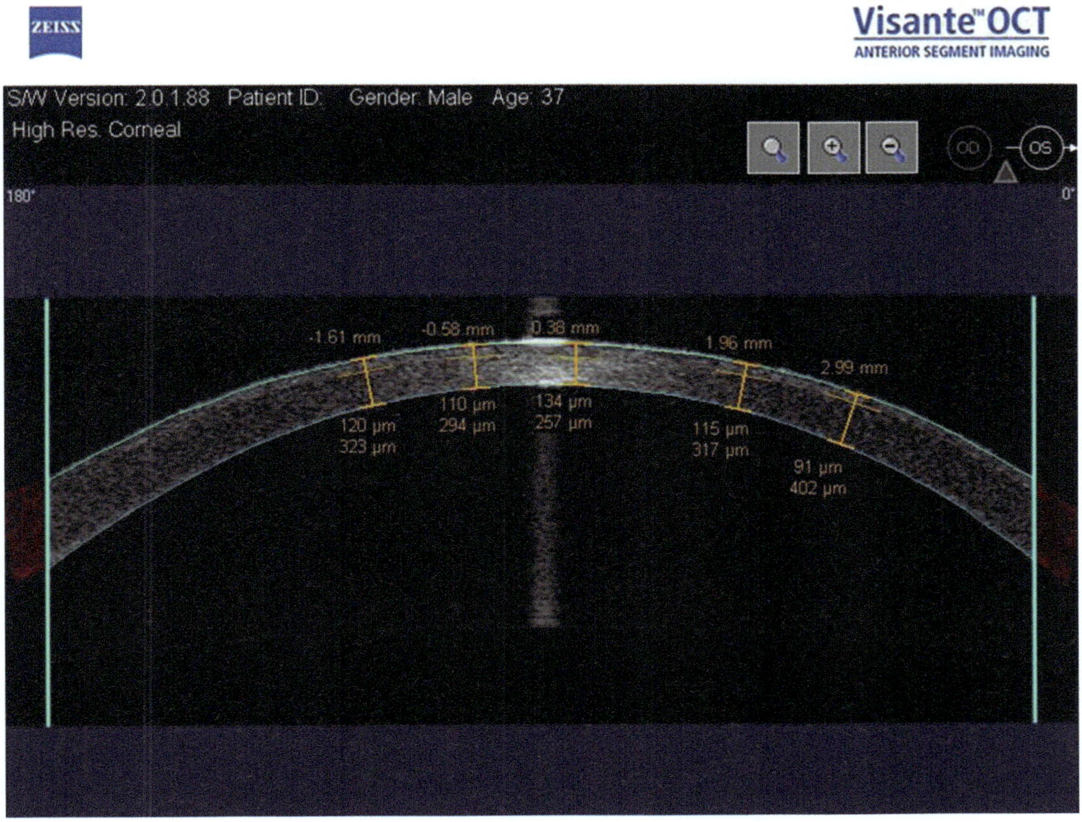

Fig. 31.2 Visante OCT showing flap depth in left eye

would at least smooth out the bed side of the raster pattern as had been done in the patient's left eye. The challenge was that the raster pattern was completely invisible to inspection in contrast to doing a side cut only at the time of the original surgery when the bubbles are still visible. Both the technician and the surgeon felt that the original raster pattern was well centered. Although we had the original programmed flap depth, the actual attained flap depth was unknown. We obtained OCT studies with the Visante (Figs. 31.2 and 31.3), and although we could identify the flap depth with the left eye, it could not be clearly seen in the right eye. We referred the patient to Dr. Larry Hopp to obtain confocal studies. Dr. Hopp was able to identify the flap interface on the confocal (Fig. 31.4) and he estimated the flap depth to be 113 µm with an optical pachymetry of 530 µm.

Surgical/Medical Intervention

We explained the problem to the patient and told him there was no guarantee that we would be able to find the original interface with a side cut only but that this was his best chance to reduce his rainbow glare symptoms while at the same time correcting his vision and eliminating his anisometropia. We programmed the IntraLase for side cut only with a diameter of 8.2 mm to hopefully be inside the original diameter of 9.0 mm and a depth of 140 µm to be deeper than the original raster pattern so that we would be more likely to find the original flap interface and lift the flap. At surgery, suction was easily obtained, the side cut only was accomplished, the flap was easily lifted, and the Visx Custom Wavefront-guided ablation of – 8.5 diopters was completed.

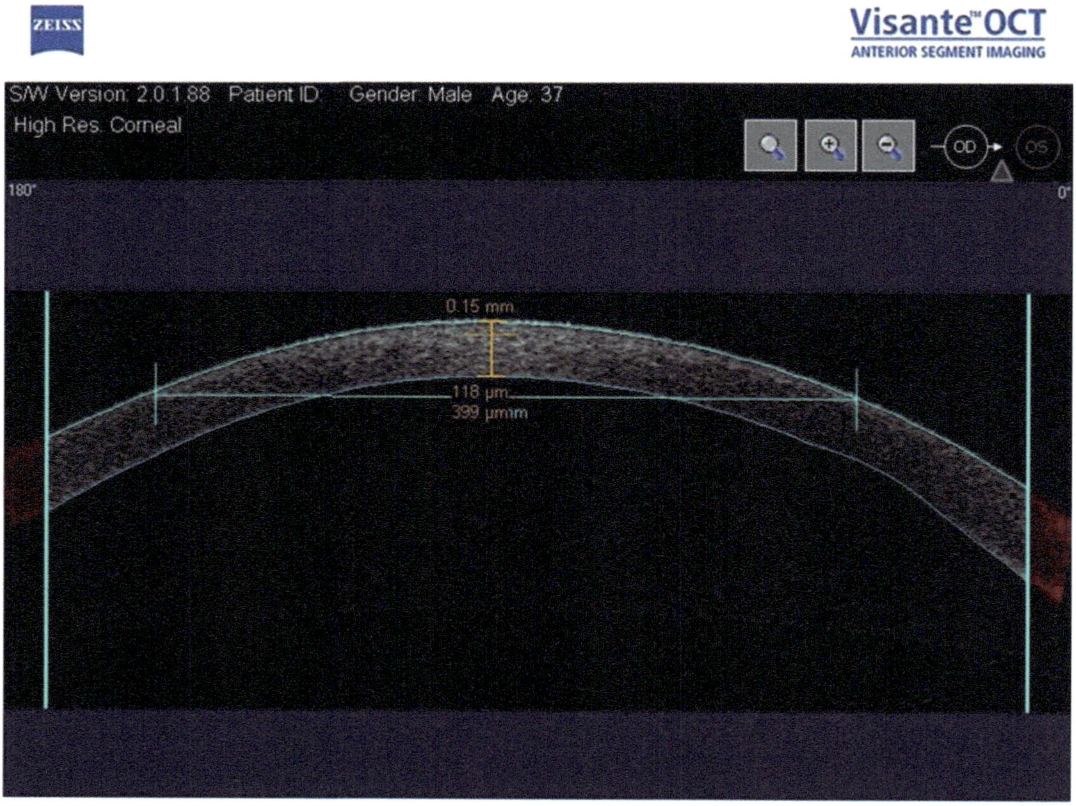

Fig. 31.3 Visante OCT of right eye and inability to clearly see flap interface

Outcome

The next day the uncorrected visual acuity was 20/25, and the patient reported that his rainbow glare was 90 % improved. Here is his detailed description of the glare 1 month after the second surgery: spectrum streaks after 2nd LASIK, "1 vertical up (1 spectrum in the middle of the glare, and a partial spectrum at the end tip): 1 vertical down (1 spectrum in the middle of the glare, and a partial spectrum at the end tip); 1 left (partial single spectrum on the tip); 1 right (partial single spectrum on the tip); also other light streaks which do not show the spectrum going right or left. – color is same as the light source." Figure 31.5 is his attempt at recreating the residual rainbow glare that he sees 1 month after the second surgery.

What to Learn from This Case

We can learn from this case that flaps can be lifted even months after the original application of the femtosecond laser. Rainbow glare is fortunately a rare complication with the newer femtosecond lasers, but when it occurs after an incomplete flap that could not be lifted at the time of surgery, an attempt at lifting the original flap might be a better way to treat the complication than performing a PRK. If the flap cannot be lifted, there is little downside to a side cut only as it is far outside the visual axis and a PRK can still be performed.

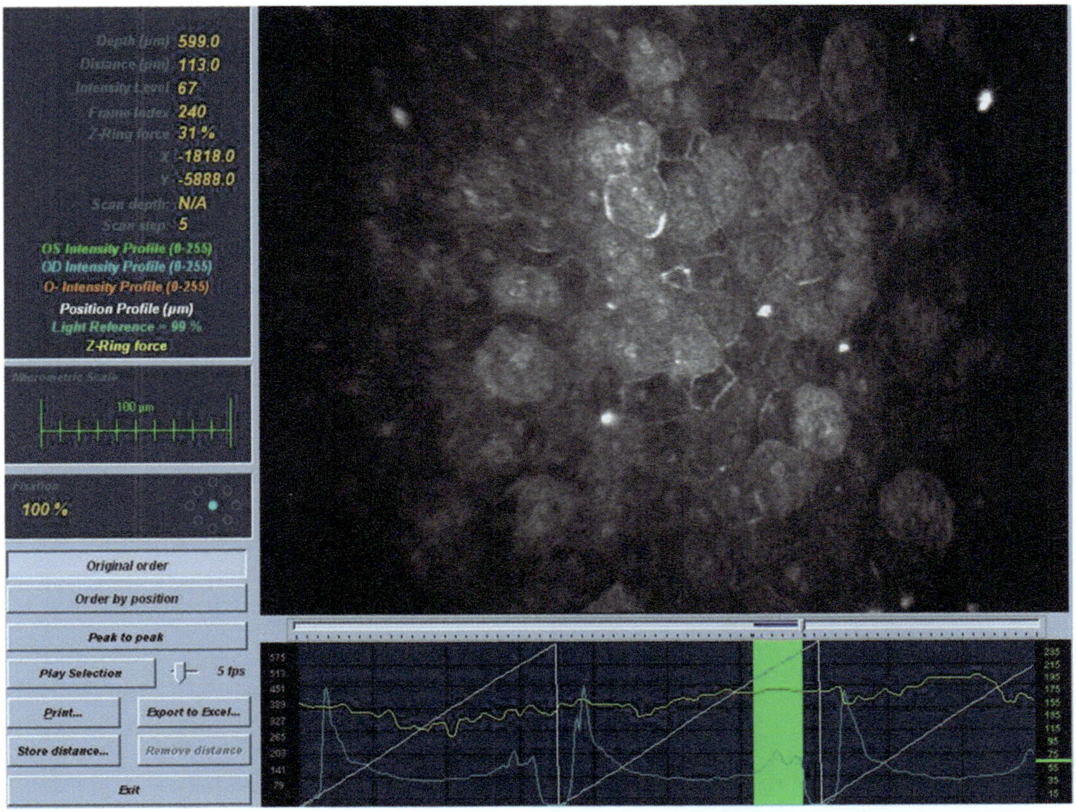

Fig. 31.4 Confocal microscopy of patient 3; *green bar* estimates depth from epithelium to interface – 113 µm (Courtesy of Dr. Larry Hopp)

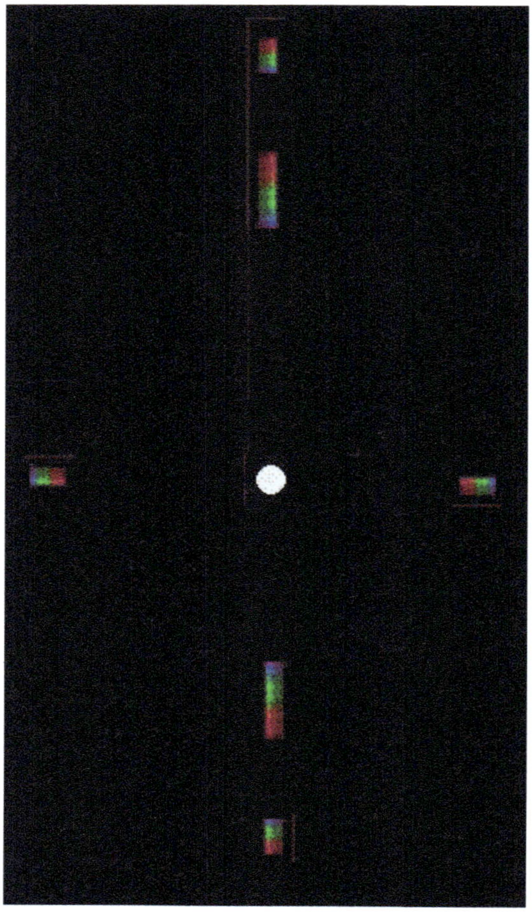

Fig. 31.5 Patient's simulation of reduction in rainbow glare after the completion of ablation

Reference

1. Krueger RR, Thornton IL, Xu M, Bor Z, van den Berg TJ (2008) Rainbow glare as an optical side effect of IntraLASIK. Ophthalmology 115:1187–1195

Part III

Lasik Early Postoperative Complications: Infection Complications and Sterile Complications

Dear reader,

This important chapter contains two sections: infection and corneal infiltrate complications.

Infections after LASIK, though rare, can cause significant visual loss. Infection sources are varied, ranging from patient eyelid to surgical instrumentation and environmental factors. Prompt identification and management are critical. In the second section you can read the case of DLK and the different diagnoses of lesser known diseases. While reading, it is important is to bear in mind the rule of inflammatory response.

Cases will cover complications such as infection, various types of keratitis, GAPP syndrome, early flap striae, marginal sterile corneal infiltrates, management of traumatic LASIK flap edge invagination, as well as other issues. Our hope is to draw attention to major early postoperative LASIK considerations and to provide guidance toward differentiation and management for these complications.

To further explore this subject, we suggest the first book of this series: J.L. Alio', D. Azar *Management of Complications in Refractive Surgery*, Chapter 4: Lasik Early Postoperative Complication Refractive Surprise (pp. 34–70).

Specific topics covered by the cases include how to manage a simple infection (Case 32), a step-by-step evolution of a severe infection (Case 33), and the importance of diagnosis in corneal infiltrates (Case 34). Other cases cover diffuse lamellar keratitis, a common complication (Case 35), extreme light sensitivity despite a completely normal slit-lamp exam and excellent visual acuity (Case 36), pressure-induced interlamellar stromal keratitis simulating infectious keratitis (Case 37), and fast recognition and recovery of flap striae (Case 38). We end with cases focused on the effects of early and late decision making in the management of recalcitrant flap macrostriae (Case 39), prophylactic treatment prior to surgery for moderate blepharitis and/or meibomian gland dysfunction (Case 40), differences between the clinical appearance and management of infections (Case 41), and how to manage traumatic flap dehiscence (Case 42).

Lesson to Learn

Case 32: Interface infection following LASIK

Infections after a LASIK procedure can lead to devastating complications. An adequate preoperative protocol may help to prevent infectious keratitis following LASIK.

Case 33: Infections after refractive surgery

How to deal with severe infection happens after LASIK and how to follow its evolution until keratoplasty is finally performed.

Case 34: Staphylococcal hypersensitivity keratitis following femtosecond LASIK

The importance to recognize the different diagnosis in the corneal infiltrates to understand the risk associated to the refractive surgery.

Case 35: DLK early

The importance of early diagnosis and adequate intervention to obtain a good visual result.

Case 36: GAPP syndrome

To remember a GAPP syndrome when the patient present an extreme light sensitivity despite a completely normal slit-lamp exam and excellent visual acuity.

Case 37: Pressure-induced interlamellar stromal keratitis

To be able to perform a differential diagnosis between pressure-induced interlamellar stromal keratitis and infectious keratitis.

Case 38: Early flap striae

Immediate intervention will yield excellent results; delay in intervention may result in recalcitrant striae that may be difficult or impossible to eliminate.

Case 39: Management of recalcitrant flap macrostriae

The option of observation versus surgical management. Flap lift and suturing to stretch and flatten the flap is an effective treatment against flap macrostriae.

Case 40: Marginal sterile corneal infiltrates

Moderate blepharitis and/or meibomian gland dysfunction should have prophylactic treatment prior to surgery to avoid postoperative complications.

Case 41: Hypersensitivity to vancomycin

To take into account the difference between an infection or lamellar keratitis and a hypersensitivity to the drug. The use of vancomycin has to alert the surgeon of the differential diagnosis.

Case 42: Management of traumatic LASIK flap edge invagination

A correct management, as proper and timely diagnosis of a traumatic flap dehiscence, can increase the chance of an optimal visual outcome.

Interface Infection Following LASIK

32

Jorge L. Alió, Angelo Rampone, and Alessandro Abbouda

Contents

J.L. Alió, MD, PhD (✉)
Department of Refractive Surgery, Vissum Corporación Oftalmológica, Alicante, Spain
e-mail: jlalio@vissum.com

A. Rampone, MD
Department of Ophthalmology, Seconda Università degli Studi di Napoli, Naples, Italy

R&D Department, Vissum Corporacion, Alicante 03016, Alicante, Spain
e-mail: angelo.rampone@gmail.com

A. Abbouda, MD
Department of Refractive Surgery, Vissum Corporación Oftalmológica, Alicante, Spain

Department of Ophthalmology-Policlinico Umberto I of Rome, University of Rome "Sapienza", Viale del Policlinico, 155, 00186, Roma, Italy

R&D Department, Vissum Corporación Oftalmológica, 03016, Alicante, Spain
e-mail: a.abbouda@gmail.com

Why Is This Case Relevant for the Refractive Surgeon?

Infections after LASIK procedures are rare, with incidence ranging from 0.02 to 1.5 % [1]. Although uncommon, when infections occur they can lead to moderate or severe reduction of visual acuity [2]. Therefore, refractive surgeons should be able to promptly diagnose and manage them in order to avoid serious consequences.

Case Background

A 49-year-old man who underwent a refractive lensectomy in his left eye attended our center for an evaluation of his residual refractive error. His manifest refraction in the left eye (LE) was −2.50, −0.75 × 80 and his BCVA was 20/20. The slit-lamp examination did not reveal any problems. The corneal topography showed a regular surface. The keratotomy reading was 46.22/47.09 × 148° and his pachymetry was 554 μm. The slit-lamp examination revealed a centered IOL. No contraindications were observed, so we decided to perform a LASIK procedure. Five days after treatment, the patient reported decreased vision, mild light sensitivity, pain, and discomfort. The slit-lamp examination revealed a paracentral epithelial defect with a stromal infiltrate (Fig. 32.1). Culture scrapping and Gram stain were performed.

J.L. Alió et al. (eds.), *Difficult and Complicated Cases in Refractive Surgery*,
DOI 10.1007/978-3-642-55238-0_32, © Springer-Verlag Berlin Heidelberg 2015

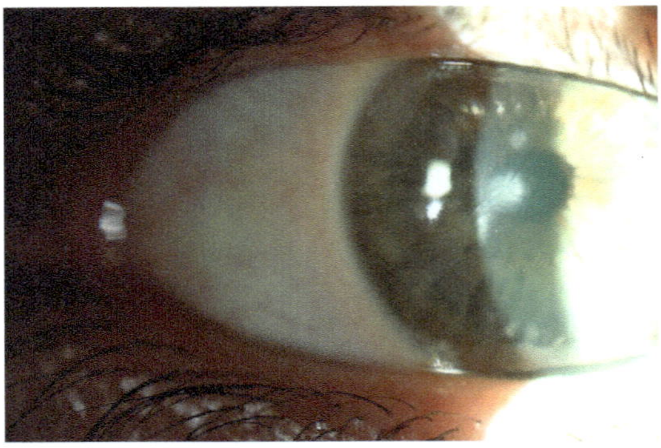

Fig. 32.1 Paracentral epithelial defect and stromal infiltrates

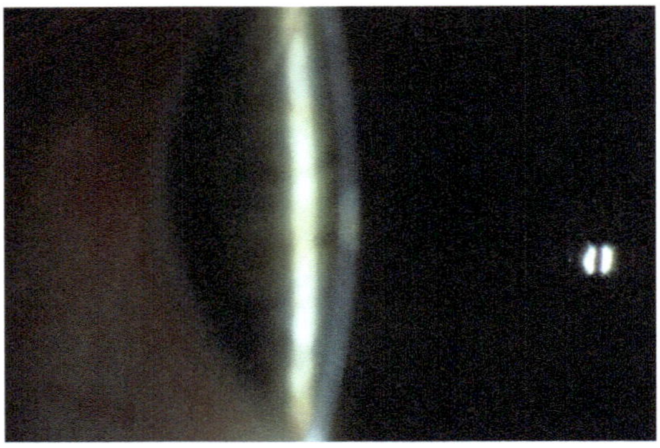

Fig. 32.2 Peripheral opacity

Main Problem to Solve

Early onset infections occurred within 1 week of surgery and an epithelial defect was present.

Ancillary Tests

Gram-positive infections are commonly associated with pain, an epithelial defect, flap separation, and anterior chamber reaction. The anterior segment appearance at the time of onset and the patient's symptoms caused us to consider the possibility of a Gram-positive infection.

Surgical/Medical Intervention

We used ciprofloxacin one drop four times per day and cycloplegic drops three times per day for 2 days. When the results of microbiological culture showed a positivity to *Streptococcus pneumoniae*, we changed the prescription to ciprofloxacin one drop every 2 h alternated with fortified drops of cefazolin (50 mg/ml) + vancomycin (50 mg/ml) and dexamethasone one drop four times per day, tapering to one drop every week for a total of 4 weeks, followed by fluorometholone one drop three times per day for 2 weeks.

Outcome

Seven days after the start of the therapy, the patient had a complete regression of pain and defect and a reduction of corneal infiltrates. Two months later, peripheral opacity was evident (Fig. 32.2). The UCVA was 20/20 in both eyes. The corneal topography showed a temporal flattening area in accordance to the location of the infection (Fig. 32.3). The pupillary zone was not modified and the aberrometry value was normal.

What to Learn from This Case

Infections after LASIK procedure can lead to devastating complications.

Several steps may help prevent infectious keratitis following LASIK. Meibomian gland disease should be treated prior to LASIK. Proper sterilization of instruments, including sterile gloves and drapes, and intraoperative sterile techniques are important preventative measures.

Gram-positive bacteria, including *S. aureus*, *Streptococcus pneumoniae*, *Streptococcus viridans*, *Staphylococcus epidermidis*, Rhodococcus, and Nocardia [3], were identified as the predominant cause of 53.7 % of infections. Fourth-generation quinolone followed by therapy based on microbiological evidence of the sample is the initial

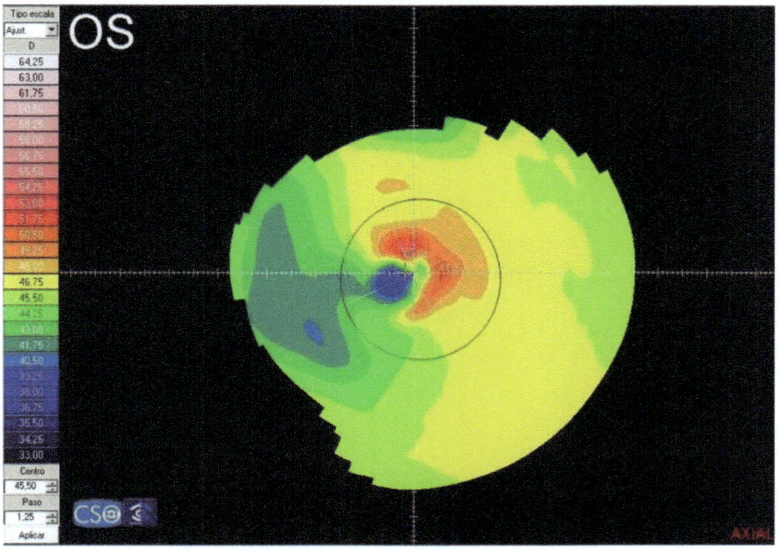

Fig. 32.3 Corneal topography showed a flattening area associated with a previous site of corneal melting

treatment in infectious keratitis. If no improvement is evident within 2 days, irrigation of the flap interface with an antibiotic solution (vancomycin 50 mg/ml and amikacin 35 mg/ml) is suggested [4].

References

1. Chang MA, Jain S, Azar DT (2004) Infections following laser in situ keratomileusis: an integration of the published literature. Surv Ophthalmol 49:269–280
2. Yang KS, Chen YF, Lin KK, Hsiao CH (2005) Mycobacterium keratitis after laser in situ keratomileusis. Cornea 24:344–346
3. De La Cruz J, Hallak J, Azar D, Jain S (2008) Chapter 4.1. Infections after refractive surgery. In: Alio JL, Azar D (eds) Management of complications in refractive surgery. Springer, Berlin/Heidelberg, pp 34–39
4. Alió JL, Pérez-Santonja JJ, Tervo T, Tabbara KF, Vesaluoma M, Smith RJ, Maddox B, Maloney RK (2000) Postoperative inflammation, microbial complications, and wound healing following laser in situ keratomileusis. J Refract Surg 16:523–538

Infections After Refractive Surgery 33

Jorge L. Alió and Alessandro Abbouda

Contents

J.L. Alió, MD, PhD (✉)
Department of Refractive Surgery, Vissum Corporación Oftalmológica, Alicante, Spain
e-mail: jlalio@vissum.com

A. Abbouda, MD
Department of Refractive Surgery, Vissum Corporación Oftalmológica, Alicante, Spain

Department of Ophthalmology-Policlinico Umberto I of Rome, University of Rome "Sapienza", Viale del Policlinico, 155, 00186, Roma, Italy

R&D Department, Vissum Corporación Oftalmológica, 03016, Alicante, Spain
e-mail: a.abbouda@gmail.com

Why Is This Case Relevant for the Refractive Surgeon?

Microbial keratitis is an infection of the cornea that is associated with the risk of permanent visual impairment [1, 2]. It can be caused by bacteria, virus, fungus, protozoa, and parasites. The prevalence of the infection after refractive surgery is reported between 0.02 and 1.5 %. Several large LASIK case series have reported no infectious complications [3, 4].

Infections caused by a single gram-positive organism are more common and include *S. aureus*, *S. pneumoniae*, *S. viridans*, *S. epidermidis*, Rhodococcus, and Nocardia. Fungus such as *Fusarium*, *Aspergillus*, *Curvularia*, and *Scedosporium*, and mycobacterial infections and *M. chelonae*, *Mycobacterium abscessus*, *M. szulgai*, *M. fortuitum*, and *Mycobacterium mucogenicum* were reported [5].

Case Background

A 29-year-old man with a history of uneventful bilateral LASIK for myopia, performed in another country, was referred to our department because of increasing keratitis in his left eye after 2 weeks of the surgery. The visual acuity had dropped from 20/20 at the early postoperative stage to 20/200. He gave a history of soap entering in his left eye which he washed with running water. After 2 weeks of the refractive treatment, the examination

J.L. Alió et al. (eds.), *Difficult and Complicated Cases in Refractive Surgery*,
DOI 10.1007/978-3-642-55238-0_33, © Springer-Verlag Berlin Heidelberg 2015

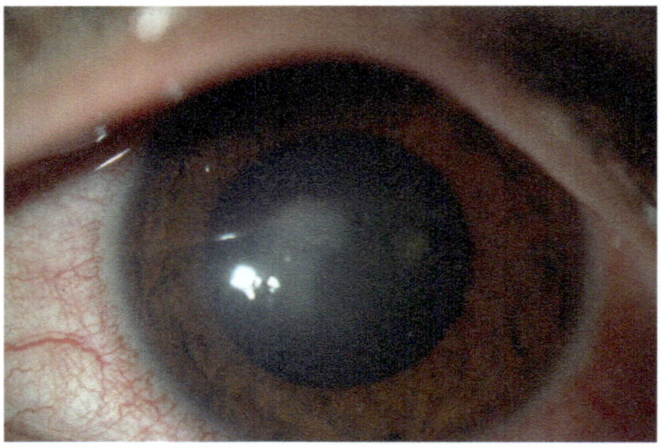

Fig. 33.1 Annular stromal infiltrate in the optic zone

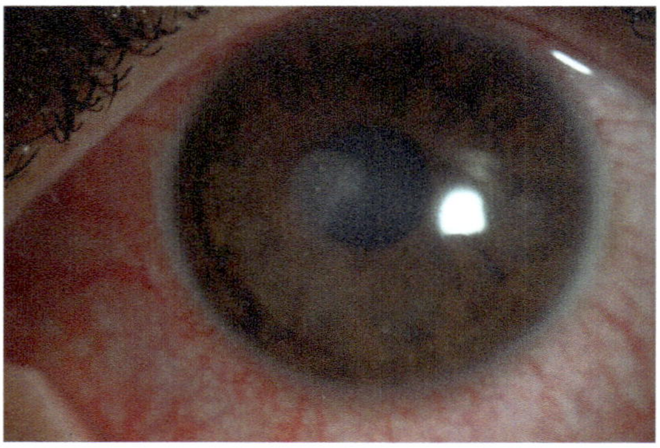

Fig. 33.2 Reduction of the corneal infiltrate but increasing of conjunctival injection after 2 weeks of treatment

revealed well-circumscribed focus of infiltration on the surface of the flap just nasal to the pupil and another infiltration in the temporal side of the flap bed junction. Ofloxacin and Okacin drops were applied every hour. After 1 week, the condition was standstill. Fluconazole, vancomycin drops, and acyclovir ointment were added. When he arrived at our department, the patient complained of having pain, photophobia, and visual loss. The slit-lamp examination revealed conjunctival injection and central white infiltrate in the interface with a small epithelial erosion over this lesion. The stroma adjacent to the opacity appeared infiltrated and edematous (Fig. 33.1).

Main Problem to Solve

The late onset of infection suggested an atypical pathogen. Microbiological cultures are recommended to help with treatment decisions.

Ancillary Tests

We performed a PCR over the corneal scraping and microbiological culture. The results of this examination showed a positivity for *Mycobacterium chelonae*. It was resistant to levofloxacin and vancomycin and sensitive to amikacin.

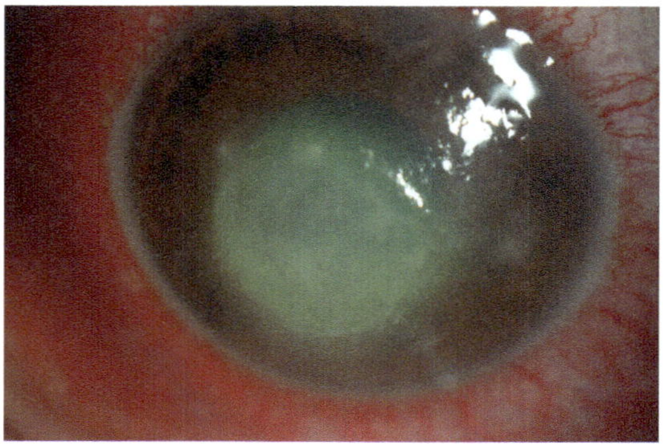

Fig. 33.3 Progression of infiltrate, melting of the flap

Surgical/Medical Intervention

The treatment was modified with clarithromycin drops 10 mg/ml one drop each hour and oral treatment with clarithromycin 500 mg two times per day. After the initial week of improvement (Fig. 33.2), the corneal infiltrate started to progress, causing an extensive corneal melting in 2 weeks (Fig. 33.3). The residual LASIK flap was amputated because most of the flap had melted. Overlying epithelium was removed across an 8.0 mm zone; PTK (10 mm) was performed to smoothen the bed. At the end of the procedure, a silicone–hydrogel bandage contact lens was placed on the eye.

Outcome

The patient followed amikacin and clarithromycin drops three times per day for 3 weeks. The corneal melting and ulcer progressed. He went back to his country and performed two penetrating keratoplasties. After the first one, the infection developed in the graft and it was necessary to perform a second graft.

At 2 years from the last surgery, 8 months after suture removal, his best correct visual acuity was 20/32.

What to Learn from This Case

Although infection after LASIK is a rare complication, serious consequences such as moderate or severe reductions in visual acuity are common. Treatment should not be empirical. Cultures and smears should be performed after flap lifting and aggressive topical antibiotic therapy initiated. The initial treatment should be modified based on the culture and scraping results and the clinical response to therapy.

References

1. Keay L, Edwards K, Naduvilath T, Taylor HR, Snibson GR, Forde K, Stapleton F (2006) Microbial keratitis predisposing factors and morbidity. Ophthalmology 113:109–116
2. Bourcier T, Thomas F, Borderie V, Chaumeil C, Laroche L (2003) Bacterial keratitis: predisposing factors, clinical and microbiological review of 300 cases. Br J Ophthalmol 87:834–838
3. Seedor JA, Shapiro DE, Ritterband DC et al (2001) LASIK complication rates. ARVO abstract no. 2668
4. Miller D, Newton J, Alfonso E (2000) Surveillance and infection control standards for refractive surgery centers? ARVO abstract no. 1679 2000
5. De La Cruz J, Hallak J, Azar D, Sandeep J (2008) Chapter 4.1. Infections after refractive surgery. In: Alio J, Azar D (eds) Management of complications in refractive surgery. Springer, Berlin, pp 34–39

Staphylococcal Hypersensitivity Keratitis Following Femtosecond LASIK

34

Roberto Pineda II, J.P. Frangie, and Jnanankar Medhi

Contents

R. Pineda II, MD (✉) • J.P. Frangie
Department of Refractive Surgery, Massachusetts Eye and Ear Infirmary, Harvard Medical School, Boston, MA, USA
e-mail: roberto_pineda@meei.harvard.edu

J. Medhi, MD
Department of Refractive Surgery, Massachusetts Eye and Ear Infirmary, Boston, MA, USA
e-mail: jmedhimail@gmail.com

Why Is This Case Relevant for the Refractive Surgeon?

Keratitis after refractive surgery is relatively uncommon but a potentially sight-threatening complication. Its incidence may vary widely from 0 to 1.5 % [1]. Surveys reveal the incidence of keratitis as 2.5 times more common with photorefractive keratectomy (PRK) than with a keratome, six times more common with PRK than with the femtosecond laser, and 2.4 times more common with a keratome than with the femtosecond laser [2]. Literature show noninfectious keratitis occurs more frequently than infectious keratitis [3]. It is important to identify infection early as the line of management differs significantly between these two clinical entities.

Case Background

A 47-year-old man presented to the clinic with complaints of overnight burning sensation and teary, red, swollen eyes following femtosecond LASIK surgery in both eyes the previous day for a refraction of −5.75 D (OU). He returned to his surgeon on the first postoperative day with the above symptoms and was subsequently referred to our institution. Medical history was unremarkable. Slit lamp examination showed presence of infiltrates at the flap margin and in the interface (involving around 270° in scattered

J.L. Alió et al. (eds.), *Difficult and Complicated Cases in Refractive Surgery*,
DOI 10.1007/978-3-642-55238-0_34, © Springer-Verlag Berlin Heidelberg 2015

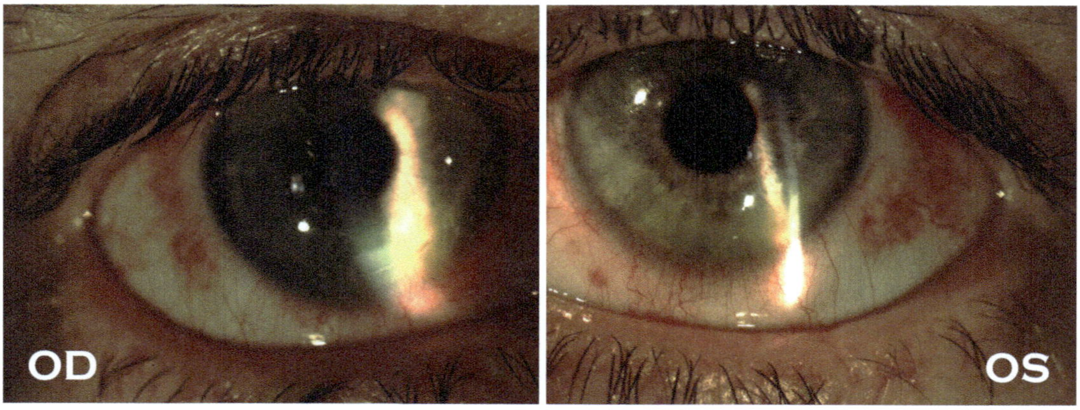

Fig. 34.1 Postoperative day 1: epithelial edema and corneal infiltrates seen along the flap margin and adjacent peripheral cornea outside the flap margin (both eyes). *OD* oculo dextro, *OS* oculo sinistro

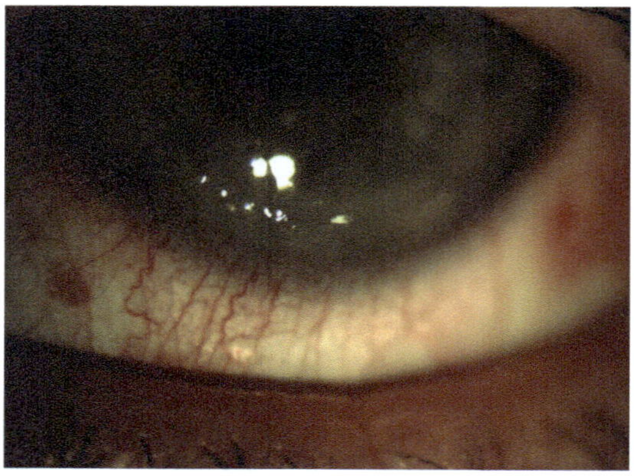

Fig. 34.2 Close-up picture showing corneal infiltrates at the flap margin

patches), including the peripheral cornea beyond the flap margin in both the eyes. Fluorescein stain-positive epithelial defects were noted and the epithelium around the affected areas was edematous. The flap interface was quiet on postoperative day 1 (Figs. 34.1, 34.2, and 34.3). There was no reaction in the anterior chamber. Eyelid examination revealed Meibomian gland disease in both sides.

Main Problem to Solve

1. To rule out infective etiology
2. To look for other probable causes

Ancillary Tests

Smear and culture of the corneal scraping samples obtained from the LASIK flap edges.

Surgical/Medical Intervention

Corneal scraping revealed the presence of coagulase-negative staphylococcus and alpha-hemolytic streptococcus. There was no growth in broth till 72 h. The patient was started on topical steroids (prednisolone) 1 hourly and topical moxifloxacin four times a day with careful follow-up. The patient presented on the 4th postoperative day with a visual acuity of 20/40 in right eye and 20/50 in the left eye. Examination revealed diffuse lamellar keratitis with aggregate clumping of white blood cell with involvement of the visual axis in both eyes (left more than right). An interface washout was performed on the left eye. Postoperatively topical prednisolone (tapered down), moxifloxacin, polymyxin B/trimethoprim, and vancomycin were continued along with oral steroids.

Outcome

The patient was diagnosed with staphylococcal hypersensitivity keratitis and responded well to topical prednisolone and antibiotic therapy along

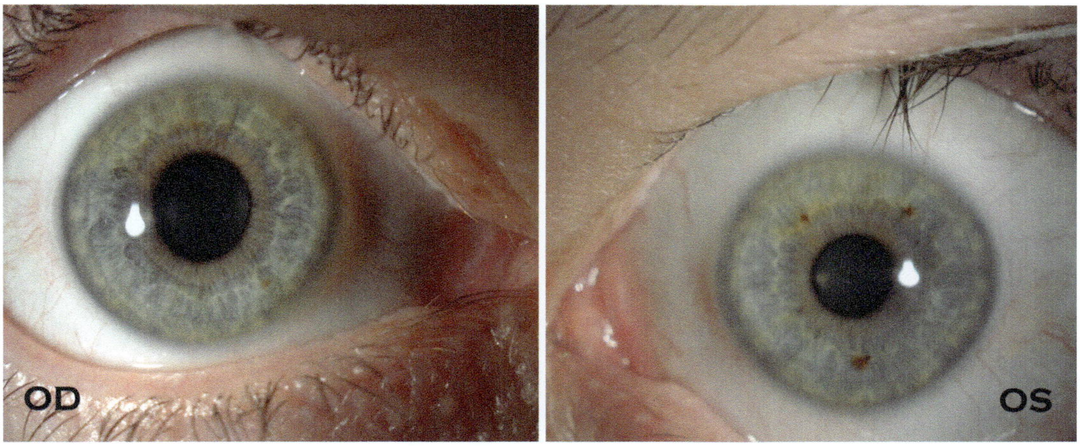

Fig. 34.3 Complete resolution of diffuse lamellar keratitis and flap margin infiltrates (both eyes). *OD* oculo dextro, *OS* oculo sinistro

with the interface washout with recovery of vision to 20/20 (right eye) and 20/25 by 1 month's time.

What to Learn from This Case

Infection following femtosecond LASIK is rare [4]; however, noninfective inflammation, especially lid margin-related hypersensitivity reaction, is not uncommon. Management of lid disease is essential before undertaking refractive surgery. It is important to consider history of atopy and its preoperative treatment before refractive surgery. Noninfective inflammation can be well controlled with topical steroids, whereas in case of infective keratitis, it is recommended to start fourth-generation topical fluoroquinolones like moxifloxacin as first-line management.

References

1. Chang MA, Jain S, Azar DT (2004) Infections following laser in situ keratomileusis: an integration of the published literature. Surv Ophthalmol 49:269–280
2. Leaming DV, Duffey RJ. Leaming 2011 survey of American Society of Cataract and Refractive Surgery Members. http://www.analeyz.com/AnaleyzASCRS2011.htm. Accessed 25 Jan 2013
3. Moshirfar M, Welling JD, Feiz V, Holz H, Clinch TE (2007) Infectious and non-infectious keratitis after laser in situ keratomileusis. Occurrence, outcomes and visual outcomes. J Cataract Refract Surg 33:474–483
4. Bucci MG, McCormick GJ (2012) Idiopathic peripheral necrotizing keratitis after femtosecond laser in situ keratomileusis. J Cataract Refract Surg 38:544–547

DLK Early

35

Michael Weisberg

Contents

M. Weisberg, MD
Department of Ophthalmology,
Midwest Eye Center SC, Calumet City, IL, USA
e-mail: michaelweisberg@gmail.com

Why Is This Case Relevant for the Refractive Surgeon?

Diffuse lamellar keratitis (DLK) is an inflammatory condition that occurs in up to 4 % of LASIK treatments. It is characterized by the presence of white granular noninfectious sterile infiltrates in the LASIK flap interface. The condition usually presents postoperatively on days 1–5 and typically starts at the periphery of the flap and progresses centrally. The syndrome is also known as "Sands of the Sahara," as the shifting wavelike progression of the cellular infiltrates simulates shifting sands. The syndrome was first described by Maloney in 1998 and later classified into stages by Linebarger et al. in 2000 based on the location and severity of inflammation [1, 2].

Early diagnosis and treatment of DLK is essential in order to avoid adverse outcomes and loss of vision. In one study, this condition resulted in the loss of two lines of best spectacle-corrected visual acuity (BSCVA) in 5.6 % of patients and at least one line in 22.2 % [3]. The advanced stages of DLK have a higher likelihood of causing loss of best-corrected visual acuity, emphasizing the importance of early diagnosis and intervention.

Case Background

A 42-year-old woman with mild myopia presented for a LASIK consultation. Manifest refraction was −1.75 sph in the right eye and

J.L. Alió et al. (eds.), *Difficult and Complicated Cases in Refractive Surgery*,
DOI 10.1007/978-3-642-55238-0_35, © Springer-Verlag Berlin Heidelberg 2015

−1.75 sph in the left eye with a visual acuity of 20/20 in both eyes. Slit-lamp exam was significant only for mild punctate staining inferiorly in both eyes from dry eye. Her right eye was dominant, and after discussion, the patient decided to have monovision LASIK surgery in her right eye only, leaving her left eye focused for near vision. Surgery using the Moria One-Use microkeratome 90 μm flap and Allegretto Wavelight laser was uneventful. The patient was placed on prednisolone 1 % every hour and gatifloxacin 4×/day. On postoperative day 1, the patient complained of mild foreign body sensation. Uncorrected visual acuity was 20/30 in the right eye with slit-lamp exam, revealing granular cellular infiltrates in the flap interface both centrally and peripherally.

Main Problem to Solve

DLK is ideally diagnosed early within the first postoperative week and treated immediately. Treatment is almost always indicated, and the stage of DLK will determine whether medical or surgical intervention is needed.

Ancillary Tests

Meticulous slit-lamp biomicroscopy and a good history are essential when diagnosing DLK. Stage 1 DLK (Fig. 35.1) occurs in about 4 % of cases and is characterized by the development of cellular infiltrates involving only the peripheral LASIK flap interface. If DLK develops, it is usually present on the first day. Visual acuity is usually good with stage 1 DLK, but patients may describe foreign body sensation and photosensitivity. Stage 2 DLK (Fig. 35.2) occurs in 0.5 % of cases and is characterized by the central progression of the leukocytic infiltrates, usually seen on day 2 or 3. Visual acuity may or may not be affected, with some patients noting cloudiness or haziness since the central visual axis is involved. In stage 3 DLK (Fig. 35.3), which occurs in 1 out of every 500 cases, clustering of the infiltrates in the central visual axis occurs most commonly on days 2 or 3 [2]. Once the syndrome has progressed to stage 3, the situation is more dire, with increased chances of corneal scarring and opacification. Linebarger et al. described stage 4 DLK (Fig. 35.4) as the end-stage result of this exuberant inflammatory process that releases collagenases

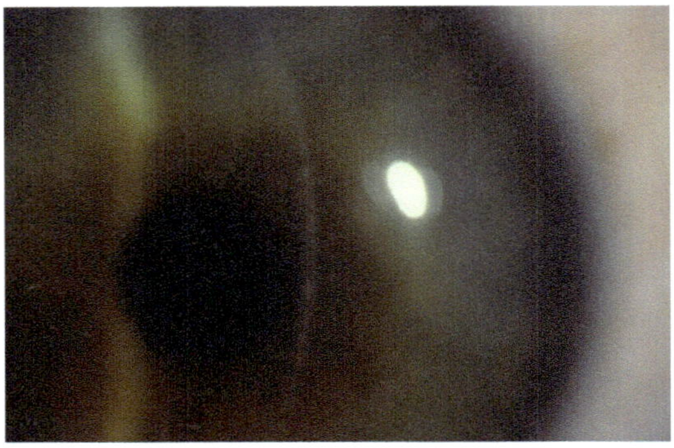

Fig. 35.1 DLK stage 1. Cells are mainly in the periphery and in the stroma

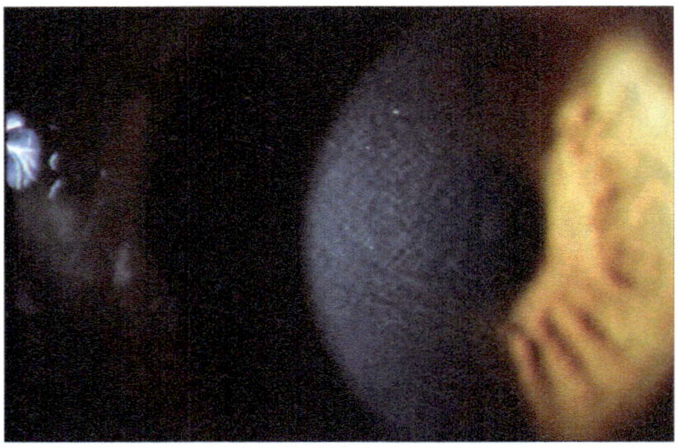

Fig. 35.2 DLK stage 2. Cells are distributed throughout the cornea, including centrally, and yet are still in the stroma

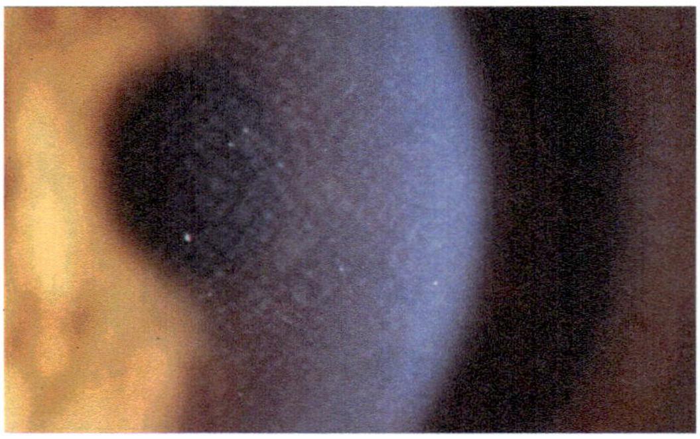

Fig. 35.3 DLK stage 3. Cells are clumped paracentrally and are found in the LASIK flap interface

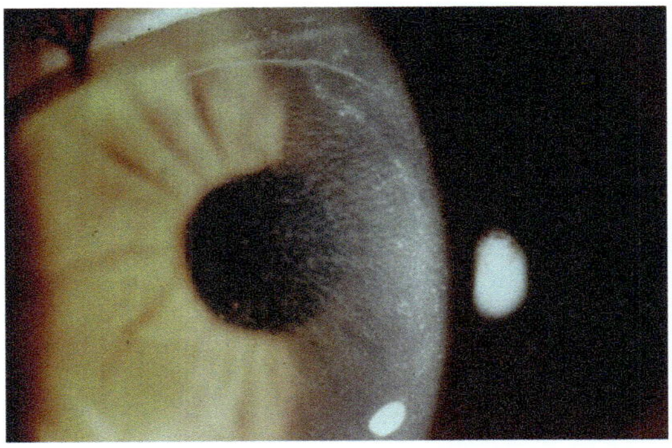

Fig. 35.4 DLK stage 4. Scarring and loss of stromal volume

from the aggregated inflammatory cells, leading to stromal melting with central corneal opacification, striae, and a hyperopic shift from the stromal loss. This stage typically presents on days 3–7 and occurs in only 1 out of 5,000 cases.

There is some controversy about whether stage 4 DLK is the same process that occurs in stages 1–3 or a different process entirely. What Linebarger et al. called stage 4 DLK, Sonmez and Maloney labeled as central toxic keratopathy (CTK) [4]. Sonmez and Maloney describe CTK as a noninflammatory syndrome that appears between days 3 and 6 with central corneal opacification, striae, posterior stromal collapse, hyperopic shift, loss of best-corrected visual acuity, and gradual clearing over 2–18 months. The fact that CTK is rare in eyes with PRK supports the hypothesis that it is a different process from DLK, which theoretically cannot occur in PRK because there is no interface. However, CTK is frequently preceded by DLK, suggesting that the two conditions may share a common etiology and that CTK is just a severe stage of DLK [4].

In addition, Hainline et al. describe a similar clinical syndrome to stage 4 DLK or central toxic keratopathy called central lamellar flap necrosis, in which there is diffuse central inflammation leading to central opacification and the "Mercedes Benz" sign of cracked folds central in the flap. Unlike in DLK, there is little inflammation in the interface and the posterior surface of flap remains intact. In central lamellar flap necrosis, the anterior stroma becomes necrotic and assumes a jellylike consistency [5].

It is important to distinguish DLK from an infectious etiology as well as from a rare condition called pressure-induced interlamellar stromal keratitis (PISK). Most cases of DLK occur in the first postoperative week. Although there have been cases of late-onset DLK associated with large epithelial defects, collagen cross-linking, and SLT, other diagnoses need to be considered when there is a delay in onset of symptoms. In PISK, there is a rise in intraocular pressure often related to the use of topical steroids, thus the onset is typically after 1 week. This IOP rise causes transudation of fluid that collects in the flap interface. A fine haze forms in the interface, and a clear space between the stromal bed and flap due may form to the collection of fluid. IOP by applanation will remain normal or may even be low due to the fluid in the interface causing a false reading, and measurements in the periphery outside the flap will reveal the elevated IOP. If PISK is mistaken for DLK, it will only be worsened by increasing the frequency of topical steroids when in fact PISK demands discontinuation of topical steroids and initiation of IOP-lowering agents [6].

Surgical/Medical Intervention

Our patient was diagnosed with grade 2 diffuse lamellar keratitis (DLK) and continued on prednisolone 1 % every hour. When she returned the following day, uncorrected visual acuity in the right eye was 20/50, and the central cellular infiltrates were slightly more clustered. Grade 3 DLK was diagnosed and the patient was brought to the operating room. The flap was relifted, and BSS on a cannula was used to irrigate both the stromal bed and posterior surface of the flap. The patient was again placed on prednisolone 1 % hourly and gatifloxacin 4×/day.

Once a patient is diagnosed with DLK, he or she must be monitored every 24 h because the condition can progress rapidly to stages with more adverse outcomes. Treatment for stage 1 and 2 DLK involves escalating topical steroid drop frequency to every hour with a steroid ointment at night, and in some cases a short course of oral steroids such as Medrol dose pack or prednisone. Typically, stages 1–2 DLK will resolve over 3–4 days with treatment. Stage 3 DLK treatment is more aggressive and involves surgical intervention by relifting the LASIK flap and irrigating both the stromal bed and undersurface of the LASIK flap with BSS. After flap irrigation, patients are maintained on high-frequency topical steroids until the stromal infiltrates have regressed; afterward, the steroids are tapered appropriately. Stage 3 DLK resolves over 9–10 days once treated. Once DLK has progressed to stage 4, Linebarger et al. do not advocate lifting and irrigating the LASIK flap, since this stage typically involves significant stromalysis and further manipulation and irrigation could hasten additional stromal loss. Stage 4 DLK may take months to resolve. Similarly, the natural course of lamellar flap necrosis seems to be spontaneous clearing of the cornea and regression of the hyperopic shift due to epithelial remodeling over several months. As with stage 4 DLK, treatment with steroids or flap lift did not seem to affect the natural course of lamellar flap necrosis.

Outcome

On postoperative day 3 (day 1 after flap irrigation), the patient's stromal interface reaction had lessened and uncorrected visual acuity was 20/30. The patient remained on the same frequency of drops, and 3 days after flap irrigation, the stromal interface infiltration was gone, with uncorrected visual acuity improved to 20/20 in the right eye. The prednisolone 1 % drops were tapered slowly over 2 weeks with no recurrence of DLK, and the patient was happy to be independent from glasses.

What to Learn from This Case

DLK seems to be an exaggerated inflammatory response due to a multifactorial constellation of exogenous environmental and endogenous patient-specific etiologies that could be related to the deposition of some inciting antigen in the flap interface during surgery. Cases of DLK can be classified as either sporadic, occurring in isolation, or as epidemic, a clustering of cases. This case was sporadic. Epidemic cases may be related to problems in the surgical environment, like debris on the microkeratome, ink from surgical markers, talc from gloves, or autoclave bacterial endotoxin contamination [7–10].

One group noticed a dramatic increase in DLK rates when there was a switch from a steam sterilizer to a cassette sterilizer with reservoir. It was hypothesized that a biofilm developed in the reservoir, endotoxins were released into the steam which coated instruments, and when these instruments were used, the endotoxins were deposited in the flap interface, causing DLK [9]. Sporadic cases may be related to epithelial defects which increase the risk of DLK by a factor of 13–26, blood in the interface, meibomian secretions in the interface, or dry eye [3]. Other cases of late-onset DLK have been reported to occur after collagen cross-linking, selective laser trabeculoplasty (SLT), conductive keratoplasty, and uveitis flare-ups [11–13]. Increased rates of DLK have also occurred since the advent of the femtosecond laser to create LASIK flaps. This phenomenon has been attributed to the degree of energy used by the femtosecond laser; lower laser energy settings are associated with lower rates of DLK. Some studies have also found a higher incidence of DLK with larger flap diameters, higher raster and side cut energy, and possibly thinner flaps [14, 15]. No correlation has been found with patient age, patient gender, or ablation depth [9].

DLK is a rare postoperative LASIK complication that requires vigilance in diagnosis and initiation of treatment in order to avoid adverse outcomes. Prevention may be achieved by meticulous cleaning of instruments, avoiding epithelial defects, maintaining good air quality in the operative suite, using non-powdered gloves, treating lid margin disease and meibomian gland secretions preoperatively, and ensuring that no debris are left in the flap interface. In our case, dry eye and preoperative punctate staining may have predisposed the patient to developing DLK. Treating the ocular surface beforehand may have been prudent.

References

1. Smith RJ, Maloney RK (1998) Diffuse lamellar keratitis. A new syndrome in lamellar refractive surgery. Ophthalmology 105:1721–1726
2. Linebarger EJ, Hardten DR, Lindstrom RL (2000) Diffuse lamellar keratitis: diagnosis and management. J Cataract Refract Surg 26:1072–1077
3. Johnson JD, Harissi-Dagher M, Pineda R, Yoo S, Azar DT (2001) Diffuse lamellar keratitis: incidence, associations, outcomes, and a new classification system. J Cataract Refract Surg 27:1560–1566
4. Sonmez B, Maloney RK (2007) Central toxic keratopathy: description of a syndrome in laser refractive surgery. Am J Ophthalmol 143:420–427
5. Hainline BC, Price MO, Choi DM, Price FW Jr (2007) Central flap necrosis after LASIK with microkeratome and femtosecond laser created flaps. J Refract Surg 23:233–242
6. Belin MW, Hannush SB, Yau CW, Schultze RL (2002) Elevated intraocular pressure-induced interlamellar stromal keratitis. Ophthalmology 109: 1929–1933
7. Lazaro C, Perea J, Arias A (2006) Surgical-glove-related diffuse lamellar keratitis after laser in situ keratomileusis: long-term outcomes. J Cataract Refract Surg 32:1702–1709
8. Hadden OB, McGhee CN, Morris AT, Gray TB, Ring CP, Watson AS (2008) Outbreak of diffuse lamellar keratitis caused by marking-pen toxicity. J Cataract Refract Surg 34:1121–1124
9. Stulting RD, Randleman JB, Couser JM, Thompson KP (2004) The epidemiology of diffuse lamellar keratitis. Cornea 23:680–688
10. Villarrubia A, Palacín E, Gómez del Río M, Martínez P (2007) Description, etiology, and prevention of an outbreak of diffuse lamellar keratitis after LASIK. J Refract Surg 23:482–486
11. Kymionis GD, Bouzoukis DI, Diakonis VF, Portaliou DM, Pallikaris AI, Yoo SH (2007) Diffuse lamellar keratitis after corneal crosslinking in a patient with post-laser in situ keratomileusis corneal ectasia. J Cataract Refract Surg 33:2135–2137
12. Davis EA, Fahmy AM (2009) Stage III diffuse lamellar keratitis following conductive keratoplasty over a LASIK flap. J Cataract Refract Surg 35:1141–1143
13. Holz H, Pirouzian A (2010) Bilateral diffuse lamellar keratitis following consecutive selective laser trabeculoplasty in LASIK patient. J Cataract Refract Surg 36:847–849
14. de Paula FH, Khairallah CG, Niziol LM, Musch DC, Shtein RM (2012) Diffuse lamellar keratitis after laser in situ keratomileusis with femtosecond laser flap creation. J Cataract Refract Surg 38:1014–1019
15. Choe CH, Guss C, Musch DC, Niziol LM, Shtein RM (2010) Incidence of diffuse lamellar keratitis after LASIK with 15 KHz, 30 KHz, and 60 KHz femtosecond laser flap creation. J Cataract Refract Surg 36:1912–1918

GAPP Syndrome

36

Michael Weisberg

Contents

M. Weisberg, MD
Department of Ophthalmology,
Midwest Eye Center SC, Calumet City, IL, USA
e-mail: michaelweisberg@gmail.com

Why Is This Case Relevant to the Refractive Surgeon?

Good acuity plus photosensitivity (GAPP) syndrome is a relatively new syndrome that has been seen with the introduction of the femtosecond laser for creating LASIK flaps. It has also been called transient light-sensitivity syndrome. This syndrome typically presents 2–6 weeks following LASIK with the femtosecond laser and involves extreme light sensitivity despite a completely normal slit-lamp exam (no dryness, injection, cell, flare, infiltrates, striae, epithelial ingrowth) and excellent visual acuity. The rate of GAPP can range from 0.2 to 1.3 % and is more common when higher femtosecond laser energy levels are used to create the LASIK flap [1, 2]. The light sensitivity can be incapacitating to the patient and can make for a very unhappy patient.

Case Background

A 30-year-old woman with moderate myopia presented for LASIK consultation. Best-corrected visual acuity was 20/20 in both eyes with refraction in the right eye −3.00 +0.50×090 and in the left eye −3.50 +0.50×085. Corneal topography and slit-lamp exam were unremarkable, and the patient underwent bilateral LASIK with 60 kHz IntraLase femtosecond laser using a 110 μm flap and Visx excimer laser. The patient was started on prednisolone 1 % every hour and gatifloxacin

J.L. Alió et al. (eds.), *Difficult and Complicated Cases in Refractive Surgery*,
DOI 10.1007/978-3-642-55238-0_36, © Springer-Verlag Berlin Heidelberg 2015

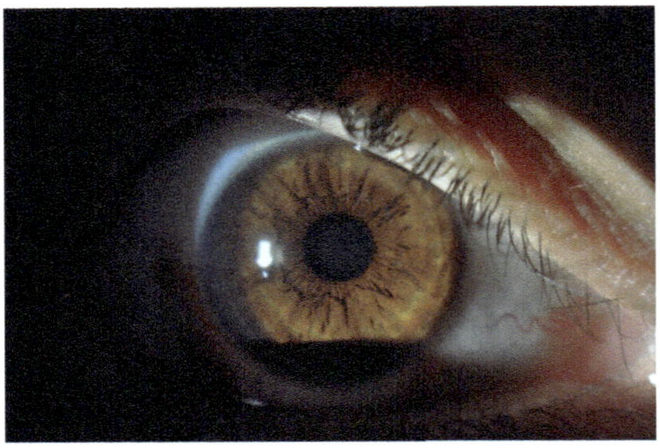

Fig. 36.1 Slit-lamp examination revealed well-centered flaps with no evidence of striae, infiltrates, drying, iritis, scleritis, or epithelial ingrowth

4×/day. On postoperative day 1, the patient had uncorrected visual acuity of 20/20, with well-centered flaps showing no striae, DLK, or drying. The prednisolone 1 % was decreased to 4×/day. Findings were similar at postoperative week 1 when the gatifloxacin was discontinued and prednisolone 1 % was tapered to 2×/day for 1 week before stopping. At postoperative week 4, the patient was doing well with uncorrected visual acuity of 20/20 and an unremarkable slit-lamp exam. On postoperative week 6, the patient returned complaining of extreme photophobia, especially when working around computers. Uncorrected visual acuity remained 20/20, and slit-lamp exam remained unremarkable, showing well-centered flaps with no evidence of striae, infiltrates, drying, iritis, scleritis, or epithelial ingrowth (Fig. 36.1).

Main Problem to Solve

GAPP syndrome is a unique syndrome because often the patient will have intense symptoms but no clinical findings on exam. It is important to listen the patient's symptoms and treat them appropriately.

Ancillary Tests

A good history and detailed slit-lamp exam are fundamental in diagnosing GAPP syndrome. A plethora of other ocular diseases can present with photophobia as their main complaint. Using slit-lamp biomicroscopy, it is essential to rule out other conditions including epithelial ingrowth, iritis, ocular surface disease, dryness, infiltrates, diffuse lamellar keratitis, flap striae, scleritis/episcleritis, and conjunctivitis. Once a completely normal slit-lamp exam is confirmed, then one can treat for GAPP syndrome.

Surgical/Medical Intervention

Our patient was diagnosed with GAPP and started on prednisolone 1 % 4×/day. The patient showed improvement in symptoms after 1 week, and the steroid was tapered one drop per week. The patient remained off steroids with no recurrence of symptoms. Most patients with GAPP syndrome respond well to a brief course of topical steroids that is titrated to the degree of their symptoms and tapered accordingly.

Outcome

The outcome of our case was excellent with complete resolution of symptoms over 1 week and a slow taper of topical steroids over 1 month. The patient remained free of symptoms and off treatment after discontinuation of her topical steroids.

What to Learn from This Case

The etiology of this syndrome remains unclear, but some have hypothesized that it is a response to the shockwaves generated by the femtosecond laser on corneal nerve endings or stromal keratocytes [1]. In addition, it could be related to ciliary body irritation from migrated cavitation bubbles during flap creation or an inflammatory reaction to cellular debris created by the femtosecond laser. One study found that rates of GAPP were not associated with iris color or formation of an outer bubble layer. They did find, however, that patients treated with heavier doses of topical steroids postoperatively were less likely to develop GAPP compared with those with lighter doses of steroids. In addition there was a tenfold increased risk of developing GAPP among patients who had previously developed DLK postoperatively, suggesting that increased postoperative inflammation made patients more susceptible to developing GAPP [3]. Prevention of this syndrome can be achieved by using the lowest femtosecond laser energy settings that allow for easy flap dissection and perhaps a heavier course of immediate postoperative steroids. If GAPP syndrome does develop, treatment consists of topical steroids like prednisolone 1 % 4×/day tapered over a month according to symptomatic improvement.

References

1. Stonecipher KG, Dishler JG, Ignacio TS, Binder PS (2006) Transient light sensitivity after femtosecond laser flap creation: clinical findings and management. J Cataract Refract Surg 32:91–94
2. Haft P, Yoo SH, Kymionis GD, Ide T, O'Brien TP, Culbertson WW (2009) Complications of LASIK flaps made by the IntraLase 15- and 30-kHz femtosecond lasers. J Refract Surg 25:979–984
3. Muñoz G, Albarrán-Diego C, Sakla HF, Javaloy J, Alió JL (2006) Transient light-sensitivity syndrome after laser in situ keratomileusis with the femtosecond laser Incidence and prevention. J Cataract Refract Surg 32:2075–2079

37 Pressure-Induced Interlamellar Stromal Keratitis

Alberto Artola

Contents

A. Artola, MD, PhD
Department of Refractive Surgery, Universidad Miguel Hernández de Elche, Alicante, Spain

Oftalmar, Medimar Hospital Internacional, Alicante, Spain
e-mail: alberto.artola@umh.es; albertoartola@coma.es

Why Is This Case Relevant for the Refractive Surgeon?

With recent advances and global practice of LASIK, the incidence of interface fluid syndrome is increasing [1–3]. Slit-lamp microscopy during early postoperative follow-up is essential in differentiating interface fluid syndrome from DLK or infectious keratitis [1].

Case Background

A 32-year-old male underwent a myopic LASIK procedure in 2002. His refraction was −8.00 (−2.50) 15° for the right eye (RE) and −7.00 (−2.00) 20° for the left eye (LE) and his BCVA was 20/25 bilaterally. Full ophthalmological evaluation of the patient revealed a typical myopia profile. One week after an uneventful LASIK, UCVA was 20/25 bilaterally and the topical steroids were instilled for three more weeks per the postoperative protocol.

One month after the procedure, the patient developed corneal haze and infiltration that was diagnosed as late-onset DLK, and a topical antibiotic/steroid combination (Tobradex®) of one drop per hour was prescribed (Fig. 37.1). As the UCVA continued to drop, the decision was made to perform flap lifting and interface wound debridement and biopsy 10 days after the provisional diagnosis of DLK. After the procedure, the patient was discharged with a prescription of

J.L. Alió et al. (eds.), *Difficult and Complicated Cases in Refractive Surgery*,
DOI 10.1007/978-3-642-55238-0_37, © Springer-Verlag Berlin Heidelberg 2015

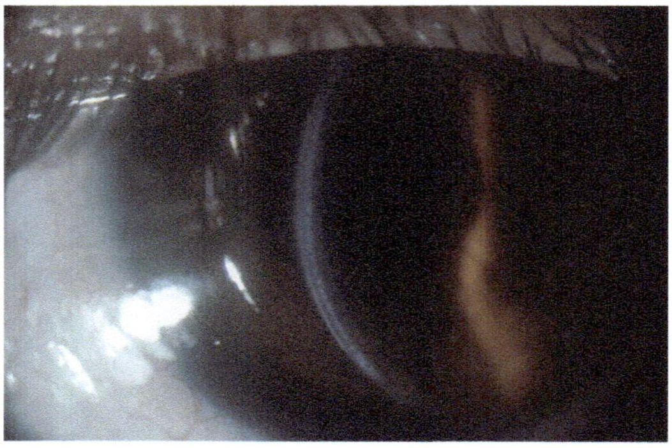

Fig. 37.1 Slit-lamp microscopy showing diffuse corneal interface infiltrate edema, including the inferior two-thirds of the flap

topical steroids (prednisolone acetate) one drop per hour along with topical antibiotics. One month later, the DLK reaction continued without responding to topical steroid therapy.

The patient underwent another flap lifting and interface wound debridement and biopsy. Two weeks later, the UCVA was 20/160 RE and 20/50 LE. An ocular examination at week 8 revealed a corneal infiltration and IOP measured via central corneal tonometry was found within normal limits (16 and 15 mmHg for right and left eyes, respectively). Topical beta-blockers were added to the treatment schedule for a few days by the treating ophthalmologist, together with continuation of the topical steroid (prednisolone acetate) drops every 4 h and ointment by night. However, no improvement was noted after 10 days. The IOP measuring the central cornea showed 10 mmHg bilaterally. The infiltration progressed and UCVA decreased to 20/200 in the RE. The topical steroids were changed to fluorometholone every hour; other medications were stopped and the patient was admitted to the surgery room for the third time for the possibility of microbial keratitis.

Biopsy and culture results were taken during the intervention (later shown negative) and the interface was irrigated with fortified antibiotic solution. The procedure was complicated after 24 h by flap dislocation which necessitated suturing the corneal flap of the right eye. During the next 2 weeks, various treatment modalities with antibiotics and steroids were prescribed, but visual acuity improved only slightly to 20/63 in spite of intense medical therapies. The case was referred to our center after 3 months. Goldmann tonometry was used to measure the central and peripheral IOP. Elevated IOP (central cornea 17, 20 mmHg and peripheral cornea 32, 44 mmHg for right and left eyes, respectively) was confirmed and thought to be the cause of interface fluid syndrome, which masqueraded as infective keratitis. Antiglaucoma therapy in the form of systemic carbonic anhydrase inhibitors (CAI) 250 mg/6 h and topical beta-blocker (Betagan 0.5 %) were started. The dose of fluorometholone was reduced (1 drop/12 h) and finally eliminated after 3 days.

Main Problem to Solve

Determining the differential diagnoses of DLK, pseudo-DLK, and infectious keratitis after LASIK.

Ancillary Tests

Measuring central and peripheral IOP and performing the microbial culture.

Surgical/Medical Intervention

The treatment of choice is topical antiglaucoma therapy with the elimination of topical steroids.

Outcome

One week later, the UCVA had improved to 20/40 bilaterally and IOP measurements were 10 and 12 mmHg (central and peripheral readings respectively, bilaterally). Ophthalmological examination showed corneal astigmatism, central faint corneal leukoma, interface cicatrization with flap edge fibrosis (Fig. 37.2), and optic nerve damage together with visual-field glaucomatous damage.

What to Learn from This Case

Pressure-induced interlamellar stromal keratitis simulating infectious keratitis should be regarded as a differential diagnosis for those eyes that develop late DLK and are unresponsive to topical steroidal therapy [4, 5].

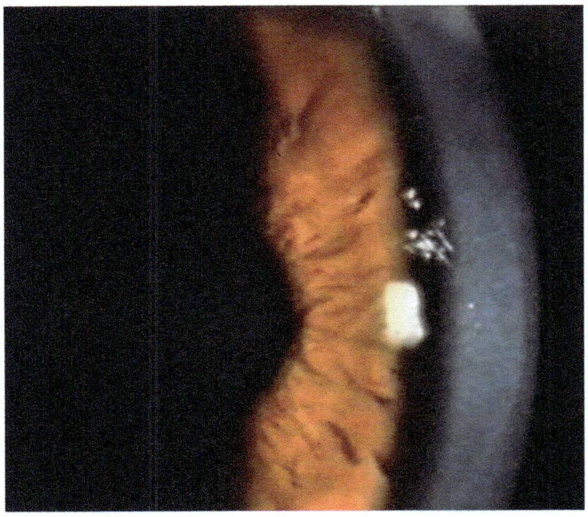

Fig. 37.2 Improvement of the interface fluid. Yet, haze at the borders of the flap persists even after successful syndrome treatment

References

1. Galal A, Artola A, Belda J, Rodriguez- Prats J, Claramonte P, Sánchez A, Ruiz-Moreno O, Merayo J, Alió JL (2006) Interface corneal edema secondary to steroid-induced elevation of intraocular pressure simulating diffuse lamellar keratitis. J Refract Surg 22:441–447
2. Belin MW, Hannush SB, Yau CW, Schultze RL (2002) Elevated intraocular pressured-induced interlamellar stromal keratitis. Ophthalmology 109:1929–1933
3. Davidson RS, Brandt JD, Mannis MJ (2003) Intraocular pressure-induced interlamellar keratitis after LASIK surgery. J Glaucoma 12:23–26
4. Nordlund ML, Grimm S, Lane S, Holland EJ (2004) Pressure-induced interface keratitis: a late complication following LASIK. Cornea 23:225–234
5. Najman-Vainer J, Smith RJ, Maloney RK (2002) Interface fluid after LASIK: misleading tonometry can lead to end-stage glaucoma. J Cataract Refract Surg 26:471–472

Early Flap Striae

38

Roger F. Steinert

Contents

R.F. Steinert, MD
Department of Refractive Surgery, Gavin Herbert Eye Institute, University of California, Irvine, CA, USA
e-mail: steinert@uci.edu

Why Is This Case Relevant for the Refractive Surgeon?

Flap striae can reduce corrected distance visual acuity (CDVA). When recognized and treated immediately, striae generally can be reduced to a level that is clinically insignificant [1, 2].

Case Background

Patient presents at an early exam (typically the first post-op exam, unless there is later trauma to the cornea) with suboptimal CDVA and with striae visible at the slit-lamp examination.

Main Problem to Solve

Treat the striae to allow full CDVA and maximal uncorrected distance visual acuity (UDVA). Differential diagnosis is between microstriae and macrostriae. Microstriae are fine "lacquer" cracks, random in orientation, and due to the compression of the anterior cornea when the flap is forced into place on a flatter corneal bed after moderate to high myopic correction, and/or due to compression and reverse curling damage to the Bowman layer by a microkeratome. Not all microstriae are optically significant (Fig. 38.1). Macrostriae are larger folds, semi-parallel, and usually greater on one side of the flap,

J.L. Alió et al. (eds.), *Difficult and Complicated Cases in Refractive Surgery*,
DOI 10.1007/978-3-642-55238-0_38,

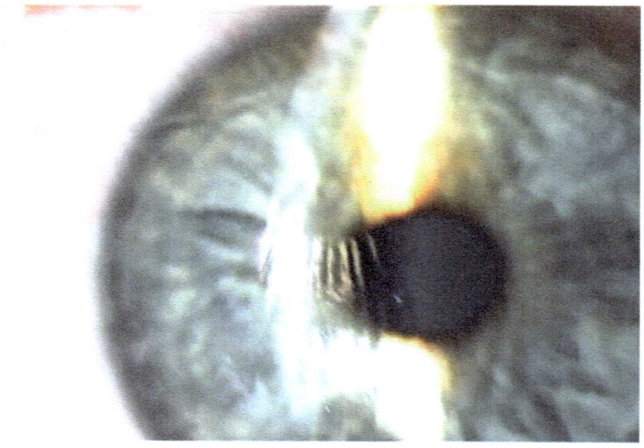

Fig. 38.1 Microstriae

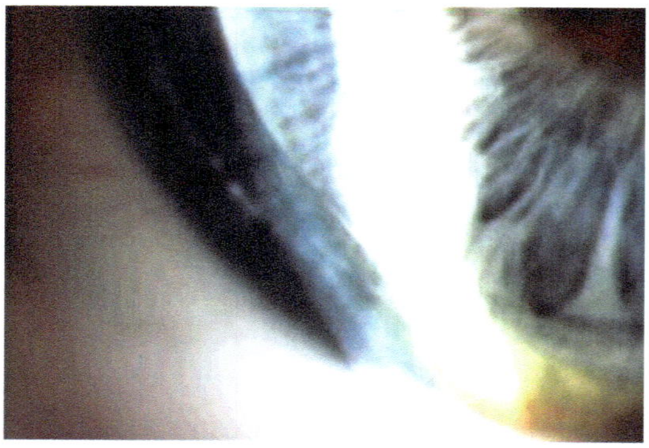

Fig. 38.2 Macrostriae

as macrostriae are due to slippage and subsequent compression of a portion of the flap (Fig. 38.2).

Ancillary Tests

1. Assess the tear film and cornea with fluorescein. If microstriae are optically significant, the tear film would be disrupted over the elevated microstriae ("negative staining" as shown in Fig. 38.3). A smooth tear film indicates that the microstriae may not be optically significant. With macrostriae, the tear film will always be disrupted over the large corneal folds. Moreover, the fluorescein will pool and/or frankly stain the gutter where the flap has shifted away from the proper position.
2. Corneal topography with a Placido ring pattern will show disruption of the corneal surface.

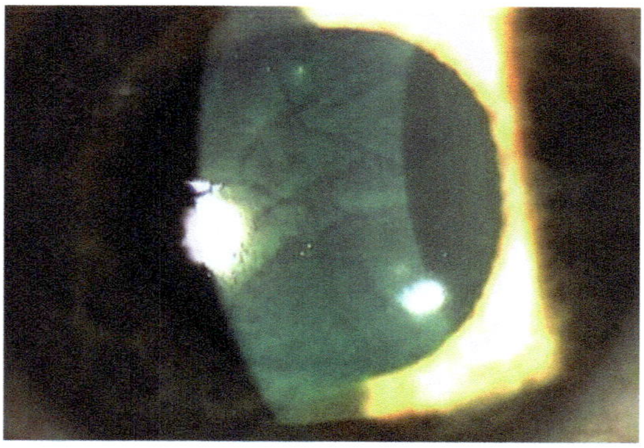

Fig. 38.3 Negative staining

3. Rigid contact lens placement will resolve any visual disturbances.

Surgical/Medical Intervention

The flap is refloated and repositioned. A bandage soft contact lens is applied for 24 h.

Outcome

Excellent UDVA and CDVA

What to Learn from This Case

Immediate intervention will yield excellent results; delay in intervention may result in recalcitrant striae that are difficult or impossible to eliminate.

References

1. Steinert RF, Ashrafzadeh A, Hersh PS (2004) Results of phototherapeutic keratectomy in the management of flap striae after LASIK. Ophthalmology 111:740–746
2. Ashrafzadeh A, Steinert RF (2007) Results of phototherapeutic keratectomy in the management of flap striae after LASIK before and after developing a standardized protocol: long term follow-up in an expanded patient population. Ophthalmology 114:1118–1123

Management of Recalcitrant Flap Macrostriae

39

Scott Kelly and Dimitri T. Azar

Contents

S. Kelly (✉) • D.T. Azar, MD, MBA
Department of Ophthalmology and Visual Sciences
Illinois Eye and Ear Infirmary,
University of Illinois at Chicago,
Chicago, IL, USA
e-mail: scottkellyy@gmail.com; dazar@uic.edu

Why Is This Case Relevant for the Refractive Surgeon?

Flap macrostriae are relatively rare but can be a very challenging complication of LASIK surgery [1]. This case demonstrates early and late decision-making paradigm for managing flap macrostriae.

Case Background

Our patient is a 29-year-old male who presented for evaluation for laser vision correction. He was intolerant to contact lenses and wanted to get out of his glasses. He had no past ocular or medical history. He took no medications and is allergic to penicillin.

Wearing his current prescription, his vision was $20/20^{-1}$ in the right eye with −8.50 + 1.00 × 079 and $20/20^{-2}$ in the left eye with −8.50 + 1.00 × 084. Auto refraction showed −8.25 +1.00 × 092 in the right eye and −8.00 +1.00 × 093 in the left eye. He saw 20/15 in the right eye with −8.00 +0.50 × 092 and 20/15 in the left eye with −8.00 +1.00 × 095. Stability in refraction was confirmed by comparing the patient's current glasses to a prescription he brought from 5 years earlier.

Slit lamp exam revealed clear corneas, deep anterior chambers, and clear lenses in both eyes. Pachymetry was 596 in the right eye and 605 in the left eye. Tonometry was 17 mmHg OD and 16 mmHg OS. Scotopic pupil diameters were

J.L. Alió et al. (eds.), *Difficult and Complicated Cases in Refractive Surgery*,
DOI 10.1007/978-3-642-55238-0_39, © Springer-Verlag Berlin Heidelberg 2015

5.9 mm OD and 5.7 mm OS. Schirmer test was normal. Dilated fundus exam was normal OU.

The risks and benefits of LASIK versus Epi-LASIK with mitomycin C were discussed with the patient. Given good pachymetry and Schirmer test result and reasonable expectations, he decided to proceed with femtosecond and wavefront-guided LASIK in both eyes.

His treatment application was −7.03 +0.61 × 090 in the right eye and −7.32 +0.69 × 093 in the left eye.

The postoperative day 1 visit was uneventful, with uncorrected visual acuity of $20/25^{-2}$ in the right eye and 20/20 in the left eye. He did have extensive punctate epithelial changes. There was no evidence of cell or flare in the anterior chambers OU. He was placed on prednisolone acetate and Zymaxid four times daily and artificial tears every hour.

At postoperative day 10, the patient returned with decreased vision in the right eye that was worse at near vision. He maintained good subjective vision in the left eye. He was still using prednisolone acetate four times daily and frequent artificial tears. Uncorrected visual acuity was $20/25^{-2}$ in the right eye and 20/20 in the left eye. Slit lamp exam revealed large central flap "wrinkles" in both corneas, but more severe in the right. Steroids were tapered, and the patient was brought back 1 week later.

Main Problem to Solve

The issue in this case is how to manage flap macrostriae. Our initial management was conservative, namely, continuing frequent artificial tears and then attempting correction with spectacles. What are the other options we may try in this case? The patient was given the option of observation versus surgical management.

Ancillary Tests

Corneal topography is necessary to evaluate for corneal astigmatism. OCT may be valuable because it can allow direct visualization of striae. In our patient, the OCT was non-revealing (Fig. 39.1).

Outcome

Three weeks following LASIK surgery, his vision was slightly improved in the right eye, but was subjectively worse binocularly at night and at near vision. His uncorrected visual acuity was $20/20^{-2}$ in the right eye and 20/20 in the left eye. His vision improved to 20/20 in both eyes with −0.50 +0.75 × 170 in the right eye and +0.25 +0.25 × 076 in the left eye. Slit lamp examination showed flap wrinkles were mildly improved OU. He was still using prednisolone acetate four times daily and frequent artificial tears. The decision was made to give corrective lenses to see if the symptoms improve in the right eye.

Three months after the surgery, the patient was more symptomatic and unsatisfied with his spectacles. He was still having trouble with his night vision and near vision in his right eye more than his left eye.

The patient was given, again, the option of observation versus flap lift and flap suturing. He elected the flap OD lift and suture.

The flap edge was marked and lifted, and the stromal bed was irrigated profusely. The flap was then stretched, refloated, and laid back into place. Seven interrupted 10-0 nylon sutures were then used to stretch and hold the flap in place. The suture knots were buried, and a bandage contact lens was placed over the eye.

One day later, the patient's uncorrected vision was 20/200 in the right eye with seven sutures in place and a few macrostriae still present; however, the central cornea was free of striae. High with-the-rule astigmatism was noted on Pentacam photography (Fig. 39.2). The patient continued to improve, and at the 3-week postoperative visit, his uncorrected vision was 20/100 in the right eye with sutures in. Corrected visual acuity was 20/20 with −2.75 +1.00 × 158. The flap sutures were removed at this point.

Over the next few months, the patient's recovery was complicated by anterior uveitis of unknown etiology and elevated intraocular pressure in the right eye. He was treated with prednisolone acetate and timolol. Once resolved (approximately 5 months after flap suturing), the patient's uncorrected visual acuity was $20/25^{-2}$ in

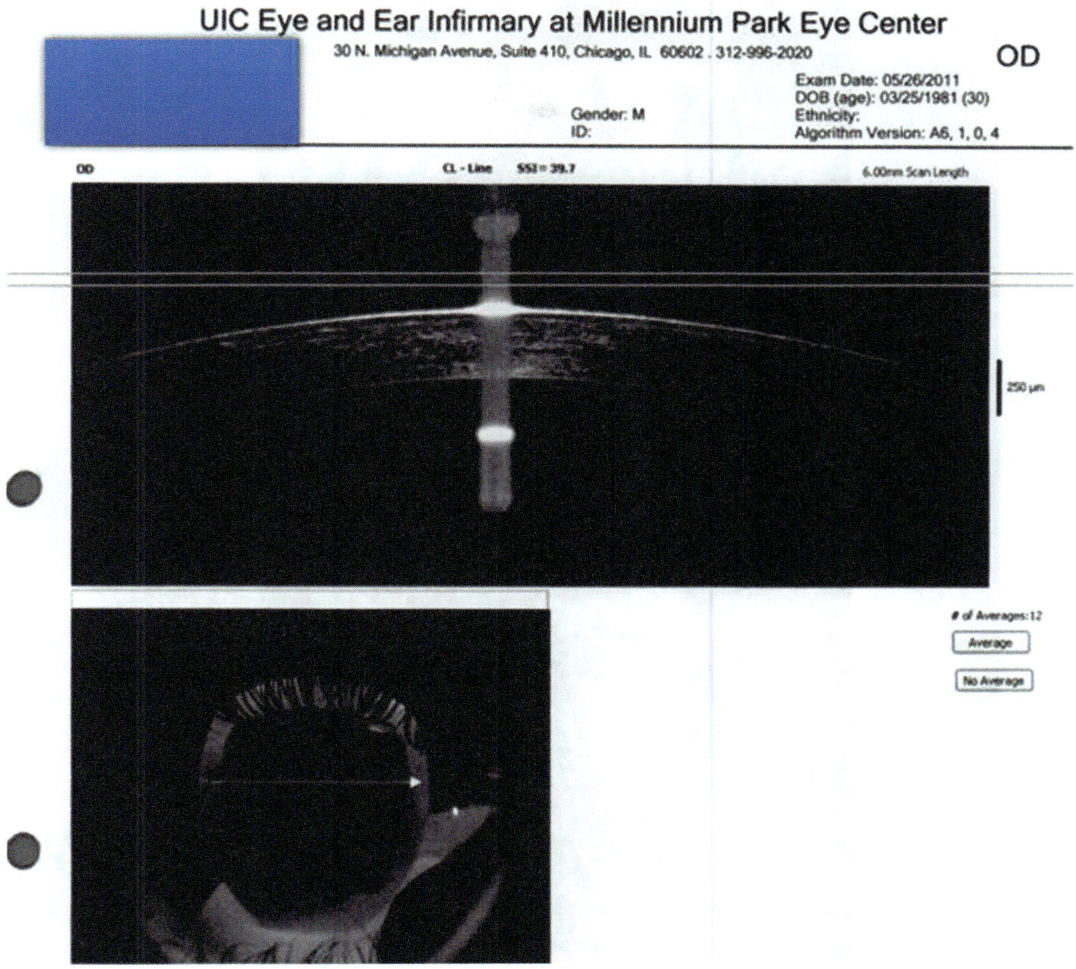

Fig. 39.1 OCT of striae

the right eye and corrected to 20/15^{-2} with −0.50 +0.50 × 160. There were a few macrostriae still present in both eyes, but both central corneas were clear and free of striae. Over several months, however, the striae slowly reformed in the central cornea, but were not associated with a decrease in visual acuity OD or topographical abnormalities (Fig. 39.3).

What to Learn from This Case

Flap macrostriae can be a difficult problem to solve. They are most common in patients who squeeze their eyes postoperatively. They cause varying degrees of visual symptoms when present, mostly depending on size, location, and individual patient awareness [1]. Flap lift and suturing to stretch and flatten the flap is an effective treatment against macrostriae, but it should be performed relatively early in the postoperative course [1, 2]. A higher incidence of flap folds is found in high myopes due to reduced central convexity of the stromal bed resulting in central flap redundancy and a tenting effect over the central cornea. Striae may occur intraoperatively from misalignment of the flap to the globe. These may be seen in the immediate postoperative period. This case exhibits striae that occur in the early postoperative period from sliding or dislodgement of the flap,

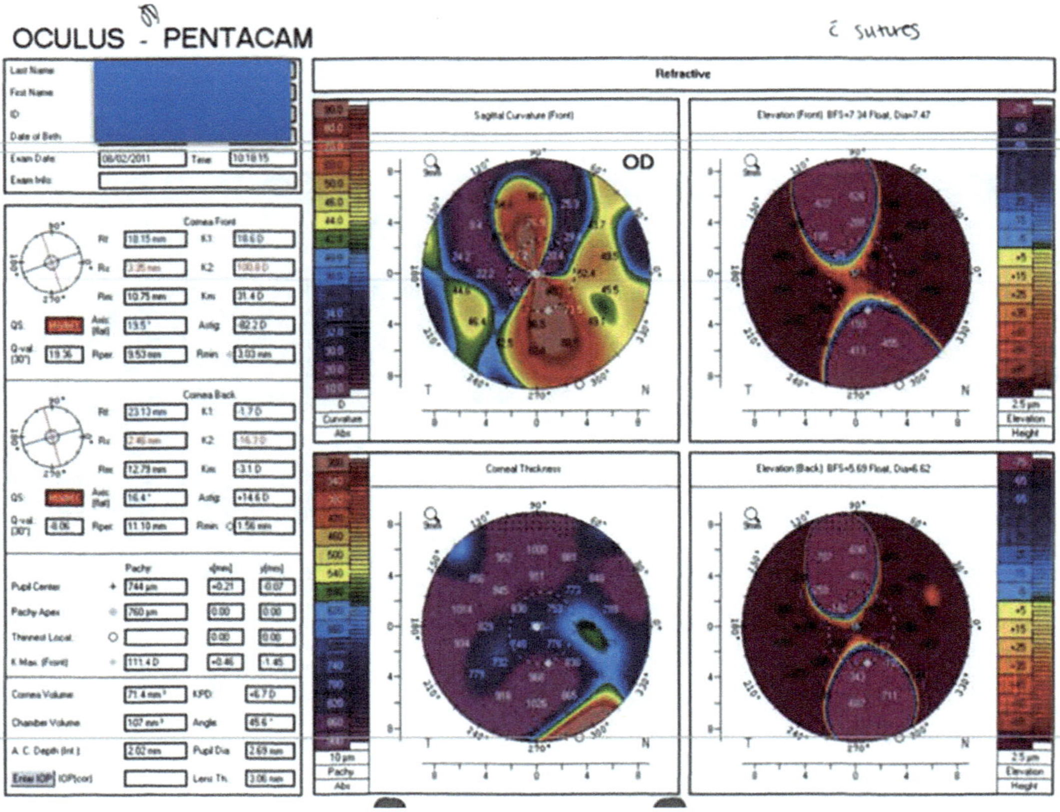

Fig. 39.2 Pentacam with K sutures

likely caused by eye rubbing or eyelid pressure during blinking. Flap folds may induce irregular astigmatism and optical aberrations along with glare and reduced visual acuity. The folds are best visualized with sodium fluorescein showing negative-staining lines.

The earlier flap folds are attended to, the better the chance for resolution. In the early postoperative period, the flap may be lifted and refloated into proper position. Deionized water has also been shown to help hydrate the flap and reduce postoperative folds. With time these folds may become fixed when epithelial hyperplasia occurs. Once the folds become fixed, lifting and flattening of the flap may be attempted with sutures or even with a LASIK flap iron.

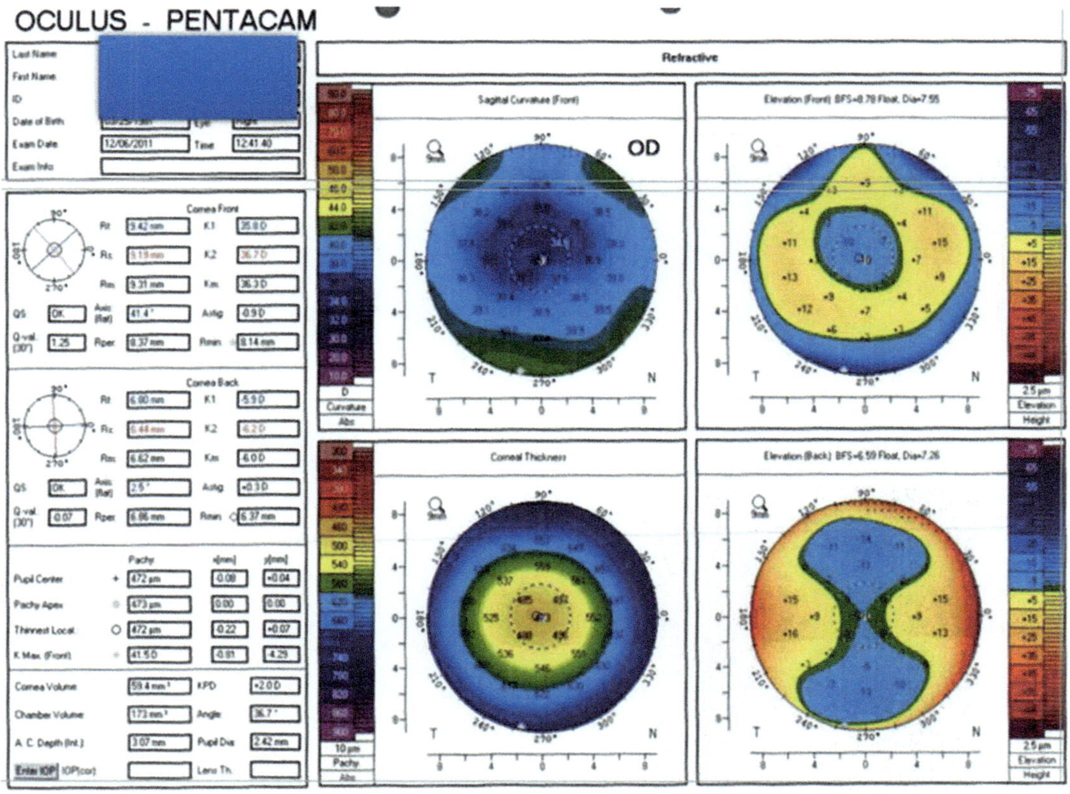

Fig. 39.3 Pentacam after suture removal

References

1. Steinert RF (2008) Prevention and management of flap striae after LASIK. In: Alio JL, Azar DT (eds) Management of complications in refractive surgery. Springer, Berlin/Heidelberg, pp 49–54
2. Lichter H, Russell GE, Waring GO III (2004) Repositioning the laser in situ keratomileusis flap at the slit lamp. J Refract Surg 20:166–169

40 Marginal Sterile Corneal Infiltrates

Renato Ambrósio Jr., I. Ramos, and F.F. Correia

Contents

R. Ambrósio Jr., MD, PhD (✉) • I. Ramos
F.F. Correia
Instituto de Olhos Renato Ambrósio
& VisareRIO Refracta Personal Laser,
Rio de Janeiro, Brazil

Department of Ophthalmology, Pontific Catholic University, Rio de Janeiro, Brazil

Federal University of São Paulo, São Paulo, Brazil
e-mail: dr.renatoambrosio@gmail.com

Why Is This Case Relevant for the Refractive Surgeon?

Acute, culture-negative, peripheral catarrhal infiltrates of the cornea can occur in the early postoperative period following LASIK. This complication typically occurs in patients with chronic blepharitis and meibomian gland dysfunction (MGD) [1]. Bilateral involvement is common if both eyes undergo operation on the same day. In this case, multiple whitish stromal infiltrates occurred in both eyes the first day after LASIK. The patient also had acne rosacea and hypercholesterolemia, which are significant risk factors [2, 3].

Case Background

A 49-year-old male presented for correction of myopic astigmatism. The patient denied past ocular disease and surgery denied atopic diseases. His cycloplegic refraction was −6.50 +1.75 × 5° RE and −7.00 +2.25 × 135° LE, and his corrected distance visual acuity (CDVA) was 20/20^{+} in each eye. Preoperative ophthalmologic examination was remarkable for moderate blepharitis and meibomian gland dysfunction (MGD). The remainder of the examination was within normal limits in both eyes. Bilateral LASIK was performed with the goal of full correction. On the first postoperative day, uncorrected distance visual acuity (UDVA) was 20/40 in each eye.

J.L. Alió et al. (eds.), *Difficult and Complicated Cases in Refractive Surgery*,
DOI 10.1007/978-3-642-55238-0_40, © Springer-Verlag Berlin Heidelberg 2015

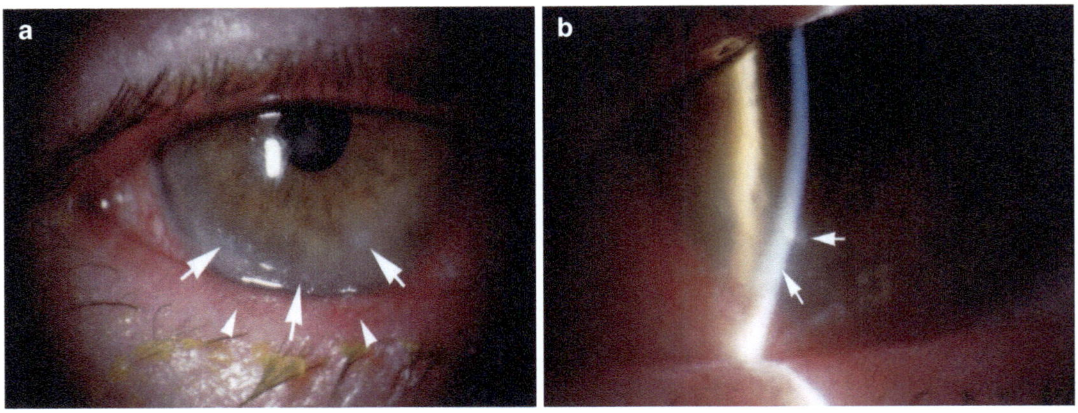

Fig. 40.1 (**a**) Numerous peripheral infiltrates located just outside the flap edge (*arrows*) on the first day after LASIK. (**b**) High magnification demonstrates the clear zone (also called the lucid interval) between the infiltrates and the limbus

Slit-lamp cornea examination was remarkable for clear flaps but with numerous peripheral infiltrates located just outside the flap edge, with a clear zone between the infiltrates and the limbus (Fig. 40.1). The infiltrates resembled marginal catarrhal keratitis infiltrates.

Main Problem to Solve

It is important to inform the patient regarding the potential of marginal sterile corneal infiltrates and the likely need for a second surgical intervention. The primary treatment goal is to minimize the sequelae induced by inflammation. Clinically, it is important to exclude an infectious process, and the culture is essential in order to exclude bacteria or fungus. Herpes virus peripheral keratitis should be also considered as a differential diagnosis.

Ancillary Tests

Bacterial and fungal cultures were obtained. Because of the peripheral location of multiple infiltrates, the condition was thought to be noninfectious. However, treatment with fortified antibiotics was continued until the cultures were verified.

Surgical/Medical Intervention

On the first postoperative day, the patient was started on fortified vancomycin (50 mg/ml) and tobramycin (50 mg/ml) every hour in addition to prednisolone acetate 1 % every hour. There was marked improvement of the infiltrates over the next 3 days and prednisolone acetate 1 % was tapered to four times per day.

Three days after surgery, the patient developed small peripheral epithelial defects and 5 days after surgery stage III diffuse lamellar keratitis (DLK) developed in both eyes. Both flaps were lifted for irrigation and cleaning. The patient was started on doxycycline 100 mg twice a day and received lid hygiene instructions. Prednisolone acetate 1 % was increased to eight times per day. Significant improvement was noted over the next 2 days. Vancomycin and tobramycin were tapered to four times per day. Prednisolone acetate 1 % was tapered to six times per day. Meanwhile, cultures were negative for bacteria and fungus. Based on these findings, vancomycin and tobramycin were discontinued and the prednisolone acetate was slowly tapered over 1 month. The patient was asked to continue doxycycline 100 mg each day, lid hygiene, and to use FML QID OU for 2 more weeks. At 3 months after surgery, his cycloplegic refraction demonstrated regression to -3.25 $+1.25 \times 46°$ with

20/20⁻ in the right eye and −2.75 +0.75 × 155° with 20/20⁻ in the left eye. Corneal topography showed centered ablations with flattening. The patient had stopped using oral doxycycline due to gastric intolerance.

The patient requested LASIK enhancement and was warned of possible recurrence of the infiltrates. He was instructed to restart doxycycline 100 mg twice a day for 2 weeks prior to enhancement and prednisolone acetate 1 % four times a day, 3 days prior to enhancement. LASIK enhancement was performed in one eye at a time with an increase to prednisolone acetate 1 % to six times a day on a taper over 1 month. After the enhancement in each eye, there was mild recurrence of the peripheral infiltrates without signs of DLK. At the 1-week postoperative examination, UCVA was 20/20⁻ in his right eye and 20/25⁻ in his left eye with clear corneas on slit-lamp examination.

Outcome

The infiltrates resolved with intensive high-penetration topical corticosteroid treatment. The clinical findings, clinical courses, and response to corticosteroid treatment were highly reminiscent of classic marginal catarrhal keratitis, suggesting a similar pathophysiologic mechanism.

What to Learn from This Case

Preoperative screening is a key factor for success in keratorefractive surgery. In order to reduce the likelihood of marginal sterile corneal infiltrates, we recommend that [1] patients with moderate blepharitis and/or meibomian gland dysfunction receive prophylactic treatment prior to surgery. Classically, lid scrubs, hygiene, omega-3-type essential fatty acid nutritional supplementation, and doxycycline treatment (100 mg BID) should be considered. Prophylactic pretreatment with high-penetration corticosteroids for 2–3 days prior to LASIK may be helpful for eyes with residual signs of blepharitis and meibomian gland dysfunction despite lid hygiene and doxycycline. These patients should be monitored carefully following surgery, with more intensive corticosteroid treatment initiated if peripheral catarrhal infiltrates appear in the early postoperative period. Recurrence is likely with LASIK enhancement but is attenuated with treatment of high-penetration corticosteroids prior to reoperation [4, 5].

References

1. Ambrósio R Jr, Wilson SE (2001) LASIK complications: etiology, prevention, and treatment. J Refract Surg 17:350–379
2. MacRae S, Macaluso DC, Rich LF (1999) Sterile interface keratitis associated with micropannus hemorrhage after laser in situ keratomileusis. J Cataract Refract Surg 25:1679–1681
3. Macaluso DC, Rich LF, MacRae S (1999) Sterile interface keratitis after laser in situ keratomileusis: three episodes in one patient with concomitant contact dermatitis of the eyelids. J Refract Surg 15:679–682
4. Johnson JD, Harissi-Dagher M, Pineda R, Yoo S, Azar DT (2001) Diffuse lamellar keratitis: incidence, associations, outcomes, and a new classification system. J Cataract Refract Surg 27:1560–1566
5. Wilson SE, Ambrósio R Jr (2002) Sporadic diffuse lamellar keratitis (DLK) following LASIK: contrast with epidemic (exogenous) DLK. Cornea 21:560–563

Hypersensitivity to Vancomycin

41

Jorge L. Alió and Alessandro Abbouda

Contents

J.L. Alió, MD, PhD (✉)
Department of Refractive Surgery,
Vissum Corporación Oftalmológica,
Alicante, Spain
e-mail: jlalio@vissum.com

A. Abbouda, MD
Department of Refractive Surgery,
Vissum Corporación Oftalmológica, Alicante, Spain

Department of Ophthalmology-Policlinico Umberto I of Rome, University of Rome "Sapienza", Viale del Policlinico, 155, 00186 Roma, Italy

R&D Department, Vissum Corporación Oftalmológica, 03016, Alicante, Spain
e-mail: a.abbouda@gmail.com

Why Is This Case Relevant for the Refractive Surgeon?

Vancomycin, a glycopeptide antibiotic, is effective in treating methicillin-resistant *Staphylococcus aureus* (MRSA) infections. A topical application of vancomycin solution prepared by in-house prescription is used to treat ocular infections [1]. However, this application can cause patient compliance problems [2]. We describe a case of vancomycin hypersensitivity after refractive surgery. The refractive surgeon's awareness of complicating factors in vancomycin treatment is important in supporting optimum patient outcomes.

Case Background

A 30-year-old man came to our center 48 h after an iLASIK procedure. The flap in his left eye was lifted after 24 h due to the presence of meibomian secretion in the interface and was scraped by vancomycin. The patient was treated with a topical steroid (dexamethasone one drop every 2 h), vancomycin, and ceftazidime (one drop every hour). He presented complaining of reduced vision, pain, and redness. Ophthalmological examination showed a best-corrected visual acuity (BCVA) of 20/125, a perikeratic reaction, and a central fluorescein-positive ulcer (Fig. 41.1a).

We decided to stop the topic treatment and tape the eye. The next day, the ulcer appeared

J.L. Alió et al. (eds.), *Difficult and Complicated Cases in Refractive Surgery*,
DOI 10.1007/978-3-642-55238-0_41, © Springer-Verlag Berlin Heidelberg 2015

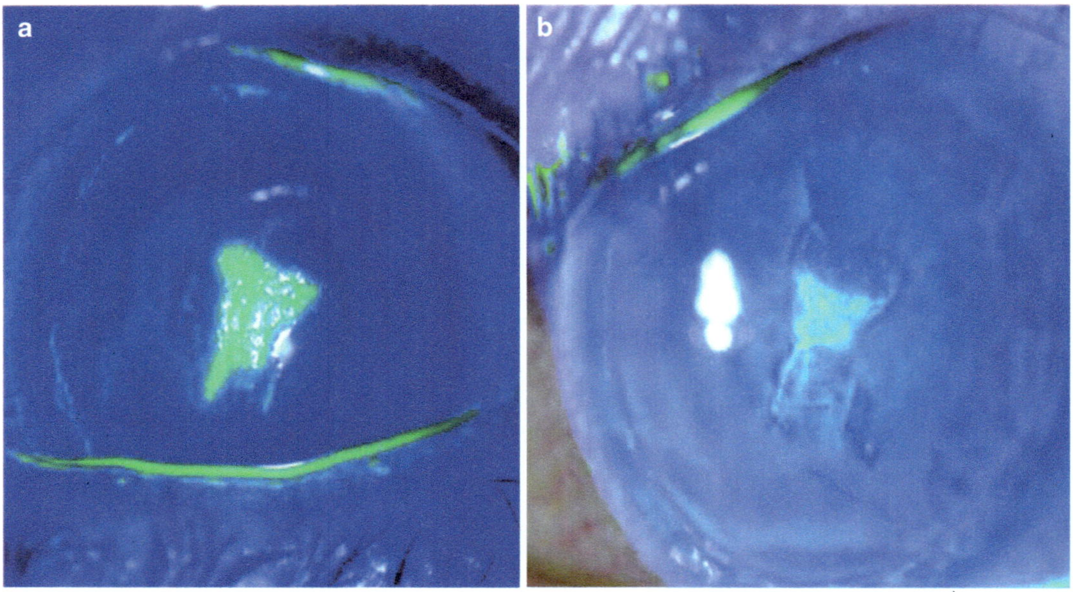

Fig. 41.1 (**a**) Slit-lamp photography at the first visit. Central ulcer staining fluorescein and corneal edema. (**b**) Slit-lamp photography a day later, showing reduction of corneal edema and ulcer and a clear margin

smaller with a clear margin (Fig. 41.1b) and the patient started prednisone, one drop eight times a day, and ofloxacin, one drop two times a day, tapering off to one drop of steroids per week. After 3 weeks, BCVA was 20/32, the ulcer was completely resolved, but epithelial in growth appeared near the margin of the lesion (Fig. 41.2a). At 5 months, BCVA was 20/25 and we decided to perform YAG laser. Following steroid therapy and YAG laser treatment, the slit-lamp examination showed a tender interface opacity in the area of the previous ulcer (Fig. 41.2b). At 9 months we performed a PTK, and 1-month post BCVA was 20/20 (Fig. 41.2c).

Main Problem to Solve

In this case, the slight interface opacity created by the meibomian secretion did not justify scraping and lifting of the flap with vancomycin. The use of this antibiotic must alert the surgeon to a differential diagnosis such as infectious or lamellar keratitis.

Ancillary Tests

Close follow-up with meticulous slit-lamp examination is critical to determine the evolution of this syndrome. Generally, hypersensitive reactions of systemic vancomycin include maculopapular rash, urticaria, drug fever, vasculitis, anaphylaxis, IgA bullous dermatosis, and Stevens-Johnson syndrome or toxic epidermal necrolysis [3]. Ocular manifestation includes periorbital skin rash, conjunctival congestion, corneal epithelial defects with stromal edema, and Descemet membrane striae [4].

Surgical/Medical Intervention

We preferred to treat the complication of epithelial ingrowth by YAG laser to avoid lifting the flap again. Nd:YAG treatment for this complication was first described in 2008 [5]. In the only series published to date, 100 % of patients treated had topographic and symptomatic improvement. After 9 months of the first event, the patient underwent PTK obtaining a good VA in 1 month.

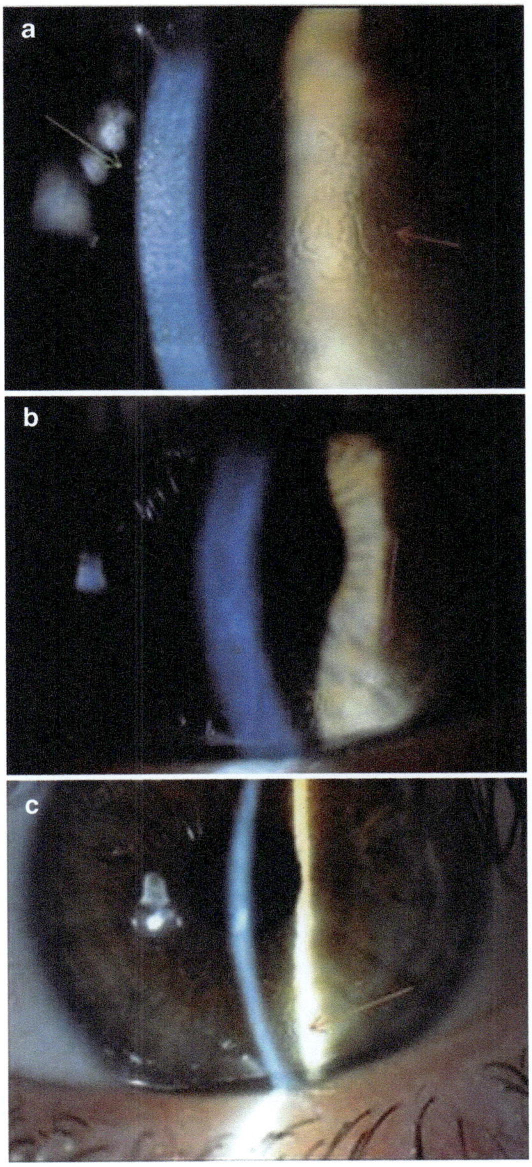

Fig. 41.2 (**a**) Slit-lamp photography 3 weeks after. *Red arrow* shows epithelial ingrowth in the interface and the *green arrow* shows opacity from the previous ulcer. (**b**) Slit-lamp photography 5 months after the YAG laser was performed. The *violet arrow* shows the persistence of the epithelial needle. (**c**) Slit-lamp photography 9 months after PTK was performed. The *orange arrow* shows a residual epithelial ingrowth and tender opacity in the central cornea

Outcome

After 1 month of PTK, the slit-lamp examination showed a clear interface with tender interface opacity. There were no epithelial cells and the flap was well positioned (Fig. 41.2c). BCVA was 20/20.

What to Learn from This Case

The surgeon must be aware of this syndrome and differential diagnoses. Ciliary reaction, conjunctival hyperemia, stromal infiltrates, and epithelial defect that stains with fluorescein are common symptoms of both hypersensitivity to vancomycin and infectious or lamellar keratitis. The correct anamnesis and use of vancomycin can help to differentiate. Although topical corticosteroid treatment (preservative-free) can resolve cornea opacity and the inflammation over a period of weeks to months, permanent sequelae such as corneal opacity do occur. Patients receiving topical treatment with vancomycin need to be informed about possible adverse complications.

References

1. Goodman DF, Gottsch JD (1988) Methicillin-resistant staphylococcus epidermidis keratitis treated with vancomycin. Arch Ophthalmol 106:1570–1571
2. Fleischer AB, Hoover DL, Khan JA (1986) Topical vancomycin formulation for methicillin-resistant Staphylococcus epidermidis blepharoconjunctivitis. Am J Ophthalmol 101:283–287
3. Bernedo N, Gonza'lez I, Gastaminza G et al (2001) Positive patch test in vancomycin allergy. Contact Dermatitis 45:43
4. Hwu J-J, Chen K-H, Hsu W-M, Lai J-Y, Li Y-S (2005) Ocular hypersensitivity to topical vancomycin in a case of chronic endophthalmitis. Cornea 24:754–756
5. Ayala MJ, Alió JL, Mulet ME, De La Hoz F (2008) Treatment of laser in situ keratomileusis interface epithelial ingrowth with neodymium:yttrium-aluminum-garnet laser. Am J Ophthalmol 145:630–634

Management of Traumatic LASIK Flap Edge Invagination

42

Samuel H. Lee, Dimitri T. Azar, and Jose de la Cruz

Contents

Why Is This Case Relevant for the Refractive Surgeon?

Refractive surgeons who perform LASIK should be familiar with how to manage a traumatic flap dehiscence, as proper and timely diagnosis and management can increase the chance of an optimal visual outcome [1].

Case Background

A 49-year-old female with a history of bilateral myopic LASIK 5 years prior to presentation was poked in her right eye by a tree branch while gardening. She was treated for a corneal abrasion but still complained of blurry vision even after the epithelial defect had healed. She was referred to a cornea specialist who subsequently referred her to our institution for management.

She had no significant past medical or surgical history, other than the previous LASIK. On presentation, she was on antibiotic eye drops and artificial tears in the affected eye.

On examination, her uncorrected vision was $20/30^{-2}$ in the right and 20/25 in the left. She was able to read 20/20 with a −0.75 +1.00×045 refraction in the right and 20/20 with +0.50 sphere in the left. Her central corneal thickness was 454 and 448. Her tonometry was 13 and 13, and her confrontation fields, extraocular movements, and pupillary exam were normal.

S.H. Lee, MD (✉) • D.T. Azar, MD, MBA
J. de la Cruz
Department of Ophthalmology and Visual Sciences
Illinois Eye and Ear Infirmary, University of Illinois at Chicago, Chicago, IL, USA
e-mail: samuel.lee.md@gmail.com; dazar@uic.edu; josedlc@uic.edu

J.L. Alió et al. (eds.), *Difficult and Complicated Cases in Refractive Surgery*,
DOI 10.1007/978-3-642-55238-0_42, © Springer-Verlag Berlin Heidelberg 2015

On slit-lamp examination, she had a superonasal flap tear in the right eye, with a portion of the flap folded in on itself, with no epithelial defect, and 1 mm of epithelial downgrowth under the fold. The rest of the examination was normal.

Main Problem to Solve

Appropriate management in this case is imperative, as the patient is at risk for multiple complications including infectious keratitis (especially fungal keratitis from the tree branch injury), epithelial downgrowth, late-onset diffuse lamellar keratitis (DLK), and irregular astigmatism. After infection and DLK have been ruled out or treated, the fold in the flap and epithelial downgrowth should be addressed, as it can have visually significant consequences.

Ancillary Tests

We obtained corneal topography using a Scheimpflug camera (Pentacam) (Figs. 42.1 and 42.2) as well as anterior segment optical coherence tomography (OCT) (Fig. 42.3). Of note, there is significant irregular astigmatism in the meridian of the dehiscence (Fig. 42.1). In the OCT image, there is an area where the flap is thicker than the rest and not uniform. It is difficult to discern the epithelium in this image, because there is also epithelial downgrowth.

Surgical/Medical Intervention

After risks, benefits, and alternatives to treatment were discussed, the patient underwent epithelial debridement and flap repositioning of the superonasal flap in the right eye. After the right eye was prepped and draped and a speculum placed, the superonasal epithelium was removed with LASIK spatula and Weck-Cel sponges. Care was used to ensure that an adequate amount of epithelium was removed in order to unfold the flap, but the entire flap was not lifted. The flap was then unfolded, and scraping was performed on the underside of the flap as well as the stromal bed to remove any epithelial cells. This portion of the stromal bed was then irrigated with balanced salt solution (BSS) and the flap ironed in place with application with a Weck-Cel sponge. Approximately 1 mm of epithelium was removed on the host side of the flap, in the area that the flap was lifted to help reduce any recurrent epithelial downgrowth. A bandage contact lens was placed as well as prednisolone acetate and a fluoroquinolone eyedrop.

Outcome

On postoperative day #1, the patient had $20/20^{-2}$ uncorrected vision in the right eye. 1 week later, she was 20/25 uncorrected. The flap remains well positioned without striae and with small islands of epithelial downgrowth.

What to Learn from This Case

Important points from this case start with effective counseling of the patient, to seek care from an eye-care professional with any concerns of potential flap trauma that may go unrecognized [2]. Diagnosis of a folded flap can be difficult to make if the epithelium had grown over, but anterior segment imaging, especially with an OCT, can help. Surgical management of this case is preferable if the flap dehiscence leads to significant striae, or serves as a nidus for epithelial downgrowth [1–3]. Local debridement of epithelium can lower risk for downgrowth, and it is preferable to lift only the affected portion of the flap.

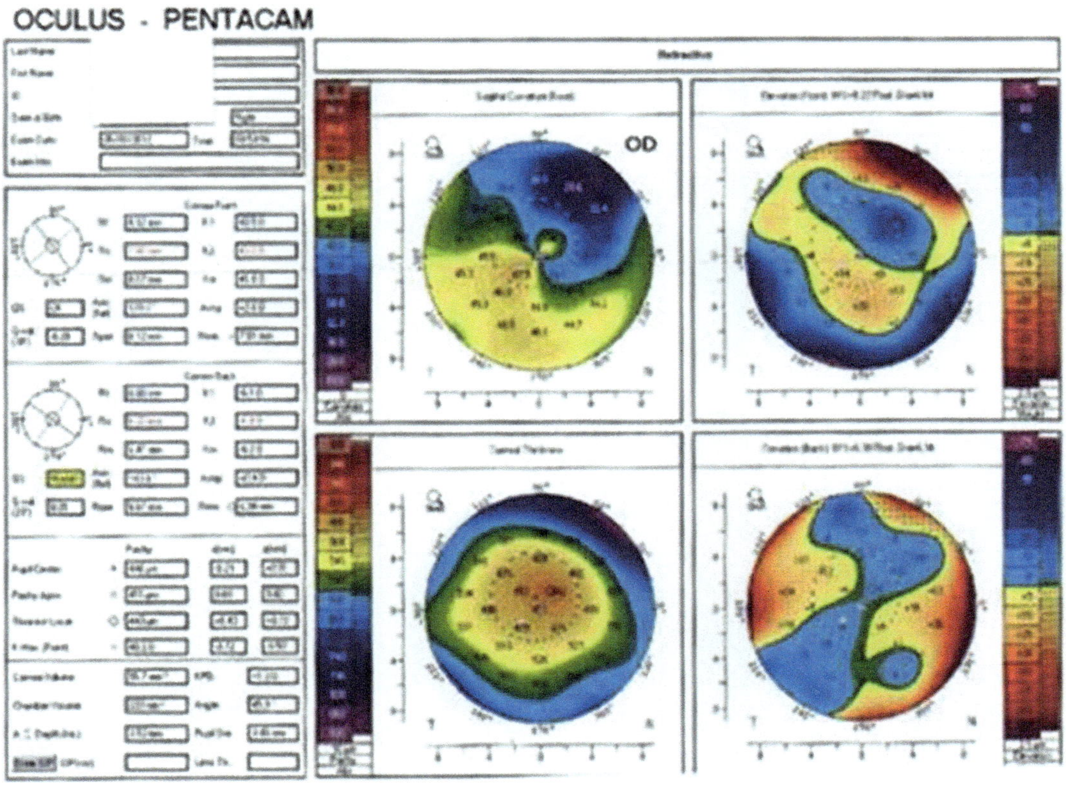

Fig. 42.1 Pentacam image, right eye

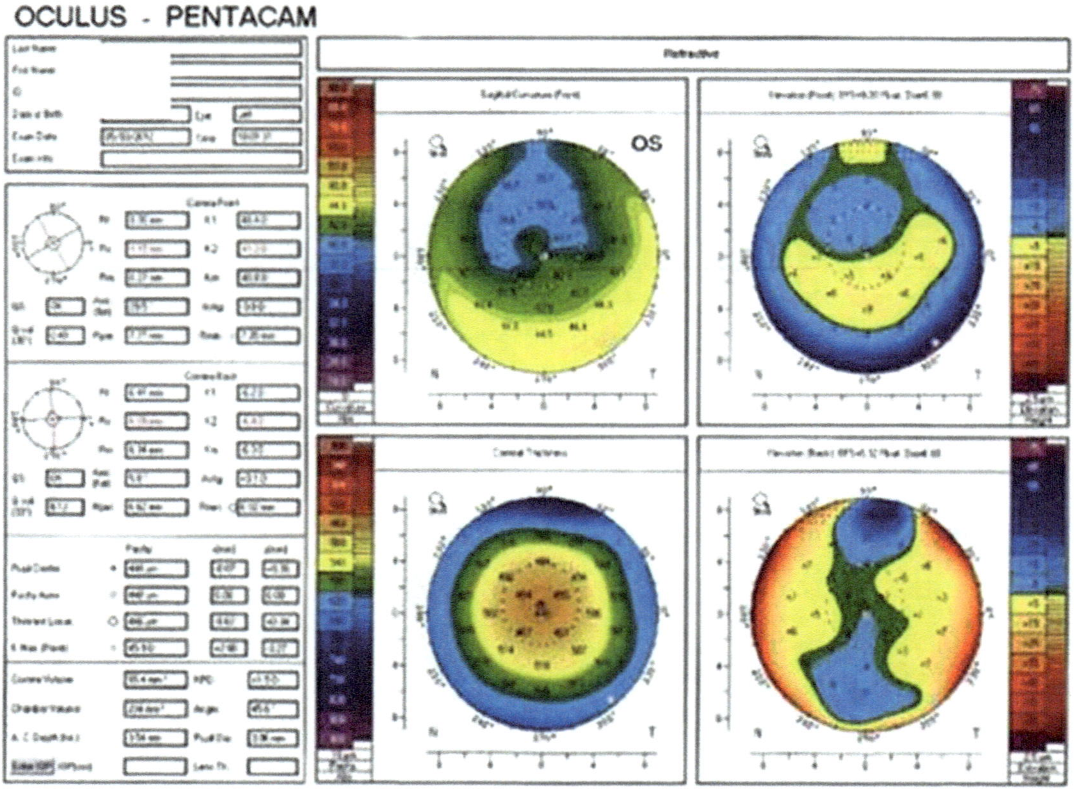

Fig. 42.2 Pentacam image, left eye

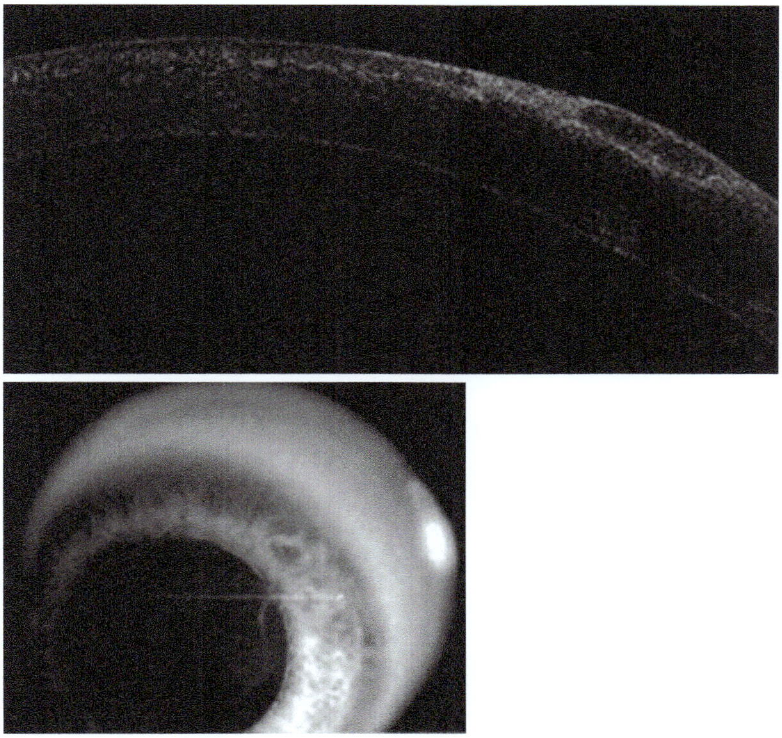

Fig. 42.3 Anterior segment OCT of traumatic flap dehiscence

References

1. Melki SA, Talamo JH, Demetriades AM, Jabbur NS, Essepian JP, O'Brien TP, Azar DT (2000) Late traumatic dislocation of laser in situ keratomileusis corneal flaps. Ophthalmology 107:2136–2139
2. Geggel HS, Coday MP (2001) Late-onset traumatic laser in situ keratomileusis (LASIK) flap dehiscence. Am J Ophthalmol 131:505–506
3. Pereira Cda R, Narvaez J, King JA, Seery LS, Gimbel HV (2006) Late-onset traumatic dislocation with central tissue loss of laser in situ keratomileusis flap. Cornea 25:1107–1110

Part IV

LASIK Late Postoperative Complications: Dry Eye Syndrome, Epithelial Ingrowth, Corneal Ectasia, and Other Complications

Dear reader,

This section includes many cases related to late LASIK postoperative complications that you will encounter during your clinical practice. We divide it into four sections.

In the first, we describe dry eye complication, the most common complication of LASIK and therefore the most relevant for patients.

The second section includes cases of epithelial ingrowth. Although incidence of epithelial ingrowth is declining due to progress of LASIK and knowledge of predisposing factors, awareness of the condition is still important. Cases cover management methods such as flap elevation, scraping, and the use of topography.

The third section includes cases of corneal ectasia and its management. New corneal measurement techniques should facilitate identification of patients at risk, but what do we currently know and do? This section provides an overview of available procedures, including transepithelial phototherapeutic keratectomy and deep anterior lamellar keratoplasty.

The fourth section covers miscellaneous cases including abnormal healing and ptosis after LASIK.

Although the incidence of late postoperative conditions in LASIK has declined thanks to growth in knowledge and technology, this section contains indispensable pearls for practice.

For further reading, we suggest the first book of this series: J.L. Alio', D. Azar *Management of Complications in Refractive Surgery*, Chapter 5: Lasik Early Postoperative Complication Refractive Surprise (pp. 74–101).

Specific topics covered by the cases include a new effective treatment for dry eye (Case 43), how to manage the most frequent complication after LASIK (Case 44), the importance of identifying epithelial membrane dystrophy before refractive surgery (Case 45), how to manage severe blepharitis and severe inflammation (Case 46), how to manage epithelial ingrowth (Case 47), how can corneal topography help us in the decision about epithelial ingrowth treatment (Case 48), and determining the clinical significance of epithelial ingrowth (Case 49). Other cases cover femtosecond penetrating keratoplasty and deep anterior lamellar keratoplasty (DALK) using a dovetail pattern for managing corneal ectasia (Cases 50 and 51), managing ectasia with DALK and transepithelial PRK with MMC (Case 52), and the use of collagen cross-linking post-LASIK ectasia with high coma aberrations (Case 53). Other topics cover ways of dealing with persistent flap striae (Case 54), with scarring following vertical breakthrough (Case 55), thin flap and keratocyte activation (Case 56), haze formation and a small depth (Case 57), late onset of DLK and trauma (Case 58), late regression (Case 59), and irregular astigmatism after 12 years from the first surgery (Case 60). We end with cases focused on lifting a flap after 15 years (Case 61), dealing with a rare complication, LASIK ptosis (Case 62), late DLK without an obvious cause (Case 63), and presurgical planning of corneal incision location before performing any intraocular procedure in patients who have previously undergone LASIK surgery (Case 64).

Lesson to Learn

Case 43: Ocular surface syndrome after LASIK treated with eye platelet-rich plasma (E-PRP)

How to use a new effective treatment eye platelet-rich plasma (E-PRP) teardrops for dry eye following LASIK.

Case 44: Management of post-LASIK dry eye disease

The most frequent complication after LASIK. How to manage this complication in a convenient way.

Case 45: Recurrent epithelial erosion after LASIK

The importance to identify epithelial membrane dystrophy before refractive surgery to adequately plan refractive surgery.

Case 46: Severe ocular surface inflammatory syndrome post-LASIK caused by blepharitis

A case of severe chronic blepharitis associated with severe inflammation. The negative culture, the absence of progression, and improvement with antibiotic drops help in the differential diagnosis.

Case 47: Epithelial ingrowth into visual axis after primary LASIK surgery treated by flap elevation and scraping.

How the quality of the flap edge and its inadequate manipulation are associated to the risk of intraoperative epithelial cell implantation leading to epithelial ingrowth.

Case 48: Use of topography in the management of epithelial ingrowth

How to use corneal topography as a good tool to follow the corneal melting related to epithelial ingrowth, leading the decisions on its treatment.

Case 49: Epithelial ingrowth after LASIK

How can you decide if epithelial ingrowth following LASIK is clinically significant and how it should be addressed?

Case 50: Management of corneal ectasia after LASIK with dovetail femtosecond penetrating keratoplasty

A case of corneal ectasia treated by penetrating keratoplasty which a good outcome.

Case 51: Ectasia post-LASIK managed by femtosecond-assisted deep anterior lamellar keratoplasty (DALK)

A case of patient suffering of post-LASIK corneal ectasia was solved by DALK.

Case 52: Management of corneal ectasia after LASIK with deep anterior lamellar keratoplasty (DALK) and transepithelial photorefractive keratectomy (PRK) with Mitomycin C

Another way to treat corneal ectasia post-LASIK using DALK. The high refractive error after the surgery was treated by topography-guided PRK.

Case 53: Transepithelial phototherapeutic keratectomy and corneal collagen cross-linking for patient affected by ectasia post-LASIK and with high coma aberration.

Simultaneous topography-guided PTK with corneal CXL appears to be an acceptable alternative for the management of some cases of post-LASIK corneal ectasia.

Case 54: Late flap striae

When striae have been present for a month or more, direct treatment of the elevations of the flap is needed to reduce the optical impact of the striae.

Case 55: Scaring

A case of vertical breakthrough who developed corneal scaring in the peripheral part of the femto flap.

Case 56: Abnormal healing in femtosecond LASIK

Thin flap and keratocyte activation. Unusual complication related to LASIK when the flap is too thin. How to manage it?

Case 57: Haze-related myopic shift after PRK on a LASIK-operated eye treated by transepithelial PTK

Haze formation induced by a small ablation depth surface treatment on a previous LASIK flap resolved by transepithelial PRK.

Case 58: Late-onset diffuse lamellar keratitis after LASIK in a patient with epithelial defect after microtrauma.

An epithelial microtrauma in a patient with previous LASIK surgery could be a risk for a late onset of DLK.

Case 59: Late-onset myopic regression 12 years following properly centered myopic LASIK

Three are the possible causes of late-onset myopic regression: worsening nuclear cataract, worsening axial myopia, or the development of corneal ectasia.

Case 60: Late-onset unilateral irregular mixed astigmatism following thick-flap LASIK

The differential diagnosis of late-onset irregular astigmatism after LASIK include preexisting keratoconus or forme fruste keratoconus, post-LASIK ectasia, PRK decentration (shift and/or drift), and deep LASIK.

Case 61: Flap lift after 15 years

Clinical examination before planning flap lift is mandatory. Lift has to be avoided if the flap does not show a good quality and if there is some doubt about the ectasia presence and residual stromal bed.

Case 62: Ptosis after LASIK

The cause of this complication is disinsertion, dehiscence, or damage to the levator aponeurosis, due to intraoperative mechanical insult to the levator during the retraction of the eyelids.

Case 63: Management of recalcitrant late-onset DLK after hyperopic LASIK
Medical and surgical options were discussed including topical steroids, systemic steroids, flap lifting and irrigation, laser retreatment, as well as keratoplasty.
Case 64: Management of corneal infiltrate after cataract surgery in a patient with previous LASIK treatment
A presurgical planning of corneal incision location is warranted before performing any intraocular procedure in patient with previous LASIK surgery.

Dry Eye Syndrome: Ocular Surface Syndrome After Lasik and Treated with Eye Platelet-Rich Plasma (E-PRP)

43

Jorge L. Alió and Alessandro Abbouda

Contents

J.L. Alió, MD, PhD (✉)
Department of Refractive Surgery, Vissum Corporación Oftalmológica, Alicante, Spain
e-mail: jlalio@vissum.com

A. Abbouda, MD
Department of Refractive Surgery, Vissum Corporación Oftalmológica, Alicante, Spain

Department of Ophthalmology-Policlinico Umberto I of Rome, University of Rome "Sapienza", Viale del Policlinico, 155, 00186 Roma, Italy

R&D Department, Vissum Corporación Oftalmológica, 03016, Alicante, Spain
e-mail: a.abbouda@gmail.com

Why Is This Case Relevant for the Refractive Surgeon?

The incidence of dry eye after LASIK ranges from 5 [1] to 52 % [2] among Caucasian patients, with a higher reported incidence among Asians [1]. This transitory condition, which typically resolves within 6–9 months after surgery [3], is neurotrophic in origin and is frequently associated with ocular surface inflammation. It can cause significant decrease in visual acuity and quality of vision.

Case Background

A 29-year-old woman came to our center complaining of pain and blurred vision in both eyes 2 years after having a LASIK procedure in another hospital for hyperopia. The ophthalmological examination showed a best-corrected visual acuity (BCVA) of 20/25 in both eyes and diffuse epithelial erosion. The Oxford scheme was IV (Fig. 43.1). The patient was treated with topical cyclosporine, steroids, and a lacrimal substitute without improvement. We decided to stop this treatment and begin "eye platelet-rich plasma" (E-PRP) [4] for 6 weeks followed by tacrolimus 0.03 %, one application overnight, and fluorometholone, one drop three times a day.

J.L. Alió et al. (eds.), *Difficult and Complicated Cases in Refractive Surgery*,
DOI 10.1007/978-3-642-55238-0_43, © Springer-Verlag Berlin Heidelberg 2015

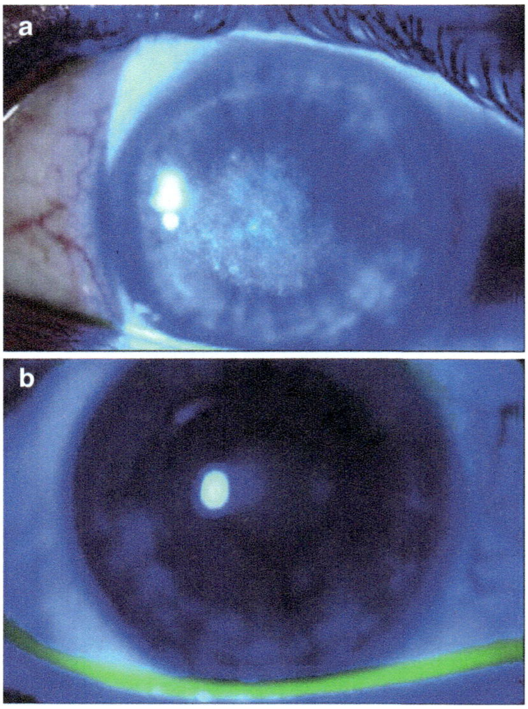

Fig. 43.1 (**a**) Severe cornea disepithelization at the beginning. (**b**) After 1 month of E-PRP treatment

Main Problem to Solve

After LASIK, the patient was affected by ocular surface syndrome that mimics Sjögren's syndrome [5]. Corneal refractive surgery should be avoided in this case because its risk factors correlate with the development of dry eye after LASIK. A refractive surgeon who understands the risk factors of dry eye will be able to select effective strategies to optimize the ocular surface prior to surgery and therefore improve outcomes.

Ancillary Tests

A diagnostic approach to patients with dry eye after LASIK includes the evaluation of tear film secretion through Schirmer's test, tear film volume using the phenol red test, tear film osmolality performed collecting the patient's tear meniscus at the slit lamp with a polyester rod, and tear film stability measuring tear breakup time. The severity of dry eye is evaluated by the Oxford scheme, which quantifies the amount of corneal and conjunctiva damaged. The OSDi (Ocular Surface Disease Index) questionnaire can help in evaluating the patient's symptoms.

Surgical/Medical Intervention

Eye platelet-rich plasma (E-PRP) provides a higher concentration of essential growth factors and cell adhesion molecules by concentrating platelets in a smaller volume of plasma compared to autologous serum. These growth factors and cell adhesion molecules have a major role in wound healing and enhance the physiological process at the site of the injury/surgery via eye drops or clot. As noted in peer-review articles, E-PRP has recently been used to achieve successful outcomes in treating dormant ulcers (epithelial defects of the cornea that fail to heal), moderate to severe dry eye syndrome, ocular surface syndrome post-laser in situ keratomileusis (LASIK), and surface reconstruction after corneal perforation associated with amniotic membrane transplantation [6]. Preparation of E-PRP in the two available formulations, eye drops and clot, is inexpensive and easy although it requires following strict sterile conditions using sterile and disposable materials and operating inside a laminar flow hood. No serious adverse effects have been described and it is generally well tolerated.

Outcome

After 6 weeks of treatment, the patient's symptoms had completely improved. Her blurred vision had disappeared and BCVA was 20/20 in both eyes. The cornea appeared completely re-epithelized. The Oxford scheme was I (Fig. 43.1b).

What to Learn from This Case

The management of dry eye after LASIK begins during the screening visit, with optimization of the ocular surface using artificial tears, warm compresses, and lid hygiene and treating the underlying ocular surface inflammation with immunomodulatory agents such as cyclosporine A 0.05 %. Refractive surgery should be avoided in patients who do not improve their tear health following this treatment.

References

1. Albietz JM, Lenton LM, McLennan SG (2005) Dry eye after LASIK: comparison of outcomes for Asian and Caucasian eyes. Clin Exp Optom 88:89–96
2. De Paiva CS, Chen Z, Koch DD et al (2006) The incidence and risk factors for developing dry eye after myopic LASIK (Exp EyeRes). Am J Ophthalmol 141:438–445
3. Toda I, Asano-Kato N, Komai-Hori Y, Tsubota K (2001) Dry eye after laser in situ keratomileusis. Am J Ophthalmol 132:1–7
4. Alio JL, Pastor S, Ruiz-Colecha J, Rodriguez A, Artola A (2007) Treatment of ocular surface syndrome after LASIK with autologous platelet-rich plasma. J Refract Surg 23:617–619
5. Ramos-Esteban J, Wilson S (2008) Chapter 5.1: Dry eye. In: Alio JL, Azar D (eds) Management of complications in refractive surgery. Springer, Berlin/Heidelberg, pp 74–83
6. Alio JL, Arnalich-Montiel F, Rodriguez AE (2012) The role of "eye platelet rich plasma" (E-PRP) for wound healing in ophthalmology. Curr Pharm Biotechnol 13:1257–1265

Dry Eye Syndrome: Management of Post-LASIK Dry Eye Disease

44

Sapna Tibrewal and S. Jain

Contents

S. Tibrewal, MD (✉) • S. Jain, MD
Department of Ophthalmology and Visual Sciences, University of Illinois at Chicago, Chicago, IL, USA
e-mail: sapna.tibrewal@gmail.com

Why Is This Case Relevant for the Refractive Surgeon?

Laser in situ keratomileusis (LASIK) has emerged as the standard surgical procedure for the correction of refractive errors [1]. During LASIK procedure, stromal nerves are transected in the flap area. Post-LASIK, the subbasal nerve plexus density decreases more than 80 % [2]. Although nerve regrowth is observed in the flap area at 6 months post-procedure, preoperative levels are not achieved even 5 years after surgery [2–4]. About 50 % patients experience some degree of dry eye symptoms during the initial postoperative period [5]. Besides symptoms of ocular discomfort, which in the most severe form can be debilitating to the patient, it can also compromise visual acuity if the central cornea develops LASIK-induced neurotrophic epitheliopathy (LINE).

Case Background

Our patient is a 28-year-old female who underwent bilateral myopic LASIK treatment 3 years ago. She presented to us with complaints of dull pain, discomfort, soreness, irritation, and FB sensation in both eyes.

On initial examination, her best-corrected visual acuity (BCVA) was 20/25 in the right eye (OD) and 20/20 in the left eye (OS). Slit-lamp examination revealed intact and clear flaps in

J.L. Alió et al. (eds.), *Difficult and Complicated Cases in Refractive Surgery*,
DOI 10.1007/978-3-642-55238-0_44, © Springer-Verlag Berlin Heidelberg 2015

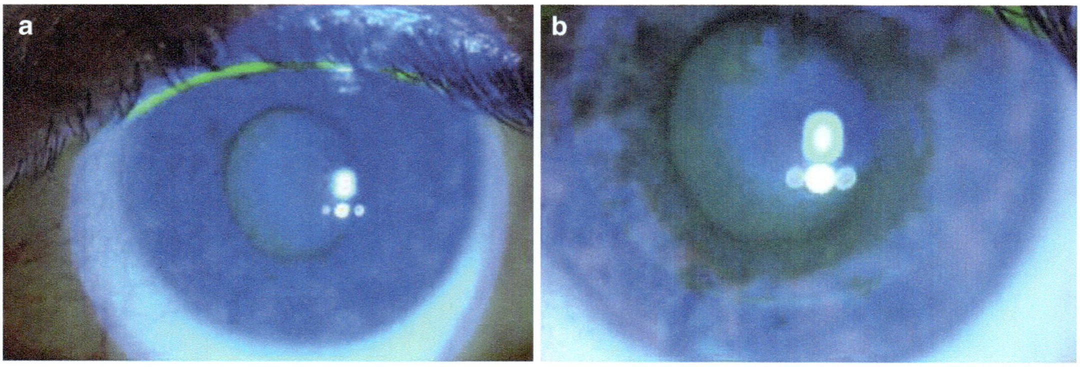

Fig. 44.1 (**a**) Fluorescein stained low magnification image of cornea showing LASIK flap with mild conjunctival injection. No staining of peripheral cornea or conjunctiva is seen. (**b**) Magnified image of the same eye showing that superficial punctate staining is limited to the flap area only

both eyes. There was no interface haze or scarring. On applying fluorescein stain, she showed mild punctate staining of both corneas, which was limited over the flap area (Fig. 44.1a, b). The surrounding cornea or conjunctiva did not show any staining. Mild conjunctival injection was present OU. No reaction in the anterior chamber or discharge was present. Schirmer I (without anesthesia) was 1 mm OD and 2 mm OS. Corneal sensations were normal in both eyes (40 mm OU) as measured by Cochet-Bonnet esthesiometer.

Our impression was that our patient had LASIK-induced neurotrophic epitheliopathy, given the timing of her disease onset, fluorescein staining pattern limited to the flap area, and the absence of prior ocular surface disease.

Main Problem to Solve

The dry eye in this case is likely caused by a loss of trophic influence to the epithelium attributable to transection of corneal nerve trunks during LASIK procedure. There is some suggestion of neuropathic pain as well. The treatment needs to be targeted at healing the corneal SPKs and to promote regeneration of corneal nerves.

Ancillary Tests

Post-LASIK dry eye disease should be evaluated using a slit lamp to perform a complete and careful assessment of the ocular surface. It is important to rule out any coexisting lid/lash abnormality or meibomian gland disease. Symptom analysis should be done using a standardized questionnaire (OSDI). Other important tests include Schirmer I without anesthesia, corneal esthesiometry, ocular surface staining with vital dyes (fluorescein/rose bengal), and tear meniscus height measurement using OCT. Additionally, tear osmolarity measurement may be done, if available.

Surgical/Medical Intervention

Based on the diagnosis, medical management was planned for the patient. Treatment included the frequent use of non-preserved artificial tears to lubricate the surface, platelet-rich plasma (PRP) eyedrops to promote nerve regeneration and epithelial healing, and daily disposable silicon hydrogel contact lens (Acuvue 1-day TruEye) for ensconcing the cornea to promote epithelial healing. Cyclosporine 0.05% eyedrops were started twice a day to promote tear production.

Outcome

The patient responded well to the above regimen. PRP and contact lenses were discontinued after 2 months. By 6 months, she was comfortable and her ocular symptoms had resolved. Current maintenance therapy includes artificial tears as needed and cyclosporine eyedrops twice a day. At the most recent follow-up visit, slit-lamp examination revealed a clear and smooth LASIK flap surface. There was no fluorescein staining of the ocular surface.

What to Learn from This Case

A multipronged approach is needed to effectively treat dry eye due to corneal nerve dysfunction after LASIK surgery. In general, patients should discontinue the use of all preserved eyedrops. One common preservative, benzalkonium chloride, can increase corneal inflammation and additionally has direct neurotoxicity [6]. Topical corticosteroid eyedrops should also be avoided, as they can excessively retard inflammation and some inflammation appears facilitative of nerve regeneration [7–10]. Corneal nerve regeneration can be stimulated by topical application of platelet-rich plasma (PRP) because platelets contain neurotrophic factors like VEGF [10, 11]. This treatment modality was first described by Alio and co-workers in the treatment of dormant corneal ulcers and ocular surface syndrome after LASIK [12, 13]. Silicone hydrogel soft contact lenses can be used as a bandage, and non-preserved artificial tears can be used for lubrication to promote healing [14]. Oral minocycline can be used for neuroprotection [15].

References

1. American Academy of Ophthalmology. Eye Health Statistics at a Glance. http://www.aao.org/newsroom/press_kit/upload/Eye_Stats_3-5-07. Accessed online Dec 2012
2. Moilanen JA, Holopainen JM, Vesaluoma MH, Tervo TM (2008) Corneal recovery after Lasik for high myopia: a 2-year prospective confocal microscopic study. Br J Ophthalmol 92:1397–1402
3. Erie JC, McLaren JW, Hodge DO, Bourne WM (2005) Recovery of corneal subbasal nerve density after PRK and LASIK. Am J Ophthalmol 140: 1059–1064
4. Darwish T, Brahma A, O'Donnell C, Efron N (2007) Subbasal nerve fiber regeneration after LASIK and LASEK assessed by noncontact esthesiometry and in vivo confocal microscopy: prospective study. J Cataract Refract Surg 33:1515–1521
5. Ambrósio R Jr, Tervo T, Wilson SE (2008) LASIK-associated dry eye and neurotrophic epitheliopathy: pathophysiology and strategies for prevention and treatment. J Refract Surg 24:396–407
6. Sarkar J, Chaudhary S, Namavari A, Ozturk O, Chang JH, Yco L, Sonawane S, Khanolkar V, Hallak J, Jain S (2012) Corneal neurotoxicity due to topical benzalkonium chloride. Invest Ophthalmol Vis Sci 53:1792–1802
7. Namavari A, Chaudhary S, Chang JH, Yco L, Sonawane S, Khanolkar V, Yue BY, Sarkar J, Jain S (2012) Cyclosporine immunomodulation retards regeneration of surgically transected corneal nerves. Invest Ophthalmol Vis Sci 53:732–740
8. Li H, Xie W, Strong JA, Zhang JM (2007) Systemic anti-inflammatory corticosteroid reduces mechanical pain behavior, sympathetic sprouting, and elevation of proinflammatory cytokines in a rat model of neuropathic pain. Anesthesiology 107:469–477
9. Lee HK, Ryu IH, Seo KY, Hong S, Kim HC, Kim EK (2006) Topical 0.1 % prednisolone lowers nerve growth factor expression in keratoconjunctivitis sicca patients. Ophthalmology 113: 198–205
10. Li Z, Burns AR, Han L, Rumbaut RE, Smith CW (2011) IL-17 and VEGF are necessary for efficient corneal nerve regeneration. Am J Pathol 178: 1106–1116
11. Fong KP, Barry C, Tran AN, Traxler EA, Wannemacher KM, Tang HY, Speicher KD, Blair IA, Speicher DW, Grosser T, Brass LF (2010) Deciphering the human platelet sheddome. Blood 117:e15–e26
12. Alio JL, Abad M, Artola A, Rodriguez-Prats JL, Pastor S, Ruiz-Colecha J (2007) Use of autologous platelet-rich plasma in the treatment of dormant corneal ulcers. Ophthalmology 114:1286–1293
13. Alio JL, Arnalich-Montiel F, Rodriguez AE (2012) The role of "eye platelet rich plasma" (E-PRP) for wound healing in ophthalmology. Curr Pharm Biotechnol 13:1257–1265
14. Gil-Cazorla R, Teus MA, Arranz-Márquez E (2008) Comparison of silicone and non-silicone hydrogen soft contact lenses used as a bandage after LASEK. J Refract Surg 24:199–203
15. Wells J, Hurlbert RJ, Fehlings MG, Yong VW (2003) Neuroprotection by minocycline facilitates significant recovery from spinal cord injury in mice. Brain 126:1628–1637

Dry Eye Syndrome: Recurrent Epithelial Erosion After LASIK

45

Jorge L. Alió, Angelo Rampone, and Alessandro Abbouda

Contents

J.L. Alió, MD, PhD (✉)
Department of Refractive Surgery, Vissum Corporación Oftalmológica, Alicante, Spain
e-mail: jlalio@vissum.com

A. Rampone, MD
Department of Ophthalmology, Seconda Università degli Studi di Napoli, Naples, Italy

R&D Department, Vissum Corporacion, 03016, Alicante, Spain
e-mail: angelo.rampone@gmail.com

A. Abbouda, MD
Department of Refractive Surgery, Vissum Corporación Oftalmológica, Alicante, Spain

Department of Ophthalmology-Policlinico Umberto I of Rome, University of Rome "Sapienza", Viale del Policlinico, 155, 00186 Roma, Italy

R&D Department, Vissum Corporación Oftalmológica, 03016, Alicante, Spain
e-mail: a.abbouda@gmail.com

Why Is This Case Relevant for the Refractive Surgeon?

Epithelial basement membrane dystrophy (EBMD) is the most common corneal dystrophy, with an estimated prevalence of 5 %. However, it is often undiagnosed because it has nonspecific symptoms [1]. The pathogenesis of EBMD involves primary synthesis of an abnormal epithelial basement membrane with intraepithelial extensions. The absence of anchoring fibrils in patients with EBMD leads to a poorly adherent epithelium and increased risk for recurrent corneal erosion (RCE). It also increases risk of a perforated flap during cutting and of diffuse lamellar keratitis (DLK) [2].

We present a case in which EBMD developed 3 months after IntraLASIK treatment.

Case Background

A 25-year-old man with no ocular history presented for a refractive surgery evaluation. His manifest refraction was −8.0, −1.75 × 10 in the right eye (RE) and −8.0, −2.50 × 170 in the left eye (LE). Keratometry reading was 41.61/42.82 × 176 in the RE and 41.71/43.54 × 107 in the LE. His best-corrected visual acuity (BCVA) was 20/20 for distance and near vision in both eyes. The slit-lamp and fundus examinations were normal. According to the topography, his cornea surface was regular, his RE pachymetry was 607 μm and his LE was 612 μm.

J.L. Alió et al. (eds.), *Difficult and Complicated Cases in Refractive Surgery*,
DOI 10.1007/978-3-642-55238-0_45, © Springer-Verlag Berlin Heidelberg 2015

The patient underwent an uneventful LASIK procedure with both eyes targeted for distance. Flap creation at depth 100–130 was performed using the IntraLase FSTM CORP Femtosecond Laser System and corneal stromal ablation by the AMARIS SCHWIND excimer laser. The postoperative evaluation was normal and the slit-lamp examination showed no anomalies. No epithelial defects at the flap edge indicated a clear interface and a well-positioned flap.

After 2 months, the patient reported discomfort and a sensation of foreign bodies in both eyes. The slit-lamp examination revealed an epithelial defect and a tender opacity in the anterior stroma in both eyes compatible with EBMD associated with DLK 2 (Fig. 45.1).

We managed this complication with topical antibiotics and steroid therapy (ofloxacin one drop four times a day, dexamethasone one drop four times a day tapering to one drop every week for a total of 4 weeks, followed by fluorometholone one drop three times a day for 2 weeks). During the following weeks, the patient noted improvement in his condition.

Main Problem to Solve

In managing EBMD after a microtrauma post-LASIK, it is important to avoid the onset of infectious keratitis and to eliminate discomfort.

Ancillary Tests

A slit-lamp examination can help identify the trend of the epithelial defect. Confocal microscopy as a diagnostic technique and prompt local therapy are important.

Surgical/Medical Intervention

The patient underwent a topical treatment with the use of a bandage contact lens, associated with preservative free corticosteroid and artificial tears (Systane Ultra). The bandage contact lens was eliminated after 2 weeks, and only the treatment with preservative free topical lubricants remained. PTK was not performed due to stability throughout the 6-month follow-up.

Outcome

At 3 and 6 months, the slit-lamp examination showed no signs of epithelial defect and stromal opacity (Fig. 45.2) despite no treatment. The uncorrected visual acuity (UCVA) was 20/20 for distance and near vision in both eyes. The keratometry reading was 35.16/35.77 × 111 in the RE and 35.00/35.34 × 53 in the LE. The topography showed a central ablation and a reduction of value of keratometry compatible to a LASIK treatment for moderate myopia.

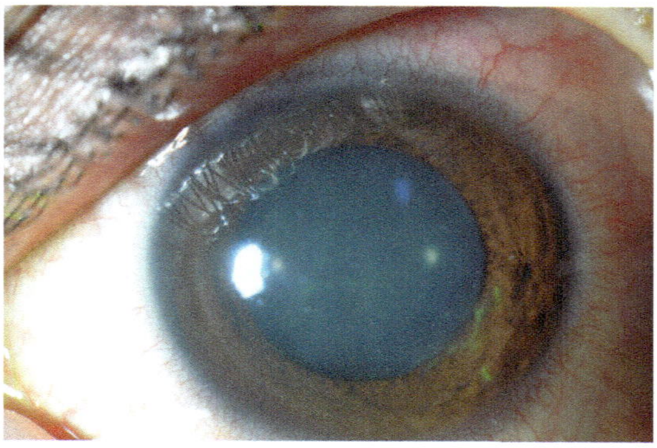

Fig. 45.1 Slit-lamp examination revealed an epithelial defect and opacity in the anterior stroma

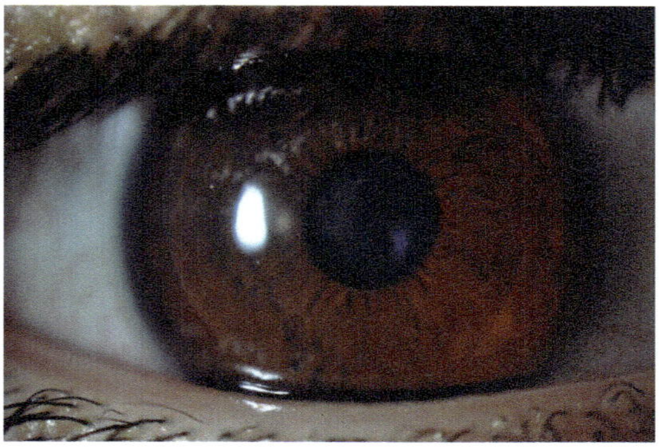

Fig. 45.2 Slit-lamp examination showed no signs of epithelial defect and stromal opacity

What to Learn from This Case

Epithelial basement membrane dystrophy is commonly asymptomatic and undiagnosed. However, it might be associated with recurrent corneal erosions and lead to severe complications after LASIK surgery [3]. Confocal microscopy can guide diagnosis and follow-up. In this case it may have been useful to perform a confocal microscopy examination before the patient underwent intraLASIK [4]. Considering conservative treatment first has successful results in many cases such as this one.

References

1. Rezende RA, Uchoa UC, Cohen EJ, Laibson PR, Rapuano CJ (2004) Complications associated with anterior basement membrane dystrophy after laser in situ keratomileusis. J Cataract Refract Surg 30:2328–2331
2. Alió JL, Pérez-Santonja JJ, Tervo T, Tabbara KF, Vesaluoma M, Smith RJ, Maddox B, Maloney RK (2000) Postoperative inflammation, microbial complications, and wound healing following laser in situ keratomileusis. J Refract Surg 16:523–538
3. Bozkurt B, Irkec M (2009) In vivo laser confocal microscopic findings in patients with epithelial basement membrane dystrophy. Eur J Ophthalmol 19:348–354
4. Kobayashi A, Yokogawa H, Sugiyama K (2012) In vivo laser confocal microscopy findings in patients with map-dot-fingerprint (epithelial basement membrane) dystrophy. Clin Ophthalmol 6:1187–1190

Dry Eye Syndrome: Severe Ocular Surface Inflammatory Syndrome Post LASIK Caused by Blepharitis

46

Jorge L. Alió, Dominika Wróbel, and Alessandro Abbouda

Contents

J.L. Alió, MD, PhD (✉)
Department of Refractive Surgery, Vissum Corporación Oftalmológica, Alicante, Spain
e-mail: jlalio@vissum.com

D. Wróbel, MD
Glaucoma Diagnostic and Microsurgery Department, Medical University of Lublin, Lublin, Poland

R&D Department, Vissum Corporacion, Alicante, Spain
e-mail: ddudzinska@interia.pl

A. Abbouda, MD
Department of Refractive Surgery, Vissum Corporación Oftalmológica, Alicante, Spain

Department of Ophthalmology-Policlinico Umberto I of Rome, University of Rome "Sapienza", Viale del Policlinico, 155, 00186 Roma, Italy

R&D Department, Vissum Corporación Oftalmológica, 03016, Alicante, Spain
e-mail: a.abbouda@gmail.com

Why Is This Case Relevant for the Refractive Surgeon?

Blepharitis and chronic meibomitis can affect the tear film composition, produce epithelial corneal defects, and lead to dangerous bacterial infections after LASIK surgery. Infection symptoms include pain, decreased vision, photophobia, irritation, or redness. As many as 10 % of cases may be asymptomatic. The refractive surgeon should identify preoperative blepharitis to avoid serious complications [1].

Case Background

A 49-year-old woman was referred to our department complaining of photophobia and blurred vision for 1 week. She underwent refractive surgery 2 years prior, and her manifest refraction before the treatment was −6.5 diopters (D). Prior to surgery, she wore contact lenses regularly and had recurrent blepharitis. The current manifest refraction was +3.0 −3.0×50° in the right eye (RE) and +0.75 −0.50×130° in the left eye (LE). Her best corrected visual acuity (BCVA) was 20/25 in the RE and 20/63 in the LE. The slit lamp examination showed blepharitis in both eyes and ciliary injection and central corneal infiltrate in the LE (Fig. 46.1). The fundus examination was normal.

J.L. Alió et al. (eds.), *Difficult and Complicated Cases in Refractive Surgery*,
DOI 10.1007/978-3-642-55238-0_46, © Springer-Verlag Berlin Heidelberg 2015

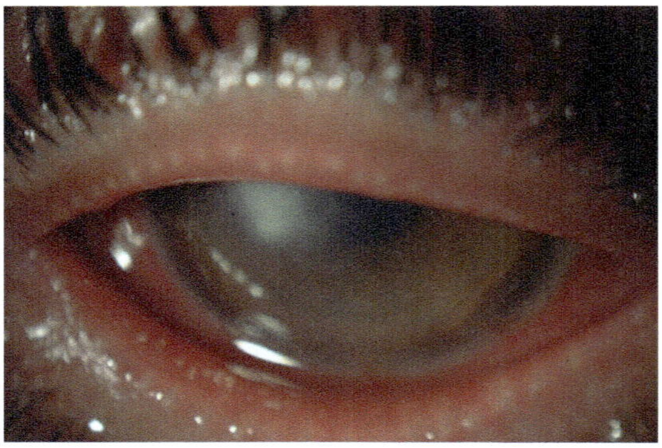

Fig. 46.1 Slit lamp examination showed blepharitis and central corneal infiltrate

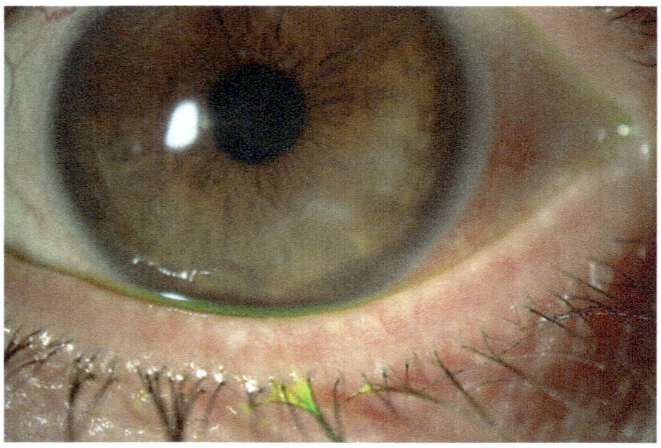

Fig. 46.2 Slit lamp examination showed a resolution of central infiltrate, but an inferior epithelial ingrowth nest was observed

Main Problem to Solve

Diagnosing blepharitis before LASIK, especially blepharitis caused by chronic meibomitis, is important in avoiding postoperative complications. Bacteria which cause corneal infections after LASIK are often found in the eyelids and conjunctiva [2]. Preoperative eyelid hygiene and antibiotic eye drops can help prevent infection. Vancomycin ophthalmic ointment 1 % is a new treatment for intractable blepharitis [3].

Ancillary Tests

A differential diagnosis for blepharitis is peripheral sterile infiltrate. A microbiological culture can help with the diagnosis.

Surgical/Medical Intervention

Microbial cultures and gram stain were negative. Due to high suspicion of staphylococcus aureus keratitis, we began the following therapy: hourly fortified vancomycin 50 mg/ml drops, hourly fortified ceftazidime 100 mg/ml drops, Pred Forte® (prednisolone acetate ophthalmic suspension 1 %; Allergan, USA) one drop three times a day, cyclopentolate one drop two times a day, and Oftacilox® (ciprofloxacin 0.3 %; Alcon) once a night. The case did not show the progressive evolution of an infection, and the treatment had no apparent anti-infectious effect. We decided to stop the treatment and introduce artificial tears.

Outcome

At 1 month, the uncorrected visual acuity (UCVA) in the LE had improved to 20/32, but the patient still complained of photophobia. The slit lamp examination showed a resolution of central infiltrate, but an inferior epithelial ingrowth nest was observed (Fig. 46.2). We decided to follow the patient without treatment to avoid the increase of inflammation. For 3 years, the patient remained stable although she complained of photophobia. At year three, the slit lamp examination showed an increasing epithelial ingrowth and a significant meibomian gland deposit. The epithelial ingrowth was removed from the stromal bed, and the thin and irregular flap was fixed in place with 10/0 nylon sutures (Fig. 46.3).

What to Learn from This Case

The surgeon should be able to distinguish noninfectious keratitis from microbial keratitis to avoid aggressive management and use of antimicrobial

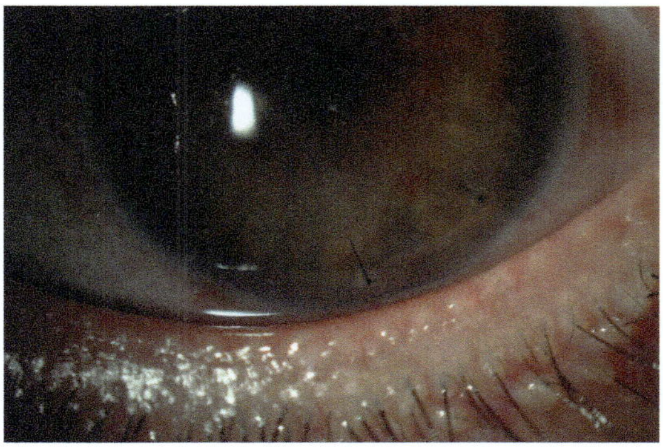

Fig. 46.3 Slit lamp examination showed a thin and irregular flap sutured by 10/0 nylon

drugs [4]. In this case, the negative culture, the absence of progression, and improvement with antibiotic drops helped us differentiate between these two syndromes.

References

1. Chang MA, Jain S, Azar DT (2004) Infections following laser in situ keratomileusis: an integration of the published literature. Surv Ophthalmol 49: 269–280
2. Ayala MJ, Alió JL, Mulet ME, De La Hoz F (2008) Treatment of laser in situ keratomileusis interface epithelial ingrowth with neodymium:yytrium-aluminum-garnet laser. Am J Ophthalmol 145:630–634
3. Sotozono C, Fukuda M, Ohishi M, Yano K, Origasa H, Saiki Y, Shimomura Y, Kinoshita S (2013) Vancomycin ophthalmic ointment 1 % for methicillin-resistant Staphylococcus aureus or methicillin-resistant Staphylococcus epidermidis infections: a case series. BMJ Open 29:1–6. pii: e001206
4. Alió JL, Pérez-Santonja JJ, Tervo T, Tabbara KF, Vesaluoma M, Smith RJ, Maddox B, Maloney RK (2000) Postoperative inflammation, microbial complications, and wound healing following laser in situ keratomileusis. J Refract Surg 16:523–538

Epithelial Ingrowth: Epithelial Ingrowth into Visual Axis After Primary LASIK Surgery Treated by Flap Elevation and Scraping

47

Florence Cabot and Sonia H. Yoo

Contents

F. Cabot, MD • S.H. Yoo, MD (✉)
Bascom Palmer Eye Institute,
University of Miami Miller School of Medicine,
900 Nw 17th St, Miami 33136, FL, USA
e-mail: florence.cabot@gmail.com

Why Is This Case Relevant for the Refractive Surgeon?

LASIK is the most common refractive surgery performed all around the world. Epithelial ingrowth is a rare complication which usually occurs by postoperative invasion rather than by intraoperative implantation, which suggests that the quality of the flap edge and its apposition are very important [1, 2]. In this case, the isolated island of epithelial ingrowth is located in the visual axis, visualized on postoperative day one, without any epithelial flap edge defect suggesting it was caused by intraoperative implantation.

Case Background

A 44-year-old woman with no ocular history presented for refractive surgery evaluation. Her manifest refraction was $-3.25+0.50\times155$ in the right eye and $-3.25+0.25\times175$ in the left eye which was her dominant eye. Her best corrected visual acuity was 20/20 for distance and near in both eyes, and slit lamp and fundus examinations were normal. According to the topography, her cornea surface was regular, her right eye pachymetry was 573 µm, and her left eye pachymetry was 571 µm. She underwent an uneventful LASIK procedure, both eyes targeted for distance. Flap creation was performed using the Alcon WaveLight® FS200 femtosecond laser and corneal stromal ablation by the Alcon Allegretto®

J.L. Alió et al. (eds.), *Difficult and Complicated Cases in Refractive Surgery*,
DOI 10.1007/978-3-642-55238-0_47, © Springer-Verlag Berlin Heidelberg 2015

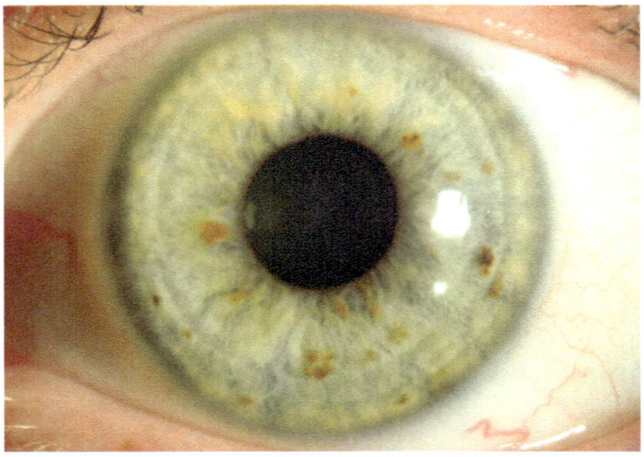

Fig. 47.1 Slit lamp photography 1 week after LASIK. Mild epithelial ingrowth into the visual axis

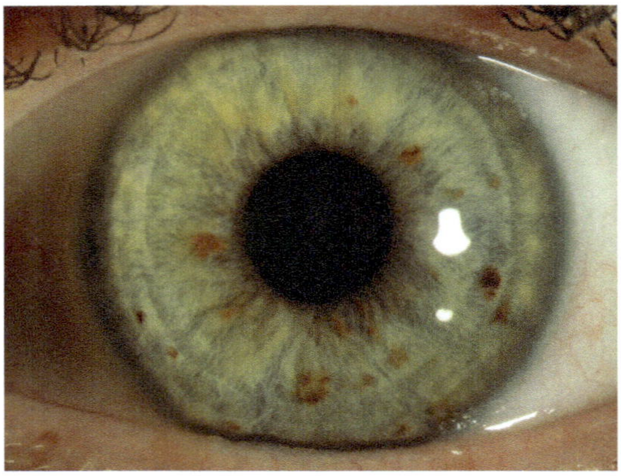

Fig. 47.2 Slit lamp photography 3 weeks after LASIK. Severe epithelial ingrowth into the visual axis

excimer laser. One hour post operatively, the slit lamp examination showed no anomalies: no epithelial defects at the flap edge, a clear interface, and well-positioned flap. One week postoperatively, the slit lamp examination showed an isolated opacity in the interface within the visual axis of the left eye (Fig. 47.1).

Main Problem to Solve

Performing a slit lamp examination the day and the week following a LASIK procedure is important to detect early postoperative complications. In this case, there is a slight interface opacity within the pupillary diameter, and although the slit lamp examination suggests the possibility of epithelial ingrowth, we do not see frank epithelial nests yet. The diagnosis of epithelial ingrowth remains uncertain, and the surgeon has to keep in mind it could be the beginning of an infectious keratitis process, an early diffuse lamellar keratitis, or haze. Close follow-up is recommended to be able to treat the patient with success as soon as we get all the clues leading to the right diagnosis. Most of the time, when epithelial ingrowth is caused by intraoperative implantation, cells have limited proliferation, and a surgical procedure is not required if the visual axis is not affected. In this case the lesion, though involving the visual axis, should be treatable by lifting and scraping the cells in order to preserve the patient's visual acuity.

Ancillary Tests

Close follow-up with meticulous slit lamp examination is the most important thing to do in order to determine the evolution of epithelial ingrowth. If cell proliferation is limited and does not affect the visual axis, the patient does not need surgical intervention. In contrast, if cell proliferation extends toward the visual axis, surgical intervention is required to remove the epithelial cells. An anterior segment OCT (optical coherence tomography) could be helpful in the case of epithelial ingrowth caused by migration of epithelial cells from the flap gutter across the flap interface, to visualize the path followed by the epithelial cells. Slit lamp photos also are helpful to determine the epithelial ingrowth progression over time. In our case, the diagnosis of epithelial ingrowth was confirmed and the cell proliferation extended into the visual axis within 3 weeks, as shown in Fig. 47.2.

Surgical/Medical Intervention

The patient underwent a flap lift and scrape. A mechanical debridement of epithelial cells was performed on the back of the flap and on the surface of the residual stromal bed. All epithelial cells were removed, and the interface was irrigated with balance salt solution (BSS). The flap was repositioned, and a bandage contact lens was used to improve flap adhesion.

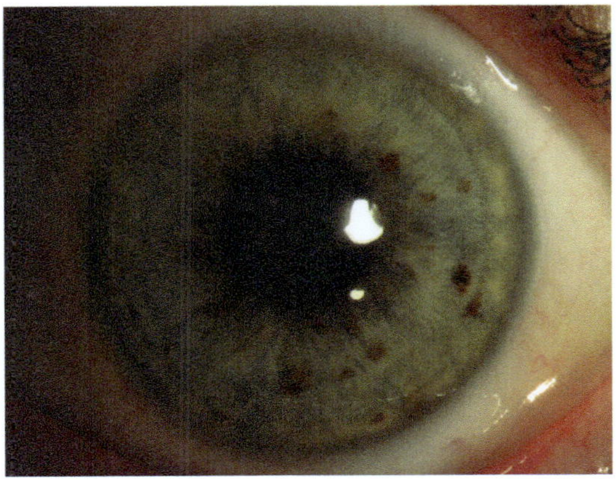

Fig. 47.3 Slit lamp photography 1 day after epithelial ingrowth removal showing a clear interface

Outcome

One day postoperatively, the slit lamp examination showed a clear interface with no epithelial cells, and the flap was well positioned (Fig. 47.3). The uncorrected visual acuity was 20/40 in the left eye and 20/20 in the right eye.

What to Learn from This Case

Epithelial ingrowth can occur after primary LASIK, but the incidence is higher in cases of retreatment [3]. Two mechanisms of epithelial ingrowth have been described: the first one is the deposition of epithelial cells by the microkeratome or other instruments during the surgical procedure. The second mechanism is the postoperative migration of epithelial cells from the flap gutter across the flap interface [4]. Usually in the cases of epithelial ingrowth caused by intraoperative implantation, the cell proliferation is limited, and a surgical procedure is not required. Nevertheless, clinically significant epithelial ingrowth affecting the patient's visual acuity or extending into the visual axis should be treated by surgical removal of the epithelial cells. Nd:YAG treatment was first described in 2008 [5] in cases of clinically significant epithelial ingrowth, but further studies are necessary to confirm the safety and the effectiveness of this technique [6].

References

1. Knorz MC (2002) Flap and interface complications in LASIK. Curr Opin Ophthalmol 13:242–245
2. Asano-Kato N, Toda I, Hori-Komai Y et al (2002) Epithelial ingrowth after laser in situ keratomileusis: clinical features and possible mechanisms. Am J Ophthalmol 134:801–807
3. Caster AI, Friess DW, Schwendeman FJ (2010) Incidence of epithelial ingrowth in primary and retreatment laser in situ keratomileusis. J Cataract Refract Surg 36:97–101
4. Henry CR, Canto AP, Galor A et al (2012) Epithelial ingrowth under LASIK flap: clinical characteristics, risk factors, and visual outcomes in patients requiring flap lift. J Refract Surg 18:1–5
5. Ayala MJ, Alio J, Mulet ME et al (2008) Treatment of laser in situ keratomileusis interface epithelial ingrowth with neodymium:yytrium-aluminum-garnet laser. Am J Ophthalmol 14:630–634
6. Lindfield D, Ansari G, Poole T (2012) Nd:YAG laser treatment for epithelial ingrowth after laser refractive surgery. Ophthalmic Surg Lasers Imaging 43:247–249

Epithelial Ingrowth: Use of Topography in the Management

48

Jaime Javaloy and Alessandro Abbouda

Contents

J. Javaloy, MD, PhD (✉)
Department of Anterior Segment and Refractive Surgery, Vissum Corporacion Oftalmológica, Alicante, Spain
e-mail: jjavaloy@coma.es

A. Abbouda, MD
Department of Refractive Surgery, Vissum Corporación Oftalmológica, Alicante, Spain

Department of Ophthalmology-Policlinico Umberto I of Rome, University of Rome "Sapienza", Viale del Policlinico, 155, 00186 Roma, Italy

R&D Department, Vissum Corporación Oftalmológica, 03016, Alicante, Spain
e-mail: a.abbouda@gmail.com

Why Is This Case Relevant for the Refractive Surgeon?

Epithelial ingrowth at the edge of the flap is one of the most significant complications of LASIK. Reports of the incidence of epithelial ingrowth have ranged from 0 to 20 % [1–4]. It usually presents in the early postoperative period and is known to be associated with loose epithelium, epithelial defects at the time of surgery, hyperopic LASIK correction, enhancement surgeries, flap instability, and corneal epithelial basement membrane dystrophy [1, 3–5]. While not always serious, it can progress to induce irregular astigmatism or melting of the overlying flap and threaten the central vision.

Background of the Case

A 34-year-old woman with no ocular history presented for refractive surgery evaluation. Her manifest refraction was −1.5 in the right eye and −4.5 in the left eye. Her best corrected visual acuity (BCVA) was 20/20 for distance and near in both eyes. Both slit lamp and fundus examinations were normal. According to the topography, her cornea surface was regular, her right eye pachymetry was 534 μm, and her left eye pachymetry was 546 μm. She underwent an uneventful LASIK procedure, both eyes targeted for distance. Flap creation was performed using the IntraLase FS laser (IntraLase Corp) and

J.L. Alió et al. (eds.), *Difficult and Complicated Cases in Refractive Surgery*,
DOI 10.1007/978-3-642-55238-0_48, © Springer-Verlag Berlin Heidelberg 2015

corneal stromal ablation by the AMARIS SCHWIND excimer laser. The postoperative evaluation was normal. The slit lamp examination showed no anomalies, no epithelial defects at the flap edge, a clear interface, and a well-positioned flap.

At the 2-year follow-up, the patient complained of a reduced vision in her left eye. Her uncorrected visual acuity (UCVA) was 20/32. According to the topography, her cornea surface was regular, and her left eye pachymetry was 490 μm. She opted to receive a re-treatment. Her residual stroma was 320 μm.

After 4 months, the slit lamp examination showed an epithelial ingrowth near the margin of the pupil. The topography showed an initial sinking area. We decided her follow-up should be without re-treatment. After 3 months, she presented frank epithelial nests. The topography didn't change with respect to previous months (Fig. 48.1a).

After 6 months, she complained of a reduced vision in the left eye. Her UCVA was 20/60, and her corrected distance visual acuity (CDVA) was 20/20. The topography showed an increase in the defect area. The slit lamp showed a white stromal oval area of 3×4 mm with indistinct margins. The lesion was fluorescein negative (Fig. 48.1b).

Main Problem to Solve

In this case, there is evident interface opacity within the pupillary diameter, and the slit lamp examination and topography suggest the possibility of stromal melting. Close follow-up is recommended to be able to treat the patient with success as soon as we get all the clues leading to the right diagnosis. A topography can help in the management.

Ancillary Tests Necessary

A corneal topography could be helpful in the case of epithelial ingrowth to show the shift versus stromal melting. The progressive increasing of the lesion area suggested a fast removal of epithelial cells.

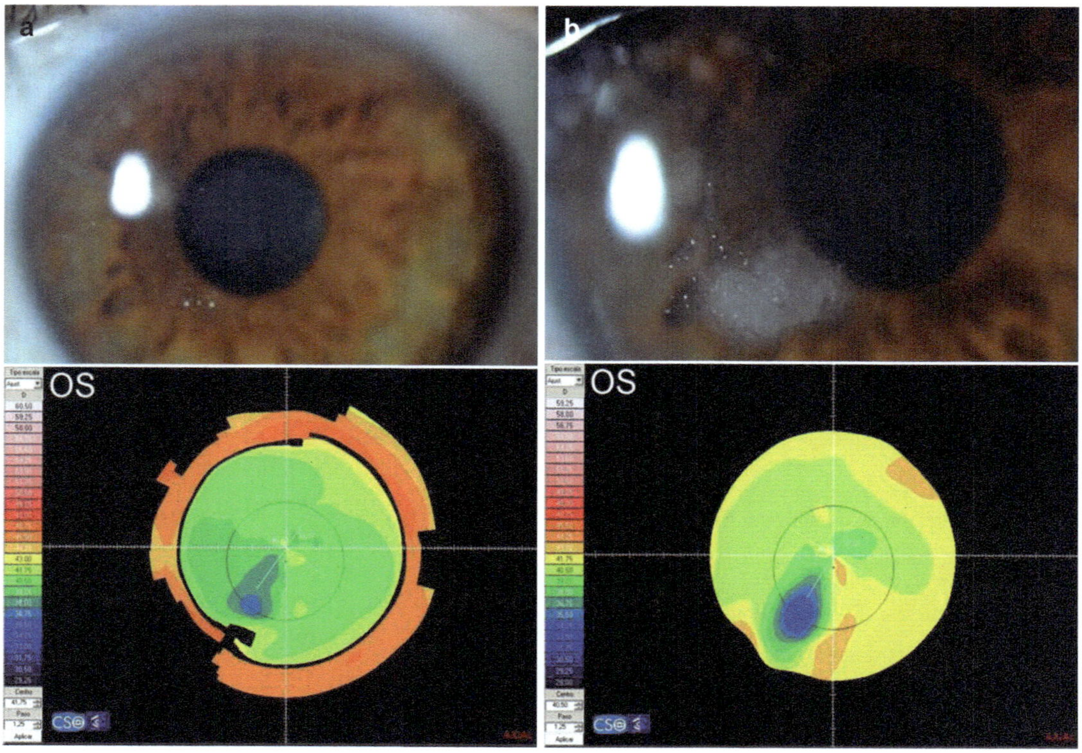

Fig. 48.1 These pictures show a topography and clinical aspect of epithelial ingrowth at the beginning (**a**) and before the re-treatment (**b**). (**c**) Shows clinical and topography resolution aspect

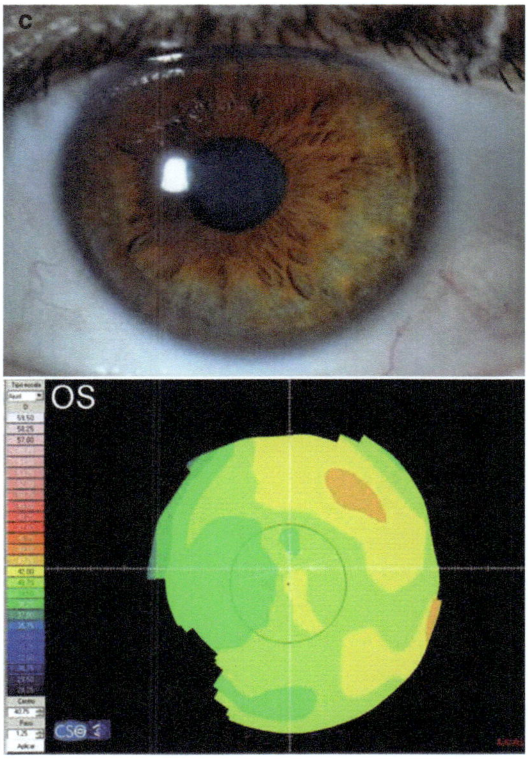

Fig. 48.1 (continued)

Surgical/Medical Intervention

The patient underwent a flap lift and scraping of the ingrowth material. A mechanical debridement of epithelial cells was performed on the back of the flap and on the surface of the residual stromal bed. All epithelial cells were removed, and the interface was irrigated with balance salt solution (BSS). The flap was repositioned and stitched with nylon 10.0.

Outcome

After 4 months postoperatively, the slit lamp examination showed a tender oval opacity with no epithelial cells with a well-positioned flap (Fig. 48.1c). In the left eye, the UCVA was 20/32, and the CDVA was 20/20.

What to Learn from This Case

Corneal topography is a sensitive test to alert us to a progression of epithelial ingrowth. In the topography the evolution towards flap melting due to collagenase release from necrotic epithelium appears as an increase of a flattening area. The patient may be asymptomatic. However, flap melts can lead to a distortion of the corneal surface with possible astigmatic changes.

References

1. Ambrósio R Jr, Wilson SE (2001) Complications of laser in situ keratomileusis: etiology, prevention, and treatment. J Refract Surg 17:350–379
2. Melki SA, Azar DT (2001) LASIK complications: etiology, management, and prevention. Surv Ophthalmol 46:95–116
3. Walker MB, Wilson SE (2000) Incidence and prevention of epithelial growth within the interface after laser in situ keratomileusis. Cornea 19:170–173
4. Wang MY, Maloney RK (2000) Epithelial ingrowth after laser in situ keratomileusis. Am J Ophthalmol 129:746–751
5. Jabbur NS, Chicani CF, Kuo IC, O'Brien TP (2004) Risk factors in interface epithelialization after laser in situ keratomileusis. J Refract Surg 20:343–348

Epithelial Ingrowth After LASIK

49

Isaac W. Porter

Contents

Why Is This Case Relevant for the Refractive Surgeon?

Ingrowth of corneal epithelial cells under the flap may occur after LASIK. When this is noticed, the surgeon must decide if it requires treatment. Peripheral epithelial ingrowth may be observed, but progressive ingrowth causing complications should be addressed promptly. This case provides an example of epithelial ingrowth that only required observation and also details the potential treatment options when intervention is necessary. Observable epithelial ingrowth occurs in less than 5 % of primary LASIK cases. Although epithelial ingrowth must be recognized, it is often clinically insignificant. In one study, some degree of epithelial ingrowth to the flap margin was detectable by histology in 53 % of LASIK cases [1]. Epithelial ingrowth results from the growth of peripheral epithelial cells into the flap interface which can be seen as pearls or nests of cells. The communication between the surface epithelium and the flap interface is the source of epithelial ingrowth and must be eliminated to adequately prevent recurrent ingrowth. Epithelial cells can be implanted into the interface at the time of surgery, but this is not thought to be a significant cause of epithelial ingrowth since these cells have limited reproductive potential. Risk factors for epithelial ingrowth include intraoperative epithelial defects, hyperopic treatments, re-treatments, and poor flap adhesion [2, 3]. The improved geometry of the flap edge in flaps

I.W. Porter, MD
Department of Ophthalmology, Cornea, Cataract, and Refractive Surgery, Lowry Porter Ophthalmology, Raleigh, NC, USA
e-mail: isaac_porter@hotmail.com

J.L. Alió et al. (eds.), *Difficult and Complicated Cases in Refractive Surgery*,
DOI 10.1007/978-3-642-55238-0_49, © Springer-Verlag Berlin Heidelberg 2015

created with a femtosecond laser could result in fewer cases of epithelial ingrowth as compared to microkeratome-created flaps. Epithelial ingrowth may occur more frequently than is commonly clinically recognized. This case will help the refractive surgeon determine if epithelial ingrowth is clinically significant and how it should be addressed.

Case Background

A 57-year-old woman had LASIK in the left eye for a planned monovision result. The preoperative refractive error was $-1.75+0.25\times155$ in the right eye and $+0.75+0.50\times045$ in the left eye. LASIK was performed using a Hansatome microkeratome and a Visx Star S4 IR excimer laser. According to nomogram adjustments, a conventional ablation of $+0.90+0.50\times045$ was completed on the left eye. Intraoperatively, there was a corneal abrasion inferonasally on the flap and loosening of the central corneal epithelium from the microkeratome. A therapeutic soft contact lens was applied at the end of the procedure, and gatifloxacin four times daily and prednisolone acetate hourly were started. On the first postoperative day, epithelial irregularity was noted at the flap edge inferiorly and nasally, and the contact lens was removed. One week after surgery, a filament was present at the inferior flap edge, and there was heavy punctate epithelial staining centrally. Gatifloxacin was stopped, and prednisolone was tapered. At the 1-month postoperative visit, epithelial ingrowth was noted inferiorly with a stream of epithelial cells extending into the interface no more than 1 mm from the flap edge. Uncorrected visual acuity was 20/25, and the patient was comfortable and pleased with her monovision result.

Main Problem to Solve

Once epithelial ingrowth is detected, the surgeon must decide if the ingrowth requires intervention or if it may be observed for signs of progression or complications. As in this case, epithelial ingrowth will usually be noticed by the 1-month postoperative visit [4].

Ancillary Tests

Biomicroscopy is the mainstay of evaluation and monitoring of epithelial ingrowth. Manifest refraction, corneal topography, and photography can also provide valuable information to help determine the stability of the area of ingrowth. If the epithelial cells remain stable in the peripheral 1–2 mm of the flap, then observation is appropriate. This case of epithelial ingrowth remained stable during monthly follow-up for the first 3 months and subsequently in 3-month intervals until 1 year postoperatively. Over this time, uncorrected visual acuity of the left eye ranged from 20/20 to 20/30, and there were low amounts of manifest refractive astigmatism (from +0.25 to +0.50 diopters).

Surgical/Medical Intervention

No intervention was required in this case. Once epithelial ingrowth is noted, serial observation is important. When any signs of progression beyond the peripheral 2 mm of the flap or complications occur, the epithelial ingrowth should be treated. Possible complications include induced astigmatism from elevation of the flap, patient discomfort from an irregular corneal surface or flap edge, glare from ingrowth near the pupil, decreased visual acuity from ingrowth into the entrance pupil, or melting of the overlying corneal flap. Primary treatment involves lifting the flap with nontoothed forceps instead of a spatula to prevent further ingrowth. Then the epithelial cells must be scraped from both the stromal bed and the underside of the flap using a blade, blunt spatula, or dry cellulose sponges. Earlier removal of epithelial ingrowth may help prevent the establishment of a more permanent fistula that can be difficult to definitively eradicate. Since epithelial ingrowth results from a communication between the surface epithelium and the flap interface, care

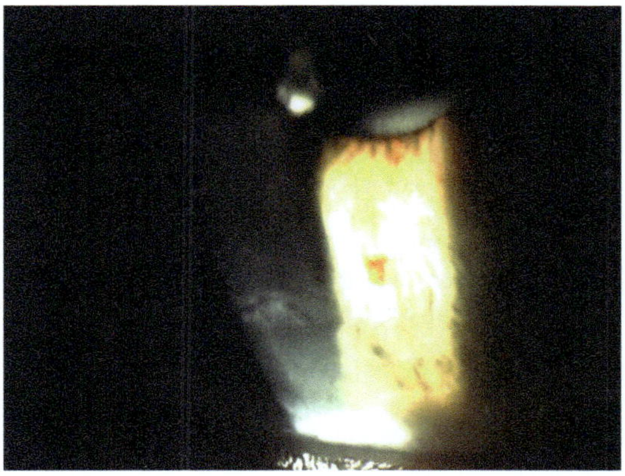

Fig. 49.1 Inferior epithelial ingrowth at the flap margin after LASIK (Photograph courtesy of Patrick W. Laber, MD)

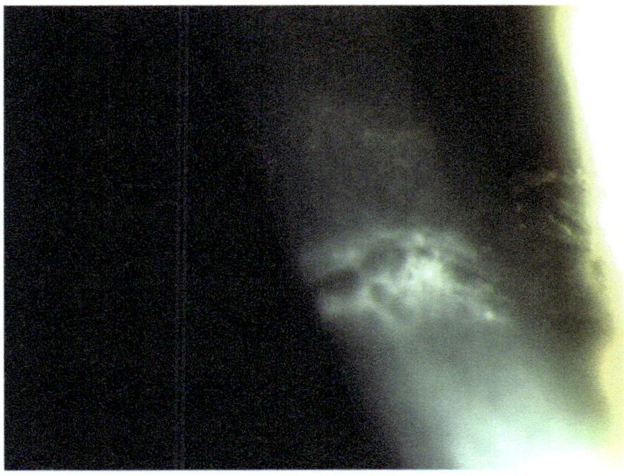

Fig. 49.2 Irregular flap edge with epithelial ingrowth (Photograph courtesy of Patrick W. Laber, MD)

must be taken to ensure appropriate apposition of the flap edge after removing the epithelial cells. This apposition can be improved with the use of sutures or fibrin glue which may be considered in primary cases and recommended for recurrent epithelial ingrowth [5]. 10-0 nylon sutures should be placed in and around the area of ingrowth at an adequate depth to secure the flap to the peripheral cornea. Fibrin glue should be placed over the flap edge and covered with a bandage contact lens until the glue dissolves.

Outcome

During observation, this case of epithelial ingrowth remained stable for 1 year without central progression more than 1–2 mm from the flap edge (Figs. 49.1 and 49.2). Peripheral remodeling of the inferior flap edge with scarring was noted in the area of ingrowth. Final uncorrected visual acuity was 20/20, and best corrected visual acuity was 20/20 with manifest refraction of −0.25+0.25×020. Corneal topography showed no signs of inferior steepening over the zone of ingrowth (Fig. 49.3).

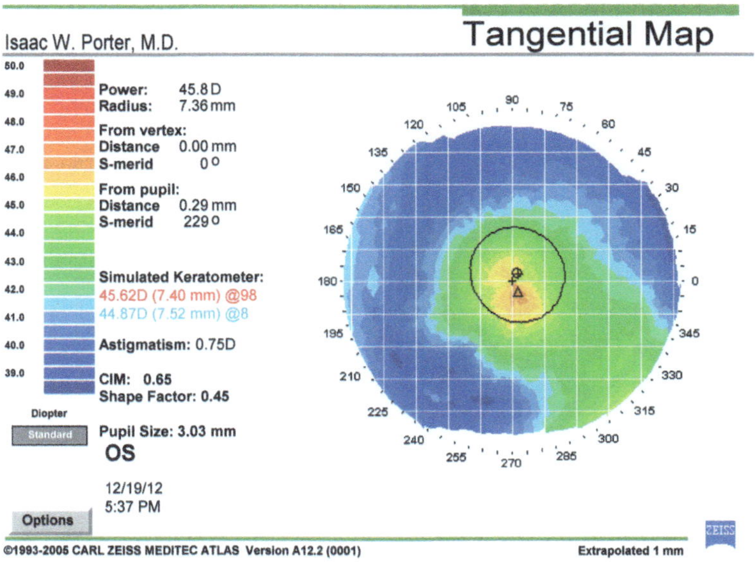

Fig. 49.3 Corneal topography with no signs of steepening inferiorly over epithelial ingrowth

What to Learn from This Case

Epithelial ingrowth may be observed as long as it remains peripheral and clinically insignificant. Lifting the flap and removing epithelial cells from the interface is indicated when the epithelial ingrowth is progressive, affects visual acuity, induces astigmatism, or compromises corneal integrity. An intraoperative epithelial defect and a hyperopic LASIK treatment increased the risk for epithelial ingrowth in this patient, but fortunately the ingrowth remained stable over the first postoperative year. By recognizing the signs of progression and the possible complications from epithelial ingrowth, surgeons may know when to observe and when to intervene.

References

1. Dawson DG, Kramer TR, Grossniklaus HE et al (2005) Histologic, ultrastructural, and immunofluorescent evaluation of human laser-assisted in situ keratomileusis corneal wounds. Arch Ophthalmol 123:741–756
2. Farah SG, Ghanem RC, Azar DT (2007) LASIK complications and their management. In: Azar DT (ed) Refractive surgery, 2nd edn. Philadelphia, USA; Mosby
3. Randleman JB, Shah RD (2012) LASIK interface complications: etiology, management, and outcomes. J Refract Surg 28:575–586
4. Wang MY, Maloney RK (2000) Epithelial ingrowth after laser in situ keratomileusis. Am J Ophthalmol 129:746–751
5. Anderson NJ, Hardten DR (2003) Fibrin glue for the prevention of epithelial ingrowth after laser in situ keratomileusis. J Cataract Refract Surg 29:1425–1429

Corneal Ectasia: Management of Corneal Ectasia After LASIK with Dovetail Femtosecond Penetrating Keratoplasty

50

Samuel H. Lee and Dimitri T. Azar

Contents

S.H. Lee, MD (✉) • D.T. Azar, MD, MBA
Department of Ophthalmology and Visual Sciences
Illinois Eye and Ear Infirmary, University of Illinois at Chicago, Chicago, IL, USA
e-mail: samuel.lee.md@gmail.com; dazar@uic.edu

Why Is This Case Relevant for the Refractive Surgeon?

A prudent surgeon will not only understand how to screen for patients that are at a high risk for developing corneal ectasia but also understand how it is treated if it develops [2].

Case Background

A 28-year-old female presented with a history of progressive corneal ectasia in both eyes 12 years after LASIK. We had performed successful deep anterior lamellar keratoplasty (DALK) and surface ablation in the left eye with an excellent visual result. The patient wanted to pursue surgical treatment in the fellow eye due to continued difficulties with her contact lenses (Fig. 50.1).

Main Problem to Solve

The patient had difficulty wearing a contact lens in her right eye. With excellent uncorrected visual acuity in her treated left eye after DALK and PRK, options were discussed to help achieve an excellent visual result in the right eye. Among the options were dovetail femtosecond keratoplasty, collagen cross-linking [3], and intracorneal ring segments.

J.L. Alió et al. (eds.), *Difficult and Complicated Cases in Refractive Surgery*,
DOI 10.1007/978-3-642-55238-0_50, © Springer-Verlag Berlin Heidelberg 2015

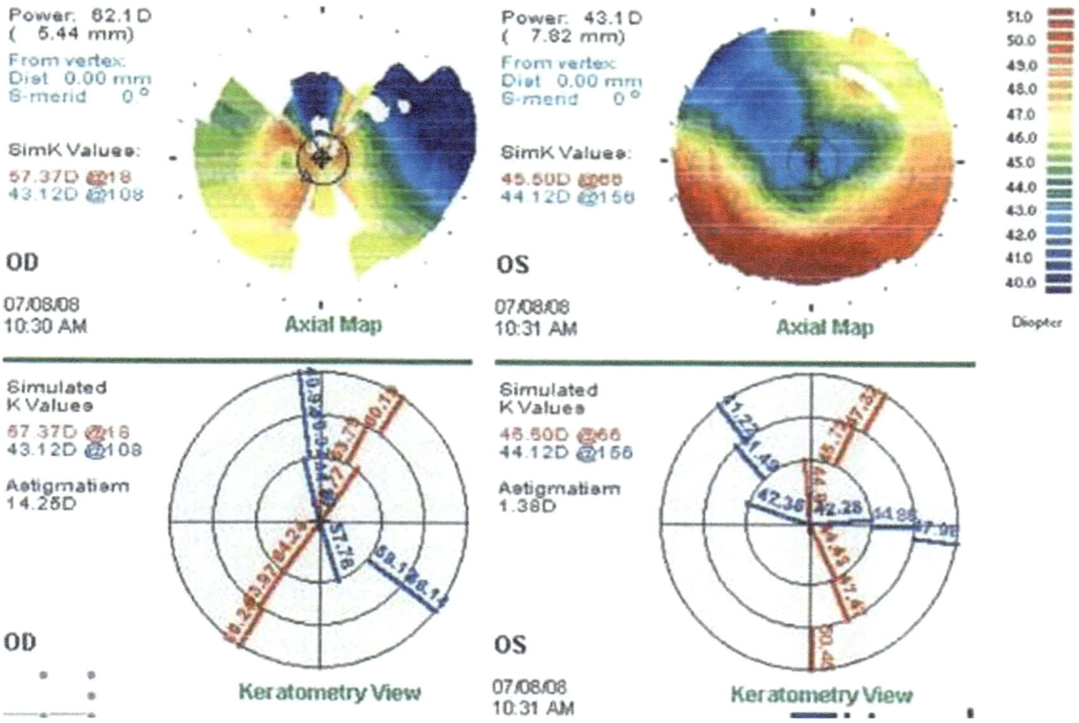

Fig. 50.1 Corneal topography of corneal ectasia, right eye

Surgical/Medical Intervention (with Video if Needed)

The patient elected to undergo dovetail keratoplasty in the right eye. A dovetail pattern was used for the side cut, and the donor tissue was cut in the same pattern and sutured into place. The plan was to attempt a DALK using pneumodissection of Descemet's membrane, but a Descemet's perforation was noted and so a full-thickness keratoplasty was performed.

Steps to perform a dovetail femtosecond keratoplasty are as follows:

1. Ultrasound pachymetry of the central cornea in anticipation of treatment 100 μm anterior to the posterior corneal surface
2. Femtosecond laser to treat the patient's cornea using a dovetail pattern (Fig. 50.2a)
3. Laser treatment of the donor cornea on an artificial anterior chamber using a dovetail pattern and oversizing by 0.2 mm
4. Removal of host cornea and option of pneumodissection for lamellar transplantation
5. Securing donor button in place with interrupted 10-0 nylon sutures ensuring proper "tongue-in-groove" alignment by placing needle through the point of the dovetail and entering the host cornea at the apex of the groove (Fig. 50.2b)

Outcome

The patient did well after dovetail femtosecond penetrating keratoplasty and was fortunate to achieve 20/30 uncorrected vision and

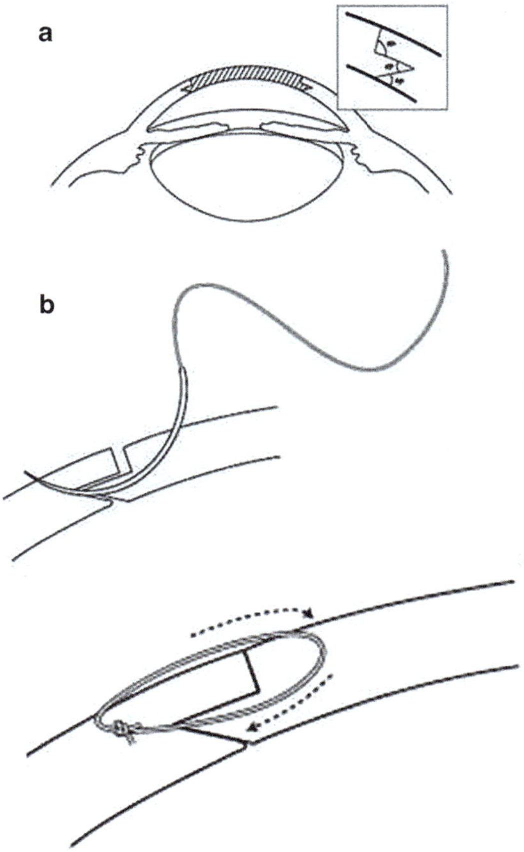

Fig. 50.2 (**a**) Illustration of the dovetail femtosecond incision pattern. (**b**) Illustration of the optimal needle entry: the needle is passed through the "point" of the dovetail in the donor tissue and is guided into the groove of the host tissue. The knot is rotated into the donor tissue to facilitate the tongue-in-groove fit and to avoid snagging the dovetail (Reproduced from Lee et al. [1] with permission from BMJ Publishing Group Ltd.)

20/20 vision with spectacles at her 2-year postoperative visit (Fig. 50.3). During her postoperative care, she underwent selective suture removal to help improve her post-keratoplasty astigmatism (Figs. 50.3, 50.4, 50.5, and 50.6).

Discussion

Management of progressive corneal ectasia after refractive surgery includes spectacles, contact lenses, intracorneal ring segments, and lamellar or penetrating keratoplasty. Lamellar keratoplasty is useful if the endothelium is healthy with or without the use of a femtosecond laser.

The femtosecond laser has proven to have multiple uses in anterior segment surgery [4]. Besides its use in LASIK and keratoplasty, it is also used to create the stromal pockets in ICRS, post-keratoplasty wedge resections, and creation of arcuate incisions for astigmatic correction. In addition to its uses in corneal surgery, it is also being used to create the capsulotomy, corneal incisions, and lens fragmentation during cataract extraction.

Potential benefits of dovetail femtosecond PK include an improved graft-host junction with more surface area, allowing for a reduction in the number of sutures. In this case, 12 interrupted sutures were used. There is the potential for a reduction in post-keratoplasty astigmatism and faster visual recovery.

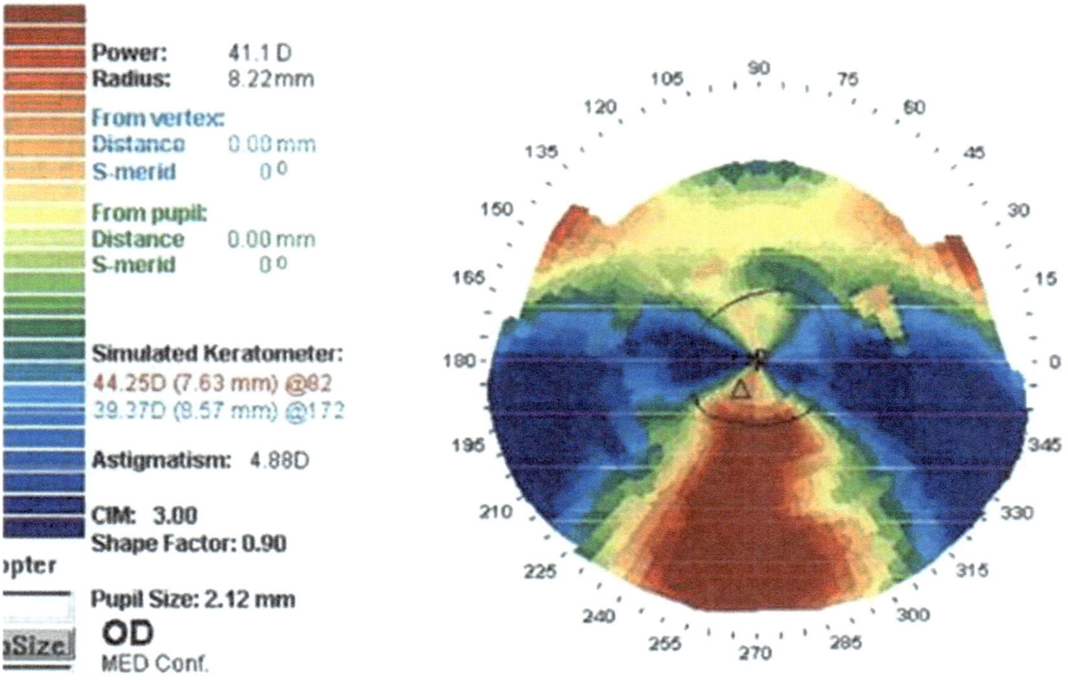

Fig. 50.3 Corneal topography 1 week after dovetail femtosecond PK, right eye

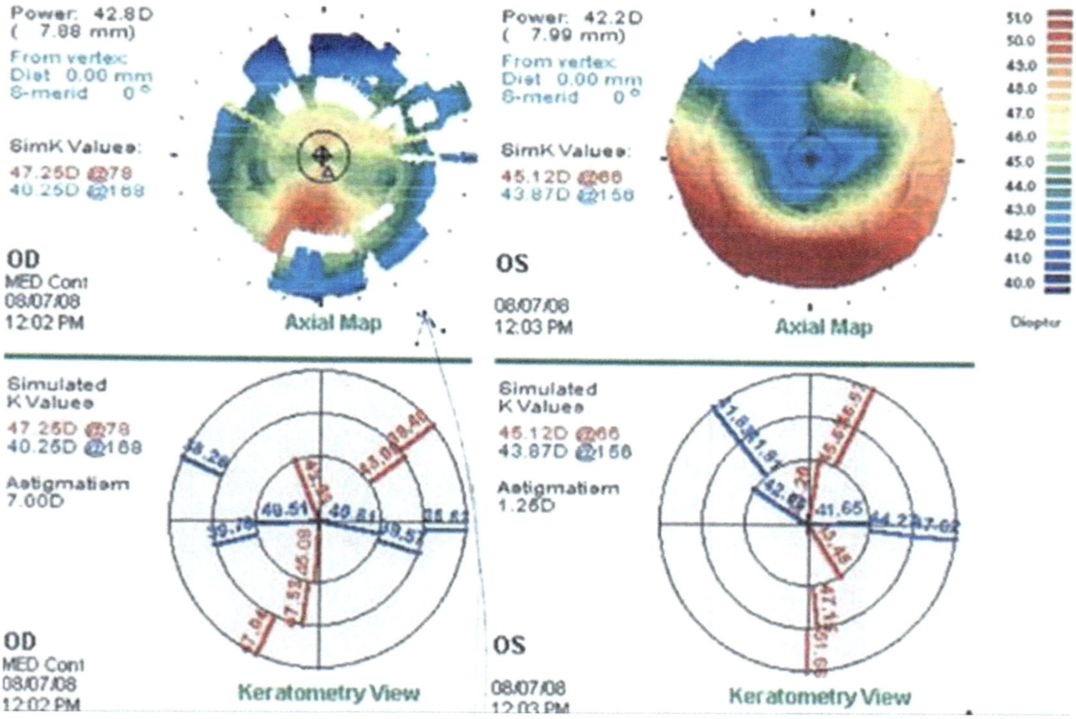

Fig. 50.4 Corneal topography 1 month after dovetail femtosecond PK, right eye

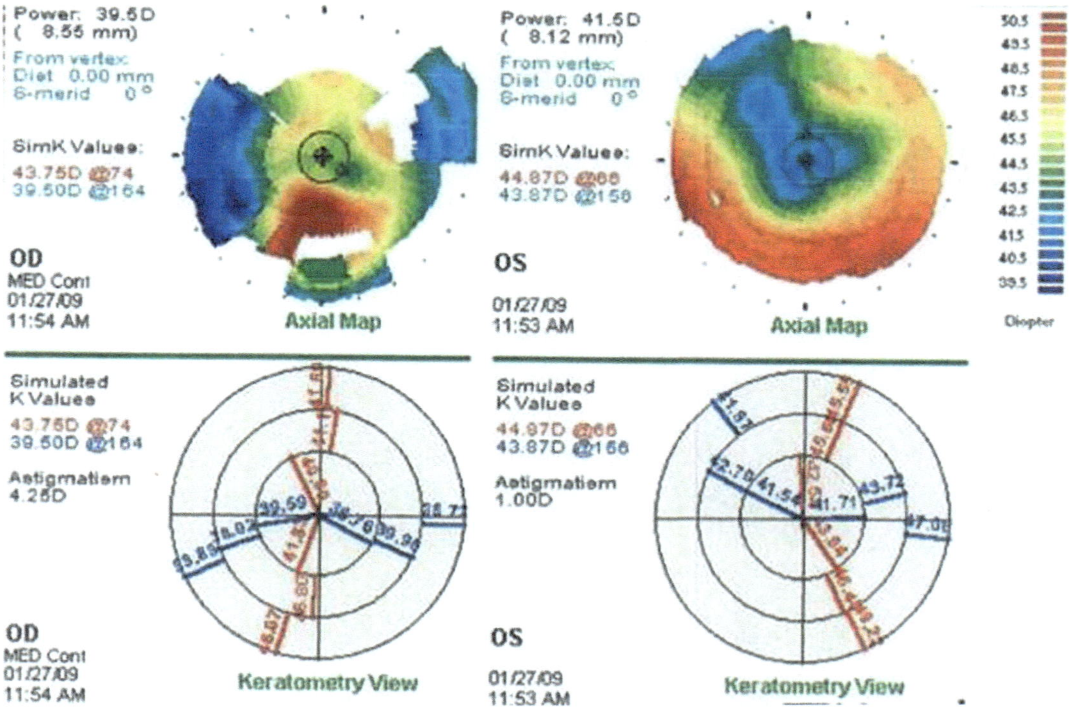

Fig. 50.5 Corneal topography 6 months after dovetail femtosecond PK, right eye

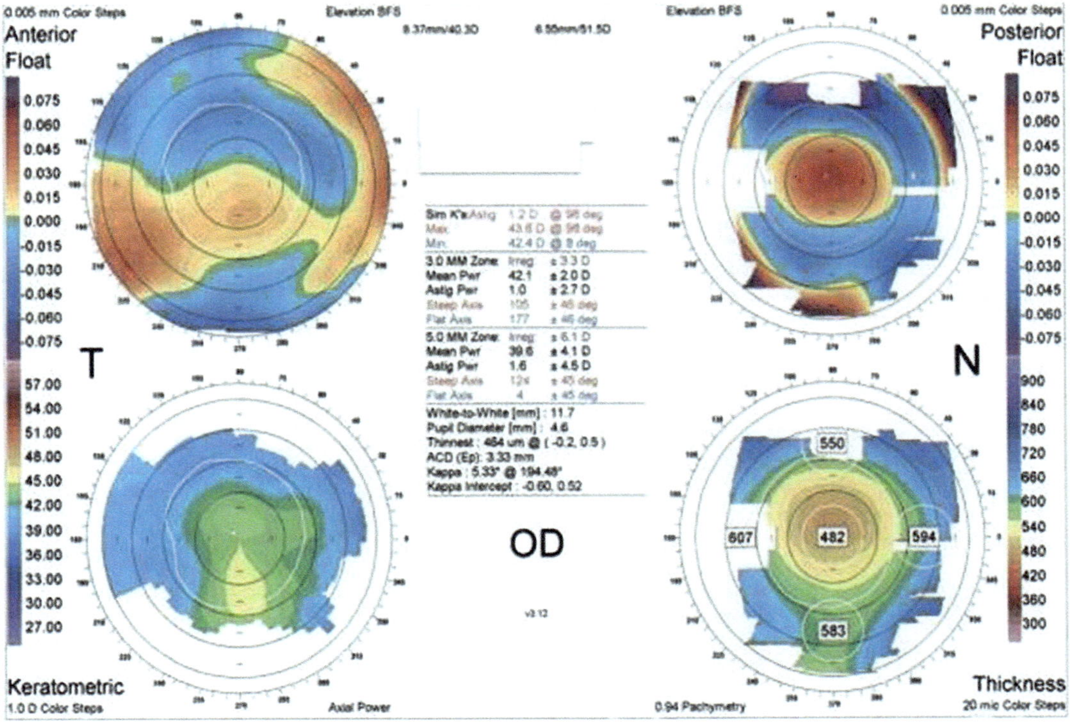

Fig. 50.6 Corneal topography 2 years after dovetail femtosecond PK, right eye

References

1. Lee J, Winokur J, Hallak J, Azar DT (2009) Femtosecond dovetail penetrating keratoplasty: surgical technique and case report. Br J Ophthalmol 93:861–863
2. Spadea L, Cantera E, Cortes M, Conocchia NE, Stewart CW (2012) Corneal ectasia after myopic laser in situ keratomileusis: a long-term study. Clin Ophthalmol 6:1801–1813
3. Poli M, Cornut PL, Balmitgere T, Aptel F, Janin H, Burillon C (2012) Prospective study of corneal collagen cross-linking efficacy and tolerance in the treatment of keratoconus and corneal ectasia: 3-year results. Cornea 32:583–590
4. Winokur J, Lee J, Kumar G, Azar DT (2011) Surgical technique of femtosecond dovetail rotational autograft. Br J Ophthalmol 95:434–436

Corneal Ectasia: Ectasia Post LASIK Managed by Femtosecond-Assisted Deep Anterior Lamellar Keratoplasty (DALK)

51

Jorge L. Alió and Alessandro Abbouda

Contents

J.L. Alió, MD, PhD (✉)
Department of Refractive Surgery, Vissum Corporación Oftalmológica, Alicante, Spain
e-mail: jlalio@vissum.com

A. Abbouda, MD
Department of Refractive Surgery, Vissum Corporación Oftalmológica, Alicante, Spain

Department of Ophthalmology-Policlinico Umberto I of Rome, University of Rome "Sapienza", Viale del Policlinico, 155, 00186 Roma, Italy

R&D Department, Vissum Corporación Oftalmológica, 03016, Alicante, Spain
e-mail: a.abbouda@gmail.com

Why Is This Case Relevant for the Refractive Surgeon?

Corneal ectasia is one of the most serious complications of laser in situ keratomileusis (LASIK), with an estimated incidence between 0.04 and 0.66 % [1–3]. The main symptoms are progressive myopia, irregular astigmatism, and loss of corrected distance visual acuity (CDVA) [4]. Risk factors for these complications are high myopia, undiagnosed forme fruste keratoconus, low residual stromal bed thickness, a large optical zone, and multiple enhancement procedures.

Case Background

A 32-year-old female patient came to our clinic complaining of low vision in both eyes. She had refractive treatment 5 years previous in a different clinic. The only available data for the previous surgery was the previous refraction status: the right eye (RE) was −5 = −2 × 30, and the left eye (LE) was −5 = −2 × 130. At her first visit to our clinic, her manifest refraction was −4 = −2 × 160 in the RE and −4 = −3 × 180 in the LE. Her BCVA was 20/30 in the RE and 20/32 in the LE. The kera-

Electronic supplementary material The online version of this chapter (10.1007/978-3-642-55238-0_51) contains supplementary material, which is available to authorized users.

J.L. Alió et al. (eds.), *Difficult and Complicated Cases in Refractive Surgery*,
DOI 10.1007/978-3-642-55238-0_51, © Springer-Verlag Berlin Heidelberg 2015

tometry reading was 40.55/54.12 × 140 in the RE and 44.19/49.12 × 37 in the LE. Corneal topography revealed inferior steepening in the LE and the RMS coma-like aberration was 2.86 μm (Fig. 51.1a, b). Pachymetry was 337 μm in the RE and 369 μm in the LE. There was a diagnosis of ectasia post LASIK.

The Main Problem to Solve

Different treatments exist for ectasia. Rigid gas permeable contact lenses are an easy treatment option; however, our patient did not tolerate them. We proposed intracorneal rings, but the patient preferred to wait to see if there was any improvement.

Ancillary Tests

When the corneal thickness is less than 300 μm centrally and/or has significant central scarring, we advise deep anterior lamellar keratoplasty (DALK). Six months after her initial visit, the patient returned to our clinic complaining of visual loss in the LE. Slit lamp examination revealed central scarring.

Surgical/Medical Intervention

Femtosecond-assisted DALK was performed. The mushroom profile was chosen because it allows excision of most of the ectatic stroma, creating a larger area of host-donor tissue interaction which improves the quality and speed of the corneal healing process. A vertical limbal-scleral incision of 1 mm with a depth of 0.5 mm was created at the limbus in order to approach the Schwalbe line. A 31G injection of air into the posterior corneal stroma created a dissection between the stroma and Descemet's membrane. Dissection of the residual stroma was performed until Descemet's membrane was completely free of stromal tissue. A corneal button was then sutured with nylon 10.0 (Video 51.1).

Outcome

On the first postoperative day, a double anterior chamber (DAC) was noted. Anterior segment optical coherence tomography (AS-OCT) showed a complete endothelium and Descemet's detachment (Fig. 51.2a). Air tamponade was injected into the AC. On the 5th postoperative day, the DAC persisted. At 2 weeks, the DAC had completely disappeared (Fig. 51.2b) with a clear corneal graft (Fig. 51.3). The patient's manifest refraction in the LE was +0.5 = −1.75 × 30. Her BCVA was 20/50. Keratometry reading in the RE was 40.55/54.12 × 140 and 42.12/47.22 × 17. The corneal topography showed a bow tie according to astigmatism with rule. RMS coma-like aberration was 1.89 μm (Fig. 51.4a, b).

What to Learn from This Case

The goal of DALK is to remove and replace the affected corneal stroma while preserving the healthy endothelium of the host; DALK eliminates the risk of endothelial graft rejection [5]. However, complications may occur during the postoperative evolution. Due to the improved anatomical donor-host profiles, modern femtosecond keratoplasty profiles allow for greater control of the induced astigmatism in DALK, including a better suturing technique.

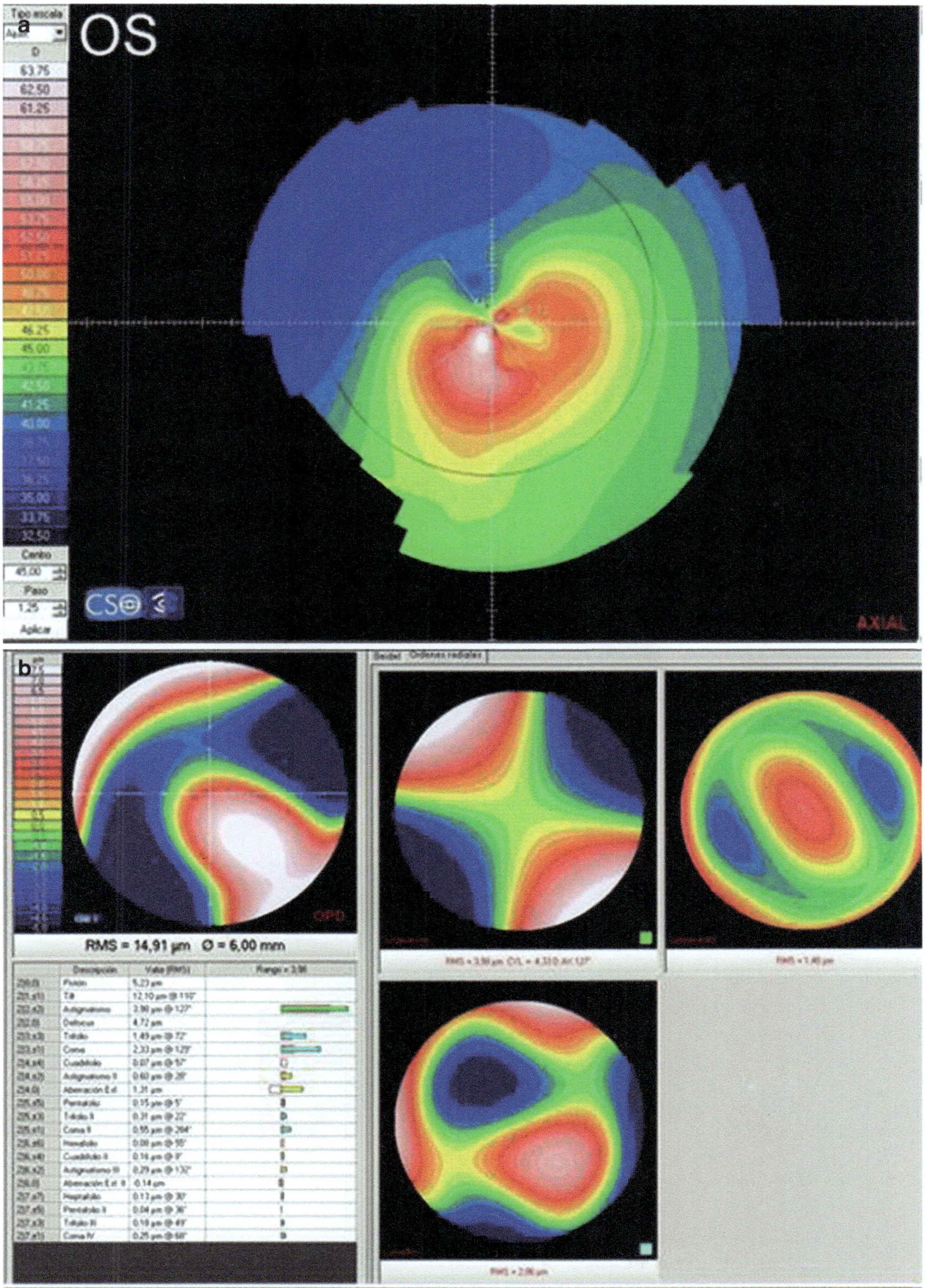

Fig. 51.1 (**a**) Corneal topography showed inferior steepening in the LE. (**b**) The RMS coma-like aberration was 2.86 µm

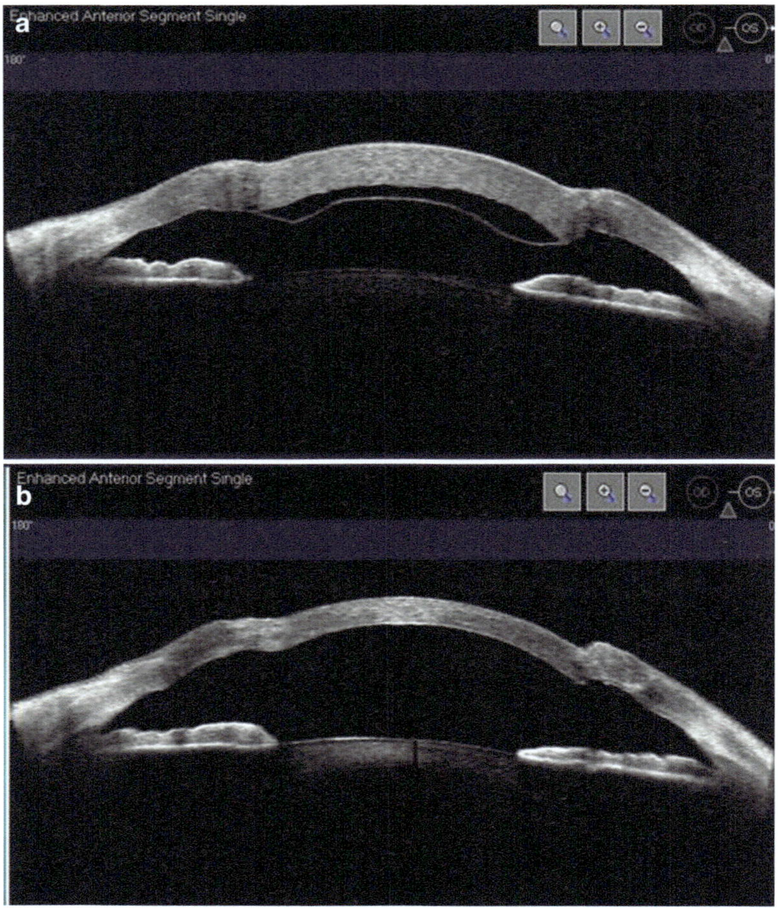

Fig. 51.2 (**a**) OCT Visante 1 day after surgery showed a double anterior chamber. (**b**) OCT Visante 2 weeks after surgery showed complete resolution

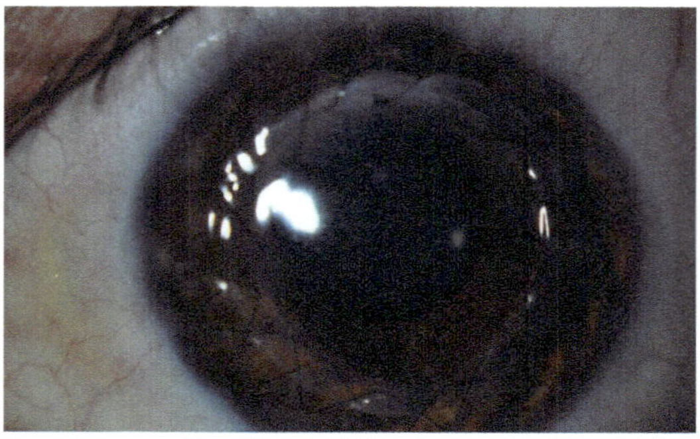

Fig. 51.3 Slit lamp examination 2 weeks after surgery showed clear corneal graft

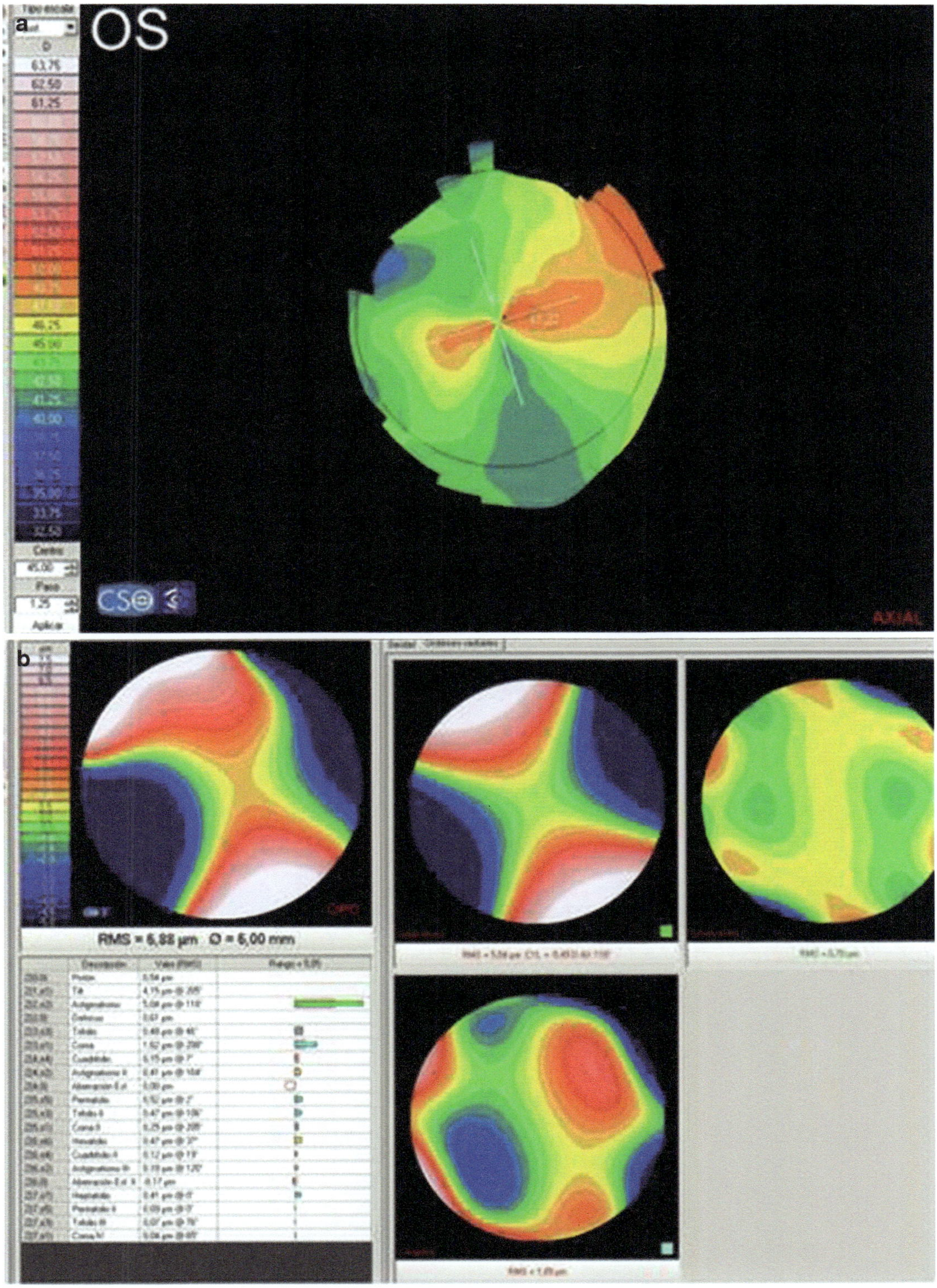

Fig. 51.4 (**a**) Corneal topography showed bow tie according to astigmatism with rule. (**b**) RMS coma-like aberration was 1.89 µm

References

1. Randleman JB, Russell B, Ward MA, Thompson KP, Stulting RD (2003) Risk factors and prognosis for corneal ectasia after LASIK. Ophthalmology 110: 267–275
2. Lyle WA, Jin GJC (2001) Laser in situ keratomileusis with the VISX Starlaser for myopia over _10.0 diopters. J Cataract Refract Surg 27:1812–1822
3. Pallikaris IG, Kymionis GD, Astyrakakis NI (2001) Corneal ectasia induced by laser in situ keratomileusis. J Cataract Refract Surg 27:1796–1802
4. Argento C, Cosentino MJ, Tytiun A, Rapetti G, Zarate J (2001) Corneal ectasia after laser in situ keratomileusis. J Cataract Refract Surg 27:1440–1448
5. Terry MA (2000) The evolution of lamellar grafting techniques over twenty-five years. Cornea 19: 611–616

Corneal Ectasia: Management of Corneal Ectasia After LASIK with Deep Anterior Lamellar Keratoplasty (DALK) and Transepithelial Photorefractive Keratectomy (PRK) with Mitomycin C

52

Samuel H. Lee and Dimitri T. Azar

Contents

S.H. Lee, MD (✉) • D.T. Azar, MD, MBA
Department of Ophthalmology and Visual Sciences
Illinois Eye and Ear Infirmary, University of Illinois
at Chicago, Chicago, IL, USA
e-mail: samuel.lee.md@gmail.com; dazar@uic.edu

Why Is This Case Relevant for the Refractive Surgeon?

A prudent surgeon will not only understand how to screen for patients that are at a high risk for developing corneal ectasia but also understand how it is treated.

Case Background

A 28-year-old female with a history of myopic LASIK 12 years ago and a "retouch" of both eyes 1 year later presents for an opinion of worsening vision and a change in her prescription. She was diagnosed with progressive corneal ectasia and eventually had difficulty tolerating contact lenses.

Main Problem to Solve

Treatment for post-LASIK corneal ectasia is similar to that of other ectatic corneal conditions, as is the decision of when to intervene [1]. In this case, the patient was intolerant to contact lenses and wished to improve her vision. Even after a successful corneal transplant, the issue of post-keratoplasty refractive error needs to be addressed.

J.L. Alió et al. (eds.), *Difficult and Complicated Cases in Refractive Surgery*,
DOI 10.1007/978-3-642-55238-0_52, © Springer-Verlag Berlin Heidelberg 2015

Surgical/Medical Intervention (With Video if Needed)

The patient underwent intracorneal ring segments (ICRS) in the left eye in hopes that it would help reduce the corneal curvature [2]. This helped for a few months, but her left eye eventually deteriorated to the point where a lamellar corneal transplant was performed. In this case a deep anterior lamellar keratoplasty (DALK) was performed. The patient did well after DALK and then underwent selective suture removal in order to improve the corneal curvature. Her refractive error after all the sutures were out was −10.0 +5.00×060. Her topography and wavefront analysis showed a steep cornea and with-the-rule astigmatism (Figs. 52.1 and 52.2).

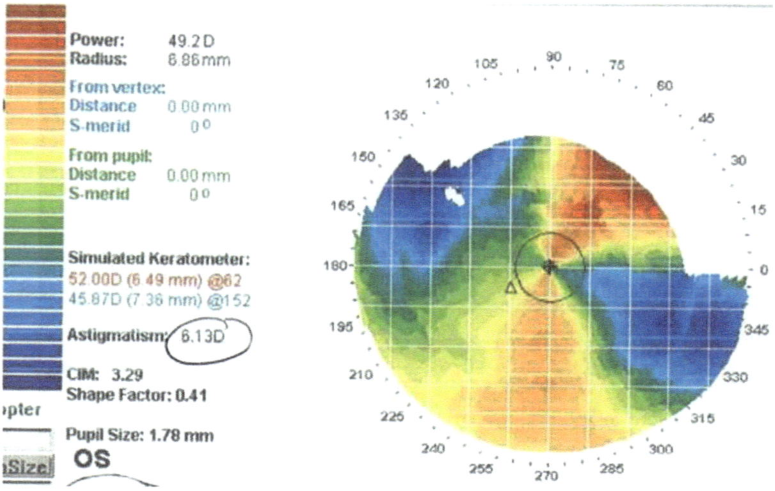

Fig. 52.1 Corneal topography after DALK, left eye showing high irregular corneal astigmatism

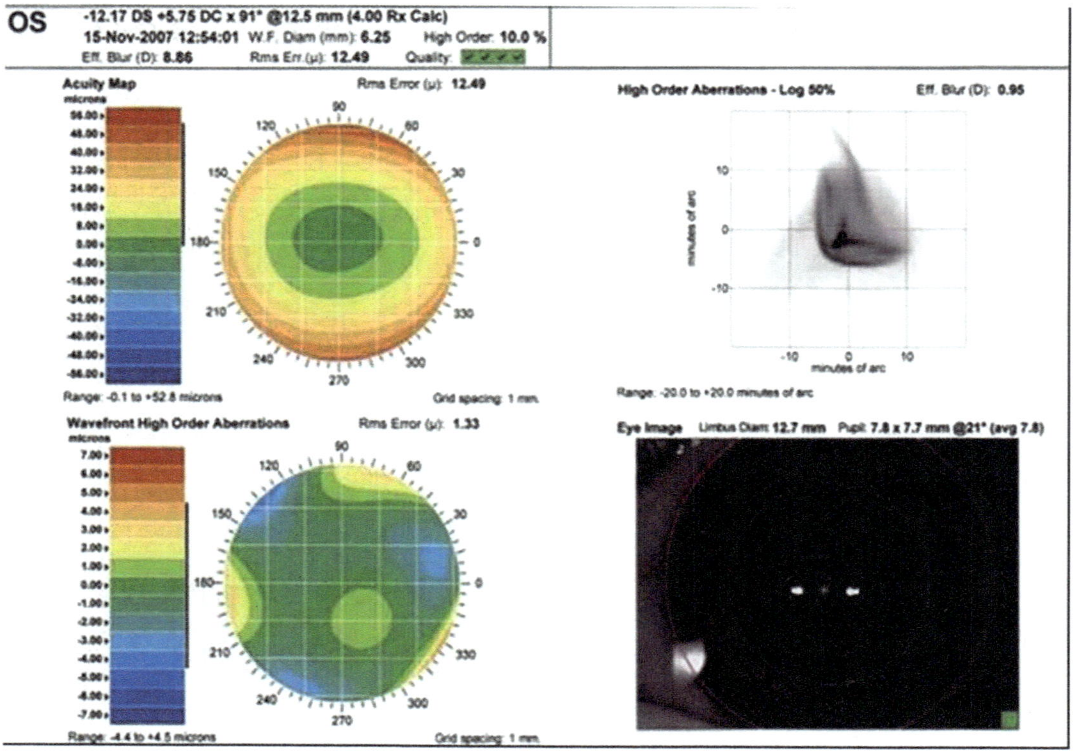

Fig. 52.2 Wavefront analysis after DALK, left eye

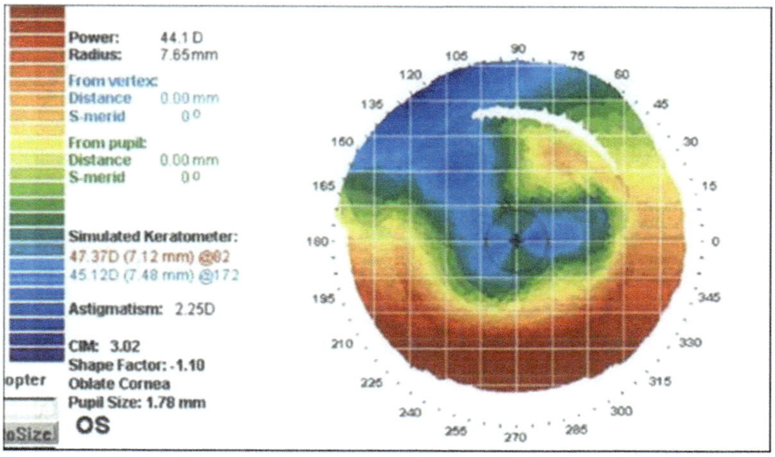

Fig. 52.3 Corneal topography after DALK and PRK, left eye

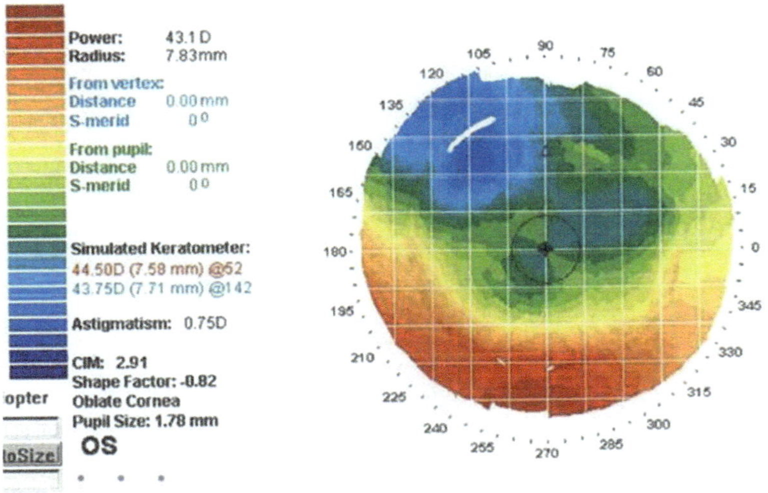

Fig. 52.4 Corneal topography after PRK re-treatment and transepithelial PRK showing 0.75 D of corneal astigmatism

Risks, benefits, and alternatives of post-keratoplasty management were discussed with the patient including spectacles, contact lenses, refractive surgery, and repeat transplantation. She underwent photorefractive keratectomy (PRK) with mitomycin C (MMC) (Fig. 52.3) and, then because of a residual refractive error of −3.50 +3.50 × 090 in the left eye, underwent transepithelial PRK with a good refractive result (Fig. 52.4).

Outcome

Two years after DALK in the left eye and 9 years after her original LASIK procedure, she is now 20/25 uncorrected in the left eye. To reach this refractive outcome, she underwent PRK with MMC and a re-treatment with transepithelial PRK with MMC. The lamellar graft is clear, and the patient is pleased.

What to Learn from This Case

1. ICRS after LASIK ectasia can be considered, but may not be sufficiently effective to halt or reverse the progression of ectasia [2].
2. Proper treatment of corneal ectasia consists of contact lenses first and consideration of corneal transplantation when deemed necessary. In the refractive population, one may also need to explore options to lower the amount of

residual refractive error after transplantation, whether a full-thickness keratoplasty or a lamellar keratoplasty is performed [3].

3. Surface ablation is a good option to treat post-keratoplasty refractive error, but requires patience after the refraction and topography, and wavefront scan has been stable.
4. Transepithelial PRK can be a useful tool to treat residual refractive error. In this case, a 54-μm PTK was performed through the epithelium, followed by PRK to alter the corneal curvature.

References

1. Randleman JB (2011) Ectasia after LASIK: new treatments, new hope. J Refract Surg 5:319–327
2. Piñero DP, Alio JL (2010) Intracorneal ring segments in ectatic corneal disease – a review. Clin Experiment Ophthalmol 38:154–167
3. Javadi MA, Feizi S (2010) Deep anterior lamellar keratoplasty using the big-bubble technique for keratectasia after laser in situ keratomileusis. J Cataract Refract Surg 36:1156–1160

Corneal Ectasia: Transepithelial Phototherapeutic Keratectomy and Corneal Collagen Cross-Linking for a Patient Affected by Ectasia Post-LASIK with High Coma Aberration

53

Jorge L. Alió and Alessandro Abbouda

Contents

J.L. Alió, MD, PhD (✉)
Department of Refractive Surgery, Vissum Corporación Oftalmológica, Alicante, Spain
e-mail: jlalio@vissum.com

A. Abbouda, MD
Department of Refractive Surgery, Vissum Corporación Oftalmológica, Alicante, Spain

Department of Ophthalmology-Policlinico Umberto I of Rome, University of Rome "Sapienza", Viale del Policlinico, 155, 00186 Roma, Italy

R&D Department, Vissum Corporación Oftalmológica, 03016, Alicante, Spain
e-mail: a.abbouda@gmail.com

Why Is This Case Relevant for the Refractive Surgeon?

Topography-guided photorefractive keratectomy (PRK) has been proposed as a palliative method for correcting irregular astigmatism in keratoconus [1]. However, this treatment needs to be associated with collagen cross-linking to avoid the risk of exacerbating the corneal ectasia.

Case Background

A 32-year-old woman diagnosed with ectasia post-LASIK and contact lens intolerance consulted us with the hope of improving her vision. She did not have any data about the previous surgery. Her best corrected visual acuity (BCVA) in the right eye (RE) was 20/30 with a manifest refraction of −1.25 = −1.5 × 120 and 20/25 in the left eye (LE) with a manifest refraction of −1 = −0.50 × 170. The corneal central thickness was 483 μm in the RE and 458 μm in the LE. Keratometry reading was 44.44/45.87 × 69 in the RE and 41.97/43.67 × 100 in the LE. The corneal topography in both eyes showed an inferior steepening (Fig. 53.1a, b). The corneal aberrometry showed an RMS coma of 1.40 μm in the RE and 1.75 μm in the LE (Fig. 53.1c, d). Because of the high coma value, we used a customized profile.

J.L. Alió et al. (eds.), *Difficult and Complicated Cases in Refractive Surgery*,
DOI 10.1007/978-3-642-55238-0_53, © Springer-Verlag Berlin Heidelberg 2015

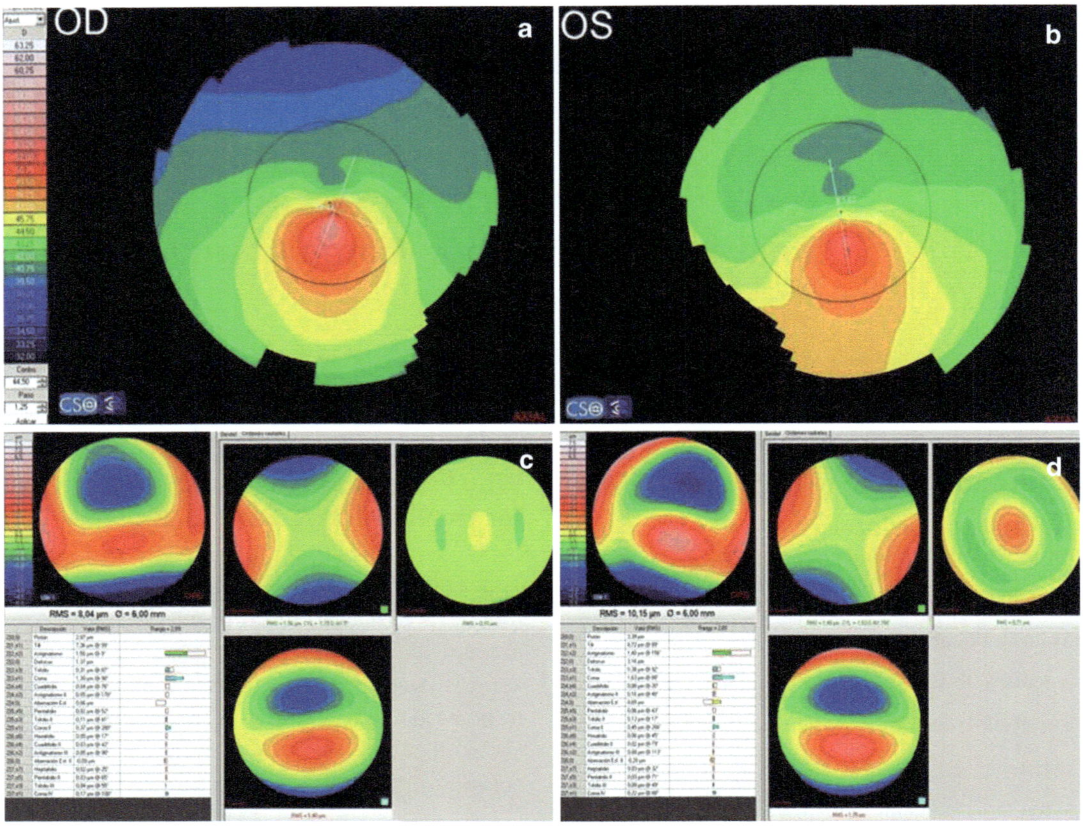

Fig. 53.1 Preoperative topography in the (**a**) right eye and (**b**) left eye. Preoperative corneal aberrometry in the (**c**) right eye and (**d**) left eye

Main Problem to Solve

The irregular astigmatism of ectasia creates highly aberrated eyes which can be minimized with customized laser ablation procedures. Topography-guided PRK is a reasonable intervention for symptomatic, highly aberrated corneas [2–5]. On the other hand, this procedure leaves the cornea vulnerable to progressive change, making it necessary to add riboflavin/UVA CXL to increase corneal stiffness and to stabilize the condition.

Ancillary Tests

Corneal topography, aberrometry, pachymetry, refraction, and BCVA

Surgical/Medical Intervention

After topical anesthesia with proxymetacaine hydrochloride 0.5 % eye drops (Alcaine; Alcon Laboratories Inc.), epithelial removal was performed by t-PTK using the PTK mode of the SCHWIND AMARIS laser. The t-PTK ablation was performed at a 7.0-mm zone with an intended depth of 50 μm. Then, the deepithelialized area was enlarged mechanically by scraping the epithelium with a beaver blade at an intended 8.0-mm zone. The tracker was engaged for topographic-guided PRK treatment. After PRK, mitomycin C (0.02 %) was applied with a sponge for 20 s and then irrigated. Following the conclusion of the MMC application, accelerated Crosslinking Avedro technique was performed. Topical riboflavin sodium phosphate 0.1 % drops were placed on the cornea every 2 min for 10 min and the surface was exposed to 370-nm UVA light with a 10-nm bandwidth at 30 mW/cm^2 for 3 min. A soft contact lens was placed on the eye with a topical antibiotic (0.3 % ofloxacin) and steroid (1.0 % prednisolone acetate) drops administered four times daily until re-epithelialization, after which the topical steroid was tapered over several weeks.

Outcome

The postoperative period was uneventful. The slit-lamp examination showed a tender haze in the center. After 3 months, the visual acuity was 20/25 in both eyes with a manifest refraction of plano in the RE and −0.75×90 in the LE. Keratometry reading was 42.83/43.37×138 in the RE and 41.04/42.4×91 in the LE. The aspect of the images showed a flattening of the previous conus (Fig. 53.2a, b). The corneal aberrometry showed a decrease of coma-like aberration. The value of coma-like aberration was RMS of 0.72 μm in the RE and 0.54 μm in the LE (Fig. 53.2c, d).

What to Learn from This Case

Simultaneous topography-guided PTK with corneal CXL appears to be an acceptable alternative for the management of ectasia post-LASIK. Innovation in this area led us to use accelerated CXL and t-PTK. This approach results in better visual and refractive outcomes [1] only in cases with good visual potential, demonstrated by a good preoperative BCVA. This procedure should always be considered before considering a more aggressive surgical treatment.

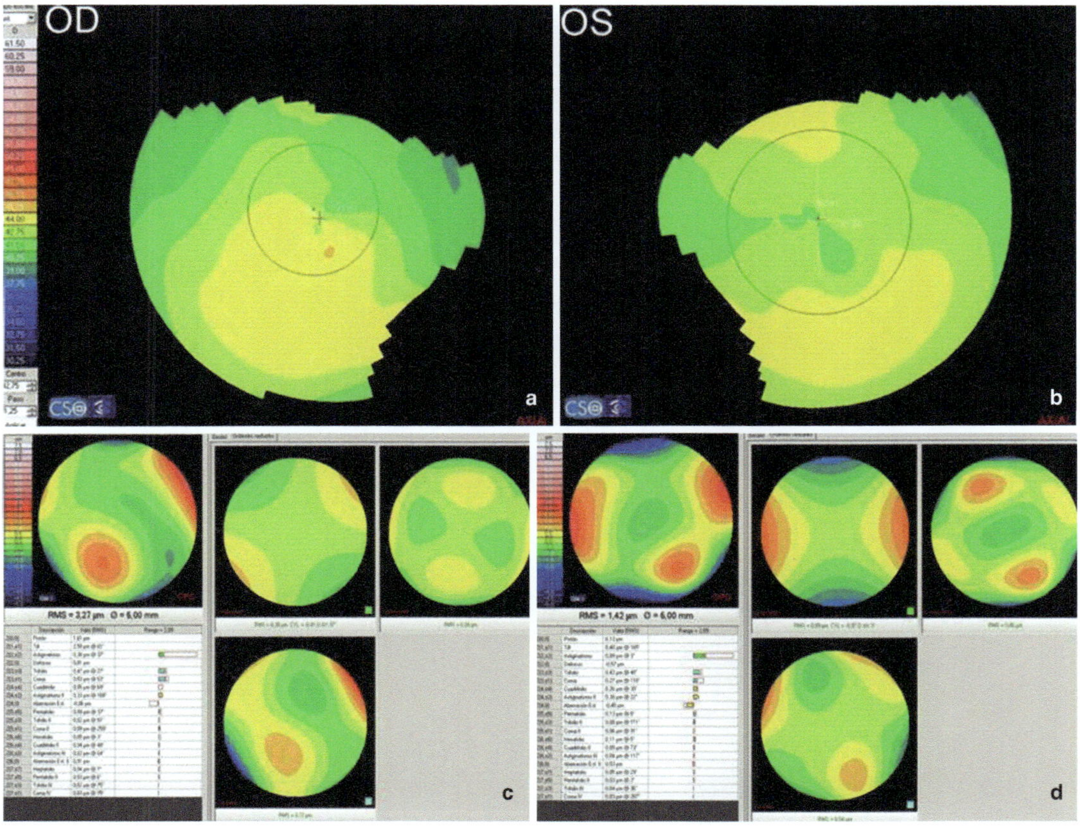

Fig. 53.2 Postoperative corneal topography after 3 months of surgery in the (**a**) right eye and (**b**) left eye and corneal aberrometry in the (**c**) right eye and (**d**) left eye

References

1. Kymionis GD, Grentzelos MA, Kounis GA, Diakonis VF, Limnopoulou AN, Panagopoulou SI (2012) Combined transepithelial phototherapeutic keratectomy and corneal collagen cross-linking for progressive keratoconus. Ophthalmology 119:1777–1784
2. Tamayo GE, Serrano MG (2003) Treatment of irregular astigmatism and keratoconus with the VISX C-CAP method. Int Ophthalmol Clin 43:103–110
3. Cennamo G, Intravaja A, Boccuzzi D, Marotta G, Cennamo G (2008) Treatment of keratoconus by topography-guided customized photorefractive keratectomy: two-year follow-up study. J Refract Surg 24:145–149
4. Lin DT, Holland SR, Rocha KM, Krueger RR (2008) Method for optimizingtopography-guided ablation of highly aberrated eyes with the ALLEGRETTO WAVE excimer laser. J Refract Surg 24:S439–S445
5. Kanellopoulos AJ, Binder PS (2007) Collagen cross-linking (CCL) with sequential topography-guided PRK: a temporizing alternative for keratoconus to penetrating keratoplasty. Cornea 26:891–895

Other Complications: Late Flap Striae

54

Roger F. Steinert

Contents

R.F. Steinert, MD
Department of Ophthalmology, Gavin Herbert Eye Institute, University of California, Irvine, CA, USA
e-mail: steinert@uci.edu

Why Is This Case Relevant for the Refractive Surgeon?

Flap striae can reduce corrected distance visual acuity (CDVA). When recognized and treated immediately, striae generally can be reduced to a level that is clinically insignificant. However, when the striae have been present for months, they are established and difficult to treat. The irregular collagen becomes fixed in position. When striae have been present for a month or more, direct treatment of the elevations of the striae is needed to reduce the optical impact of the striae.

Case Background

Patient presents at a later exam (typically not the first several post-op exams, but rather 1 month or longer) with suboptimal CDVA and with striae visible at the slit-lamp examination.

Main Problem to Solve

Treat the striae to allow full CDVA and maximal uncorrected distance visual acuity (UDVA). Options for the patient are either dependency on a

Electronic supplementary material The online version of this chapter (10.1007/978-3-642-55238-0_54) contains supplementary material, which is available to authorized users.

J.L. Alió et al. (eds.), *Difficult and Complicated Cases in Refractive Surgery*,
DOI 10.1007/978-3-642-55238-0_54, © Springer-Verlag Berlin Heidelberg 2015

rigid contact lens, which is unlikely to be appealing to a patient who underwent laser treatment to end dependency on glasses and contact lenses, or aggressive surgical intervention. The choice must then be made between flap lifting and suturing versus phototherapeutic keratectomy (PTK).

Ancillary Tests

1. Assess the tear film and cornea with fluorescein. If microstriae are optically significant, the tear film will be disrupted over the elevated microstriae ("negative staining"). A smooth tear film indicates that the microstriae may not be optically significant. With macrostriae, the tear film will always be disrupted over the large corneal folds. Moreover, the fluorescein will pool and/or frankly stain the gutter where the flap has shifted away from the proper position.
2. Corneal topography with a Placido ring pattern will show disruption of the corneal surface.
3. Rigid contact lens placement will resolve any visual disturbances.

Surgical/Medical Intervention

After optically significant striae are present for a week or longer, a refloat of the flap, with or without epithelial debridement and hydration with hypotonic water, is inadequate to resolve the striae. A more aggressive technique is required.

One option is to free up the flap then suture it very tightly with multiple interrupted sutures. While tight suturing of the flap may accomplish a release of the fixed striae, it is difficult for suturing not to induce new tension deformation of the cornea that may result in permanent irregular astigmatism, similar to the challenge of post-keratoplasty astigmatism. In addition, there is some risk of epithelial ingrowth from a late flap lift.

An alternative technique is transepithelial PTK. This requires an excimer laser with PTK capability. Because the epithelium is naturally thinner over the elevated ridges of striae and is thicker in the valleys between the ridges, the epithelium is a natural "masking" agent. By performing transepithelial ablation initially, the elevated ridges will be markedly reduced in height by the time that the epithelium is largely removed. The excimer laser should be programed to remove 50 μm of tissue over as large a diameter as possible (Fig. 54.1).

If visible striae remain, which is often the case, more smoothing can be obtained by applying further PTK pulses. Use a medium viscosity artificial tear applied in a thin film by a surgical micro-sponge as a masking agent. Use just enough moisture to make the surface shiny, but not "flooding" the surface. Run the laser for about 1 s, then re-wipe and repeat. (With the

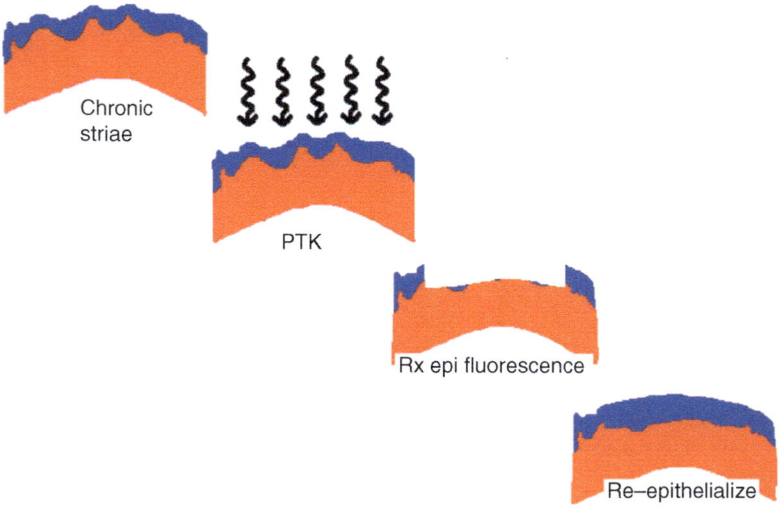

Fig. 54.1 Concept of transepithelial PTK for chronic striae

VISX laser, reduce the pulse rate to the slowest rate of 5 Hz to facilitate control.) The end point of the PTK is either a smooth surface or a maximum of 25 µm more PTK, if using a scanning laser, or 100 pulses, if using a broad beam PTK with the VISX laser. If masking fluid has been properly used, the further tissue removal will only be about 10 µm. By limiting the depth of the PTK, the risk of haze is minimal, so mitomycin is not needed. Moreover, the amount of hyperopic shift, often seen with PTK, typically will be 1 D or less. It is not necessary to remove 100 % of the striae, but just enough so that the healing epithelium can optically mask the remaining irregularities that are less elevated than the original striae.

After completion of the PTK, place a bandage contact lens for 3–4 days, accompanied by intense topical steroid and by antibiotic prophylaxis. After epithelial coverage, support further healing with aggressive lubrication using non-preserved artificial tears.

Assessment of the impact of this technique with maximal recovery of vision requires several weeks to months of epithelial healing.

Outcome

Excellent UDVA and CDVA with a maximum of 1 D of hyperopic shift [1, 2]

What to Learn from This Case

PTK offers a predictable method of striae reduction.

References

1. Steinert RF, Ashrafzadeh A, Hersh PS (2004) Results of phototherapeutic keratectomy in the management of flap striae after LASIK. Ophthalmology 111: 740–746
2. Ashrafzadeh A, Steinert RF (2007) Results of phototherapeutic keratectomy in the management of flap striae after LASIK before and after developing a standardized protocol: long term follow-up in an expanded patient population. Ophthalmology 114:1118–1123

Other Complications: Scarring

55

Jorge L. Alió, Angelo Rampone, and Alessandro Abbouda

Contents

J.L. Alió, MD, PhD (✉)
Department of Refractive Surgery, Vissum Corporación Oftalmológica, Alicante, Spain
e-mail: jlalio@vissum.com

A. Rampone, MD
Department of Ophthalmology, Seconda Università degli Studi di Napoli, Naples, Italy

R&D Department, Vissum Corporacion, 03016, Alicante, Spain
e-mail: angelo.rampone@gmail.com

A. Abbouda, MD
Department of Refractive Surgery, Vissum Corporación Oftalmológica, Alicante, Spain

Department of Ophthalmology-Policlinico Umberto I of Rome, University of Rome "Sapienza", Viale del Policlinico, 155, 00186 Roma, Italy

R&D Department, Vissum Corporación Oftalmológica, 03016, Alicante, Spain
e-mail: a.abbouda@gmail.com

Why Is This Case Relevant for the Refractive Surgeon?

The refractive surgeon who performs femtosecond LASIK should be familiar with how to manage a vertical gas breakthrough. Proper and timely diagnosis and management can increase the chance of an optimal visual outcome.

Case Background

A 25-year-old man with no ocular history presented for refractive surgery evaluation. His manifested refraction was −2.75, 0.75×180 in the right eye (RE) and −3.25, −0.75×180 in the left eye (LE). Keratometry readings were 40.32/41.62×93 in the RE and 40.59/41.67×96 in the LE. His best corrected visual acuity (BCVA) was 20/20 for distance and near in both eyes. Both slit-lamp and fundus examinations were normal. According to the topography, his cornea surface was regular. His RE pachymetry was 554 μm and his LE pachymetry was 557 μm. He underwent a LASIK procedure, both eyes targeted for distance. During the procedure we observed a vertical epithelial gas breakthrough in the peripheral part of the flap.

Main Problem to Solve

Vertical epithelial gas breakthrough is not a common complication during flap creation.

J.L. Alió et al. (eds.), *Difficult and Complicated Cases in Refractive Surgery*,
DOI 10.1007/978-3-642-55238-0_55, © Springer-Verlag Berlin Heidelberg 2015

Vertical gas breakthrough can be as the same group of buttonholed flap. The gas breakthrough can mislead the surgeon into leaving a piece of stroma intact when creating the flap. As the flap is lifted, the intact stroma will tear causing a hole [1].

Ancillary Tests

The most important thing about the possibility to follow prior to the laser procedure is the location of vertical epithelial gas breakthrough. If the vertical bubble is peripheral, the procedure can follow, while in central cases the surgery should be abandoned.

Surgical/Medical Intervention

In this case, the rupture was peripheral and the procedure was completed. The flap depth was set at 100–130 μm using the IntraLase FS™ CORP Femtosecond Laser System.

Outcome

At 1 month follow-up, the UCVA was 20/20. The slit-lamp examination only showed the presence of a tender opacity in the same place where the vertical gas breakthrough was (Fig. 55.1).

What to Learn from This Case?

Scarring is a natural part of the wound healing process, with the exception of very minor lesions. Every wound, including surgical wounds, results in some degree of scarring. Scar tissue is not identical to the tissue it replaces and is usually of inferior functional quality.

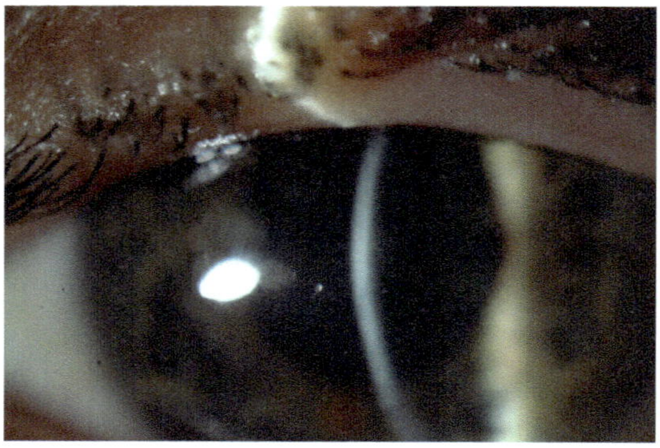

Fig. 55.1 Epithelial scar in the same place where the vertical gas breakthrough was

Transparency, regular shape, and a smooth surface are the main properties that allow the cornea to function as the first diopter of the eye. The worldwide popularity of LASIK refractive surgery is largely due to its rapid and stable refractive and visual outcome. However, even with the assistance of femtosecond lasers, the surgery is not free from complications when corneal transparency is not perfect. Thin flap, steep cornea, and epithelial basal membrane dystrophy (EBMD) are the principal causes of a vertical gas breakthrough [2]. In this case a partial loss of corneal transparency seems to be the main outcome. It is also important to remember that in case of a central vertical bubble breakthrough, the procedure should be abandoned.

References

1. Moshirfar M, Gardiner JP, Schliesser JA, Espandar L, Feiz V, Mifflin MD, Chang JC (2010) Laser in situ keratomileusis flap complications using mechanical microkeratome versus femtosecond laser: Retrospective comparison. J Cataract Refract Surg 36: 1925–1933
2. Melki SA, Azar DT (2001) LASIK complications: etiology, management, and prevention. Surv Ophthalmol 46:95–116

Other Complications: Abnormal Healing in Femtosecond LASIK

56

Jaime Javaloy, Alessandro Abbouda, and Angelo Rampone

Contents

J. Javaloy, MD, PhD (✉)
Department of Anterior Segment and Refractive Surgery, Vissum Corporacion Oftalmológica, Alicante, Spain
e-mail: jjavaloy@coma.es

A. Abbouda, MD
Department of Refractive Surgery, Vissum Corporación Oftalmológica, Alicante, Spain

Department of Ophthalmology-Policlinico Umberto I of Rome, University of Rome "Sapienza", Viale del Policlinico, 155, 00186 Roma, Italy

R&D Department, Vissum Corporación Oftalmológica, 03016, Alicante, Spain
e-mail: a.abbouda@gmail.com

A. Rampone, MD
Department of Ophthalmology, Seconda Università degli Studi di Napoli, Naples, Italy

R&D Department, Vissum Corporacion, 03016, Alicante, Spain
e-mail: angelo.rampone@gmail.com

Why Is This Case Relevant for the Refractive Surgeon?

Corneal wound healing is a complex process mediated by autocrine and paracrine interactions between cytokines, growth factors, and chemokines produced by epithelial, stromal, and immune cells, lacrimal gland, and corneal nerves [1].

The abnormal healing response may be attributable to an increased release of epithelium-derived cytokines, resulting in increased keratocyte apoptosis, keratocyte proliferation, and myofibroblast generation or basement membrane damage.

A refractive surgeon should be aware that when the thin flap is performed, keratocyte activation can occur.

Case Background

A 26-year-old woman with no ocular history presented for a refractive surgery evaluation. Her manifest refraction was −8.0, −0.50 × 90° in the right eye (RE) and −8.50, −0.50 × 115° in the left eye (LE). Keratometry readings were 47.46/47.46 × 180° in the RE and 47.51/47.51 × 180° in the LE. Her best corrected visual acuity (BCVA) was 20/20 for distance and near vision in both eyes. Slit-lamp and fundus examinations were normal. According to the topography, her cornea surface was regular. Her RE pachymetry was 573 μm and LE pachymetry was 576 μm.

J.L. Alió et al. (eds.), *Difficult and Complicated Cases in Refractive Surgery*, DOI 10.1007/978-3-642-55238-0_56, © Springer-Verlag Berlin Heidelberg 2015

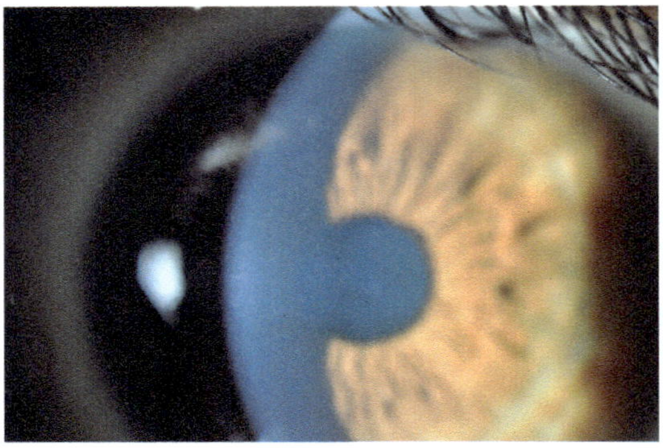

Fig. 56.1 Slit-lamp examination 1 week postoperative showed keratocyte activation

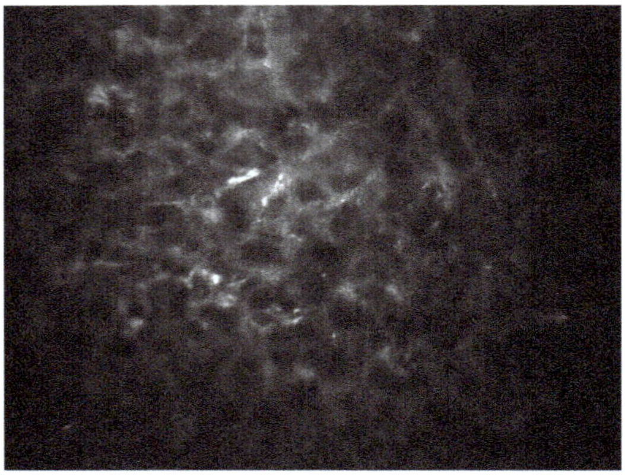

Fig. 56.2 Confocal microscopy shows increase in anterior stroma reflectivity

According to the pachymetry values and ablation depth, we decided to perform LASIK treatment with the flap setting at 100 µm. The patient started the following treatment: ofloxacin (5 times a day for 7 days) and dexamethasone 0.1 % (3 times a day for 7 days). One week after surgery, UCVA was 20/20 in both eyes. Slit-lamp examination showed a subtle white-dotted pattern located in the anterior third of the corneal stroma (Fig. 56.1).

Main Problem to Solve

Keratocyte activation induced by LASIK has a shorter duration than PRK. Flap thickness may influence corneal transparency [2]. The keratocyte population located in the anterior stroma is at particular risk to suffer activation and transformation into myofibroblasts, producing a haze.

Ancillary Test

Confocal microscopy is the most adequate examination to evaluate this alteration. The amount of reflectivity in the anterior stroma appears as a peak after the epithelium. The confocal microscopy examination showed keratocyte activation in the stromal ablation zone (Fig. 56.2). The slit-lamp examination is useful in examining subclinical haze.

Surgical/Medical Intervention

The patient underwent an uneventful LASIK procedure; both eyes were targeted for distance. Flap creation at a depth of 100 µm was performed using the Intralase™ FS (IntraLase Corp) and corneal stromal ablation by the AMARIS SCHWIND excimer laser. Postoperative evaluation was almost normal. The slit-lamp examination showed a clear interface and well-positioned flap.

Outcome

After 1 month, the slit-lamp examination showed a very tender opacity. Uncorrected visual acuity (UVCA) was 20/20 in both eyes. The keratometric reading was 40.10/40.65 × 41° in RE and 39.39/39.84 × 142° in LE (Fig. 56.3).

What to Learn from This Case

LASIK is an effective and safe treatment for moderate myopia [3]. Keratocyte activation after LASIK may be a natural defense mechanism in response to corneal trauma, attempting to reconstruct and preserve the original conformation of the corneal tissue. Even if a thin flap permits LASIK treatment in a thin cornea, keratocyte

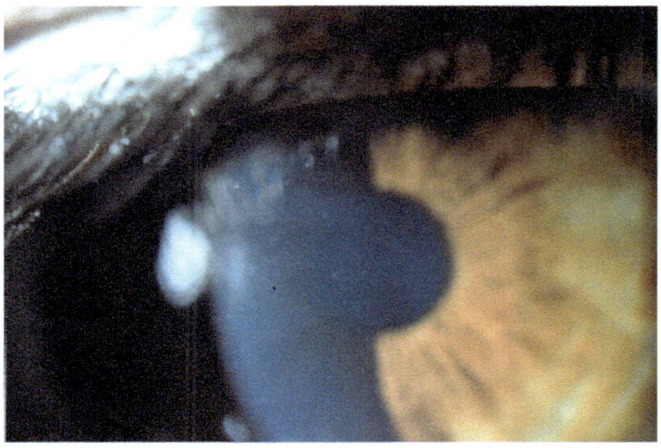

Fig. 56.3 Slit-lamp examination 1 month postoperative shows tender oval opacity

activation can frequently occur on the other side. Prophylactic effect of MMC 0.2 % may also be used for patients with a thin flap; however, it is often unnecessary because keratocyte activation does not normally affect the visual performance of the eyes [4].

References

1. Netto MV, Mohan RR, Ambrósio R Jr, Hutcheon AE, Zieske JD, Wilson SE (2005) Wound healing in the cornea: a review of refractive surgery complications and new prospects for therapy. Cornea 24:509–522
2. Alio JL, Javaloy J (2013) Corneal inflammation following corneal photoablative refractive surgery with excimer laser. Surv Ophthalmol 58:11–25
3. Melki SA, Azar DT (2001) LASIK complications: etiology, management, and prevention. Surv Ophthalmol 46:95–116
4. Teus MA, de Benito-Llopis L, Alió JL (2009) Mitomycin C in corneal refractive surgery. Surv Ophthalmol 54:487–502

Other Complications: Haze-Related Myopic Shift After PRK on a LASIK-Operated Eye Treated by Transepithelial PTK

57

Jaime Aramberri

Contents

J. Aramberri, MD
Begitek, San Sebastian, Spain

Okular, Vitoria, Spain
e-mail: jaimearamberri@telefonica.net

Why Is This Case Relevant for the Refractive Surgeon?

A refractive surgeon should be aware that haze formation can be induced by even a small ablation depth surface treatment on a LASIK flap, with myopic shift the most relevant clinical consequence [1].

Case Background

A 50-year-old man who had undergone LASIK surgery 13 years prior for −7 D presented at our clinic. The refraction on his RE was −1.00 sph −2.00 cyl × 80°. His BCVA was 20/32. Central US pachymetry was 475 μ. Scotopic pupil size was 7 mm. Scheimpflug tomography was within normal limits for all relevant parameters. The flap diameter was 7.5 mm.

PRK was performed with an Allegretto 400 Eye-Q Laser. Programmed central ablation depth was 40 μm with a target refraction of −0.50 sph. The epithelium was debrided after absolute ethanol 20 % solution was applied for 20 s. Two months post-op, BCVA was 20/30 with −1 sph with central haze +/−. Four months after surgery, BCVA was 20/30 with −2.25 sph −0.50 cyl × 130°. The patient complained of decreased distance UCVA and starbursts with artificial lights at night. Haze ++ was found on the slit-lamp exam. Corneal topography showed the curvature irregularity of an increase in the central

J.L. Alió et al. (eds.), *Difficult and Complicated Cases in Refractive Surgery*,
DOI 10.1007/978-3-642-55238-0_57, © Springer-Verlag Berlin Heidelberg 2015

area with a central island pattern. Fourier domain OCT showed subepithelial thickening with an irregular stroma-epithelium interface.

Main Problem to Solve

Our treatment goals were to eliminate haze, improve stroma-epithelium interface, correct haze-induced refraction, and prevent new haze formation.

Ancillary Tests

Fourier domain corneal OCT is the most helpful tool for measuring epithelium and haze thicknesses. In this case, peak-to-valley epithelium thickness in the central 5 mm area was 8 μm, with 48 μm in the thinnest point and 56 in the thickest. Average haze thickness in the same area was 22 μm (Fig. 57.1).

Surgical/Medical Intervention

Transepithelial PRK was performed. First plano PTK was used with a programmed 60 μm depth. Epithelium elimination was carefully monitored by the operating microscope to determine whether additional ablation was necessary, which in this case it was. Afterward, the refractive pattern was ablated with a target refraction of −0.75 sph. 0.02 % Mitomycin C (MMC) was applied on the ablated stroma for 40 s.

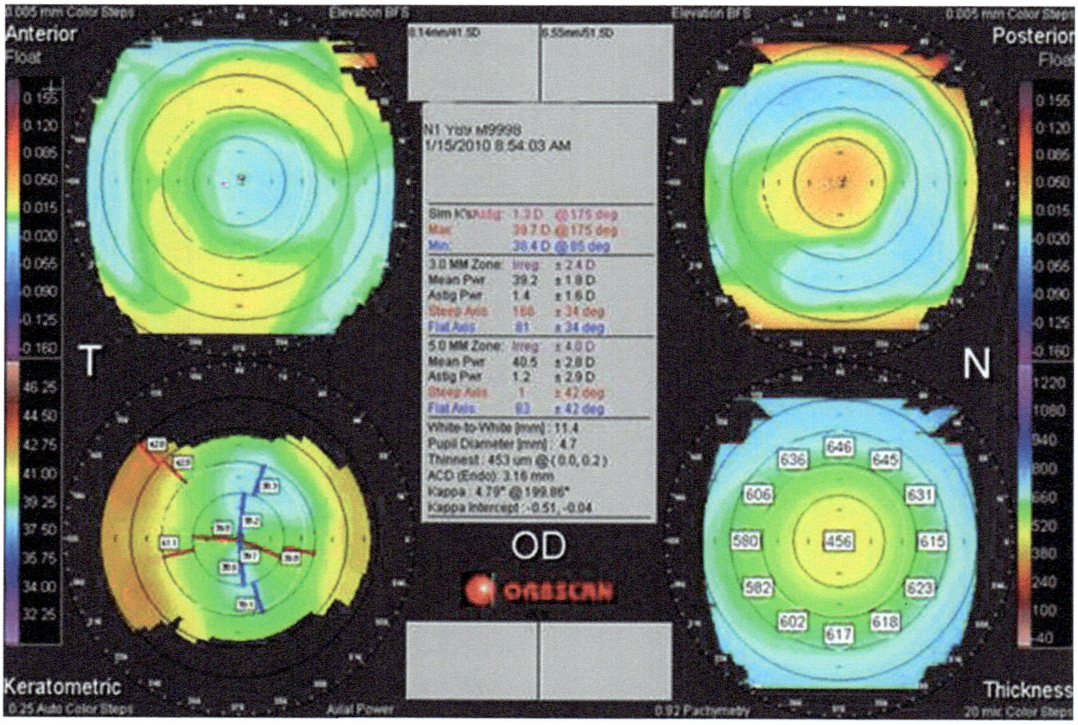

Fig. 57.1 Preoperative Orbscan corneal tomography: centered LASIK ablation with some regular astigmatism. Elevation parameters within normal limits

Outcome

Four months after surgery the patient's BCVA was 20/25 with −0.75 sph. Haze +/− was graded on the slit lamp and corneal topography displayed a regular and centered myopic ablation. The improvement of stroma-epithelium interface was clear on the corneal OCT and consequently the patient's visual perception was normalized with the elimination of light scatter-related symptoms (Figs. 57.2, 57.3, 57.4, and 57.5).

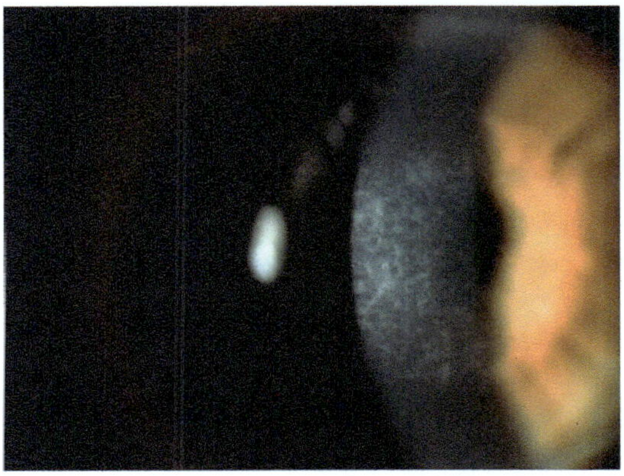

Fig. 57.2 Four months post-PRK: haze ++ with myopic shift

What to Learn from This Case

Haze-related myopia can occur even with low depth surface ablations performed on LASIK flaps in older patients. MMC should be used in such cases to prevent this complication. A transepithelial PRK approach is appropriate to improve what is frequently irregular stroma-epithelium interface in post-PRK haze cases [2–5].

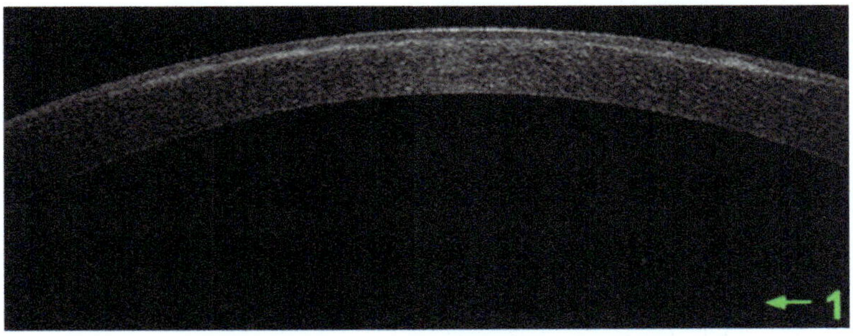

Fig. 57.3 Fourier domain corneal OCT: irregular thickening of anterior stroma due to haze formation

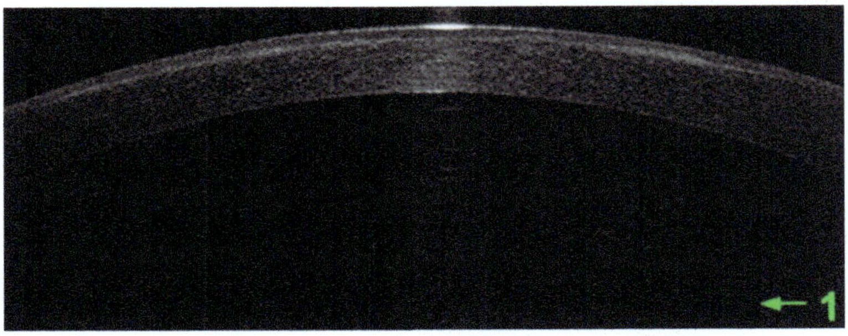

Fig. 57.4 Fourier domain corneal OCT after transepithelial PRK with MMC: improvement of the stroma-epithelium interface with elimination of haze and irregularity

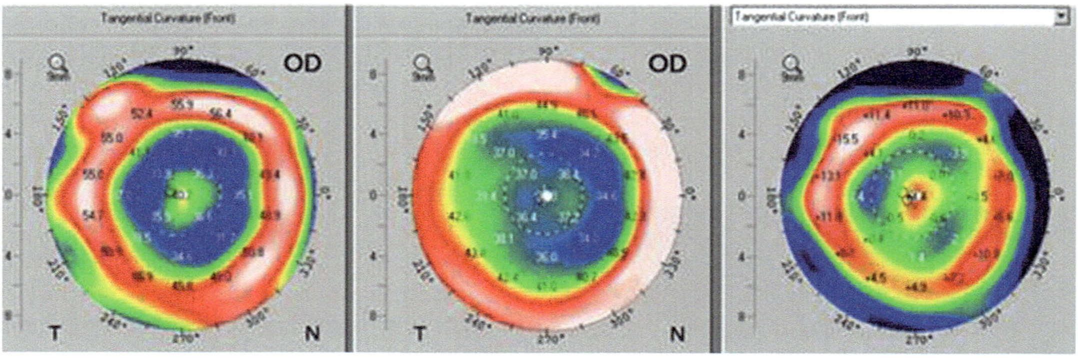

Fig. 57.5 Pentacam HR anterior cornea tangential differential map: first map is before and second map is after transepithelial PRK with MMC. Third map is the differential map

References

1. Fahd DDJ, Jain S, Azar D (2008) Corneal haze after refractive surgery. In: Alio J, Azar DT (eds) Management of complications in refractive surgery. Springer, Berlin, pp 179–186
2. Muller LT, Candal EM, Epstein RJ, Dennis RF, Majmudar PA (2005) Transepithelial phototherapeutic keratectomy/photorefractive keratectomy with adjunctive mitomycin-C for complicated LASIK flaps. J Cataract Refract Surg 31:291–296
3. Kapadia MS, Wilson SE (1998) Transepithelial photorefractive keratectomy for treatment of thin flaps or caps after complicated laser in situ keratomileusis. Am J Ophthalmol 126:827–829
4. Shaikh NM, Wee CE, Kaufman SC (2005) The safety and efficacy of photorefractive keratectomy after laser in situ keratomileusis. J Refract Surg 21:353–358
5. Teus MA, de Benito-Llopis L, Alio JL (2009) Mitomycin C in corneal refractive surgery. Surv Ophthalmol 54:487–502

Other Complications: Late-Onset Diffuse Lamellar Keratitis After LASIK in a Patient with Epithelial Defect After Microtrauma

58

Jorge L. Alió and Alessandro Abbouda

Contents

Why Is This Case Relevant for the Refractive Surgeon?

A refractive surgeon should be able to diagnose and manage uncommon cases of late-onset diffuse lamellar keratitis (DLK) in patients with epithelial defects after microtrauma. DLK is characterized by an inflammatory cellular response at the interface after lamellar corneal surgery, particularly LASIK [1]. It usually occurs during the first week following surgery. Various factors act as etiologic agents including blade debris, bacterial endotoxins on instruments, meibomian gland secretions, and epithelial defects during surgery [2–6]. Late-onset DLK is also associated with anterior segment inflammatory conditions such as allergic and adenoviral conjunctivitis or iritis [7].

Case Background

A 25-year-old male was referred for refractive surgery. Cycloplegic refraction in the right eye was $-8.5 = -1.75 \times 5°$ and in the left eye $-8.5 = -2.5 \times 170°$ diopters (D), achieving the best spectacle corrected visual acuity (BSCVA) of 20/20. Ultrasound pachymetry was 605 μm in both eyes, and the mean central keratometric value was 42.8D. No signs of previous inflammatory reaction in the cornea or anterior segment of either eye were noted. Intraocular pressure was 15 mmHg in both eyes. Flap creation was performed by the Alcon Wavelight® FS200

J.L. Alió, MD, PhD (✉)
Department of Refractive Surgery, Vissum Corporación Oftalmológico, Alicante, Spain
e-mail: jlalio@vissum.com

A. Abbouda, MD
Department of Refractive Surgery, Vissum Corporación Oftalmológica, Alicante, Spain

Department of Ophthalmology-Policlinico Umberto I of Rome, University of Rome "Sapienza", Viale del Policlinico, 155, 00186 Roma, Italy

R&D Department, Vissum Corporación Oftalmológico, 03016, Alicante, Spain
e-mail: a.abbouda@gmail.com

J.L. Alió et al. (eds.), *Difficult and Complicated Cases in Refractive Surgery*, DOI 10.1007/978-3-642-55238-0_58, © Springer-Verlag Berlin Heidelberg 2015

femtosecond laser and corneal stromal ablation by the Alcon Allegretto® excimer laser. One hour postoperative, the slit lamp examination showed no anomalies, no epithelial defects at the flap edge, a clear interface, and a well-positioned flap.

The Main Problem to Solve

Three months after LASIK, the patient complained of blurred vision in both eyes. He referenced rubbing his eyes at night. His best visual acuity was 20/32. The slit lamp examination revealed a perikeratic reaction, an epithelial defect and aggregates of white cells at the paracentral and mid-peripheral interface affecting the visual axis (Fig. 58.1a). Tender inflammatory signs at the anterior chamber were noted. Diffuse lamellar keratitis stage III and epithelial defect were diagnosed. Intensive topical corticosteroid and antibiotic therapy (Pred Forte, Allergan Inc, Irvine, CA, and Vigamox, Alcon) was started hourly. A bandage soft contact lens was placed in each eye. After 2 days, corneal infiltration decreased, but we still observed some epithelial defect fluorescence positive (Fig. 58.1b). We added intensive lubrication. Topical medications were tapered up to day 9, and the patient started fluorometholone (FML® 0.1 % Allergan) 1 drop 3–4 times a day for 3 weeks.

Ancillary Tests

Considering the association of DLK with overlying epithelial defects, it is appropriate to institute measures to prevent and treat epithelial defects, while closely monitoring for the development of interface inflammation. Mahnaz N. Shah [4] suggested these measures:

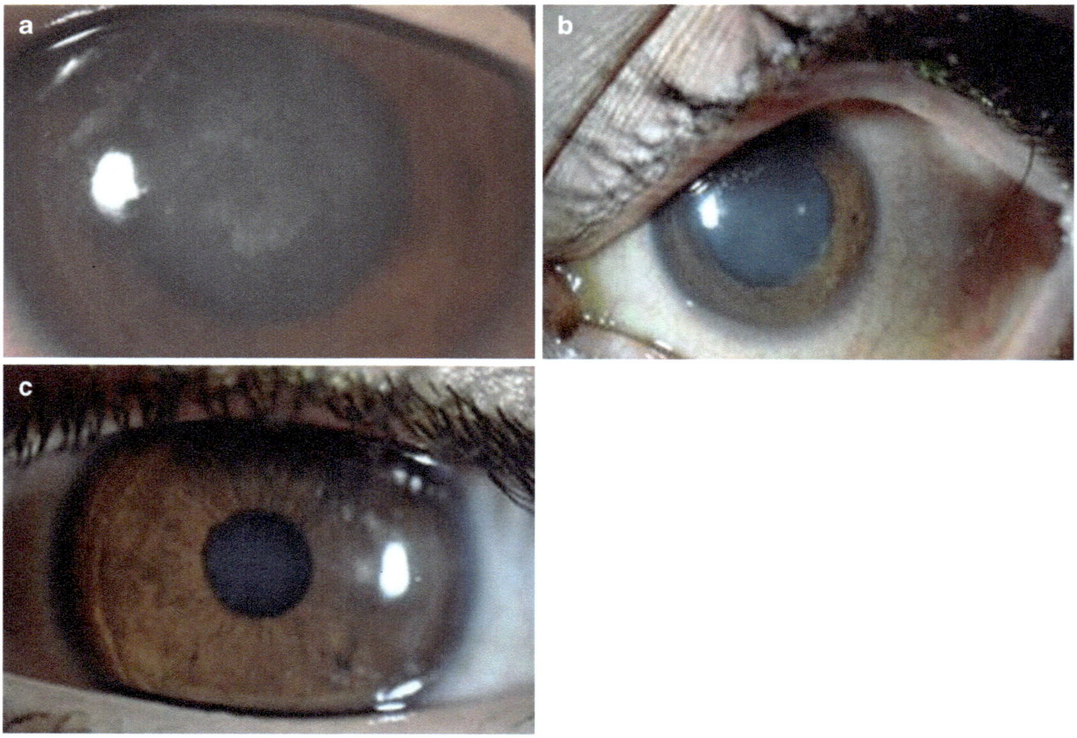

Fig. 58.1 (**a**) Slit lamp photography at the onset of DLK. (**b**) Epithelial defect at the margin of flap at 2 days. (**c**) Clear cornea at 2 months

1. Minimize the occurrence and magnitude of surgically induced epithelial injury. Use preventive measures including identifying and treating dry eye patients preoperatively, limiting the use of topical anesthetics and drops with preservatives, avoiding epithelial dehydration, minimizing intraoperative corneal manipulation, and using the suction ring carefully.
2. Treat epithelial defects with generous amounts of lubrication, and possibly bandage soft contact lenses. Severe cases of post-LASIK dry eye may require punctal plugs.
3. Limit administration of topical antibiotics to 4 times daily to minimize epithelial toxicity.
4. Consider prophylactic corticosteroid therapy in patients with epithelial defects.

Surgical/Medical Intervention

Common treatment for stage III DLK is lifting the flap and irrigating the stromal bed. In our case, the patient demonstrated rapid improvement after 1 day of topical steroids and antibiotics, allowing us to avoid flap lifting. Furthermore, lifting the flap with an epithelial defect could be dangerous.

Outcome

After 2 months, BCVA was 20/20 in both eyes (both eyes with +1 spherical correction). The epithelial irregularity and lamellar keratitis were resolved (Fig. 58.1c).

What to Learn from This Case

Typical DLK develops during postoperative days 1–6 as a diffuse infiltrate confined to the flap interface and has been tied to several etiologic agents [1–5]. Late-onset DLK is an uncommon condition associated with circumstances able to generate surface or intraocular inflammation such as epithelial defects [5, 6]. The presence of an epithelial defect increases an individual's risk of developing DLK by 24 times [4]. Other causes of DLK involve the presence of inciting factors in the interface. The association of epithelial defects with DLK implies the release of inflammatory stimulants distal to the actual site of inflammation. Flap elevation and cleaning of the interface speeds the evolution of these cases and prevents stromal scarring [8].

References

1. Smith RJ, Maloney RK (1998) Diffuse lamellar keratitis. A new syndrome in lamellar refractive surgery. Ophthalmology 105:1721–1726
2. Alió JL, Pérez-Santonja JJ, Tervo T, Tabbara KF, Vesaluoma M, Smith RJ, Maddox B, Maloney RK (2000) Postoperative inflammation, microbial complications, and wound healing following laser in situ keratomileusis. J Refract Surg 16:523–538
3. Holland SP, Mathias RG, Mork DW, Chiu J, Salde SG (2000) Diffuse lamellar keratitis related to endotoxins released from sterilizer reservoir biofilms. Ophthalmology 107:1227–1233
4. Shah MN, Misra M, Wihelmus KR, Koch DD (2000) Diffuse lamellar keratitis associated with epithelial defects after laser in situ keratomileusis. J Cataract Refract Surg 26:1312–1318
5. Harrison DA, Periman LM (2001) Diffuse lamellar keratitis associated with recurrent corneal erosions after laser in situ keratomileusis. J Refract Surg 17:463–465
6. Keszei VA (2001) Diffuse lamellar keratitis associated with iritis 10 months after laser in situ keratomileusis. J Cataract Refract Surg 27:1126–1127
7. Gris O, Güell JL, Wolley-Dod C, Adan A (2004) Diffuse lamellar keratitis and corneal edema associated with viral keratoconjunctivitis 2 years after laser in situ keratomileusis. J Cataract Refract Surg 30:1366–1370
8. Javaloy J, Alió JL, El Kady B, Muñoz G, Barraquer RI, Maldonado MJ (2011) Refractive outcomes and quality of vision related to an outbreak of diffuse lamellar keratitis. J Refract Surg 27(11):804–810

Other Complications: Late-Onset Myopic Regression 12 Years Following Properly Centered Myopic LASIK

59

Scott Kelly and Dimitri T. Azar

Contents

S. Kelly • D.T. Azar, MD, MBA (✉)
Department of Ophthalmology and Visual Sciences
Illinois Eye and Ear Infirmary,
University of Illinois at Chicago,
Chicago, IL, USA
e-mail: scottkellyy@gmail.com; dazar@uic.edu

Why Is This Case Relevant for the Refractive Surgeon?

Myopic regression following myopic LASIK is a common long-term outcome of refractive surgery [1, 2]. High degrees of myopic changes raise red flags that something more serious might be occurring.

Case Background

The patient is a 45-year-old man who had myopic LASIK in both eyes at the age of 31 (in 1996). He presented complaining of worsening vision in the left eye worse than the right eye occurring gradually over the last 4 years, but rapidly worsening over the last 2 weeks. He was also complaining of glare and haloes at night and was requesting LASIK re-treatment.

He denied past medical or family history. Significant past ocular history included a "lazy" left eye requiring patching as a child. He was currently using artificial tears as needed.

Prior to LASIK in 1996, his refractive error was −3.00 sphere OD and −7.00 sphere OS. His uncorrected vision was good for the first 10 years following LASIK.

J.L. Alió et al. (eds.), *Difficult and Complicated Cases in Refractive Surgery*,
DOI 10.1007/978-3-642-55238-0_59, © Springer-Verlag Berlin Heidelberg 2015

On exam, his uncorrected vision was 20/40 in the right eye and 20/250 in the left eye. Manifest refraction revealed a best corrected visual acuity of 20/25 in both eyes with $-1.50+0.50\times 180$ in the right eye and $-4.50+1.25\times 180$ in the left eye.

Motility and confrontational fields were full in both eyes. Pupils were briskly reactive with no afferent pupillary defect. Intraocular pressure measured 14 mmHg OD and 16 mmHg OS. His pachymetries were 433 and 444 μm.

Slit lamp exam showed nasally hinged LASIK flaps with trace haze in both corneas and minimal symmetric incipient trace nuclear sclerotic cataracts in both eyes.

Fundoscopic exam revealed a PVD in the left eye only and moderate myopic changes in each fundus with tilted optic nerves and peripapillary atrophy. No posterior staphylomas were seen. The remainder of the retinal exam was normal.

Main Problem to Solve

The patient has developed significant myopia following myopic LASIK, regressing almost to his presurgical level of myopia. Investigations must be done to determine possible causes of his refractive change. In the absence of progressive cataracts, PRK or LASIK re-treatment would be considered if there is no corneal ectasia.

Ancillary Tests

Corneal topography and pachymetry were preformed. They showed evidence of properly centered photorefractive ablation OU (Figs. 59.1 and 59.2). There was no evidence of corneal ectasia. The central corneas OU were thinner and flatter than the periphery. Careful slit lamp examination

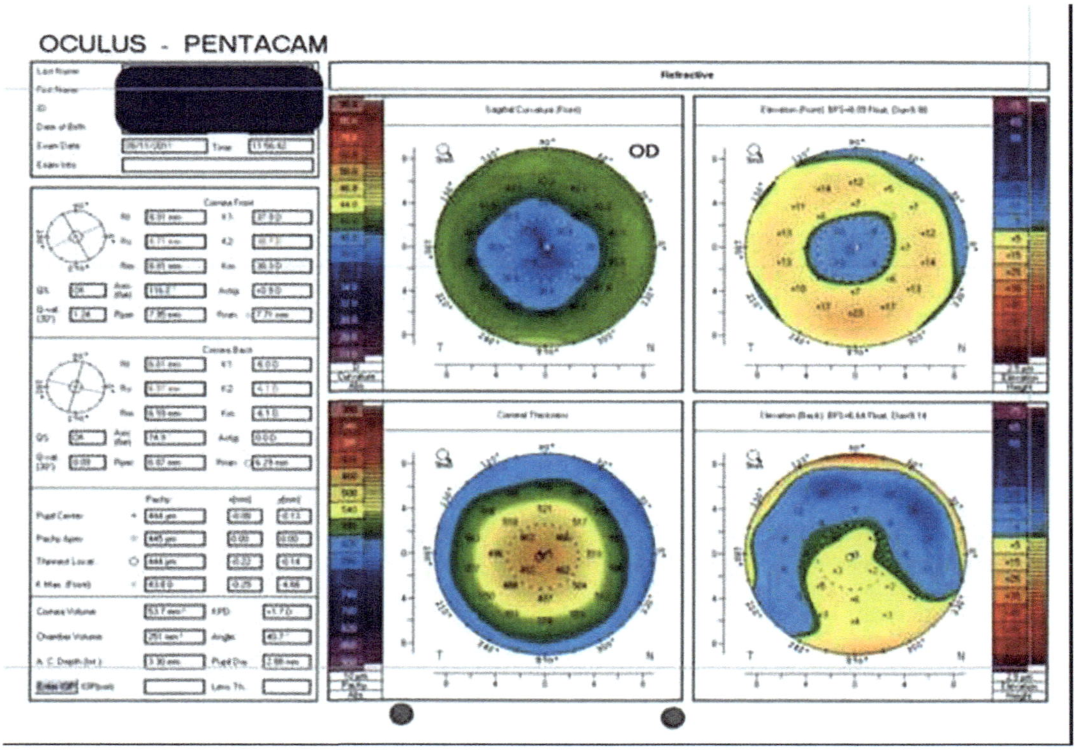

Fig. 59.1 Pentacam of the right eye shows stable corneal topography with central flattening. The topographical map features are also not suggestive of post-LASIK ectasia. The treatment zone is properly centered and does not show a central island. The flattest corneal zone also corresponds to the thinnest part of the cornea. These features do not occur in post-LASIK ectasia

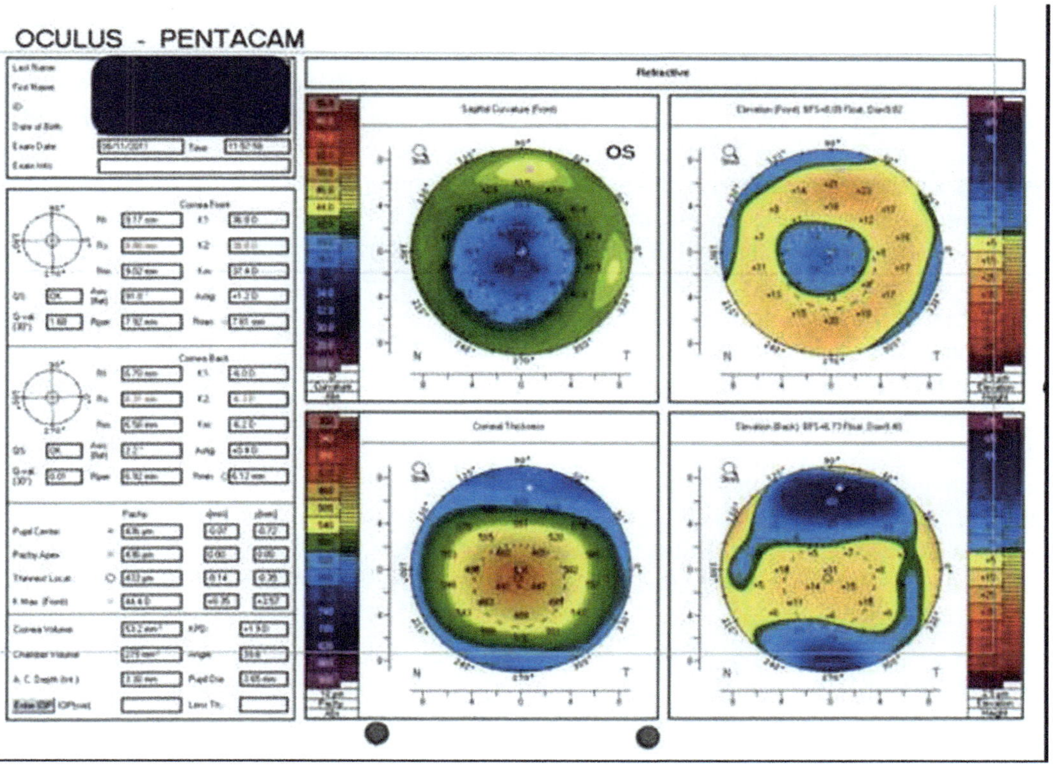

Fig. 59.2 Pentacam of the left eye shows stable corneal topography with central flattening

of the lens and careful examination of the fundus were also performed. The degree of nuclear sclerosis was minimal, so we could not attribute the progressive myopia to his incipient nuclear sclerotic changes.

We evaluated three possible causes of late-onset myopic regression that must be considered. First is worsening cataracts in each eye. This is the most common cause of myopic shift in the older age group. Our examination did not support this diagnosis in this 45-year-old patient.

The second cause of late-onset myopic regression is worsening axial myopia. Given our patient's moderate myopic fundus changes, this is a likely cause of our patient's refractive shift.

The third potential cause of myopic regression is corneal ectasia. As ectasia worsens, increasingly divergent light is needed to neutralize the increasing refractive power of the cornea. This diagnosis was not supported by the topographical maps. Additionally, with pachymetries in the 430 um range, even if the LASIK flaps were on the thick side of the spectrum at 150 um, the residual stromal bed under the flap would be in the 280 um range, above the acceptable minimum required thickness range of 250 um.

Outcome

The decision was made to observe the patient for 6 months to 1 year and consider LASIK surgery if his refraction remains stable. He was happy with his spectacle correction. One year later, the patient was reevaluated to determine if there is progressive increase in his refractive error or in his cataracts. We observed minimal changes on follow-up the following year. LASIK re-treatment was considered, but the patient reported that he was happy wearing glasses and preferred to defer surgery.

What to Learn from This Case

Late-onset myopic regression following myopic LASIK may be due to (1) worsening axial myopia [3], (2) worsening cataract, or (3) corneal ectasia [1].

In the absence of pre- and post-LASIK axial length measurements, the diagnosis of increased axial myopia is reached by elimination. We did not have the immediate post-LASIK topography, so we used indirect topographical evidence, including the absence of central steepening and postoperative central pachymetry, to rule out ectasia.

One important feature used to rule out corneal ectasia is the co-localization of the thinnest corneal pachymetry with the flattest corneal zones OU. The accepted pathogenesis of post-LASIK ectasia is progressive steepening of the cornea in the thinnest corneal region (usually centrally), which was not seen in our case.

We advised the patient to return in 6 months to 1 year to ascertain stability of the residual refractive error. We have performed LASIK re-treatment a decade after primary LASIK, which was offered to our patient. Despite the observation of stable refraction 1 year later, the patient elected to defer, or avoid, surgical intervention.

References

1. Melki SA, Azar DT (2001) LASIK complications: etiology, management, and prevention. Surv Ophthalmol 46:95–116
2. González-Pérez J, Villa-Collar C, González-Méijome JM, Porta NG, Parafita MÁ (2012) Long-term changes in corneal structure and tear inflammatory mediators after orthokeratology and LASIK. Invest Ophthalmol Vis Sci 535:301–311
3. Saka N, Ohno-Matsui K, Shimada N, Sueyoshi S, Nagaoka N, Hayashi W, Hayashi K, Moriyama M, Kojima A, Yasuzumi K, Yoshida T, Tokoro T, Mochizuki M (2010) Long-term changes in axial length in adult eyes with pathologic myopia. Am J Ophthalmol 150:562–568.e1

Other Complications: Late-Onset Unilateral Irregular Mixed Astigmatism Following Thick-Flap LASIK

60

Daoud Fahd, Joelle Hallak, and Dimitri T. Azar

Contents

D. Fahd, MD (✉)
Department of Ophthalmology and Visual Sciences, University of Illinois at Chicago, Chicago, IL, USA
e-mail: davidaliasdf@gmail.com

J. Hallak, MS, PhD
College of Medicine, University of Illinois at Chicago, Chicago, IL, USA

D.T. Azar, MD, MBA
Department of Ophthalmology and Visual Sciences Illinois Eye and Ear Infirmary, University of Illinois at Chicago, Chicago, IL, USA
e-mail: dazar@uic.edu

Why Is This Case Relevant for the Refractive Surgeon?

Irregular mixed astigmatism can be seen after LASIK surgery [1–3]. In this case the clue for proper treatment was the realization of the excessively large flap thickness of LASIK performed 12 years earlier.

Case Background

The patient is a 47-year-old woman s/p LASIK 12 years prior to presentation. She presented with the complaint of contact lens intolerance and decreased vision in the left eye. UCVA was 20/20 in OD and 20/200 in OS. With a hybrid (hard/soft shell) contact lens, she corrects to 20/20 in the left eye. She had a LASIK performed in 1998, and she reported that she saw well OD after surgery, but her vision OS was never clear. She went to have contact lenses fitted, saw fine with them, but reported that she felt her eyes were very dry when she had them on, and she was therefore unable to tolerate her contact lenses. Her wavefront analysis showed a refraction of $-3.90+6.30\times 19$ in the left eye (Figs. 60.1 and 60.2). Her slit-lamp examination showed evidence of a thick LASIK flap OS. Her SimK by Orbscan was 39.10/44.30 at 31, and her CCT was 544 OS (Fig. 60.3). The ocular response analysis showed symmetric findings OU (Fig. 60.4).

J.L. Alió et al. (eds.), *Difficult and Complicated Cases in Refractive Surgery*,
DOI 10.1007/978-3-642-55238-0_60, © Springer-Verlag Berlin Heidelberg 2015

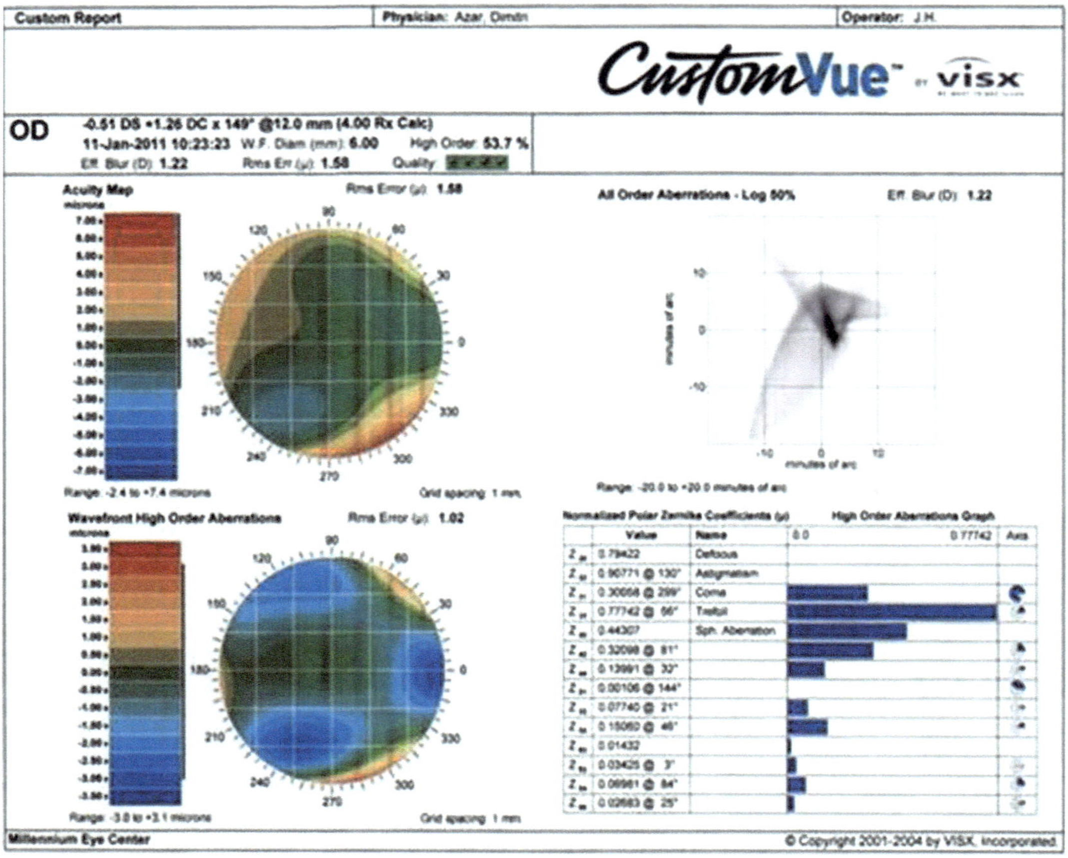

Fig. 60.1 Wavefront analysis OD

Main Problem to Solve

This is a case of late-onset irregular astigmatism following LASIK surgery done 12 years earlier, at the time when the potential for subclinical post-LASIK ectasia was not widely recognized. The records from the operating LASIK surgeons were not available. The most important questions are related to etiology and to stability of the refractive status. The most likely cause of late-onset post-LASIK irregular astigmatism is ectasia, which is often a progressive condition. Therefore the surgical intervention should be deferred in our patient until stability is ascertained.

If the refractive status is unstable, consideration should be given to collagen cross-linking, intracorneal ring segments, or keratoplasty. If the refractive status is stable and nonprogressive, the options would include, additionally, LASIK and PRK. LASIK would be ill-advised given that one may not be able to rule out the possibility of latent ectasia, even with the passage of time.

Ancillary Tests

The Orbscan topography (Fig. 60.3) showed a claw-shaped pattern OS, but the inferior zone was not measurable. Pentacam was obtained OS (Fig. 60.5) and confirmed the findings of central flattening with 6.40 D of astigmatism 12 years following surgery. The thinnest central zone (500 μm), located 1.1 mm below the pupillary center, corresponded to a relatively flat corneal

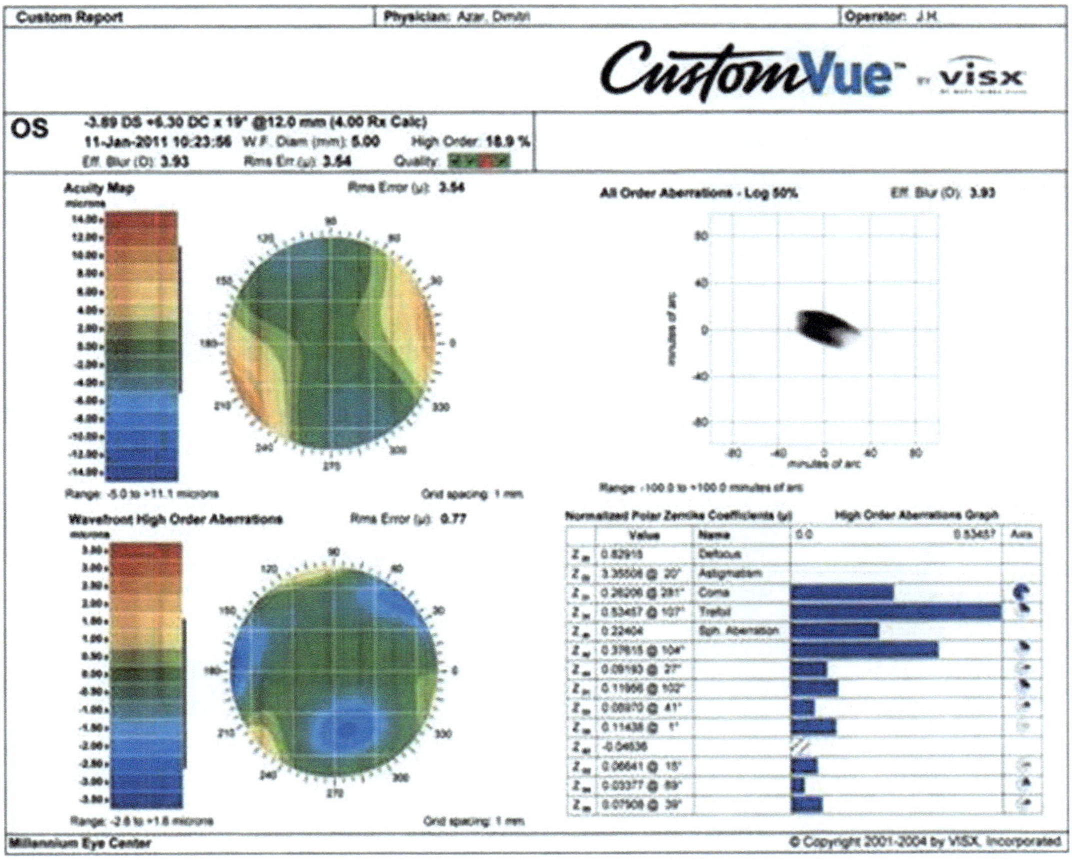

Fig. 60.2 Wavefront analysis OS

curvature (37.00 D). This was in contradistinction to the steepest corneal zone (52.80 D), which corresponded to corneal pachymetry >650 μm. These findings were not consistent with a diagnosis of post-LASIK ectasia or preexisting keratoconus. These conditions, however, could not be ruled out.

OCT was performed at a later date and the findings of a thick-flap LASIK were confirmed.

Outcome

Follow-up examinations over 1 year showed stability of the refractive error and topography. Slit-lamp examination was consistent with a 250 μm flap and no evidence of holes or irregularities.

Visante OCT pachymetry confirmed the Pentacam findings of the thinnest corneal location being inferior (and inferotemporal) to the corneal center (Fig. 60.6). Multiple corneal scans were used to estimate the Visante flap thickness OS. The LASIK flap thickness measurements ranged from 185 to 260 μm (Fig. 60.7).

Wavefront aberrometry OS measured −2.81 + 5.49 × 19 (Fig. 60.8). This was consistent with the trial lens refraction of −2.75 + 5.00 × 19, with which the patient was content.

The patient underwent a transepithelial PRK treatment of −2.75 + 5.00 × 19°, with which she was content.

The non-custom approach was associated with substantial tissue saving (26 μm treatment

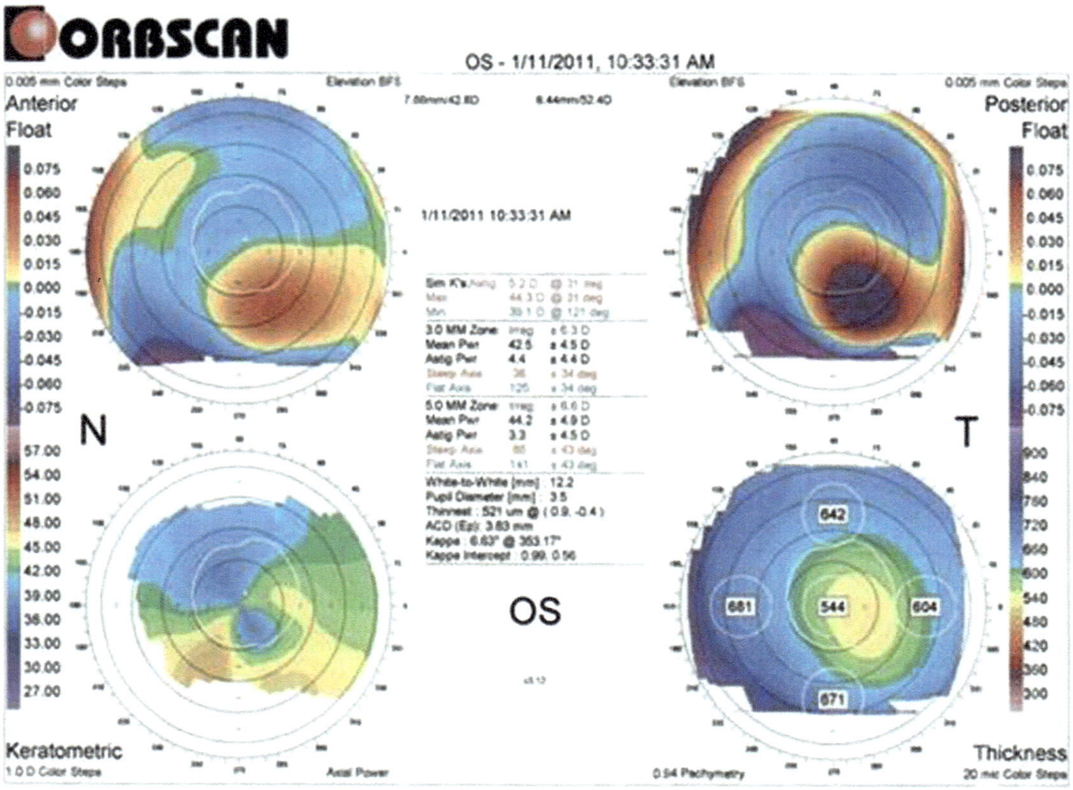

Fig. 60.3 Orbscan topography showing a claw-shaped pattern OS

depth as compared to the corresponding custom treatment depth of 69 μm).

Two months postoperatively UCVA was 20/25, and the refraction was −2.50 + 2.50 × 99.

What to Learn from This Case

The differential diagnosis of late-onset irregular astigmatism after LASIK includes preexisting keratoconus or forme fruste keratoconus, post-LASIK ectasia, PRK decentration (shift and/or drift), and deep LASIK flaps [1–3].

In this patient, the retreatment OS may have been decentered inferiorly. Given the localization of thin pachymetry with corneal flattening, it is unlikely that the thinnest corneal zone is associated with progressive ectasia, although this cannot be ruled out.

Given the fact that we cannot rule out a biomechanical etiology for the irregular astigmatism, the safest surgical treatment would be to treat the LASIK flap and to use a tissue-saving (non-custom) algorithm. This is what was done in our case. The thick LASIK flap facilitated the decision making. In the immediate postoperative period, the LASIK flap does not contribute to the biomechanical stability. It is not clear, however, whether the flap's contribution to corneal stability becomes significant 12 years postoperatively.

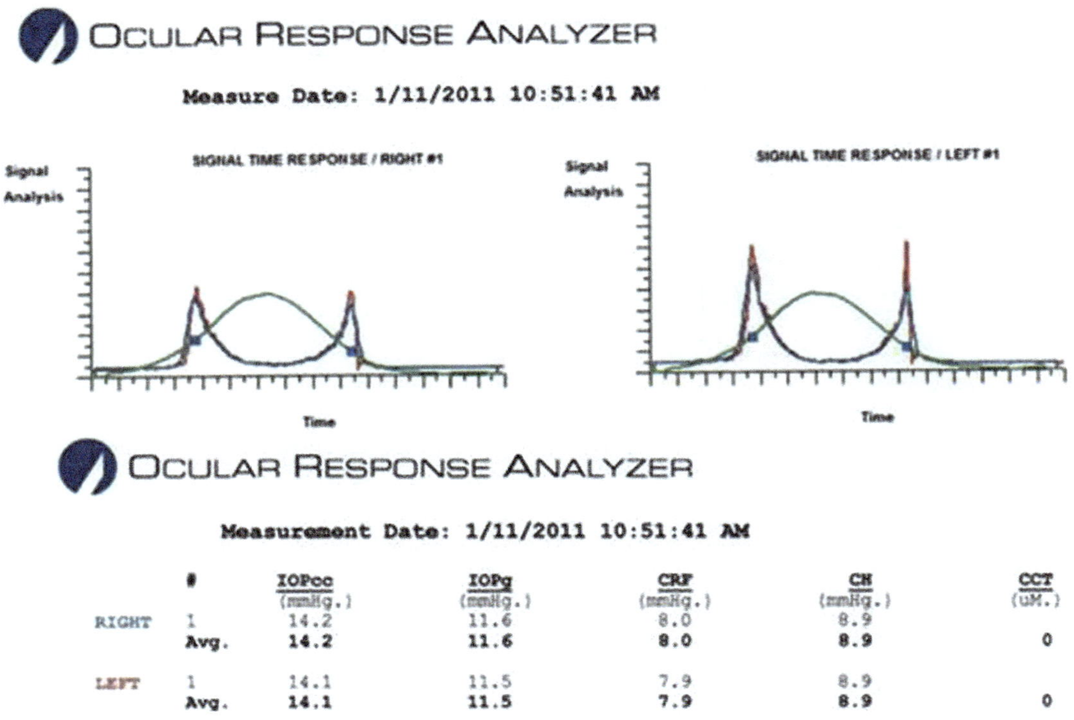

	#	IOPcc (mmHg.)	IOPg (mmHg.)	CRF (mmHg.)	CH (mmHg.)	CCT (uM.)
RIGHT	1	14.2	11.6	8.0	8.9	
	Avg.	14.2	11.6	8.0	8.9	0
LEFT	1	14.1	11.5	7.9	8.9	
	Avg.	14.1	11.5	7.9	8.9	0

Fig. 60.4 Ocular response analysis OS

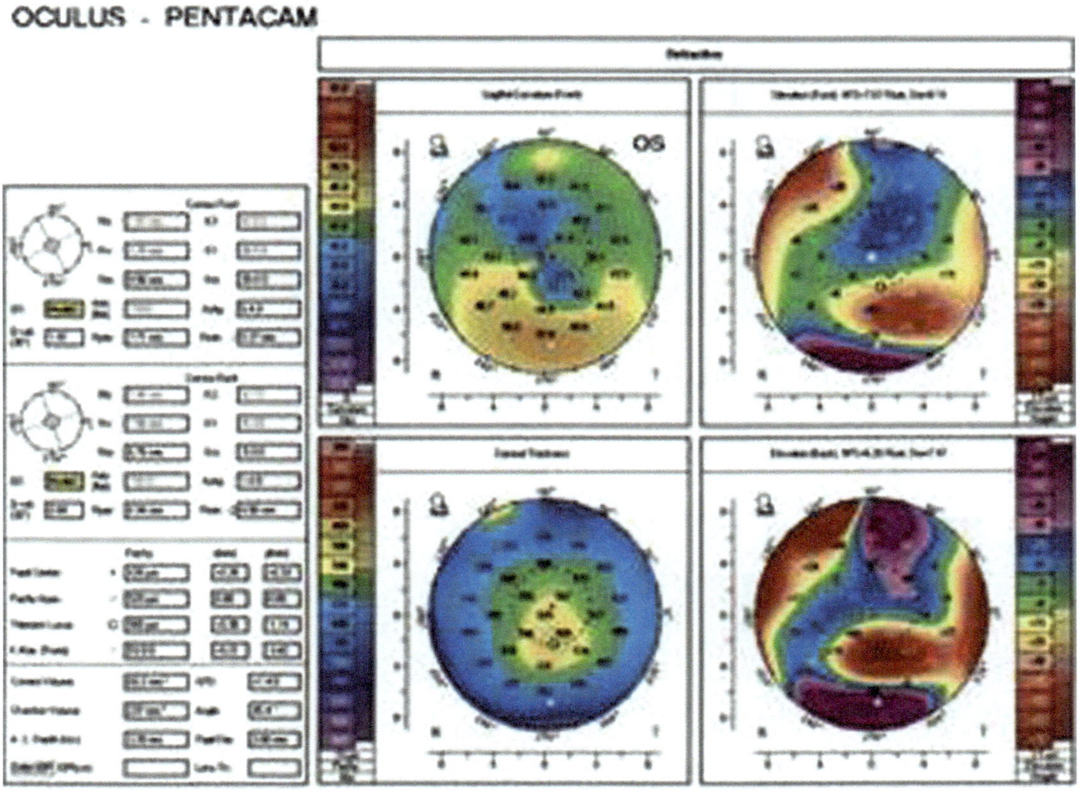

Fig. 60.5 Pentacam OS (Fig. 60.4) showing central flattening with 6.40 D of astigmatism

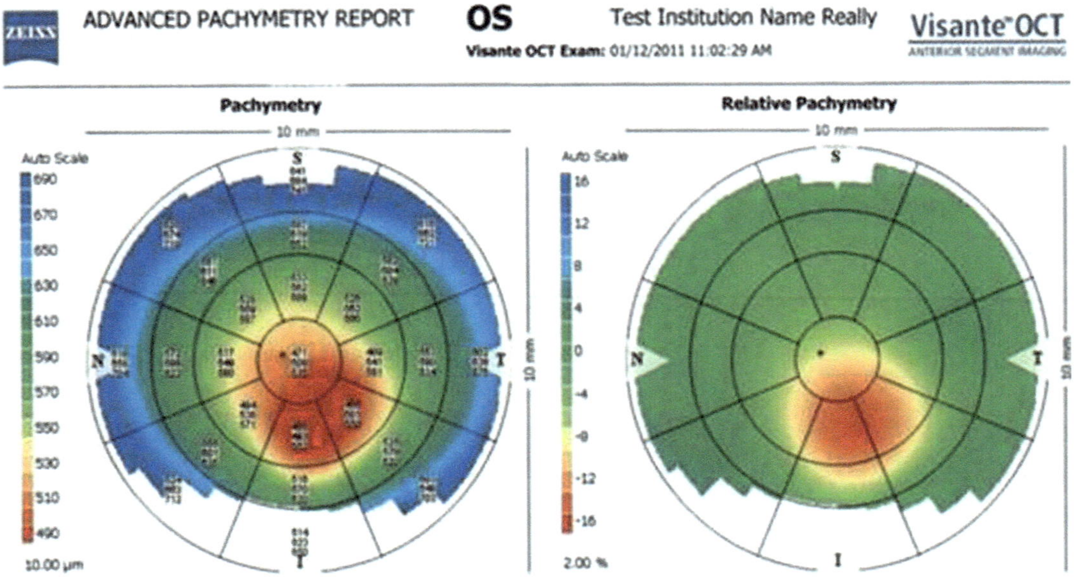

Fig. 60.6 Visante OCT pachymetry OS showing the thinnest corneal location being inferior (and inferotemporal) to the corneal center

Fig. 60.7 Multiple corneal scans (**a**–**c**) estimating the Visante flap thickness OS. The LASIK flap thickness measurements ranged from 185 to 260 µm

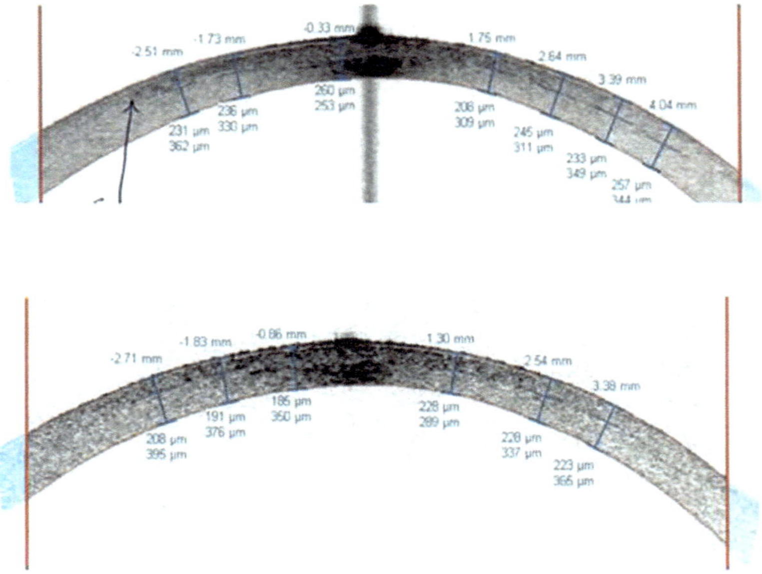

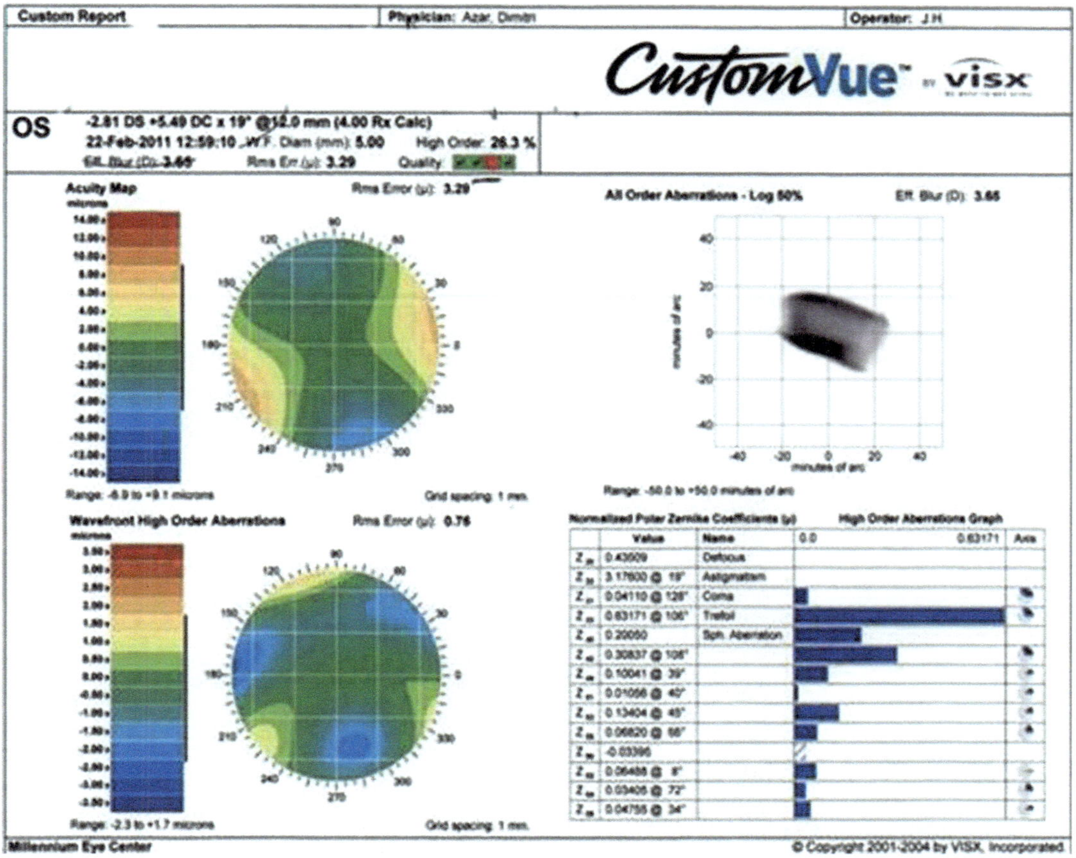

Fig. 60.8 Wavefront aberrometry OS measuring −2.81 + 5.49 × 19

References

1. Jarade EF, Azar DT (2003) Management of irregular astigmatism after laser in situ keratomileusis. Int Ophthalmol Clin 43:141–156
2. Johnson JD, Azar DT (2001) Surgically induced topographical abnormalities after LASIK: management of central islands, corneal ectasia, decentration, and irregular astigmatism. Curr Opin Ophthalmol 12: 309–317
3. Melki SA, Azar DT (2001) LASIK complications: etiology, management, and prevention. Surv Ophthalmol 46:95–116

Other Complications: Flap Lift After 15 Years

61

Jorge L. Alió and Alessandro Abbouda

Contents

J.L. Alió, MD, PhD (✉)
Department of Refractive Surgery, Vissum Corporación Oftalmológica, Alicante, Spain
e-mail: jlalio@vissum.com

A. Abbouda, MD
Department of Refractive Surgery, Vissum Corporación Oftalmológica, Alicante, Spain

Department of Ophthalmology-Policlinico Umberto I of Rome, University of Rome "Sapienza", Viale del Policlinico, 155, 00186 Roma, Italy

R&D Department, Vissum Corporación Oftalmológica, 03016, Alicante, Spain
e-mail: a.abbouda@gmail.com

Why Is This Case Relevant for the Refractive Surgeon?

Depending on the patient's clinical features, there are multiple options for LASIK retreatment: create a new flap, lift the old flap or perform surface ablation [1]. Here we present the case of a patient whose flap was lifted after 15 years.

Background

A 55-year-old man who had LASIK treatment 15 years prior presented to our department interested in refractive surgery. A flap cut was performed using microkeratome. His manifest refraction at the first procedure was −5 sph in both eyes. After 15 years, his best corrected visual acuity (BCVA) was 20/30 in both eyes with a manifest refraction of −1.25 −0.75 × 30° in the right eye (RE) and −1.25 −0.75 × 180° in the left eye (LE). The ultrasound central thickness was 465 μm in the RE and 463 μm in the LE. Keratometry readings were 41.23/42.35 × 120° in the RE and 40.33/41.80 × 77° in the LE. The corneal topography showed a flattening area according to myopic ablation profile (Fig. 61.1). OCT Visante was performed to evaluate the flap thickness and residual stromal bed (Fig. 61.2). The slit lamp examination revealed a clear cornea, and the line of the gutter was barely visible. We decided to reelevate the original flap in the LE to induce monovision in the non-dominant eye.

J.L. Alió et al. (eds.), *Difficult and Complicated Cases in Refractive Surgery*,
DOI 10.1007/978-3-642-55238-0_61, © Springer-Verlag Berlin Heidelberg 2015

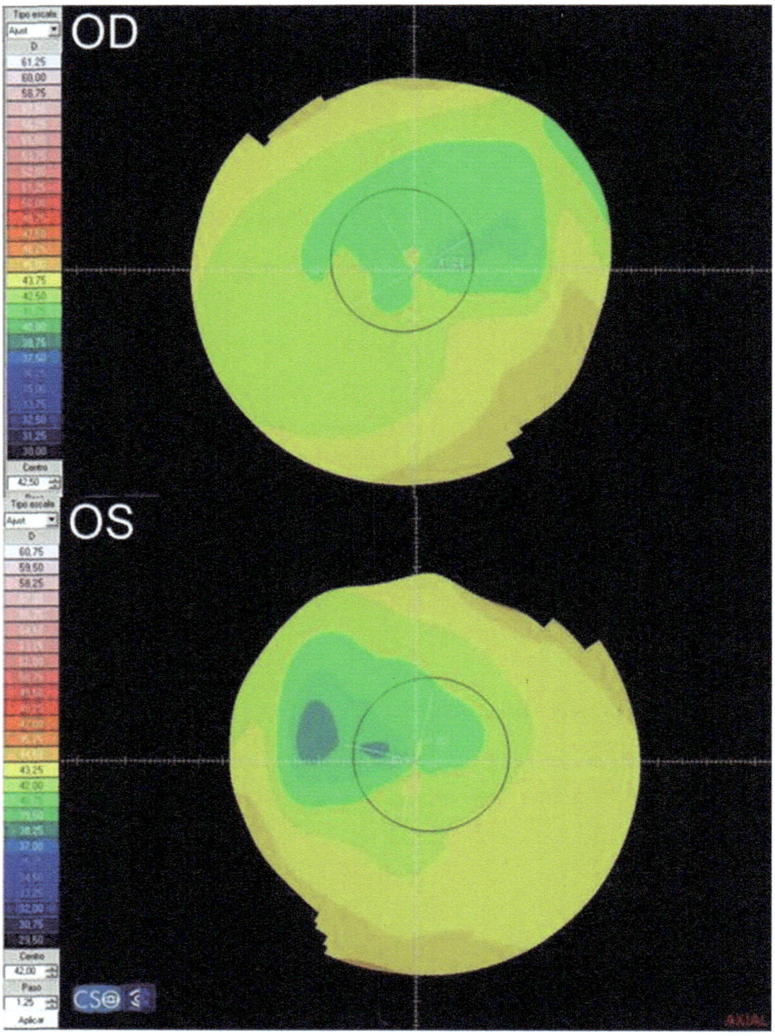

Fig. 61.1 Corneal topography showed a central flattening area according to the first treatment

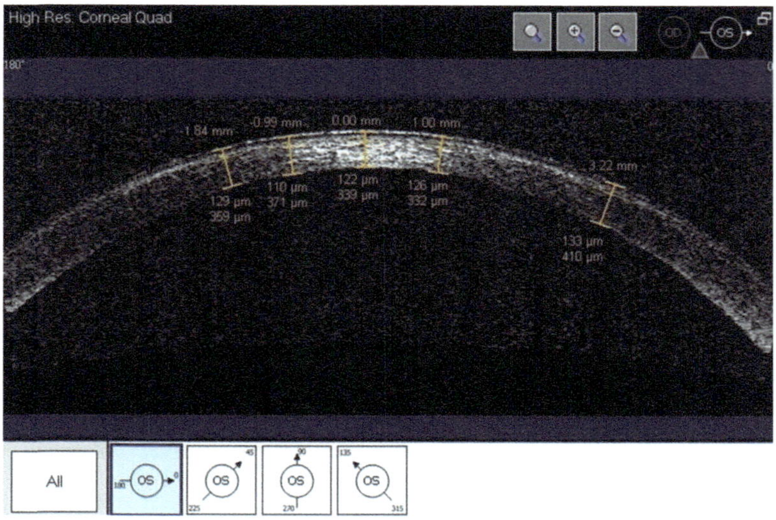

Fig. 61.2 OCT Visante (left eye). Horizontal scan shows the depth of the previous flap

Main Problem to Solve

Stretching the flap edge during surgery can create an entry point for epithelial ingrowth [2]. The spatula must engage the flap edge in the same plane as the flap interface. It is important to know if the previous flap was performed with the IntraLase femtosecond laser or microkeratome. No descriptions about long-term flap elevation following FS flap are described, but stronger healing presumably makes it more difficult than microkeratome in which the adhesion is weaker and lifting is easier.

Ancillary Tests

When considering flap lift in a patient treated elsewhere, one must perform a careful clinical examination [3]. Lifting the flap should be avoided when:

- Biomicroscopy shows evidence of previous buttonholes, scarring of the flap edge or a decentered, incomplete or severely striated flap.
- Topography indicates an incomplete ablation, suggesting an incomplete flap.
- There is doubt about adequate depth of the residual stromal bed (anterior segment optical coherence tomography can be valuable here).
- There is any doubt about the presence of ectasia.

Surgical/Medical Intervention

The flap was lifted using a Sinskey hook. The hook was pressed into the epithelium at the limbus approximately opposite the hinge and dragged, with posterior pressure, towards the centre of the flap until the instrument tip fell into the potential space at the flap edge. The tip of the Sinskey hook was used to open the flap margin for 1 h at this location. The edge of the flap was grasped gently with a sponge and retracted across the superior conjunctiva. Standard ablation through Schwind Amaris laser excimer was performed, and the remainder of the procedure and postoperative care were identical to the normal LASIK procedure.

Outcome

Three months after the procedure, the patient's UDVA was 20/20 in the LE. Binocular vision allowed the patient complete independence from glasses for distance and near vision. The slit lamp examination revealed a clear cornea. The keratometric index in the LE was 39.48/40.46 × 79°. The topography showed an increasing central flattening area (Fig. 61.3).

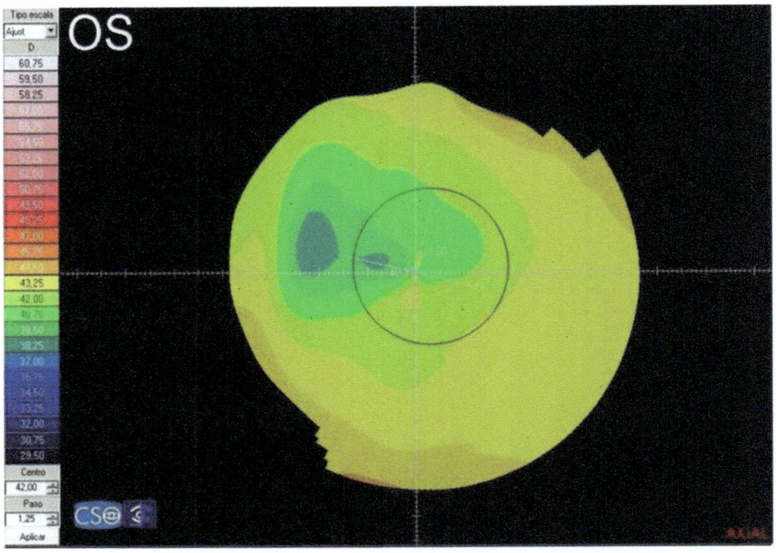

Fig. 61.3 Corneal topography (left eye) after the second treatment shows an increase in the central flattening area

What to Learn from This Case

Re-lifting the flap is the most common retreatment procedure. Studies suggest that flap re-lifting has advantages over recutting the flap–lamellar interface for LASIK retreatment, including increased safety [4, 5]. When femtosecond flap re-lift is difficult and the surgeon decides not to proceed out of concern that the flap will be damaged, the preference is to use PRK with MMC for retreatment. In this case, a flap performed after femtosecond LASIK was lifted after 15 years with excellent safety measures, yielding a good visual acuity result.

References

1. Santhiago MR, Smadja D, Zaleski K, Espana EM, Armstrong BK, Wilson SE (2012) Flap relift for retreatment after femtosecond laser-assisted LASIK. J Refract Surg 28:482–487
2. Caster AI, Friess DW, Schwendeman FJ (2010) Incidence of epithelial ingrowth in primary and retreatment laser in situ keratomileusis. J Cataract Refract Surg 36:97–101
3. Cummings AB, Frohn A, Muller MA, Sallet G, Jerry Tan Tiang Hin. LASIK retreatments: create a new flap, lift the old, or perform Surface Ablation? http://bmctoday.net/crstodayeurope/2012/04/article.asp?f=lasik-retreatments-create-a-new-flap-lift-the-old-or-perform-surface-ablation. Accessed Apr 2012
4. Domniz Y, Comaish IF, Lawless MA, Rogers CM, Sutton GL (2001) Recutting the cornea versus lifting the flap: comparison of two enhancement techniques following laser in situ keratomileusis. J Refract Surg 17:505–510
5. Davis EA, Hardten DR, Lindstrom M, Samuelson TW, Lindstrom RL (2002) LASIK re-treatments: a comparison of lifting to recutting the flap. Ophthalmology 109:2308–2313

Other Complications: Ptosis After LASIK

62

Marco Sales, Dominika Wróbel, and Alessandro Abbouda

Contents

M. Sales, MD, PhD (✉)
Oculoplastic and Orbital Surgery Department, Hospital Universitario Ramón y Cajal, Madrid, Spain

VISSUM Corporación Oftalmológica, Alicante, Spain
e-mail: salessanz@yahoo.es

D. Wróbel, MD
Glaucoma Diagnostic and Microsurgery Department, Medical University of Lublin, Lublin, Poland

R&D Department, Vissum Corporacion, Alicante, Spain
e-mail: ddudzinska@interia.pl

A. Abbouda, MD
Department of Refractive Surgery, Vissum Corporación Oftalmológica, Alicante, Spain

Department of Ophthalmology-Policlinico Umberto I of Rome, University of Rome "Sapienza", Viale del Policlinico, 155, 00186 Roma, Italy

R&D Department, Vissum Corporación Oftalmológica, 03016, Alicante, Spain
e-mail: a.abbouda@gmail.com

Why Is This Case Relevant for the Refractive Surgeon?

Ptosis after refractive surgery is a complex topic. The type of ptosis that occurs after refractive surgery is usually aponeurotic dehiscence but can also be mechanical or traumatic. The anatomic etiology of this complication is disinsertion, dehiscence, and attenuation of the elevator aponeurosis. We need to consider many factors present before, during, and after refractive surgery that influence the formation of ptosis including using hard contact lenses, mechanical insult to the levator during the retraction of the eyelids (especially in patients with narrow fissures and tight eyelids), patient's age, dry eye, side effects of local corticosteroid application, and decreased amounts of antioxidants in the pre-aponeurotic fat [1–4].

Case Background

The patient came to our department 8 months after having undergone a LASIK procedure in another center. She complained of difficulty in the visual field and her right lid was falling down.

In the first examination in our clinic, the patient showed an uncorrected visual acuity (UCVA) of 20/20 in both eyes. The external examination revealed a ptosis in the RE with a margin reflex distance (MRD) of 0.5 mm with normal superior elevator function (Fig. 62.1a).

J.L. Alió et al. (eds.), *Difficult and Complicated Cases in Refractive Surgery*, DOI 10.1007/978-3-642-55238-0_62, © Springer-Verlag Berlin Heidelberg 2015

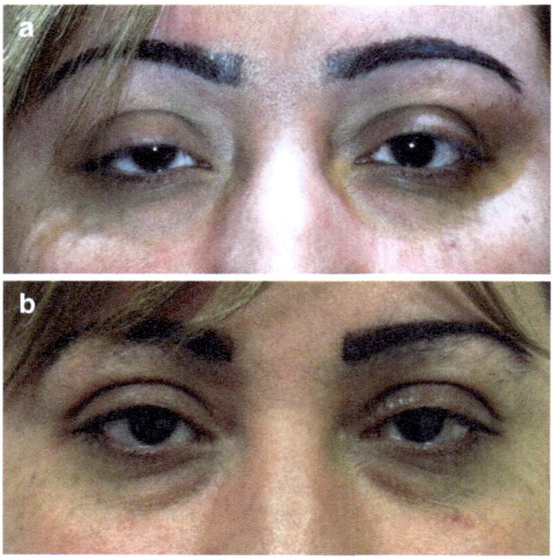

Fig. 62.1 (**a**) Preoperative right eye ptosis. (**b**) 1 month after 9 mm conjunctival-Müller resection

The superior eyelid crease was higher, and the distance from the upper eyelid to the lower eyelid margin in maximum down gaze was smaller on the ptotic side. On the LE, the MRD was 3 mm. The slit lamp examination revealed a corneal flap of 8 mm size with temporal hinge. The visual field in the RE evidenced a superior scotoma according to the ptosis. Otherwise, the examination was normal.

Main Problem to Solve

Can mild trauma to levator aponeurosis during the first LASIK procedure result in mild ptosis? How do we manage ptosis after a LASIK procedure?

Ancillary Tests

Aponeurotic ptosis includes a low MRD with good elevator function (LF) and an elevated eyelid crease. A lift test of the droopy eyelid by using 2.5 % phenylephrine showed a positive result, normalizing RE position and no contralateral secondary ptosis.

Surgical/Medical Intervention

Based on the examination, oculoplastic surgery was indicated. Müller's muscle conjunctival resection of 9 mm was performed in the RE. After local transcutaneous infiltration with lidocaine, the eyelid was everted over a Desmarres retractor. A Putterman's clamp grasped 9 mm of conjunctiva and the Müller muscle. A 5/0 nylon suture was passed through the skin to the conjunctiva at one side of the forceps. The suture was passed along the forceps side to side securing all the tissues grasped (conjunctiva-Müller-Müller-conjunctiva) in 4–5 points. On the other side of the forceps, the suture was passed again to exit through the skin and tied. The tissue grasped with the forceps was cut with a n° 15 blade.

Outcome

The patient's evolution was good. After 1 month, the patient showed a good lid aspect and she was satisfied. MRD was similar in both eyes (Fig. 62.1b).

What to Learn from This Case

Ptosis after refractive surgery is not very common. However, when this complication does occur, it can be caused by many factors including contact lens use, lid speculum and drape use, patient predisposition, and age. Performing a meticulous examination to determinate the type of ptosis and risk factors is essential. Aponeurotic surgical repair can be achieved with Müller's muscle conjunctival resection in mild aponeurotic ptosis that responds to phenylephrine drops.

References

1. Cheng ACK, Young AL et al (2004) Ptosis after laser in situ keratomileusis. J Cataract Refract Surg 30:1572–1574
2. Wasserman BN, Bigler B et al (2005) Unexpected outcomes associated with laser in situ keratomileusis: ptosis, anisocoria and curing of exotropia. J Cataract Refract Surg 31:1238–1241

3. Wantanabe A, Araki B, Noso K et al (2006) Histopathology of blepharoptosis caused by prolonged hard contact lens wear. Am J Ophthalmol 141:1092–1096
4. Perry JD, Kadakia A, Foster JA (2002) A new algorithm for ptosis repair using conjunctival Müllerectomy with or without tarsectomy. Ophthal Plast Reconstr Surg 18:426–429

Other Complications: Management of Recalcitrant Late-Onset DLK After Hyperopic LASIK

63

Joelle Hallak and Dimitri T. Azar

Contents

J. Hallak, MS, PhD
College of Medicine, University of Illinois at Chicago, Chicago, IL, USA
e-mail: joelle@uic.edu

D.T. Azar, MD, MBA (✉)
Department of Ophthalmology and Visual Sciences, Illinois Eye and Ear Infirmary, University of Illinois at Chicago, Chicago, IL, USA
e-mail: dazar@uic.edu

Why Is This Case Relevant for the Refractive Surgeon?

Diffuse lamellar keratitis (DLK), also known as Sands of the Sahara, is one of the most common early postoperative complications of laser-assisted in situ keratomileusis (LASIK). It was first described by Smith and Maloney in 1998 as a granular, white cell infiltrate within the LASIK flap interface [1]. The incidence of DLK has been shown to increase with the use of the earlier models of femtosecond laser for creating LASIK flaps.

DLK represents an inflammatory reaction, usually in the immediate postoperative period. However, some cases have been reported to occur later in the postoperative period [2]. Given the serious vision-threatening effects of DLK, proper management and treatment are required.

Case Background

Our patient is a 42-year-old male who underwent bilateral hyperopic femtosecond LASIK treatment on May 23, 2008, 9 months prior to referral to our clinic. The patient presented to our clinic with symptoms of foreign body sensation and blurred vision in the left eye (OS). He reported progressively blurred vision since the LASIK procedure with foreign body sensation OS beginning January 17, 2009. He had a history of foreign bodies (glass OU in 1992).

J.L. Alió et al. (eds.), *Difficult and Complicated Cases in Refractive Surgery*,
DOI 10.1007/978-3-642-55238-0_63, © Springer-Verlag Berlin Heidelberg 2015

His uncorrected visual acuity (UCVA) was 20/200 in the right eye (OD) and 20/400 in the left eye. His best corrected visual acuity (BCVA) was 20/40- OD with manifest refraction of $-2.50+1.00\times085$ and 20/400- with manifest refraction of $-2.50+1.50\times180$. Central corneal thickness, as measured by ultrasound pachymetry, was 537 OD and 543 OS.

Slit-lamp examination revealed intact flaps in both eyes. Focal areas of haze were noted in the right eye, and central dense scarring (2.2 mm height × 2.3 mm width) with subflap thinning and haze, resulting in flattening, was shown in the left eye. The haze was confined to the interface without stromal edema or interface fluid and was reminiscent of stage 3–4 DLK. No conjunctival injection, fluorescein staining on the corneal surface or at the flap edge, reaction in the anterior chamber, or discharge was present. Schirmer test results were <1 mm OU (after anesthetic application).

Ocular medication at time of presentation included VIGAMOX® (moxifloxacin hydrochloride ophthalmic solution 0.5 %) four times per day OS and Omnipred four times per day OS.

Our impression was late-onset DLK after LASIK OS. The DLK OS was associated with subflap thinning. The exact etiology was unknown, given the remote timing from the LASIK procedure (9 months ago).

Main Problem to Solve

The issues to focus on in this case are to decrease inflammation and scarring, improve vision, and relieve the patient from foreign body sensation and dry eye symptoms. Medical and surgical options were discussed including topical steroids, systemic steroids, flap lifting and irrigation, laser retreatment, as well as keratoplasty.

Ancillary Testing

DLK should be evaluated using slit-lamp examination, and the decreased vision should be evaluated with corneal topography using an Orbscan and a Humphrey system (Fig. 63.1) as well as custom view VISX report for higher-order aberrations. Ultrasound pachymetry must be performed to measure corneal thickness to rule out other complications. Tear production was measured using the Schirmer test.

Surgical/Medical Intervention

Medical and surgical options were presented to the patient. Medical treatment was with PRED FORTE® (prednisolone acetate 1 %).

1. Retrial of CL (e.g., HCL because the patient reports that SCL may have caused the problem) with antibiotic coverage and lubrication

Surgical

2. Surgical/laser correction of residual refractive error
3. Consideration of flap removal – WH – then CL to fix refractive error
4. LK surgery with subsequent PTK to correct and reduce refractive error

Medical intervention included Pred Forte h and increased antibiotic drops (Vigamox). The post-LASIK dry eye was managed with artificial tears.

Outcome

At 5 Months Follow-Up

UCVA was 20/60 OD and 20/80 OS (PH 20/30 and 20/60). Manifest refraction was −0.50 sph with BCVA of 20/25 OD and $-0.75+0.75\times167$ with BCVA of 0/60 OS.

Improvement of subepithelial scarring was noted. The inflammatory component subsided with residual scarring (linear and haze). Continue artificial tears OU 1–2 × /day with repeat topography next visit. Hard contact lens or soft contact lens fitting was considered.

At 9 Months Follow-Up

A mild area of scarring in visual axis OS was shown on slit-lamp examination, which was

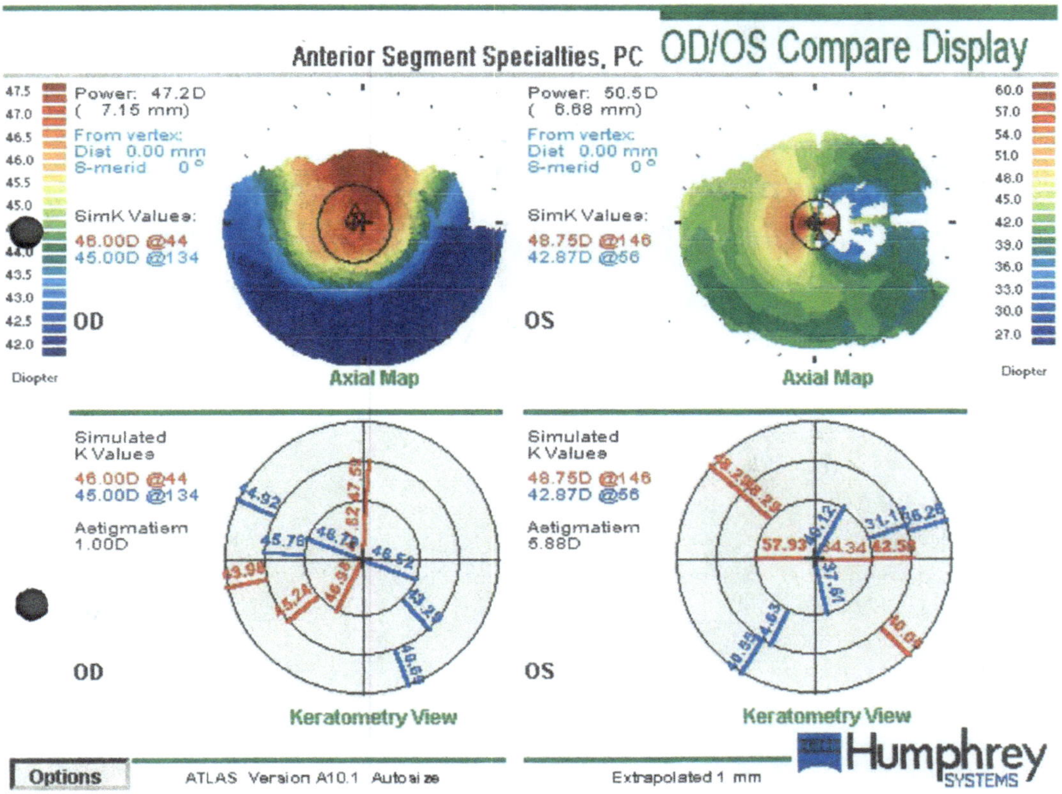

Fig. 63.1 Orbscan OS/OD 9 months following femtosecond hyperopic LASIK. Astigmatism was 1.00 D in the right eye and 5.88 in the left eye

dramatically better than prior visit. Scarring was stable and fading. The above treatment options were further discussed in addition to DALK and PK.

The patient was referred for contact lens fitting.

What to Learn from This Case

The most important consideration in late-onset DLK is to avoid overlooking an infectious etiology. In our case, the referring physician had started topical antibiotics for a possible corneal infection, and, by the time we saw the patient, we were unable to use a corneal infiltrate. We continued the topical antibiotics and increased the steroid regimen to control the DLK.

DLK can occur following microkeratome flap creation or following femtosecond laser flap creation. The incidence of DLK following femtosecond laser flap creation has been reported to be higher (estimated range from 0.2 to 19.4 %) than flaps created with microkeratomes (estimated range from 0.1 to 7.7 %) [3]. Although multiple factors associated with DLK have been proposed, the exact etiology is unknown. The presence of dry eye may also be a contributing factor. Proper corneal surface lubrication and medical treatment with topical antibiotics and corticosteroids are key to controlling this complication.

In most cases, DLK usually occurs within the first postoperative month. Late-onset DLK has been reported 2–14 months after LASIK. Reported causes associated with late-onset DLK are trauma, epithelial defects, recurrent corneal

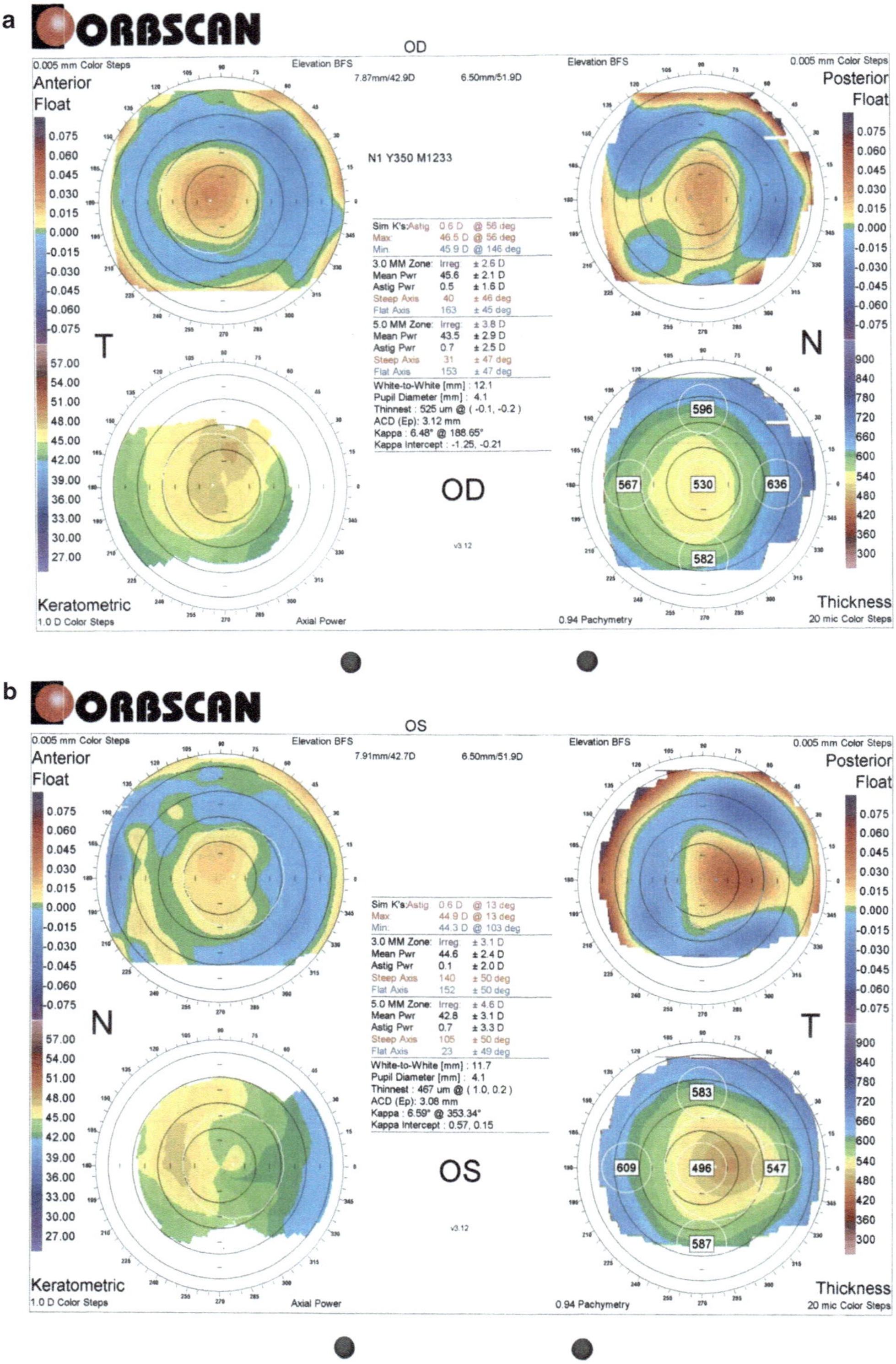

Fig. 63.2 Orbscan OD (**a**) and OS (**b**) 5 months following diagnosis of DLK and treatment

a

b

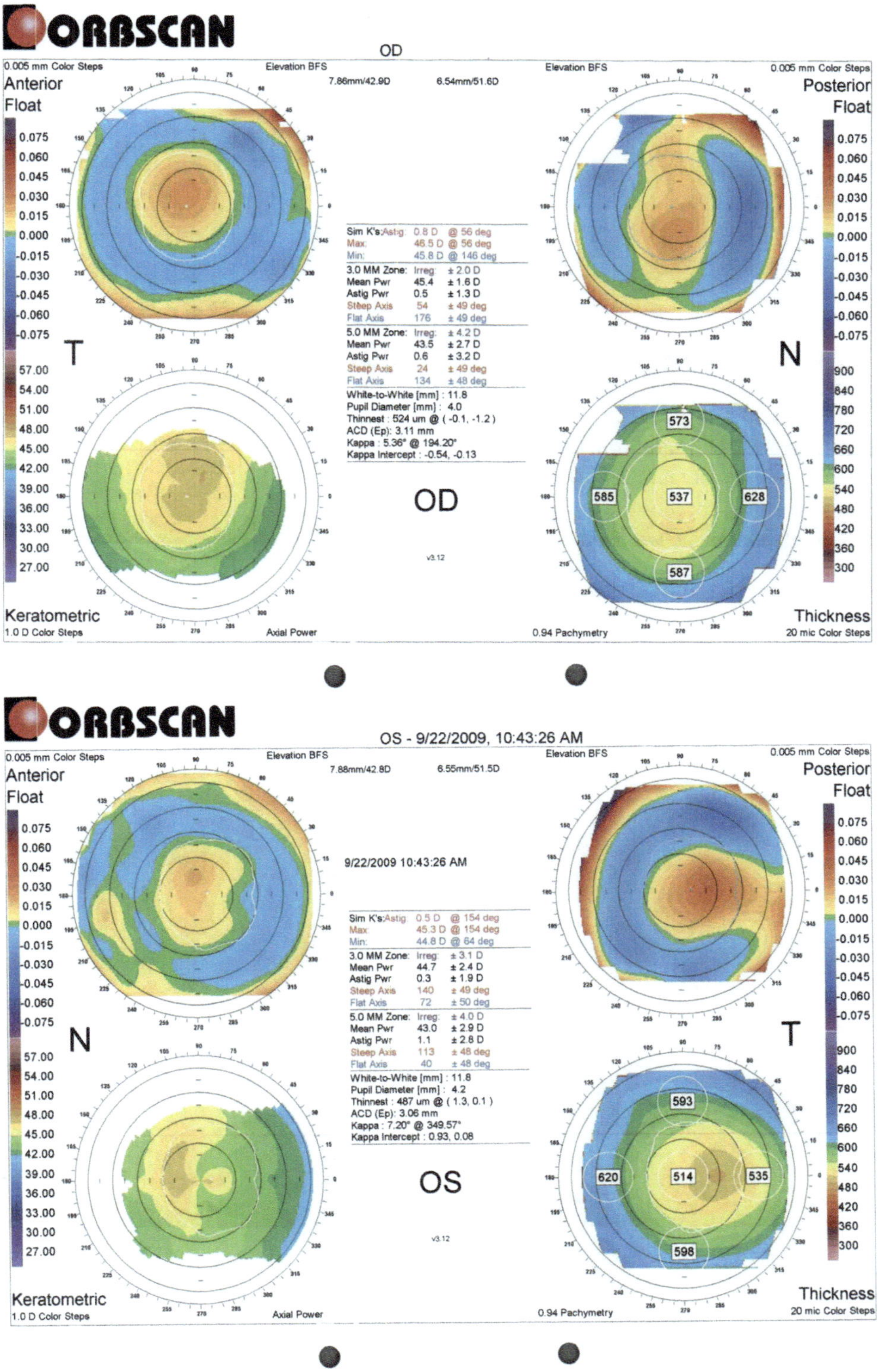

Fig. 63.3 Orbscan OD (**a**) and OS (**b**) 9 months following DLK diagnosis and treatment

erosions, and iritis. However, some DLK cases have been reported 3 years after LASIK without an obvious cause [2]. The underlying cause of DLK in this case also appears to be unknown.

The energy level for femtosecond flap creation has been shown to play a role in the risk of DLK. Some studies have shown no difference in the occurrence of DLK at different energy levels. However, in a recent case-control study, higher energy level (60 kHz) for flap creation and larger flap diameter were associated with an increased risk for DLK [3]. In our case, we could not ascertain whether the laser energy was a contributing factor.

Important points to learn from this case are the proper management of late-onset DLK with medical intervention, corticosteroids, and careful follow-up. Pretreatment with topical antibiotics and corticosteroids is encouraged to reduce the incidence of DLK. The diagnosis and management of an infectious etiology is of paramount importance. In addition, the diagnosis and management of chronic dry eye is valuable in managing the associated DLK.

References

1. Smith RJ, Maloney RK (1998) Diffuse lamellar keratitis. A new syndrome in lamellar refractive surgery. Ophthalmology 105:1721–1726
2. Jin GJ, Lyle WA, Merkley KH (2005) Late-onset idiopathic diffuse lamellar keratitis after laser in situ keratomileusis. J Cataract Refract Surg 31:435–437
3. de Paula FH, Khairallah CG, Niziol LM, Musch DC, Shtein RM (2012) Diffuse lamellar keratitis after laser in situ keratomileusis with femtosecond laser flap creation. J Cataract Refract Surg 38:1014–1019

Other Complications: Management of Apparent Corneal Infiltrates After Cataract Surgery in a Patient with Previous LASIK Treatment

64

Miguel J. Maldonado

Contents

M.J. Maldonado, MD, PhD
Ophthalmology, Refractive Surgery Unit, University of Valladolid/IOBA-Eye Institute, Valladolid, Spain
e-mail: maldonado@ioba.med.uva.es

Why Is This Case Relevant for the Refractive Surgeon?

Managing apparent corneal infiltrates after cataract surgery in a patient with past LASIK treatment will become an increasingly common scenario for refractive surgeons. This chapter provides insights about how to manage and prevent such a case.

Case Background

A 52-year-old patient sought consultation after significant deterioration of his sight in the last 2 months. He complained of blurred vision and monocular diplopia in his right eye despite cataract surgery and IOL implantation. Some degree of photophobia was also present. He underwent myopic LASIK surgery 12 years ago and cataract surgery 2 months ago.

Main Problem to Solve

The primary problem the patient presented with was poor vision after LASIK and subsequent phacoemulsification in his eye, showing mid-peripheral corneal grayish-white opacities. Uncorrected distance visual acuity in this eye was 20/80. Corrected distance vision was 20/50 with −1.25, −5.00 × 150°. Slit lamp examination disclosed hazy grayish areas in

J.L. Alió et al. (eds.), *Difficult and Complicated Cases in Refractive Surgery*,
DOI 10.1007/978-3-642-55238-0_64, © Springer-Verlag Berlin Heidelberg 2015

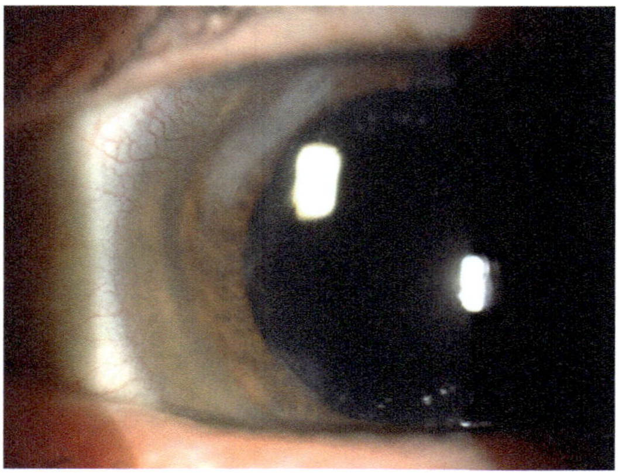

Fig. 64.1 Anterior segment photograph demonstrating corneal opacities in mid-peripheral stroma of the LASIK eye presenting with poor vision

the mid-peripheral cornea just inside the corneal flap edge (Fig. 64.1). A detailed examination showed that the infiltrate appearance corresponded to the corneal phaco incision and paracentesis wounds, which were surrounded by flap edema, but no obvious interface fluid pocket was present (Fig. 64.2a, b). Involvement of the paracentesis ruled out phaco wound burn. The LASIK flap was nasally hinged. An anterior chamber reaction and a typical diffuse lamellar keratitis were both absent. The patient showed moderate blepharitis with very scarce superficial punctate keratopathy.

Ancillary Tests

Tangential corneal topography showed grossly irregular and regular astigmatism, the latter corresponding to the manifest refraction. Particularly, the flattened meridian orientation was very close to the corneal phaco incision area. Anterior corneal elevation topography disclosed marked corneal bulging in agreement with corneal incision size and location. The prominence was higher in the main incision and the surrounding area of corneal edema. Central applanation tonometry yielded 8 mmHg and central pachymetry was 420 μm. However, the Reichert Ocular Response Analyzer corneal-compensated intraocular pressure was 21.5 mmHg (Goldman-correlated IOP was 18.4, corneal resistance factor was 8.5 mmHg, and corneal hysteresis was 7.3 mmHg). A prescription of sodium chloride hypertonicity ophthalmic ointment was given, 5 %, twice daily (daytime and nighttime) in addition to unpreserved artificial tears and eyelid hygiene. Also, timolol maleate eyedrops BID were prescribed to prevent potential intraocular pressure spikes which would possibly influence corneal edema.

Outcome

Ten weeks after initiating the medical treatment, uncorrected distance visual acuity in the right eye had improved to 20/40, and corrected distance vision was 20/32 with −0.25, −1.00 × 140°.

The grayish-white opacities corresponding to the main phaco incision and particularly the paracentesis had diminished notably (Fig. 64.3a, b). In addition, corneal edema extending centrally had completely disappeared. Consequently, tangential corneal topography and anterior corneal elevation topography showed improved corneal regularity over the pupil entrance. Central applanation tonometry yielded 14 mmHg, whereas corneal-compensated IOP with the Ocular Response Analyzer was 16 mmHg. The patient expressed satisfaction with the visual improvement. Medications were discontinued except for routine eyelid hygiene that helped minimize the blepharitis.

What to Learn from This Case

1. Presurgical planning of the corneal incision location is warranted before performing any intraocular procedure in an eye that has previously undergone LASIK. If the exact flap hinge and flap edge locations are unknown or unclear, fluorescein should be instilled onto the cornea to delineate the flap limits (Fig. 64.4). A scheme should be devised such that all the incisions are planned and performed outside the flap edge, with the incision tunnel roof running under the LASIK flap to avoid intersection with the flap interface.

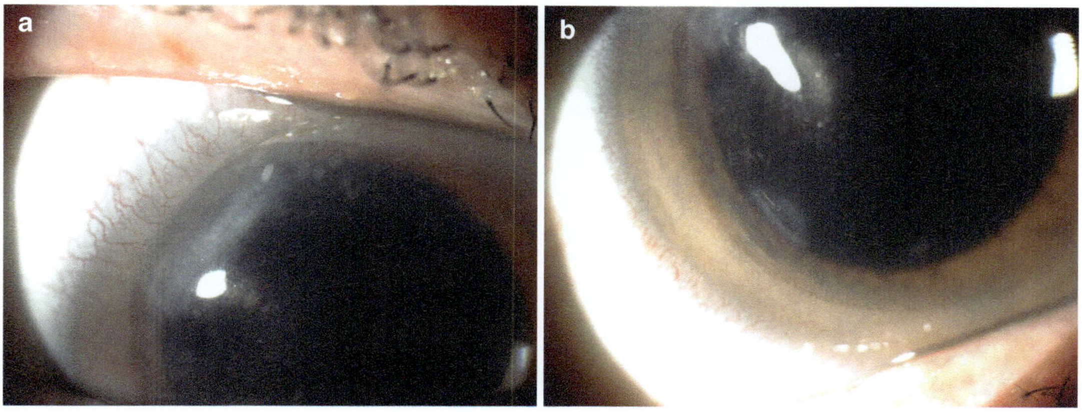

Fig. 64.2 Detailed view of the corneal opacities inside the LASIK flap margin showing transparency loss in the wound and edema in the adjacent corneal tissue extending centripetally at (**a**) the main phaco incision and (**b**) paracentesis. Blepharitis and pannus are also rather noticeable

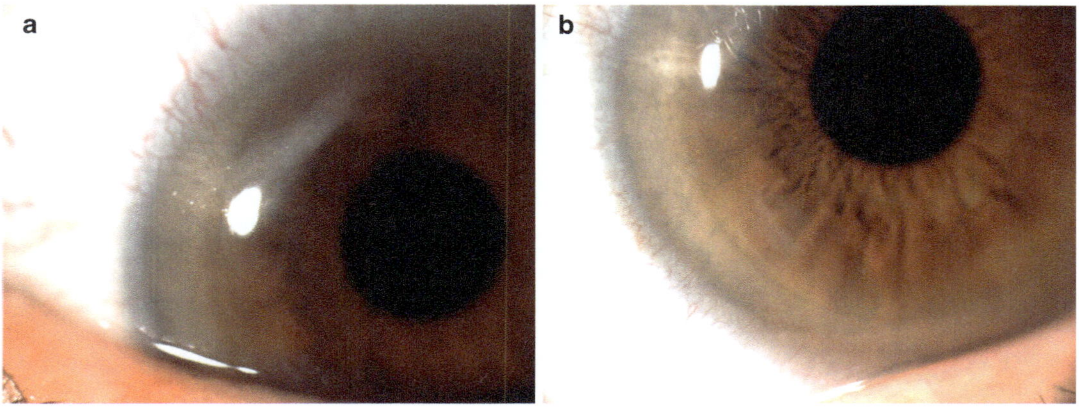

Fig. 64.3 Pictures showing improvement after 10 weeks of medical treatment. Corneal opacification in the wound is less dense, and the adjacent corneal edema has resolved at (**a**) the main phaco incision and (**b**) paracentesis

2. If the external portion of the main phaco incision or the paracentesis [1], or both, is unsuitably located anteriorly or if the incision tunnel is too shallow and intersects with the LASIK flap interface [2], two phenomena will likely occur: (1) Visibility through the cornea will be impaired due to the fluid misdirecting into the flap interface, with increasing degrees of corneal edema developing intraoperatively. This will jeopardize the intraocular procedure safety. (2) Postoperative corneal edema adjacent to the incisions extending centrally will cause long-standing disturbance to the patient, as in this case. Blurred vision and monocular diplopia will result from high irregular and regular astigmatism, with variable degrees of discomfort and photophobia delaying the visual rehabilitation of the phacoemulsification procedure despite appropriate intraocular lens power calculations after LASIK.
3. In a LASIK cornea with grayish-white opacities simulating peri-incisional sterile inflammatory infiltrates [3], the differential diagnosis should include corneal edema due to fluidics and/or intraoperative solution misdirection.

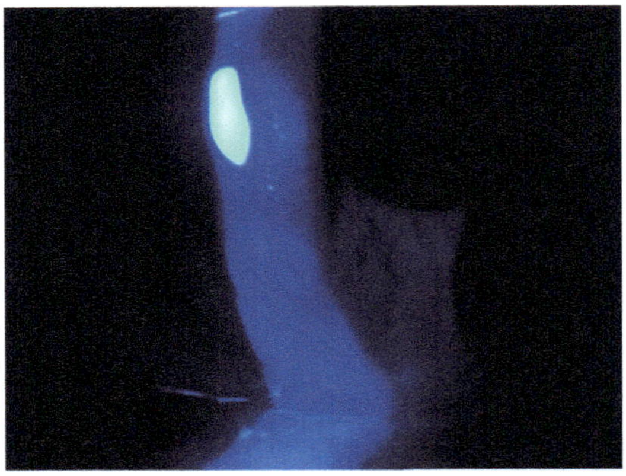

Fig. 64.4 Identification of the long-standing LASIK flap edge can be improved by examination with fluorescein and blue cobalt light at the slit lamp. Alternatively, delicate indentation of the limbal cornea may be performed under the microscope. In this case, the external incision of the paracentesis (shown) and main corneal phaco wound were performed inadequately within the flap area and thus intersected with the flap interface

4. In a cornea with a previous LASIK flap showing some degree of transparency loss, first the intraocular pressure should be controlled by administering antiglaucoma medications to prevent potential intraocular pressure spikes [4, 5]. Moreover, in a cornea with a LASIK flap and some edema, the intraocular pressure readings obtained by conventional tonometry are likely to grossly underestimate the real intraocular pressure [4, 5]. Only after the intraocular pressure is confirmed under control can steroids be considered. However, avoiding corticosteroid use in cases of corneal transparency loss from fluidic misdirection and/or in the absence of elevated intraocular pressure may help prevent steroid-induced interface fluid syndrome after LASIK [4, 5].

References

1. Alió J, Rodríguez-Prats JL, Galal A, Ramzy M (2005) Outcomes of microincision cataract surgery versus coaxial phacoemulsification. Ophthalmology 112:1997–2003
2. Maldonado MJ, Ruiz-Oblitas L, Munuera JM, Aliseda D, García-Layana A, Moreno-Montañés J (2000) Optical coherence tomography evaluation of the corneal cap and stromal bed features after laser in situ keratomileusis for high myopia and astigmatism. Ophthalmology 107:81–87
3. Singhal S, Sridhar MS, Garg P (2005) Bilateral peripheral infiltrative keratitis after LASIK. J Refract Surg 21:402–404
4. Carreño E, Portero A, Galarreta DJ, Merayo JM (2012) Interface fluid syndrome associated with cataract surgery. J Refract Surg 28:243–244
5. Ortega-Usobiaga J, Martin-Reyes C, Llovet-Osuna F, Damas-Mateache B, Baviera-Sabater J (2012) Interface fluid syndrome in routine cataract surgery 10 years after laser in situ keratomileusis. Cornea 31: 706–707

Part V
PRK Complications

Dear reader,

This section describes complications associated with one of the traditional techniques in the excimer laser refractive surgery: photorefractive keratectomy, or PRK. PRK is a refractive procedure which reduces risks such as dry eye and interference with the cornea's biomechanics. Because PRK does not require the expensive or sophisticated equipment associated with LASIK surgery and is considered an easier procedure, it is performed around the world.

Why do we include PRK in this book? Every surgical procedure had complications and PRK is no exception. In this chapter, we include discussions of epidemic keratoconjunctivitis, infection post-PRK, and a case of late-onset consecutive hyperopia. We include the most significant cases, such as corneal haze to a rarer case of ectasia.

For further reading, we suggest the first book of this series: J.L. Alio', D. Azar *Management of Complications in Refractive Surgery*, Chapter 10: Corneal Haze After Refractive Surgery (pp. 179–185).

Specific topics covered by the cases include is the absence of bowman membrane a risk for epidemic keratoconjunctivitis (Case 65), how to manage infection after PRK (Case 66), and epithelial delay or abnormal healing using Mitomycin C (Case 67). Other cases describe how to manage dry eye after PRK (Case 68), the two-stage transepithelial PRK: a useful surgical technique for treating the haze (Case 69), treating severe haze after PRK (Case 70). We end with cases focused on how PRK can cause a corneal ectasia (Case 71), managing consecutive hyperopia following myopic laser vision (Case 72), and long follow-up and refractive stability in extreme high myopia (Case 73).

Lesson to Learn

Case 65: PRK and epidemic keratoconjunctivitis

The damages in the Bowman's layer and hyperactiveness of keratocytes induced by PRK may cause an abnormal healing response in a patient who suffers from epidemic keratoconjunctivitis.

Case 66: Monolateral *Streptococcus pneumoniae* keratitis after photorefractive keratotomy (PRK)

Even if PRK is considered a safe treatment, the infectious keratitis is one of the most important complications that can affect the visual quality. The way to promote a faster reepithelialization would be achieved to reduce this risk.

Case 67: Abnormal healing

The epithelial delay or abnormal healing in a PRK in patient treated with Mitomycin C may be a significant complication. A rapid treatment gave back to this patient a good visual acuity.

Case 68: Dry eye and PRK

Even that this complication is less frequent than in LASIK, it might happen and we should know how to manage it.

Case 69: Treatment of post-PRK or post-RK haze by two-stage transepithelial PRK with Mitomycin C

Two-stage topography-guided PRK is a useful tool for the treatment of visually significant haze after RK or PRK and addresses refractive error at the same time.

Case 70: A case of severe haze after PRK in a patient treated by a 6th generation of excimer laser

The risk of haze post-PRK is still real. A case of severe haze in a patient with moderate myopia treated by new laser generation without Mitomycin C.

Case 71: Ectasia post-PRK at delayed onset

Is the corneal ectasia a risk after PRK? What are the possible risk factors associated?

Case 72: Late-onset consecutive hyperopia following decentered myopic PRK

A case of consecutive hyperopia following PRK. How to proceed? LASIK or PRK. If PRK is attempted, should MMC be used?

Case 73: Twelve years of follow-up of PRK in a patient with −22 diopter of myopia

A case of long follow-up after PRK in a patient with high myopia. An example of long-term safety and stability.

PRK and Epidemic Keratoconjunctivitis

65

Jaime Javaloy, Dominika Wróbel, and Alessandro Abbouda

Contents

J. Javaloy, MD, PhD (✉)
Department of Anterior Segment and Refractive Surgery, Vissum Corporacion Oftalmológica, Alicante, Spain
e-mail: jjavaloy@coma.es

D. Wróbel, MD
Glaucoma Diagnostic and Microsurgery Department, Medical University of Lublin, Lublin, Poland

R&D Department, Vissum Corporacion, Alicante, Spain
e-mail: ddudzinska@interia.pl

A. Abbouda, MD
Department of Refractive Surgery, Vissum Corporación Oftalmológica, Alicante, Spain

Department of Ophthalmology-Policlinico Umberto I of Rome, University of Rome "Sapienza", Viale del Policlinico, 155, 00186 Roma, Italy

R&D Department, Vissum Corporación Oftalmológica, 03016 Alicante, Spain
e-mail: a.abbouda@gmail.com

Why Is This Case Relevant for the Refractive Surgeon?

As photorefractive keratectomy became a popular refractive surgery procedure, Talamo theorized that the destruction of Bowman's layer during uneventful photorefractive keratectomy (PRK) causes abnormal healing, subepithelial infiltrates, and associated scarring [1]. Recurrent adenoviral stromal keratitis is thought to express a delayed hypersensitivity immune response to viral antigens in the corneal stroma [2].

Refractive surgeons should be aware that damages in Bowman's layer and hyperactiveness of keratocytes induced by PRK may cause an abnormal healing response in a patient who suffers from epidemic keratoconjunctivitis (EKC) [3].

Case Background

A 33-year-old woman underwent bilateral uneventful PRK for moderate myopia of −5.50 −0.50 20° in the right eye and −5.75 −0.50 20° in the left eye. The best corrected visual acuity (BCVA) was 20/20 in both eyes. Preoperative corneal pachymetry was 515 μm in both eyes. Keratometry readings before surgery were 44.21 /45.12×24 ° in the right eye and 44.35 /45.13×10° in the left eye. According to the topography, her corneal surface was regular. The slit lamp and fundus examinations were normal. She had worn soft contact lenses for many

J.L. Alió et al. (eds.), *Difficult and Complicated Cases in Refractive Surgery*, DOI 10.1007/978-3-642-55238-0_65, © Springer-Verlag Berlin Heidelberg 2015

years. Before surgery, our patient had not had a clinical history of adenoviral keratoconjunctivitis in either eye. Uneventful transepithelial photorefractive keratectomy was performed in both eyes. MMC 2 % was applied for 30 sec. The total calculated ablation depth was 170 μm in the right eye and 157 μm in the left eye (residual stoma in the right eye 345 and 358 μm in the left). Postoperative treatment was ciprofloxacin (Oftacilox®, Alcon, Spain) one drop three times a day for 7 days, dexamethasone (Maxidex®, Alcon, Spain) one drop five times a day for 7 days followed by fluorometholone (FML®, Allergan Inc., USA) one drop four times a day tapering to one drop every 3 weeks, soft bandage contact lenses while healing, and analgesic pills orally if necessary. Postoperative evaluation at 1 week was normal, the slit lamp examination showed a complete reepithelialization in both eyes. After 1 month the uncorrected visual acuity (UCVA) was 20/20. According to the topography, her corneal surface was regular and pachymetry was 430 μm in both eyes. The slit lamp examination showed no anomalies and intraocular pressure (IOP) was 18 mmHg in both eyes. Corneal haze and scarring were absent. After 4 years she presented at the emergency ophthalmology department with acute left eye redness, blurry vision, foreign body sensation, and photophobia. The patient reported left eye injury (a scratch from her child). UCVA was 20/50 in the left eye. The slit lamp examination revealed corneal erosion. The treatment was ciprofloxacin (Oftacilox®) ointment three times a day, cycloplegic drops three times a day, and dexpanthenol (Recugel®, Allergan Inc., USA) overnight. The next control appointment showed a clear and smooth cornea without a fluorescein staining and infiltration, with the patient reporting improved vision (Fig. 65.1). Ten days after the injury, the patient complained of severe pain of the left eye and a watery mucoid discharge. The slit lamp examination revealed in the left eye eyelid edema, reddening and swelling of the plica semilunaris and lacrimal caruncle, conjunctival injection, chemosis, follicular conjunctivitis and ecchymosis, cornea without fluorescein staining, and no anterior chamber reaction. The right eye was normal. IOP was 14 mmHg in both eyes. There was preauricular and submandibular adenopathy. The treatment was ciprofloxacin (Oftacilox®), artificial tears, and a cool compress. Four days later the slit lamp examination of the left eye showed eyelid edema, swelling and conjunctival injection, the cornea without fluorescein staining with multifocal subepithelial infiltrates, and no membranes and pseudomembranes on the tarsal conjunctiva. Fluorometholone (FML®) 1 drop three times per day was added. A few days later the patient complained of photophobia and permanent glare. Her UCVA was 20/80 in the right eye and 20/70 in the left eye. The slit lamp examination in both eyes revealed corneas stained with a fluorescein solution, and coin-like infiltrates (keratitis nummularis or Dimmer's keratitis) covered the entire corneal surface (Fig. 65.2 and 65.3). IOL was 18 mmHg in the right eye and 16 mmHg in the left eye. We diagnosed the epidemic keratoconjunctivitis; the diagnosis was based on the history, signs, and symptoms.

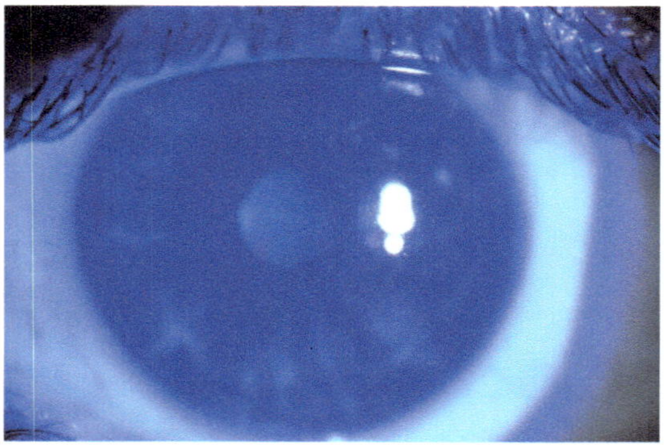

Fig. 65.1 The smooth cornea without a fluorescein staining

Main Problem to Solve

How do we manage an abnormal corneal reaction following PRK? Should we expect an abnormal corneal reaction after PRK (exaggerated corneal infiltration) in the context of KCE? What is an appropriate treatment for subepithelial infiltrates associated with KCE after PRK?

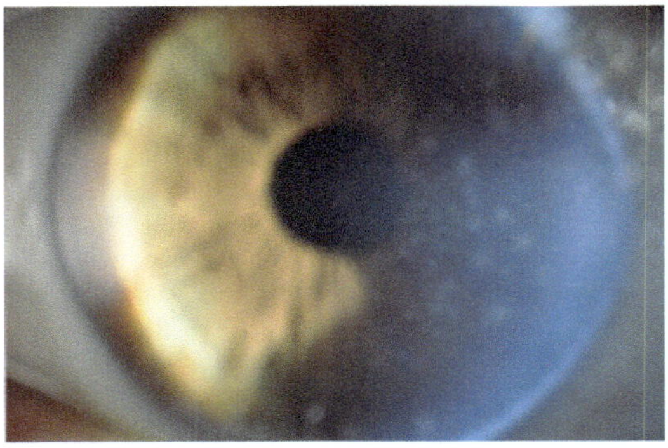

Fig. 65.2 Subepithelial infiltrates after EKC

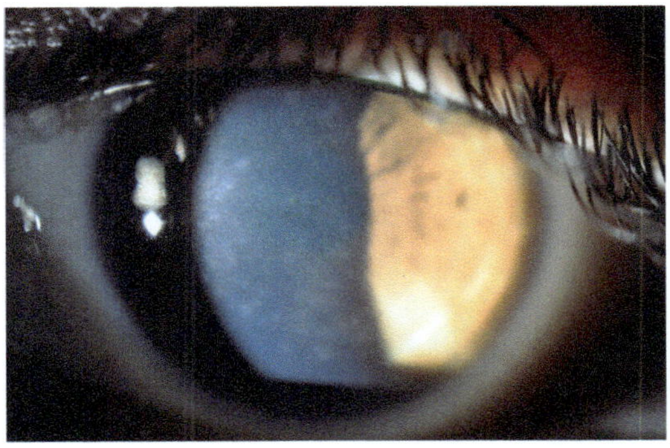

Fig. 65.3 Subepithelial infiltrates after EKC

Ancillary Tests

BCVA, UCVA, pachymetry, topography, slit lamp examination, and intraocular pressure measurement. We did not perform a cell culture in combination with immunofluorescence staining (CC-IFA) and antigen detection or polymerase chain reaction (PCR) because the diagnosis was based on the history and characteristic/pathognomonic signs.

Surgical/Medical Intervention

Fluorometholone (FML Forte®) four times a day was prescribed tapering to one drop a week. Although the destruction of the Bowman's layer during PRK may cause a problem with subepithelial infiltrates [1], some authors describe the same treatment (topical MMC in conjunction with PRK) for subepithelial infiltrates because of EKC's production of positive visual and refractive results [4]. Other authors describe a positive outcome after using cyclosporine A (CSA) 1 % to reduce subepithelial infiltrates resistant to corticosteroid eyedrops [5].

Outcome

After 4 months of treatment, UCVA was 20/20 in both eyes. Slit lamp examination revealed no secretion, no conjunctiva injection, coin-like infiltrates, and a cornea without a fluorescein staining.

What to Learn from This Case

PRK with mitomycin C is a promising treatment for moderate myopia, but a surgeon should be meticulous in selecting patients. It is important to keep the patient's clinical history in mind, especially those involving viral keratoconjunctivitis. EKC is a serious complication after excimer laser photorefractive procedure. As reported in the literature, EKC reoccurrence after PRK is more frequent in the eye without refractive surgery [3]. The cornea's response to EKC can be abnormal after PRK due to the keratocytes' hyperactivation and a loss of Bowman's layer after the refractive procedure [3, 6]. It is widely known that corneal infiltrates are an immune response to suspected adenoviral antigens deposited in corneal stroma during the primary adenoviral infection, and this is a cause of frequent relapses [3, 7]. The prompt diagnosis and the use of topical steroids seem to be effective in managing EKC after refractive surgery [3]. CSA 1 % eyedrops may be an effective corticosteroid-sparing agent in subepithelial infiltrates resistant to corticosteroid therapy.

References

1. Pineda R, Talamo JH (1998) Late onset of haze associated with viral keratoconjunctivitis following photorefractive keratectomy. J Refract Surg 14: 147–151
2. Fite SW, Chodosh J (1998) Photorefractive keratectomy for myopia in the setting of adenoviral subepithelial infiltrates. Am J Ophthalmol 126:829–831
3. Park SJ et al (2011) Development of EKC after excimer laser photorefractive surgery and subsequent recurrence of EKC-like keratitis. Korean J Ophthalmol 25:443–446
4. Alevi D, Barsam A (2012) Photorefractive keratectomy with mitomycin-C for the combined treatment of myopia and subepithelial infiltrates after epidemic keratoconjunctivitis. J Cataract Refract Surg 38:1028–1033
5. Jeng BH, Holsclaw DS (2011) Cyclosporine A 1 % eye drops for the treatment of subepithelial infiltrates after adenoviral keratoconjunctivitis. Cornea 30:958–961
6. Jabbur NS, O'Brien TP (2003) Recurrence of keratitis after excimer laser keratectomy. J Cataract Refract Surg 29:198–201
7. Arcieri ES, Arcieri RS (2004) Subepithelial infiltrates associated to viral keratoconjunctivitis following photorefractive keratectomy. Eye 18:1010–1012

Monolateral *Streptococcus pneumoniae* Keratitis After Photorefractive Keratotomy (PRK)

66

Jorge L. Alió, Alessandro Abbouda, and Angelo Rampone

Contents

J.L. Alió, MD, PhD (✉)
Department of Refractive Surgery, Vissum Corporación Oftalmológica, Alicante, Spain
e-mail: jlalio@vissum.com

A. Abbouda, MD
Department of Refractive Surgery, Vissum Corporación Oftalmológica, Alicante, Spain

Department of Ophthalmology-Policlinico Umberto I of Rome, University of Rome "Sapienza", Viale del Policlinico, 155, 00186 Roma, Italy

R&D Department, Vissum Corporación Oftalmológica, 03016, Alicante, Spain
e-mail: a.abbouda@gmail.com

A. Rampone, MD
Department of Ophthalmology, Seconda Università degli Studi di Napoli, Naples, Italy

R&D Department, Vissum Corporacion, 03016, Alicante, Spain
e-mail: angelo.rampone@gmail.com

Why Is This Case Relevant for the Refractive Surgeon?

Infectious keratitis after photorefractive keratectomy (PRK) is a devastating complication [1]. The risk factors for infectious keratitis are breakdown of the barrier function of the corneal epithelium, the use of a bandage contact lens, and topical steroid drops to control wound healing. The refractive surgeon should be prepared to recognize and manage this complication in order to achieve an optimal visual outcome.

Case Background

A 52-year-old woman presented to our department for a refractive surgery evaluation to correct myopic astigmatism in both eyes. She had no relevant ocular history. Her manifest refraction was −3.25, −1.0 × 20° in the right eye (RE) and −4.0, −0.75 × 145° in the left eye (LE). Keratometry readings were 44.44/46.09 × 103° in the RE and 44.92/45.79 × 80° in the LE. Her best corrected visual acuity (BCVA) was 20/20 for distance and near vision in both eyes. Both slit lamp and fundus examinations were normal. According to the topography, her corneal surface was regular, her RE pachymetry was 481 µm, and her LE pachymetry was 434 µm. We decided to perform a PRK in both eyes. On the third day postoperatively, the patient reported decreased vision and mild light sensitivity in her left eye (LE) with pain and discomfort. The

J.L. Alió et al. (eds.), *Difficult and Complicated Cases in Refractive Surgery*,
DOI 10.1007/978-3-642-55238-0_66, © Springer-Verlag Berlin Heidelberg 2015

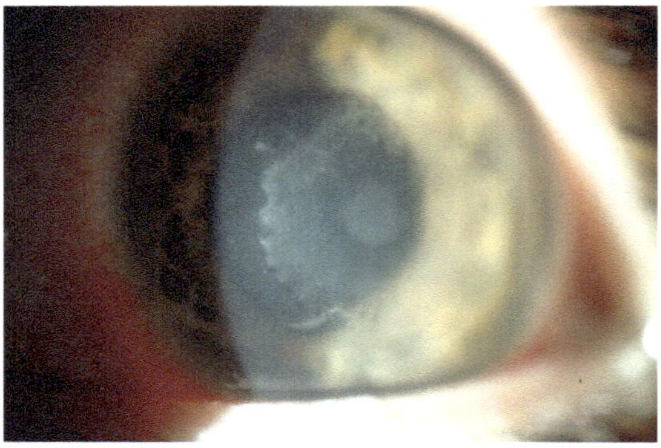

Fig. 66.1 Paracentral epithelial defect, an annular stromal infiltrate without hypopyon

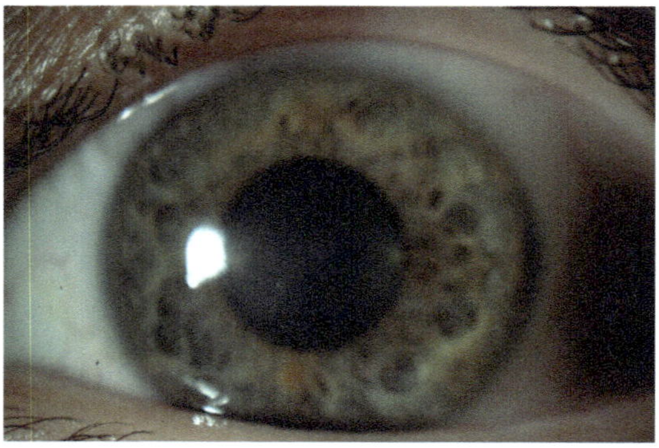

Fig. 66.2 Annular corneal haze as an outcome

slit lamp examination showed the presence of a paracentral epithelial defect, an annular stromal infiltrate without hypopyon (Fig. 66.1).

We decided to do a corneal Gram stain and contact lens. We started an empiric therapy with ofloxacin 1 drop four times per day, dexamethasone 1 drop four times per day, and cycloplegic drops (1 drop three times for 2 days). The Gram stain and cultures were positive to *Streptococcus pneumoniae*.

Main Problem to Solve

Early identification and treatment of this complication can promote a positive outcome. De Oliveira et al. [2] reported a rate of 10 % of streptococcus culture verified in infectious keratitis after a PRK.

Ancillary Tests

Fourth-generation fluoroquinolone is recommended. If this therapy is not clearly responsive in 48 hours, it could be useful for corneal scraping. Meanwhile, Gram stain and cultures of the scraped tissue should be performed to establish an effective therapy. A topical fortified combination of tear-drops could be selected when the microbiologist offers a confirmed diagnosis.

Surgical/Medical Intervention

After the results were provided, the therapy was modified as follows: ofloxacin 1 drop every 2 hours alternated with cefazolin drops, steroid drops (dexamethasone 1 drop four times per day tapering 1 drop every week for a total of 4 weeks followed by fluorometholone 1 drop three times per day for 2 weeks). Platelet-rich plasma (PRP) eyedrops were added to promote a faster reepithelialization.

Outcome

Ten days after the start of the therapy, the patient had a complete regression of pain and discomfort in the LE. The slit lamp examination showed a reduction of corneal infiltrates. At 3 months, the corneal epithelium was intact with only a ringlike haze (Fig. 66.2). The UCVA was 20/20 for distance and near vision in both eyes. Keratometry reading were 41.63/42.73 × 71° in the RE and 41.89/42.61 × 87° in the LE. The topography showed a normal ablation profile compatible to a PRK treatment myopic astigmatism.

What to Learn from This Case

Increased risk after PRK is associated with inherent creation of a large epithelial defect and the therapeutic use of a contact lens in the early postoperative period. Most postoperative infections are caused by Gram-positive organisms including *S. aureus*, coagulase-negative *Staphylococcus* species, and *Streptococcus* species [3]. The reported risk for keratitis is between 0.01 and 0.8 % after PRK and between 0.01 and 0.1 % after LASIK [4]. Although PRK is considered a safe treatment, infectious keratitis can compromise visual quality. Trans-PRK is a new technique that can reduce the risk of infectious keratitis and promote faster reepithelialization.

References

1. Donnenfeld ED, O'Brien TP, Solomon R´e, Perry HD, Speaker MG, Wittpenn J (2003) Infectious keratitis after photorefractive keratectomy. Ophthalmology 110:743–747
2. De Oliveira GC, Solari HP, Ciola FB, Lima AL, Campos MS (2006) Corneal infiltrates after excimer laser photorefractive keratectomy and LASIK. J Refract Surg 22:159–165
3. Wroblewski KJ, Pasternak JF, Bower KS, Schallhorn SC, Hubickey WJ, Harrison CE, Torres MF, Barnes SD (2006) Infectious keratitis after photorefractive keratectomy in the United States army and navy. Ophthalmology 113:520–525
4. Woodward M, Randleman JB (2007) Bilateral methicillin-resistant Staphylococcus aureus keratitis after photorefractive keratectomy. J Cataract Refract Surg 33:316–319

Abnormal Healing

67

Jaime Javaloy, Alessandro Abbouda, and Angelo Rampone

Contents

J. Javaloy, MD, PhD (✉)
Department of Anterior Segment and Refractive Surgery, Vissum Corporacion Oftalmológica, Alicante, Spain
e-mail: jjavaloy@coma.es

A. Abbouda, MD
Department of Refractive Surgery, Vissum Corporación Oftalmológica, Alicante, Spain

Department of Ophthalmology-Policlinico Umberto I of Rome, University of Rome "Sapienza", Viale del Policlinico, 155, 00186 Roma, Italy

R&D Department, Vissum Corporación Oftalmológica, 03016, Alicante, Spain
e-mail: a.abbouda@gmail.com

A. Rampone, MD
Department of Ophthalmology, Seconda Università degli Studi di Napoli, Naples, Italy

R&D Department, Vissum Corporacion, 03016, Alicante, Spain
e-mail: angelo.rampone@gmail.com

Why Is This Case Relevant for the Refractive Surgeon?

Abnormal healing can occur during the postoperative period of PRK. The refractive surgeon should be ready to recognize and manage this complication to achieve an optimal visual outcome.

Case Background

A 31-year-old man with no ocular history presented for a refractive surgery evaluation. His manifest refraction was −5.75, −0.5 × 10 in the right eye and −6 in the left eye. The keratometry reading was 41.73/42.73 × 94 in the right eye and 41.69/42.23 × 107 in the left eye. His best corrected visual acuity (BCVA) was 20/20 for distance and near vision in both eyes. The slit lamp and fundus examinations were normal. According to the topography, his corneal surface was regular, his right eye pachymetry was 487 μm, and his left eye pachymetry was 484 μm. PRK treatment was performed. The next day, the patient felt discomfort in both eyes. The slit lamp examination showed hyperemia and areas of abnormal epithelization in the pupil areas of both eyes. After 5 days, the slit lamp examination revealed an increase of epithelial ingrowth in both eyes (Fig. 67.1). Mechanical epithelial debridement was performed. Antibiotics and corticosteroid drops were applied. At 20 days

J.L. Alió et al. (eds.), *Difficult and Complicated Cases in Refractive Surgery*,
DOI 10.1007/978-3-642-55238-0_67, © Springer-Verlag Berlin Heidelberg 2015

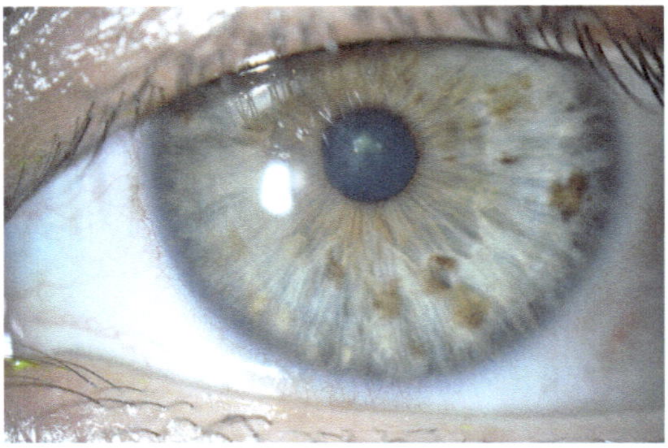

Fig. 67.1 Slit lamp examination at 5 days showed areas of abnormal epithelization in the pupil area

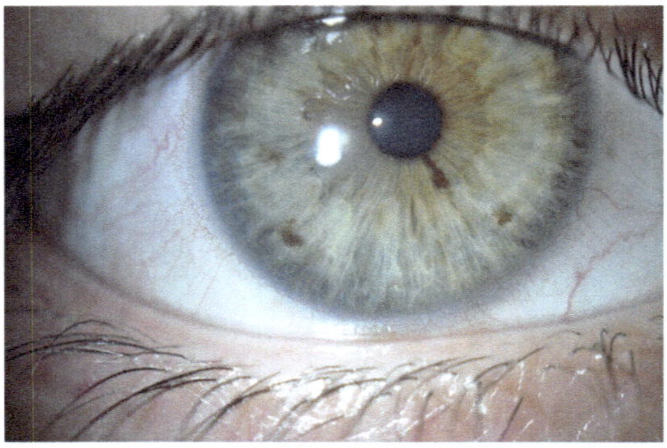

Fig. 67.2 Slit lamp examination after 1 month showed no sign of epithelial hyperplasia

post-PRK, the patient's manifest refraction was +0.50 −0.50 × 175 in the right eye and +0.50, −0.50 × 180 in the left eye. The keratometry reading was 35.97/36.43 × 101 in the right eye and 36.48/36.76 × 39 in the left eye. The BCVA was 20/20 for distance and near vision in both eyes. We noticed a regression of epithelial hyperplasia. The topography showed a framework compatible to PRK treatment.

Main Problem to Solve

Managing central epithelial hyperplasia is crucial in achieving a positive visual result. Infectious keratitis is a differential diagnosis, excluded based upon the lesion's evolution.

Ancillary Tests

Slit lamp examination can be helpful in characterizing epithelial hyperplasia. Deciding whether to treat by epithelial removal depends on the size of the aberrant epithelial hyperplasia.

Surgical/Medical Intervention

The patient followed the standard post-PRK treatment (ofloxacin five times a day for 1 week, dexamethasone 0.1 % three times a day for 1 week, fluorometholone three times a day tapering for a month, and cyclopentolate three times for 48 h). We performed a removal of the abnormal epithelial hyperplasia and extended the period of CL for 3 more days.

Outcome

After 1 month, the slit lamp examination showed a tender oval opacity with no sign of epithelial hyperplasia (Fig. 67.2). In both eyes the uncorrected visual acuity (UVCA) was 20/20.

What to Learn from This Case

Corneal wound healing is an exceedingly complex process mediated by autocrine and paracrine interactions of cytokines, growth factors, and chemokines produced by epithelial cells, stromal cells, immune cells, lacrimal gland, and corneal nerves [1]. A mitomycin C (MMC) dose at 0.02 % can prevent postoperative haze and is not associated with any clinically relevant corneal toxicity [2]. MMC blocks the transformation of keratocytes in myofibroblast, which increases corneal transparency after surface ablation. Corneal epithelial hyperplasia is related to the use of MMC, but more research is needed to determine the exact nature of the relationship. PRK for myopia greater than −6 D is a safe and effective procedure [3, 4]. In this case, the postoperative schedule prevented a permanent defect in the central corneal area, and rapid treatment helped to restore visual acuity.

References

1. Netto MV, Mohan RR, Ambrósio R Jr, Hutcheon AE, Zieske JD, Wilson SE (2005) Wound healing in the cornea: a review of refractive surgery complications and new prospects for therapy. Cornea 24:509–522
2. Teus MA, de Benito-Llopis L, Alió JL (2009) Mitomycin C in corneal refractive surgery. Surv Ophthalmol 54:487–502
3. Alió JL, Muftuoglu O, Ortiz D, Artola A, Pérez-Santonja JJ, de Luna GC, Abu-Mustafa SK, Garcia MJ (2008) Ten-year follow-up of photorefractive keratectomy for myopia of more than -6 diopters. Am J Ophthalmol 145:37–45
4. Alio JL, Artola A, Claramonte PJ, Ayala MJ, Sanchez SP (1998) Complications of photorefractive keratectomy for myopia: two year follow- up of 3000 cases. J Cataract Refract Surg 24:619–626

Dry Eye and PRK

68

Massimo Camellin, Diego Ponzin,
and Samuel Arba Mosquera

Contents

M. Camellin, MD (✉)
SEKAL Rovigo Microsurgery, Rovigo, Italy
e-mail: cammas@tin.it

D. Ponzin
The Veneto Eye Bank Foundation, Venice, Italy
e-mail: diego.ponzin@fbov.it

S. Arba Mosquera, PhD
SCHWIND Eye-Tech-Solutions,
Kleinostheim, Germany
e-mail: samuel.arba.mosquera@eye-tech.net

Why Is This Case Relevant for the Refractive Surgeon?

Dry eye is an ongoing challenge for the refractive surgeon. LASIK surgery may result in decreased corneal sensation and dry eye. PRK patients can also experience this problem, although occurrences are generally limited to the first 3 months [1].

Case Background

A 65-year-old female had previously undergone cataract surgery. She presented with dry eye and underwent surface ablation treatment in the right eye. Because of the residual mixed astigmatism, a transepithelial customized PRK was planned. Her visual acuity and refraction post-cataract surgery in the right eye was +1.25 sph/−2.5 cyl at 5 (5/10, 20/40). Six months following the cataract operation, she underwent the first customized trans-PRK. Six months later, with a right eye acuity of −1.75 sph/+3.25 cyl at 170 (4/10, 20/50), she underwent the second customized trans-PRK, with a 1-month post-acuity of −1 sph/0.75 cyl at 150 (2/10, 20/100). The patient then had a 2 punctum plug insertion in the lower puncta. One month following punctum plug insertion, her right eye acuity was −0.25 sph/−0.5 cyl at 130 (6–7/10, 20/30). The pre-op Schirmer test type 1 was 5 mm/5 min.

There was a delay in the reepithelialization. 10 days post PRK, the epithelium showed

J.L. Alió et al. (eds.), *Difficult and Complicated Cases in Refractive Surgery*,
DOI 10.1007/978-3-642-55238-0_68, © Springer-Verlag Berlin Heidelberg 2015

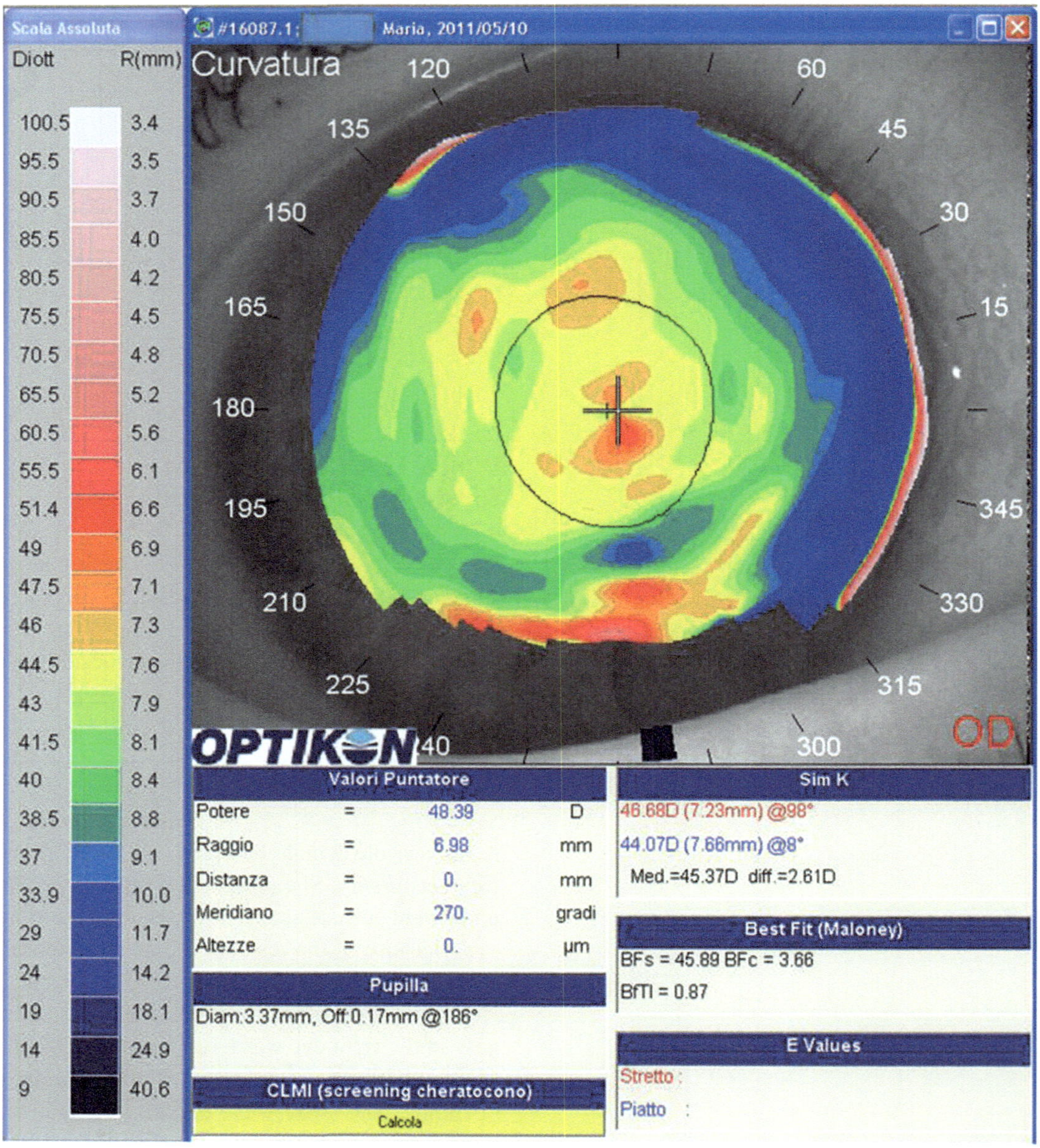

Fig. 68.1 Topography in instantaneous curvature shows a central astigmatism and some irregularities in the corneal periphery

irregularities despite the use of autologous serum eyedrops, artificial tears, and a topical steroid. After 6 months, we decided to fix the remaining irregular astigmatism by applying pure autologous serum every hour [2], and the postoperative course was uneventful. Despite the lack of delay in the reepithelialization, the quality of the surface at 1 month was not good. At this time we decided to close the lacrimal puncta by plug insertion. After 1 week, the patient's sight recovered completely (Figs. 68.1 and 68.2).

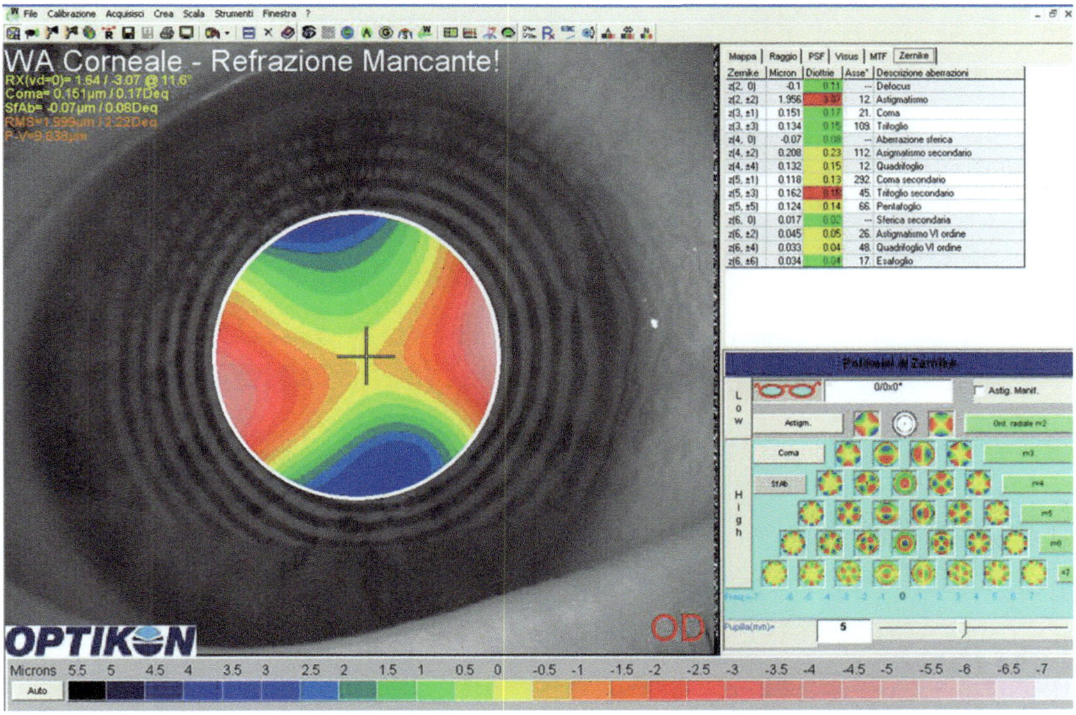

Fig. 68.2 Corneal wavefront is quite regular

Main Problem to Solve

The first challenge we faced was promoting corneal reepithelialization. We attempted this through the use of artificial tears, a soft contact lens, autologous serum eyedrops, and a weak steroid. We could obtain a complete new epithelium in 10 days, but the quality of the corneal surface was poor, with irregularities and residual astigmatism.

We waited a few months before deciding on reoperation because we feared a new epithelization delay. However, with the patient complaining of blurred vision, we were forced to reoperate. This time, we decided to use pure autologous serum every hour for the first postoperative week.

This solution prevented reepithelialization delays, but the quality of the surface was not satisfying and the BCVA remained low. At this point, we suspected that the dry eye was responsible for the low vision and inserted 2 punctum plugs in the lower puncta. The situation improved after 1 week.

Ancillary Tests

Schirmer test, topography, and corneal wavefront analysis were necessary to determine the best course of action. BCVA was the key element in the decision to reoperate.

Surgical/Medical Intervention

The programmed surgery was a topo-aberrometric link procedure in both the first and second operations, in which the topography has been converted into corneal wavefronts and these data linked to the laser [3]. The excimer laser Schwind Amaris has a particular eye tracker (6 axis) that allows a precise matching of the topography with the eye.

The procedure was a transepithelial link, in which the laser takes into account the elimination of epithelium during treatment [4]. This non-touch PRK procedure has a great advantage of perfectly

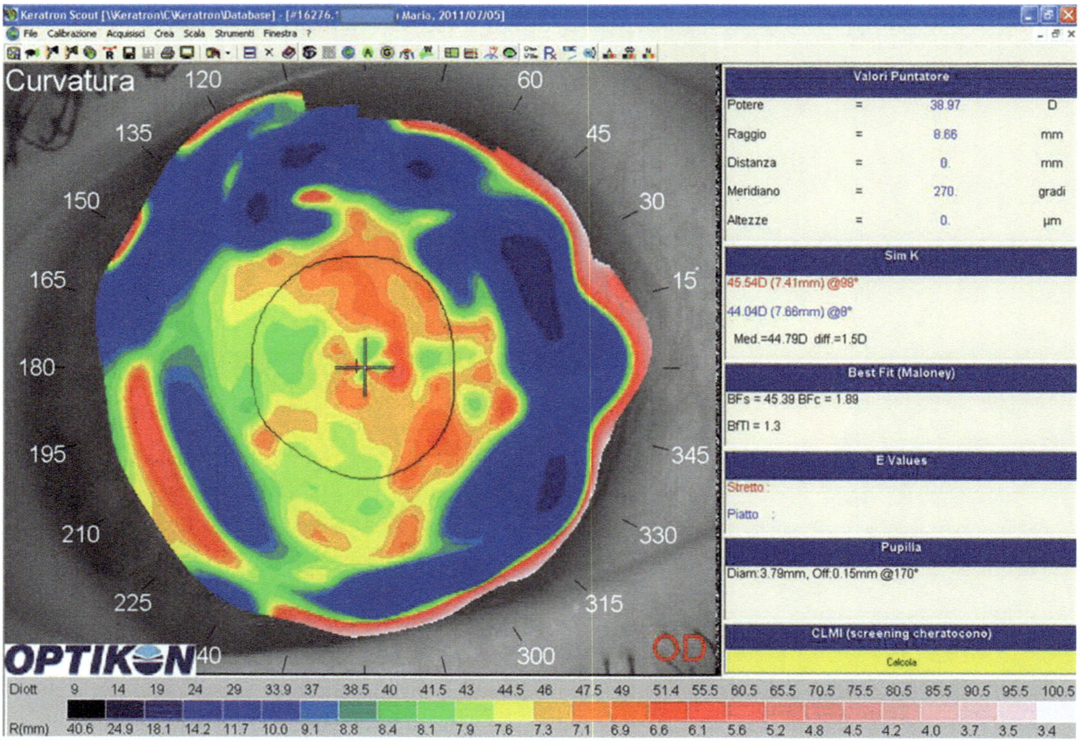

Fig. 68.3 Topography after the 1st customized trans-PRK. Despite a low astigmatism, several irregularities can be seen

matching the analyzed cornea with the laser program and the optimized epithelial ablation, determined by the diameter of the treatment.

0.02 % MMC was applied for 2 min with a Merocel sponge, as is typical in re-treatments. A contact lens was applied for 4 days. A topical treatment with gentamicin (7 days) and a steroid (clobetasone BID for 1 month) was suggested.

The insertion of the two punctum plugs (FCI S2 4002, Paris, France) was performed according to the manufacturer's instructions (Figs. 68.3 and 68.4).

Outcome

This case was a difficult one. We did not expect a delay in reepithelialization following the first customized PRK, and as we realized that the dryness was the cause of the problems, we faced the possibility of another failure with reoperation.

Fortunately, pure autologous serum had beneficial effects, and we did not experience any problems during the early recovery days after reoperation.

The ultimate visual outcome was good and corresponded to the BCVA the patient exhibited before the cataract supervened (right eye: −0.25 sph/−0.5 cyl at 130, 6–7/10, 20/30).

What to Learn from This Case

Although this case highlights the importance of autologous serum in correcting dryness during the first postoperative days, the treatment was insufficient to restore a good corneal surface. The closure of the puncta, by punctum plugs, contributed substantially in promoting the regeneration of a regular epithelium, which requires a healthy environment to regain its physiological properties (Figs. 68.5 and 68.6).

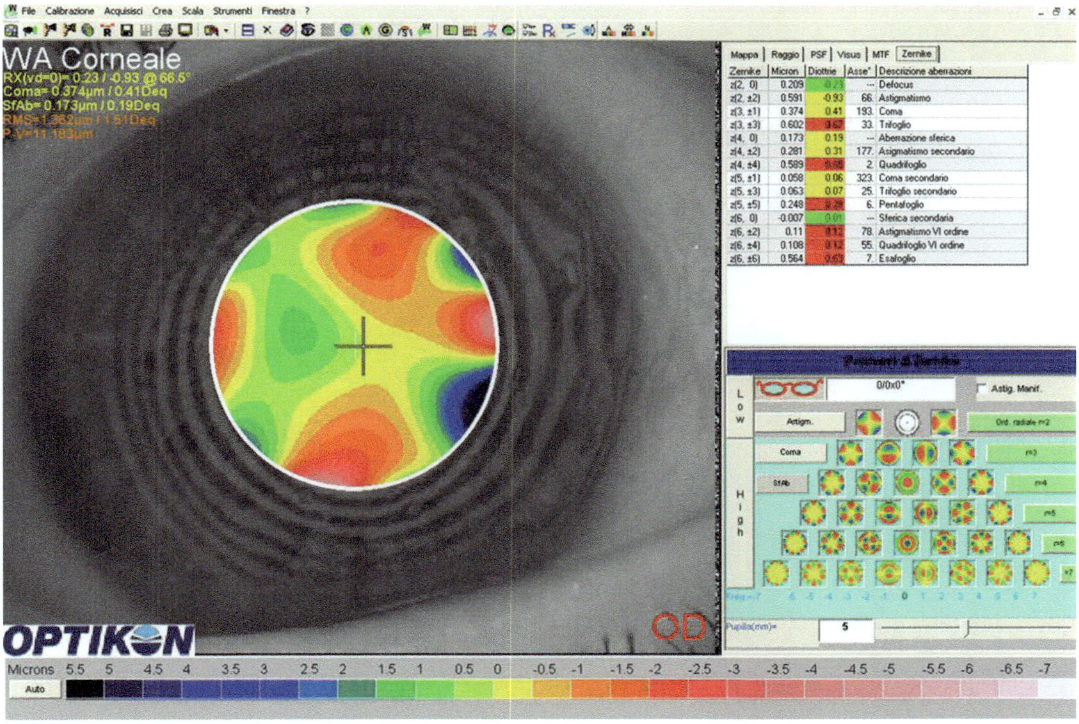

Fig. 68.4 Corneal wavefront analysis shows a pattern worse than the pre-op one, with several high-order aberrations

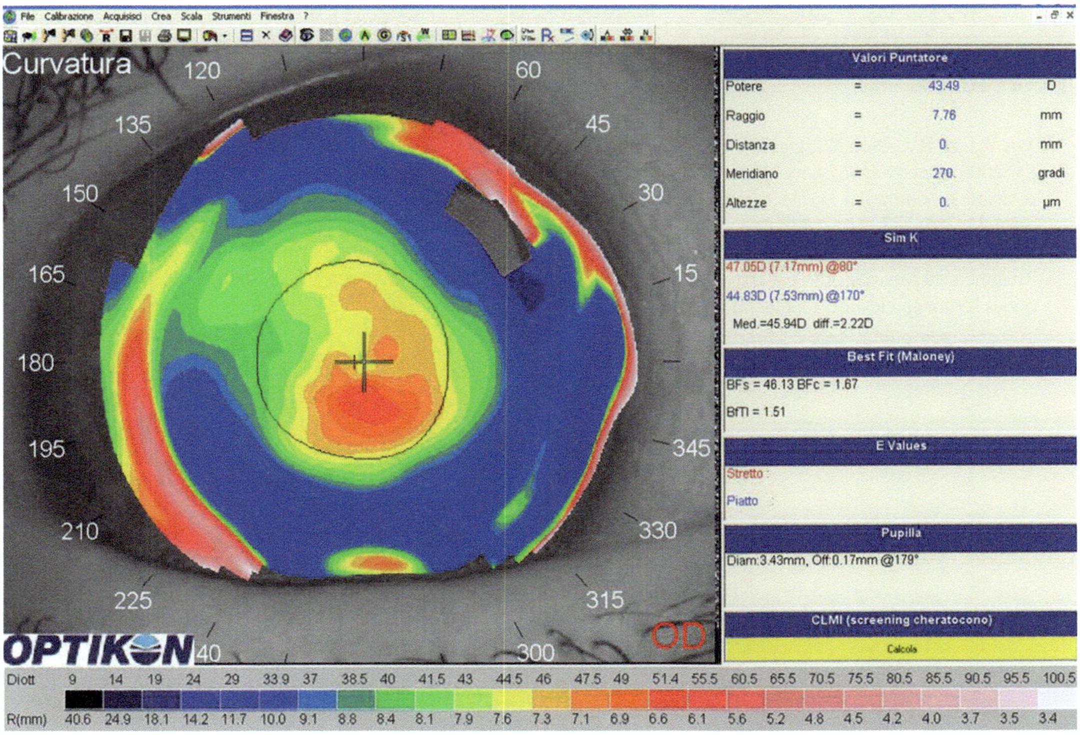

Fig. 68.5 Topography after punctum plug insertion. The surface is good with only a small amount of astigmatism

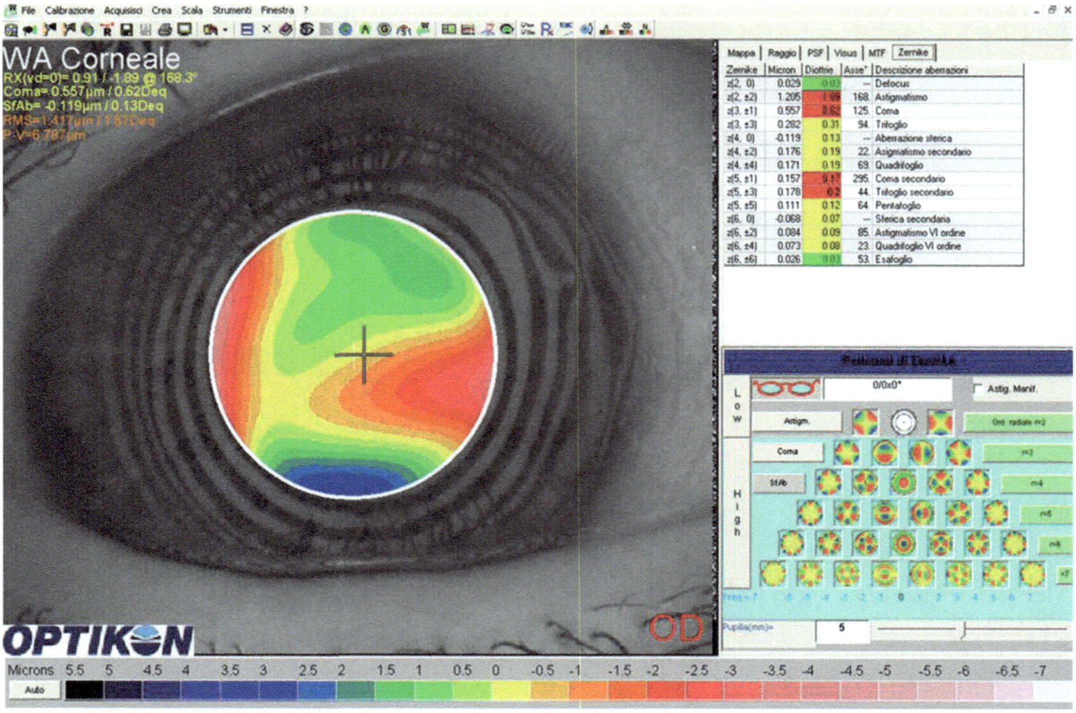

Fig. 68.6 Corneal wavefront after punctum plug insertion. Coma and trefoil are still present but high-order aberrations are greatly reduced

References

1. Wu Y, Chu RY, Zhou XT, Dai JH, Qu XM, Rao S, Lam D (2006) Recovery of corneal sensitivity after laser-assisted subepithelial keratectomy. J Cataract Refract Surg 32:785–788
2. Tsubota K, Goto E, Shimurra S, Shimazaki J (1999) Treatment of persistent corneal epithelial defect by autologous serum application. Ophthalmology 10:1984–1989
3. Camellin M, Mattioli R, Tripoli NK (2012) Topo-aberrometry with keratron onda. In: Corneal topography. Slack Incorporated, Thorofare, pp 184–190
4. Camellin M, Mosquera SA (2010) Simultaneous aspheric wavefront-guided transepithelial photorefractive keratectomy and phototherapeutic keratectomy to correct aberrations and refractive errors after corneal surgery. J Cataract Refract Surg 36: 1173–1180

Treatment of Post-PRK or Post-RK Haze by Two-Stage Transepithelial PRK with Mitomycin C

69

Daniel S. Durrie and Theodore A. Pasquali

Contents

D.S. Durrie, MD (✉)
Department of Ophthalmology, University of Kansas, Lawrence, KS, USA
e-mail: ddurrie@durrievision.com

T.A. Pasquali, MD
Durrie Vision (Clinic), Overland Park, KS, USA

Southern California Eye Physicians and Associates (Clinic), Los Alamitos, CA, USA
e-mail: theopasquali@gmail.com

Why Is This Case Relevant for the Refractive Surgeon?

Although less common with current surgical practices, corneal haze after PRK may still occur and require treatment. In addition, patients with corneal haze from procedures done in the past (RK or PRK before the use of mitomycin C) can present to the refractive surgeon with symptomatic corneal haze. Two-stage transepithelial PRK is a useful surgical technique for treating these patients [1, 2].

Case Background

A 56-year-old female status post RK and PRK OU in the mid-1990s presented for gradually worsening vision in the left eye over the last 10 years. Her manifest refraction and corresponding corrected visual acuity are as follows: OD: +1.25 −0.25 × 005 = 20/20; OS: −2.75 −0.25 × 020 = 20/30. Slit lamp examination was significant for trace corneal haze in the right eye, with 2+ central anterior corneal haze in the left eye (Fig. 69.1), and 8 incision RK scars in both eyes. Pentacam (Oculus, Wetzlar Germany) Scheimpflug imaging demonstrated increased reflectivity in the anterior cornea corresponding to the haze (Fig. 69.2a).

J.L. Alió et al. (eds.), *Difficult and Complicated Cases in Refractive Surgery*,
DOI 10.1007/978-3-642-55238-0_69, © Springer-Verlag Berlin Heidelberg 2015

Main Problem to Solve

Corneal haze producing myopia and astigmatism with reduction in best corrected visual acuity

Ancillary Tests

Pentacam Scheimpflug and topography imaging, wavefront analysis

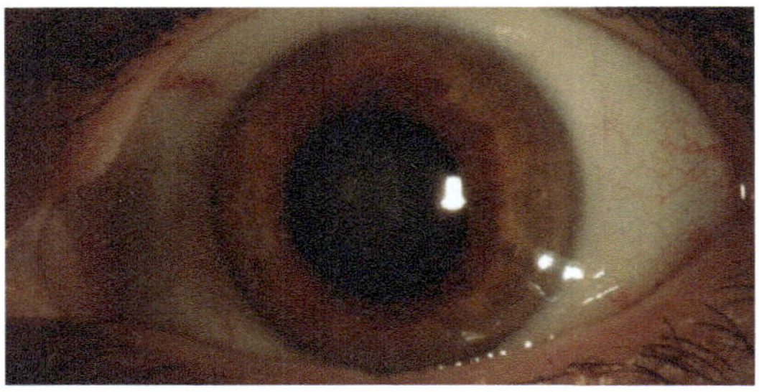

Fig. 69.1 Preoperative slit lamp photograph of the left eye demonstrating a plaque of central cornea haze and RK incisions

Surgical/Medical Intervention

Transepithelial PRK (TPRK)

In a simplified topographic model, subepithelial haze (in actuality, disordered extracellular matrix and myofibroblasts) can be thought of as a plaque-like deposit atop the stromal bed. Epithelium overlying the haze will be elevated by the "deposit," steepening the cornea in that area and thereby inducing myopic and astigmatic shifts (Fig. 69.3). In concept, by simply removing only the subepithelial haze, the overlying epithelium will no longer be propped up in this area and will again lie flat atop the stromal bed, and the refractive error will be resolved (assuming the stromal topography corresponds to a plano refraction).

Two-stage TPRK targets removal of only the layer of haze, correcting the refractive error simultaneously by the mechanism described above. In the first stage, a broad PTK ablation of 6.5 mm is applied to the entire cornea. The stroma will be reached first in the peripheral

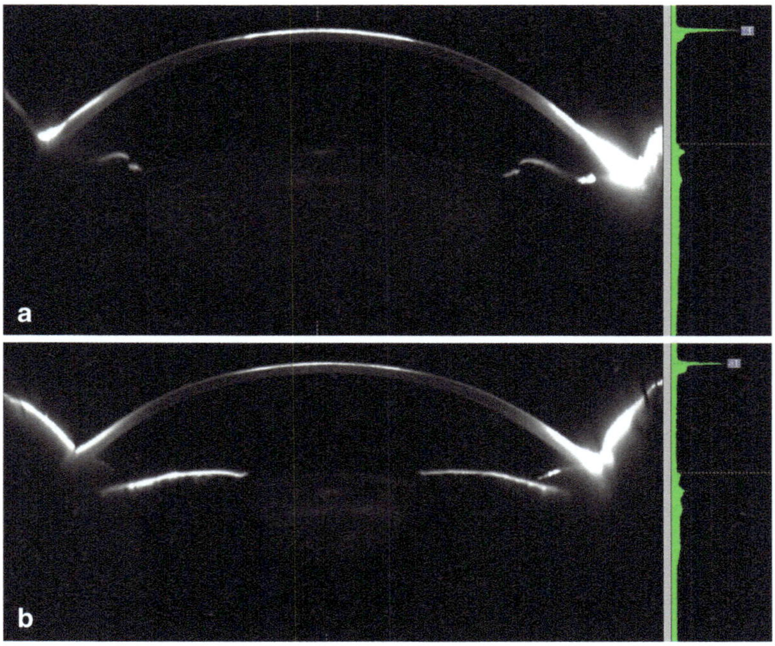

Fig. 69.2 Pentacam Scheimpflug images. (**a**) Preoperative image demonstrates increased reflectivity in the central anterior cornea corresponding to the haze noted on slit lamp examination. (**b**) Postoperative image illustrates decreased reflectivity compared with preoperative image, though the continued reflectivity represents that some haze is still present. The histograms (at right of images) confirm that the anterior corneal optical densitometry magnitude has decreased from 66.8 to 53.8

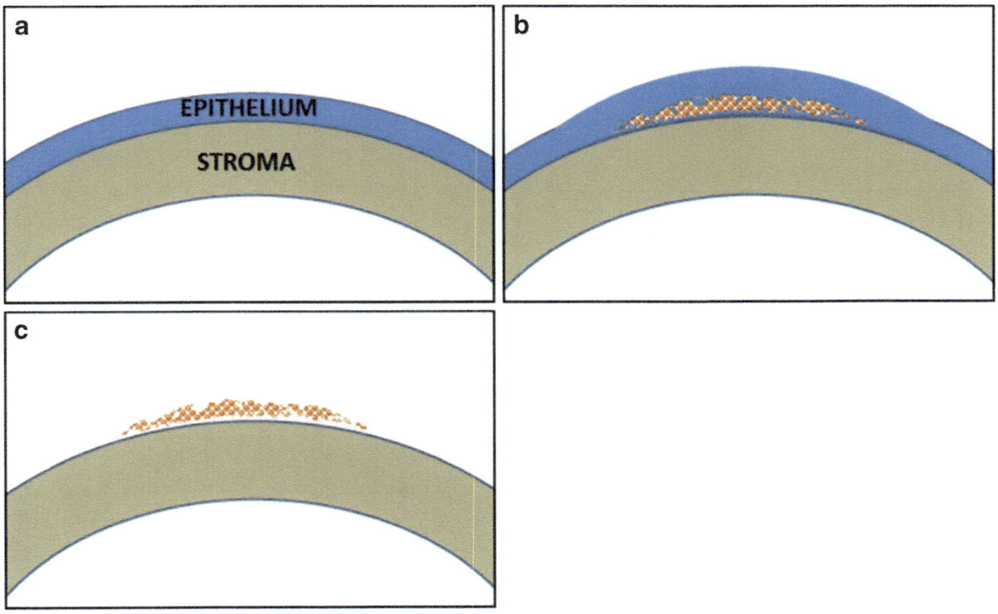

Fig. 69.3 Schematic illustration of transepithelial PRK (TPRK). (**a**) Plano cornea post RK and PRK. (**b**) Subepithelial haze develops, elevating the overlying epithelium and producing localized corneal steepening. (**c**) The epithelium has been removed by applying a uniform treatment to the cornea until the stroma is reached in the areas without haze, leaving the stroma with the areas of haze bared. Now a treatment with a profile for the induced refractive error is applied

areas without haze because the laser has only to treat through the epithelial layer, not through both the epithelial layer and the haze layer. Consequently, the surgeon watches the areas of treatment outside the haze for the color change in the laser spots that occurs when the stroma is reached and then stops this portion of the treatment. The epithelium and haze have a blue color reflection which changes to black when the epithelium has been removed by the laser. At this point a uniform amount of tissue has been removed corresponding to the thickness of the epithelial layer, leaving the haze atop the stroma.

You now have a smooth surface, and the amount of remaining haze has a thickness and shape that corresponds to the refractive error before the PTK stage. Therefore in the second stage, the desired refractive correction is programmed in the PRK mode, and a second ablation is performed. This will remove the haze and correct the refractive error (recalling that the refractive error is produced by and conjugate to the corneal elevation and steepening produced by the haze).

Finally, mitomycin C 0.02 % is applied to the cornea for 12 s to prevent the recurrence of haze.

Outcome

A follow-up visit 2 months after surgery revealed uncorrected visual acuity of 20/25 in the surgical eye with a manifest refraction of −0.25 −0.25 × 105 yielding 20/20 vision. The cornea demonstrated marked improvement of the corneal haze with slit lamp examination (Fig. 69.4). Comparison of pre- and postoperative Scheimpflug images (Fig. 69.3a, b) demonstrated a corresponding decrease in the intensity of reflectivity of the anterior cornea. Preoperative central irregularity demonstrated on the sagittal curvature map (Fig. 69.5a) appears evened out on the postoperative map (Fig. 69.5b).

What to Learn from This Case

Two-stage TPRK is a useful tool for the treatment of visually significant haze after RK or PRK and addresses refractive error at the same time. Simple PTK can also be used for the treatment of haze, but lacks the refractive precision and may produce hyperopic shifts unintentionally. Manual scraping with mitomycin C is another viable option, although older scars (>1 year old) like in our patient can be more difficult to scrape, requiring more scraping time, more force, and multiple treatments, and often produce problems with corneal regularity and smoothness. Similarly, manual scraping does not specifically address the refractive error, and irregularities produced by the scraping can have refractive consequences. Two-stage TPRK seeks to avoid these irregularities by employing the precision of a laser and specificity to the patient's refractive error.

This treatment methodology makes some assumptions (plano stromal topography, uniform epithelial thickness with no epithelial smoothing over of topographic irregularities, a spherocylindrical shape to the corneal haze) that, in addition to the normal sources of error, may lead to the necessity for subsequent enhancement in the future. Regardless, haze treated with TPRK will show significant improvement in the amount of astigmatism and myopia in addition to resolution of the haze. If an enhancement is needed at a future date, it can be performed in the surgeon's standard method because the haze is gone.

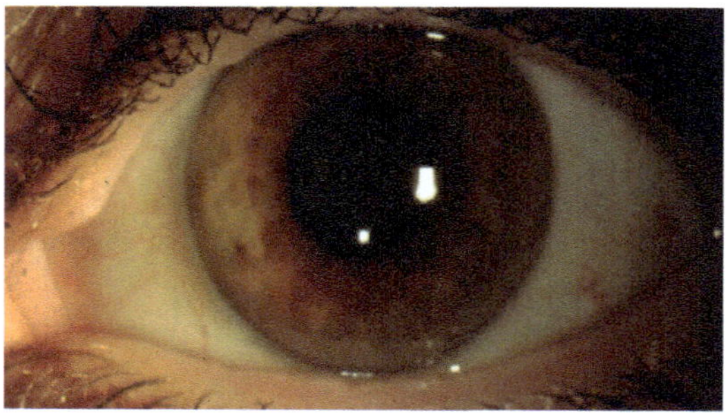

Fig. 69.4 Postoperative month 2 slit lamp photograph of the left eye. Some central corneal haze is still present; however, it is markedly improved from the preoperative haze demonstrated in Figure 1

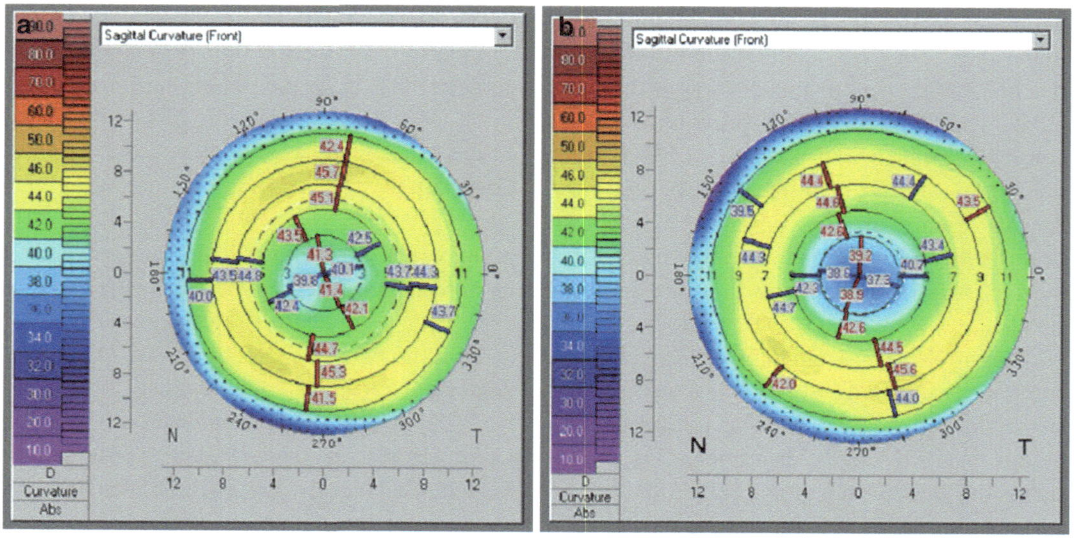

Fig. 69.5 Sagittal frontal curvature maps taken with the Pentacam. (**a**) The preoperative map details roughly 1.5 diopters of central astigmatic irregularity. (**b**) In the postoperative map the central curvature has been regularized and flattened

References

1. Netto MV, Mohan RR, Ambrosio R Jr, Hutcheon AE, Zieske JD, Wilson SE (2005) Wound healing in the cornea: a review of refractive surgery complications and new prospects for therapy. Cornea 24:509–522
2. Vigo L, Scandola E, Carones F (2003) Scraping and mitomycin C to treat haze and regression after photorefractive keratectomy for myopia. J Refract Surg 19:449–454

A Case of Severe Haze After PRK in a Patient Treated by a 6th-Generation Excimer Laser

70

Jorge L. Alió, Alessandro Abbouda, and Rana Eskndafi

Contents

Why Is This Case Relevant for the Refractive Surgeon?

It is important to be aware of the risk of corneal haze development after PRK even with a new generation of excimer laser.

Case Background

A 25-year-old woman sought refractive surgery in order to be rid of glasses. She complained of a burning sensation and dryness and had punctual closure in both eyes 4 days prior. She was uncomfortable with the plugs, so we removed them. Breakup time was 8 s in the RE and 10 s in the LE. Her examination showed the following: UCVA, RE 20/200 and LE 20/200; BCVA, RE 20/20 and LE 20/20; and, with her glasses, RE −5.00 sph −0.50 × 176° and LE −4.75 sph −.075 × 149°. She underwent PRK without MMC in both eyes. Four days after the surgery, her UCVA was RE 20/20 and LE 20/20. After 1 week, the contact lenses were removed and she was given loteprednol etabonate ophthalmic suspension 0.5 % (Lotemax® bausch and lomb) eyedrops 1 × 4, vitamin C tablets, and artificial tears. Two weeks after surgery, she returned with blurred vision. Her UCVA was RE 20/30 and LE 20/40. The slit-lamp examination revealed corneal haze in both eyes (Fig. 70.1). We increased the frequency of Lotemax® eye drops to six times per day. After 4 weeks, her UCVA was RE 20/30

J.L. Alió, MD, PhD (✉)
Department of Refractive Surgery, Vissum Corporación Oftalmológica, Alicante, Spain
e-mail: jlalio@vissum.com

A. Abbouda, MD
Department of Refractive Surgery, Vissum Corporación Oftalmológica, Alicante, Spain

Department of Ophthalmology-Policlinico Umberto I of Rome, University of Rome "Sapienza", Viale del Policlinico, 155, 00186 Roma, Italy

R&D Department, Vissum Corporación Oftalmológica, 03016, Alicante, Spain
e-mail: a.abbouda@gmail.com

R. Eskndafi, MD, MS, ABO
Department of Refractive Surgery, Beverly Hills Medical Center, Beverly Hills, CA, USA
e-mail: rscandvi@beverlyhillskuwait.com

J.L. Alió et al. (eds.), *Difficult and Complicated Cases in Refractive Surgery*, DOI 10.1007/978-3-642-55238-0_70, © Springer-Verlag Berlin Heidelberg 2015

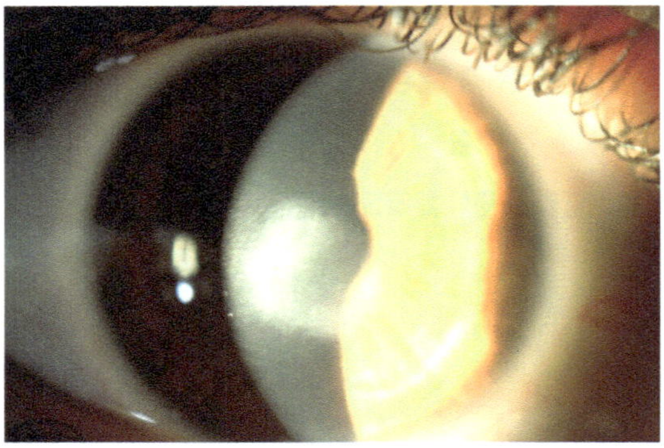

Fig. 70.1 Slit-lamp examination showed severe haze

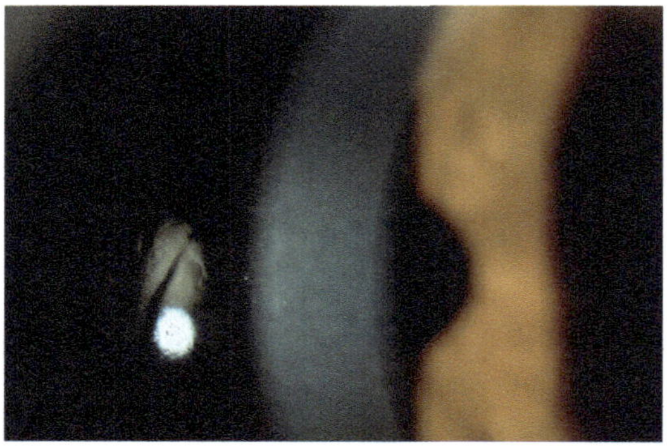

Fig. 70.2 Slit-lamp examination: detail of pupil area showed a moderate haze

and LE 20/30. The slit-lamp examination revealed a minimal corneal haze in both eyes (Fig. 70.2). Lotemax® eye drops 1 × 2 and artificial tears were continued for the following month. At the last follow-up, 3 months after surgery, her UCVA was 20/20 in both eyes and the slit-lamp examination revealed a small area of corneal haze.

Main Problem to Solve

Clinically significant haze after PRK occurs in 0.5–4 % of eyes [1]. The diameter of ablation and volume of tissue removed are considered the principle risk factors [2]. Some authors described this phenomenon as the rule of reepithelization delayed [3].

Ancillary Tests

We followed the haze evolution by slit lamp. A positive outcome allowed us to avoid more aggressive treatments.

Surgical/Medical Intervention

PRK ablation was performed using a WaveLight ALLEGRETTO WAVE™ Excimer Laser System 500. The haze was treated with a topical corticosteroid for 3 months.

Outcome

Six months after PRK, the patient's UCVA was 20/20 in both eyes and the slit-lamp examination revealed a clear cornea (Fig. 70.3). Lotemax® was stopped and artificial tears and vitamin C tablets were prescribed.

What to Learn from This Case

New-generation excimer lasers permit correction of each diopter of myopia with an ablation of less than 16 μm for a standard myopic ablation zone of 6.7 mm. The consequence is that in low-moderate myopia the amount of stromal tissue ablated is very low. According to previous studies [4], the risk of haze is greater when the ablation is greater than 80 μm, suggesting that lower ablation causes less risk of haze. Other authors [5] propose that the incidence of haze is less with use of a small flying spot laser compared to a traditional broad beam laser. This case illustrates that a patient

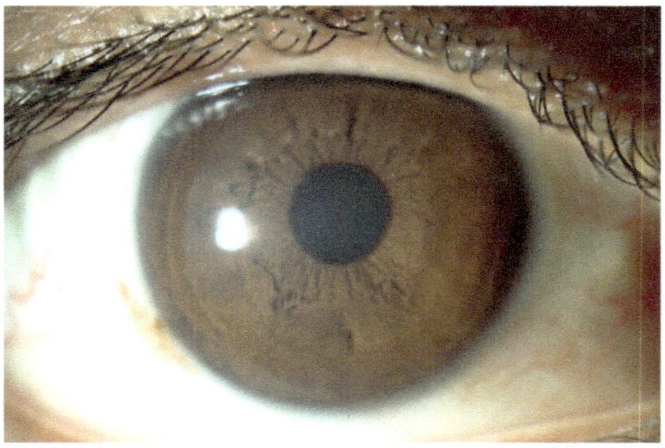

Fig. 70.3 Slit-lamp examination showed a clear cornea

treated with the new laser generation can also develop haze. The use of Mitomycin C 0.02 % for 15 s is recommended in all cases of superficial ablation regardless of the ablation depth.

References

1. Lohmann CP, Timberlake GT, Fitzke FW, Gartry DS, Muir MK, Marshall J (1992) Corneal light scattering after excimer laser photorefractive keratectomy: the objective measurements of haze. Refract Corneal Surg 8:114–121
2. Moller-Pedersen T et al (1998) Corneal haze development after PRK is regulated by volume of stromal tissue removal. Cornea 17:627–639
3. Kourenkov VV, Mytiagina ON, Kasparov AA, Pavluk AG (1999) Stimulating re-epithelialization after photorefractive keratectomy. J Refract Surg 15(2 Suppl): S234–S237
4. Braunstein RE et al (1996) Objective measurement of corneal light scattering after excimer laser keratectomy. Ophthalmology 103:439–443
5. Pallikaris IG et al (1999) Photorefractive keratectomy with a small spot laser and tracker. J Refract Surg 15:137–144

Ectasia Post PRK at Delayed Onset

71

Maria Jose Ayala, Alessandro Abbouda, and Jaime Javaloy

Contents

M.J. Ayala, MD, PHD
Department of Refractive Surgery, Vissum Corporación, Alicante, Spain

A. Abbouda, MD
Department of Refractive Surgery, Vissum Corporación Oftalmológica, Alicante, Spain

Department of Ophthalmology-Policlinico Umberto I of Rome, University of Rome "Sapienza", Viale del Policlinico, 155, 00186 Roma, Italy

R&D Department, Vissum Corporación Oftalmológica, 03016, Alicante, Spain
e-mail: a.abbouda@gmail.com

J. Javaloy, MD, PHD (✉)
Department of Anterior Segment and Refractive Surgery, Vissum Corporación Oftalmológica, Alicante, Spain
e-mail: jjavaloy@coma.es

Why Is This Case Relevant for the Refractive Surgeon?

Refractive surgeons are familiar with the risk of ectasia after LASIK. Ectasia after PRK may be due to retreatment, unrecognized keratoconus or forme fruste keratoconus [1, 2]. Koch [3] reported the case of a patient who developed bilateral corneal ectasia after an uneventful PRK. Risk factors for the development of ectasia following excimer laser include high myopia, reduced preoperative corneal thickness, a reduced residual stromal bed after laser ablation and asymmetrical corneal steepening (forme fruste keratoconus) [4]. However, none of these characteristics definitively predict the development of ectasia. We present a case in which corneal ectasia developed 14 years after PRK with no identifiable risk factors, even when a surface ablation was performed.

Case Background

A 21-year-old man was evaluated for refractive surgery to correct moderate myopia. No history of chronic eye rubbing, trauma, or atrophy was reported, and the patient had no family history of corneal ectasia. His best corrected visual acuity (BCVA) was 20/30 in both eyes with a manifest refraction of $-7.5\ -1 \times 20°$ in the right eye and $-6.5\ -1.5 \times 160°$ in the left. The preoperative central thickness was 610 μm in

J.L. Alió et al. (eds.), *Difficult and Complicated Cases in Refractive Surgery*,
DOI 10.1007/978-3-642-55238-0_71,

the right eye and 597 µm in the left. The keratometry reading was 43.24/44.39 × 110° in the right and 42.33/43.35 × 89° in the left and the corneal topography was normal in both eyes (Fig. 71.1a). In May 1995, the patient underwent PRK. The postoperative period was uneventful and the slit lamp examination showed no abnormalities. After 1 year, the patient's corrected distance visual acuity (CDVA) was 20/20 in both eyes with a manifest refraction of −0.75 −0.75 × 60° in the right eye and −0.75 −0.5 × 160° in the left eye. The keratometry reading was 38/38.3 × 94° in the right eye and 37.66/39.35 × 71° in the left eye. The aspect of the images was normal with no detectable asymmetry (Fig. 71.1b). The central corneal thickness was 530 µm in both eyes. We opted for a new PRK treatment. In August 1996, the patient's BCVA was 20/25 in the right eye and 20/20 in the left eye with a manifest refraction of −2.5 −1 × 70° in the right eye and −3.5 in the left eye. Keratometry reading was 37.7/37.96 × 89° in the right eye and 38/38.5 × 73° in the left eye, showing a symmetrical and well-centred myopic ablation (Fig. 71.1c). The slit lamp examination revealed a tender haze. The patient was not satisfied with his vision, and in December 1998, he underwent a PRK treatment. In June 1999, his BCVA was 20/32 in the right eye and 20/40 in the left eye with a manifest refraction of +2.5 in the right eye and +1.75 in the left. Keratometry reading was 36.6/36.76 × 68° in the right eye

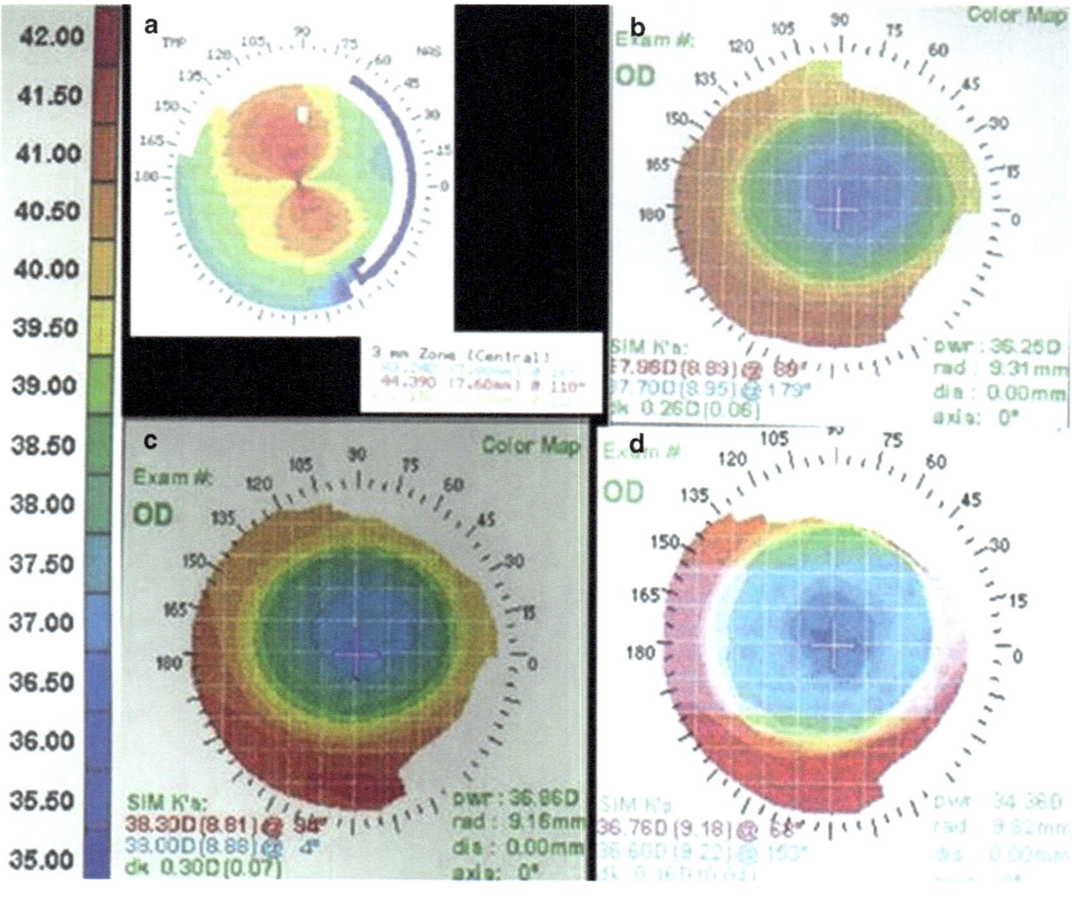

Fig. 71.1 (**a**–**d**) These pictures show a topography evolution axial scan (**a**) before the refractive treatment and (**b**) 1 year, (**c**) 2 years (**d**) and 4 years after the refractive treatment

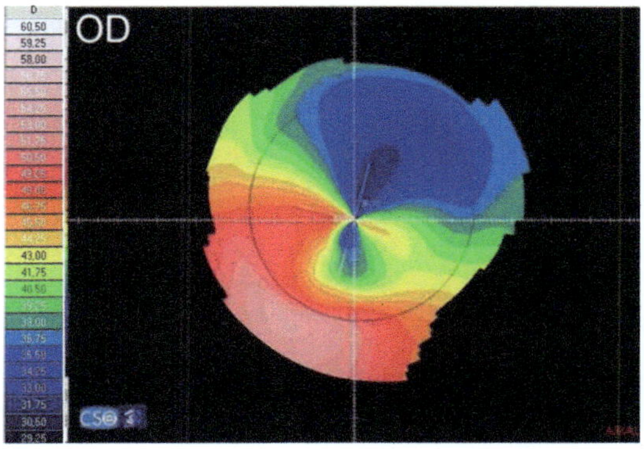

Fig. 71.2 Topography shows an inferonasal ectasia and irregular astigmatism 14 years after the primary procedure

and 35.75/35.3 × 171° in the left eye. The topography did not reveal signs of ectasia or irregular astigmatism (Fig. 71.1d). After 3 months, the refraction shifted again through a myopic value. The patient's BCVA was 20/32 in the right eye and 20/30 in the left eye with a manifest refraction of −3.5 −1 × 80° in the right eye and −4 −1 × 160° in the left. The slit lamp showed diffuse haze. The pachymetry was 480 μm in the right eye and 510 μm in the left eye. Keratometry reading was 37.9/38.3 × 104° in the right eye and 38.1/39.1 × 89° in the left eye. No surgical treatment was performed at this time. Ten years after, the patient began to complain of progressive vision reduction in the right eye. His BCVA was 20/200 in the right eye and 20/100 in the left eye with a manifest refraction of −3 −3 × 45° in the right eye and −2.5 −2 × 130° in the left. The topography showed an inferonasal ectasia with an irregular astigmatism (Fig. 71.2). The keratometry reading was 36.25/42.24 × 166°. The patient refused intracorneal ring segments and corneal collagen cross-linking (CXL). We opted for a rigid gas permeable contact lens while the patient considered the proposed surgery.

Main Problem to Solve

In this case, we did not find evident risk factors for the development of ectasia. The stromal bed residual after the last treatment was more than 400 μm. The patient did not rub his eyes. We excluded forme fruste keratoconus. The only risk factors to consider were the patient's age and retreatments with excimer laser.

Ancillary Tests

On the basis of pathophysiology of post-refractive surgery, ectasia can be explained by interlamellar biomechanical slippage (interlamellar fracture) followed by subsequent interfibrillar biomechanical slippage (interfibrillar fracture) as opposed to direct primary collagen fibril failure (fibrillar fracture) [5].

Surgical/Medical Intervention (with Video if Needed)

Traditional treatment for iatrogenic ectasia includes rigid gas permeable contact lens and an intracorneal rigid segment. Recently, several studies reported on riboflavin UVA-induced corneal collagen cross-linking (CXL) [6]. However, the most frequent choice for eyes suffering advanced ectasia is corneal transplantation (DALK). In our case, the patient refused the treatment proposed with intracorneal rings.

Outcome

One year after PRK, the patient's visual condition was worsening. His BCVA was 20/40 in the right eye and 20/25 in the left eye with a manifest refraction of −8.5 × 55° in the right eye and −0.75 −3.5 × 120° in the left. The topography showed an evident ectasia larger than the previous examination with a severe irregular astigmatism. The keratometry reading was 36.78/44.78 × 165°. The patient wanted to pursue the contact lens device, declining further surgery.

What to Learn from This Case

PRK has been proven as a safe, simple and effective procedure to correct low to moderate myopia. Alio et al. [7] reported few complications among 3,000 cases.

Refractive surgeons should be aware of the possibility of corneal ectasia occurrence in cases of low to moderate myopia, low ablation and enough residual stromal bed after ablation even when a corneal flap is not performed such as in a PRK.

References

1. Holland EJ (2005) Ectasia following laser in situ keratomileusis. J Cataract Refract Surg 31:2034
2. Malecaze F, Coullet J, Calvas P, Fournie P, Arne JL, Brodaty C (2006) Corneal ectasia after photorefractive keratectomy for low myopia. Ophthalmology 113:742–746
3. Koch DD (1999) The riddle of iatrogenic keratectasia. J Cataract Refract Surg 25:453–454
4. Randleman JB, Russell B, Ward MA, Thompson KP, Stulting RD (2003) Risk factors and prognosis for corneal ectasia after LASIK. Ophthalmology 110:267–275
5. Dawson DG, Randleman JB, Grossniklaus HE et al (2008) Corneal ectasia after excimer laser keratorefractive surgery: histopathology, ultrastructure, and pathophysiology. Ophthalmology 115:2181–2191
6. Spadea L (2012) Collagen crosslinking for ectasia following PRK performed in excimer laser–assisted keratoplasty for keratoconus. Eur J Ophthalmol 22:274–277
7. Alio JL, Artola A, Claramonte PJ, Ayala MJ, Sanchez SP (1998) Complications of photorefractive keratectomy for myopia: two year follow- up of 3000 cases. J Cataract Refract Surg 24:619–626

Late-Onset Consecutive Hyperopia Following Decentered Myopic PRK

72

Scott Kelly and Dimitri T. Azar

Contents

S. Kelly • D.T. Azar, MD, MBA (✉)
Department of Ophthalmology and Visual Sciences
Illinois Eye and Ear Infirmary, University of Illinois
at Chicago, Chicago, IL, USA
e-mail: scottkellyy@gmail.com; dazar@uic.edu

Why Is This Case Relevant for the Refractive Surgeon?

Consecutive hyperopia following myopic laser vision correction is a common problem following refractive surgery. The refractive surgeon needs to be aware of how to handle such a case.

Case Background

A 62-year-old male with a past history of myopic PRK in both eyes presented with blurry vision in the right eye more so than the left. His past medical history included hypertension, prostate cancer for which he underwent treatment, hypercholesterolemia, and a cardiac arrhythmia status post ablation. He had no other past ocular surgical history. His medications include Prevacid, Crestor, Hyzaar, and Flomax. He was allergic to sulfa and he used no ocular medications. He wanted to be able to see clearly to play tennis and golf. His uncorrected vision was 20/40 OD and 20/20+2 OS and he did not like to wear contact lenses.

His vision improved to 20/15 in both eyes with manifest refraction of +0.75+1.00×180 in the right eye and +0.25+0.75×180 in the left. The right eye was dominant, with a pachymetry of 596 in the right eye and 585 in the left eye, tonometry of 14 in both eyes, and a Schirmer test of greater than 15 mm in both eyes at 5 min without anesthesia. He had a scotopic pupil size of

J.L. Alió et al. (eds.), *Difficult and Complicated Cases in Refractive Surgery*,
DOI 10.1007/978-3-642-55238-0_72, © Springer-Verlag Berlin Heidelberg 2015

7.6 in the right eye and 6.9 in the left eye, brisk pupillary reactions, and no afferent pupillary defect. His extraocular motility and confrontational visual fields were normal in both eyes. Slit lamp biomicroscopy showed normal lids, lashes, and conjunctiva, a clear cornea with no previous LASIK flap or epithelial/basement membrane disease, a quiet anterior chamber, a normal iris, and trace nuclear sclerotic changes in the lens in both eyes. A dilated exam revealed healthy optic nerves and a normal retina in both eyes. Contact lenses were retried for monovision, with the right eye corrected for distance and the left for near vision. He underwent a monovision trial of $+0.75+1.00\times180$ OD and $+2.25+0.75\times180$ OS. The patient returned to the clinic 4 months later. He again rejected contact lenses for monovision; he preferred treating both eyes for distance and wearing reading glasses for near. He otherwise had no new visual complaints.

Main Problem to Solve

The question we were presented with was whether to proceed with LASIK or PRK. If PRK was attempted, should we use MMC? Also, should we aim for full distance correction or monovision, considering the patient's hyperopia, presbyopia, and incipient cataract?

Ancillary Tests

Corneal topography OD showed paracentral flattening OD corresponding to a region of corneal thinning measuring approximately 4 mm (Fig. 72.1). The area of previous PRK treatment was decentered inferotemporally. The pattern of topography was consistent with a small-area ablation zone, which was used at the time of PRK surgery in the mid-1990s.

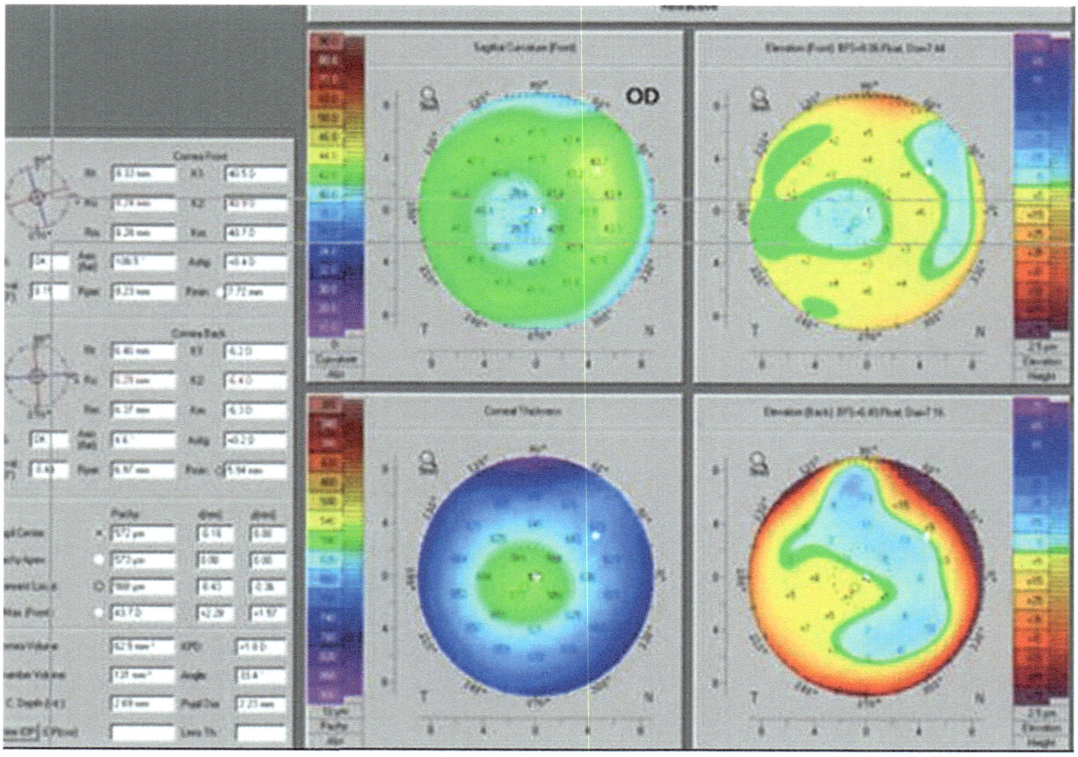

Fig. 72.1 Pretreatment topography OD 15 years following myopic PRK, showing small-central area ablation (*blue zone* in the *superior panels*) and corresponding central corneal decrease in pachymetry OD (*left inferior panel*)

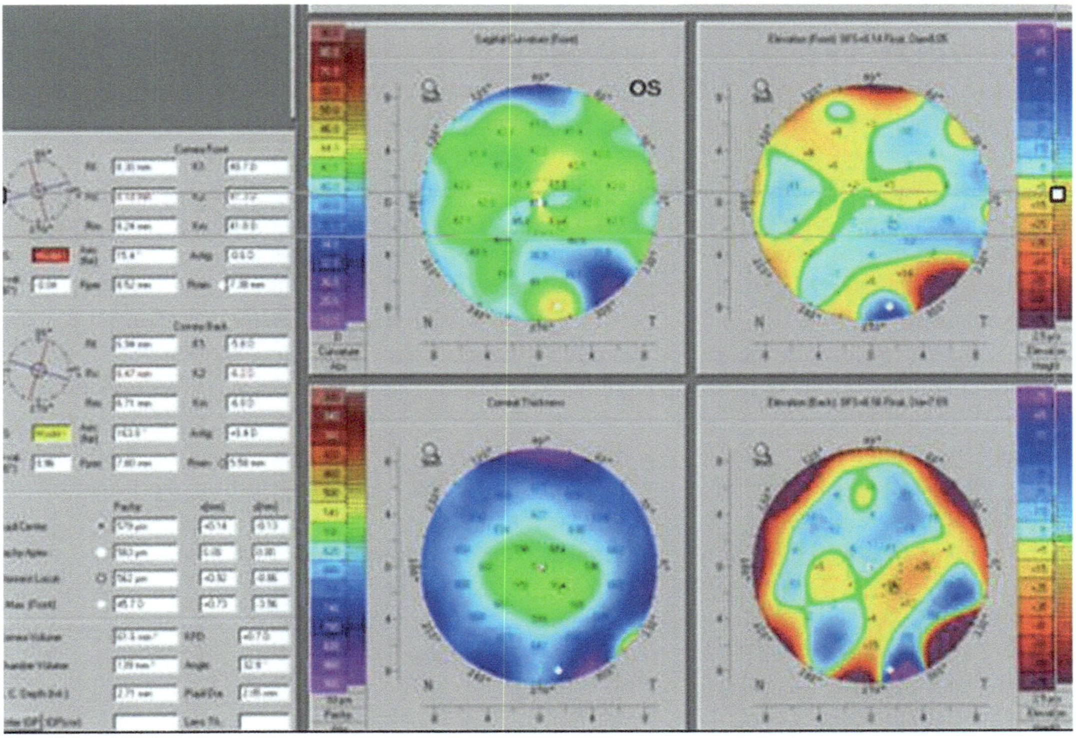

Fig. 72.2 Pretreatment topography OS showing post-PRK with-the-rule corneal astigmatism (*left superior panel*). The corresponding refractive error by wavefront aberrometry was +1.50 D at axis 175°. *Left inferior panel* shows corneal thinning consistent with small-area ablation

Corneal topography OS showed central post-PRK with-the-rule astigmatism OS (Fig. 72.2). The corneal pachymetry was also consistent with a small-area ablation.

Outcome

The patient underwent hyperopic wavefront-guided PRK with mitomycin C OS (200 μg/ml, 0.02 % for 15 s) (+0.84 + 1.49 × 175). At the 2-month post-op visit, the patient noted worsening vision and expressed interest in laser vision correction in the right eye. He was very pleased with his vision in his left eye. His preoperative vision OD was 20/40 uncorrected and improved to 20/20 with +1.25 + 1.00 × 175. His vision OS was 20/20+ uncorrected following surgery and improved slightly with plano + 0.25 × 080.

The patient opted to undergo LASIK with a femtosecond laser in the right eye, knowing that there was a possibility of overcorrection given his prior history of unstable refractive error in his right eye and the presence of cataracts OU. LASIK was performed OD, with a treatment of +1.37 + 0.80 × 002. The patient had an uneventful postoperative course. One month following LASIK OD, the patient's uncorrected vision was 20/20 + 2 in both eyes, with a refraction of plano + 0.25 × 098 OD and plano + 0.25 × 108 OS.

What to Learn from This Case

In this case of late-onset consecutive hyperopia following myopic PRK, it is unclear whether the patient was overtreated initially and used some accommodative ability to overcome his mild hyperopia or whether he had hyperopic regression in both eyes. The patient did have some degree of lenticular change in both eyes, which could have contributed to his astigmatism. Mild hyperopic shift has been reported in the early stages of nuclear sclerosis [1]. While mild cataracts were present and "clear lens exchange" was an option to improve the patient's uncorrected vision, he was correctable to 20/15 with spectacles. Laser vision correction was deemed the safer, more repeatable option given the patient's desires; however, preoperative informed consent was crucial given the risk of a cataract formation to impair vision.

One risk to consider in treating consecutive hyperopia following myopic overcorrection is residual stromal thickness. This patient had an adequate pachymetry of over 550 μm in both eyes. Additionally, he previously underwent surface ablation, eliminating the concern for flap complications caused by LASIK. Given the thick pachymetry, LASIK and PRK were both viable options. Studies by Bababeygy et al. and Rojas et al. show that both of these treatments are safe and effective for consecutive hyperopia [2, 3]. Bababeygy et al. also show that the repeatability of treatments in consecutive hyperopia is equivalent to previously untreated low hyperopes [2]. If the patient underwent LASIK initially, we would have been limited to surface ablation for his re-treatment, as flap lifts increase the risk of epithelial ingrowth and flap striae when performed 1 year beyond initial treatment. The patient underwent myopic PRK in the late 1990s, and while outcomes were generally very good, they are not as repeatable as custom and non-custom treatments today. Also of note was the patient's initial insistence upon surface ablation rather than LASIK. Surface ablation is typically not our preference in hyperopic correction, especially since the patient had adequate corneal pachymetry. His hyperopic correction was relatively mild, with the most correction for astigmatism. A positive cylinder was employed to conserve corneal tissue. Hyperopic surface ablation can lead to haze formation in the ablation area and the patient's risk is higher because of his previous surface ablation. Both of these factors led to a mitomycin C 0.2 mg/ml application of 15 s during treatment to minimize the risk.

References

1. Lee KE, Klein BE, Klein R (1999) Changes in refractive error over a 5-year interval in the Beaver Dam Eye Study. Invest Ophthalmol Vis Sci 40:1645–1649
2. Bababeygy SR (2008) Wavefront-guided laser in situ keratomileusis retreatment for consecutive hyperopia and compound hyperopic astigmatism. J Cataract Refract Surg 34:1260–1266
3. Rojas MC, Haw WW, Manche EE (2002) Laser in situ keratomileusis enhancement for consecutive hyperopia after myopic overcorrection. J Cataract Refract Surg 28:37–43

Twelve Years of Follow-Up of PRK in a Patient with −22 Diopter Myopia

73

Alessandro Abbouda and Jorge L. Alió

Contents

A. Abbouda, MD (✉)
Department of Refractive Surgery, Vissum Corporación Oftalmológica, Alicante, Spain

Department of Ophthalmology-Policlinico Umberto I of Rome, University of Rome "Sapienza", Viale del Policlinico, 155, 00186 Roma, Italy

R&D Department, Vissum Corporación Oftalmológica, 03016, Alicante, Spain
e-mail: a.abbouda@gmail.com

J.L. Alió, MD, PhD
Department of Refractive Surgery, Vissum Corporación Oftalmológica, Alicante, Spain
e-mail: jlalio@vissum.com

Why Is This Case Relevant for the Refractive Surgeon?

This case shows the possibility of treating a highly refractive defect by PRK, but it is important to remember that visual acuity is compromised with an increase in corneal aberrometry. In this case, PRK is stable over 12 years.

Case Background

The patient arrived at our department 12 years after refractive surgery to check the status of her eyes. The only data from the previous surgery was the refraction status of −22 in both eyes. At her first visit, the manifest refraction was −1 in the right eye (RE) and −2.5 in the left eye (LE). Her BCVA was 20/25 in the RE and 20/30 in the LE. The keratometry reading was 35.32/35.32 × 180 in the RE and 34.48/35.71 × 82 in the LE. The corneal topography showed a central flattening according to myopic pattern ablation (Fig. 73.1a, b). The corneal aberrometry showed high spherical aberration in the RE, with an RMS spherical-like of 2.2 μm in the RE and 2.5 μm in the LE (Fig. 73.1c, d). The ultrasonic pachymetry was 413 μm in the RE and 419 μm in the LE. The OCT Visante showed a reduction of stromal thinning in the

J.L. Alió et al. (eds.), *Difficult and Complicated Cases in Refractive Surgery*,
DOI 10.1007/978-3-642-55238-0_73, © Springer-Verlag Berlin Heidelberg 2015

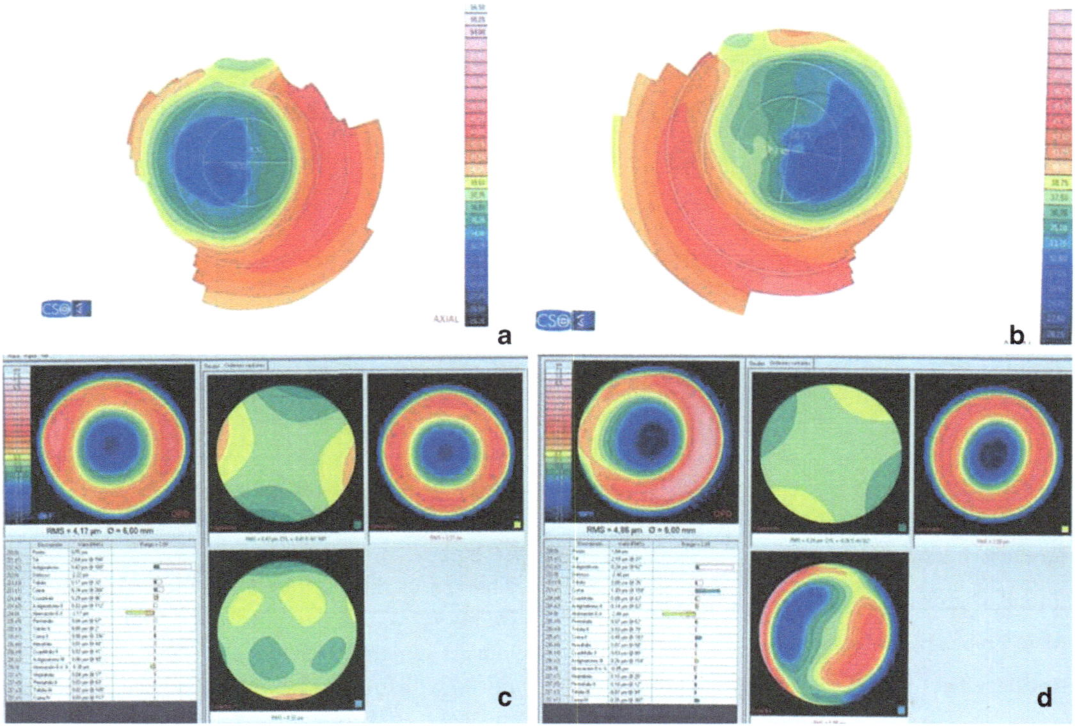

Fig. 73.1 Corneal topography after 12 years (**a**, **b**) and aberrometry (**c**, **d**)

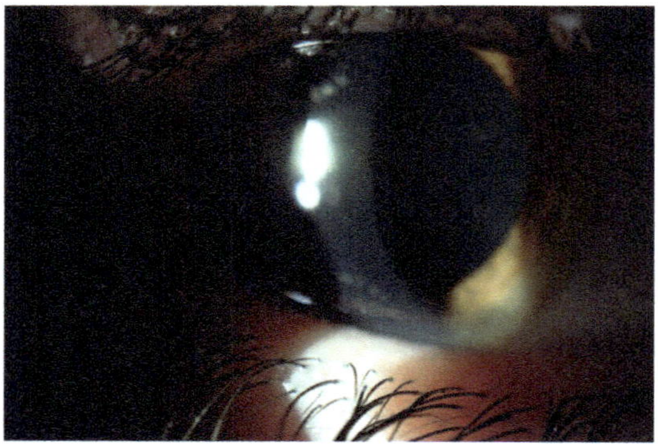

Fig. 73.2 Slit lamp examination

center of cornea according to the ablation (Fig. 73.1a, b). The slit lamp examination revealed a tender haze with an iron deposit (Fig. 73.2).

Main Problem to Solve

The most important thing in this case was to analyze the strength of the cornea.

Ancillary Tests

Corneal topography showed central flattening according to myopic pattern ablation (Fig. 73.1a, b) and corneal aberrometry showed a high spherical aberration in the RE. The RMS spherical-like was 2.2 μm in the RE and 2.5 μm in the LE (Fig. 73.1c, d). An ocular response analyzer showed a normal corneal stroma in both eyes. The index of corneal hysteresis (CH) and resistance factor (CRF) according to the huge ablation was normal (Fig. 73.3c).

Surgical/Medical Intervention

The patient was treated with a 193-nm VISX 20/20 excimer laser (software version 3.2; VISX, Inc., Santa Clara, California, USA). Ablation was achieved using a beam with a fluence of 160 mJ/cm^2 at an ablation rate of 5 Hz. 4.5, 5, and 6.0 mm-diameter multiple zone techniques were used to correct moderate and high myopia.

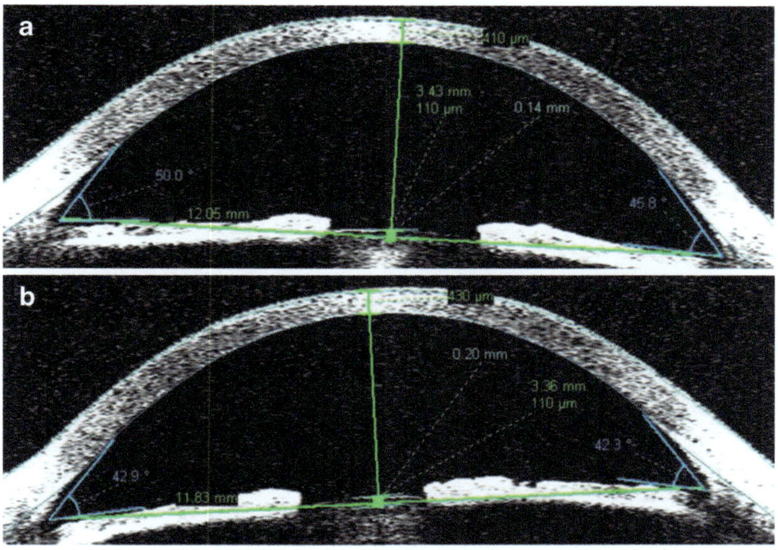

Measurement Date: 27/05/2008 21:24:39

	#	IOPcc (mmHg.)	IOPg (mmHg.)	CRF (mmHg.)	CH (mmHg.)	CCT (uM.)
RIGHT	1	11,3	8,4	7,2	9,1	
	2	11,4	8,1	6,8	8,8	
	3	10,7	8,2	7,4	9,4	
	Avg.	11,1	8,2	7,1	9,1	0
LEFT	1	13,9	10,2	6,9	8,2	
	2	12,7	9,1	6,8	8,4	
	3	11,9	9,5	7,7	9,4	
	Avg.	12,8	9,6	7,1	8,6	0

Fig. 73.3 OCT Visante (**a**, **b**), ocular response analyzer (**c**)

The optic zone was 5.90 ± 0.04 mm (range, 5.50–6.00 mm) and the mean ablation depth was 104 ± 25 µm (range, 58–157 µm). Mitomycin C was not used.

Outcome

Twelve years after PRK, the patient continued to have stable refraction and topography. Her manifest refraction was −1 in the RE and −2.5 in the LE. Her BCVA was 20/25 in the RE and 20/30 in the LE.

What to Learn from This Case

This case showed the safety of PRK in an extreme case of myopia [1–4] and illustrated the potential of corneal refractive surgery.

References

1. Rosman M, Alió JL, Ortiz D, Perez-Santonja JJ (2010) Comparison of LASIK and photorefractive keratectomy for myopia from −10.00 to −18.00 diopters 10 years after surgery. J Refract Surg 26:168–176
2. Alió JL, Ortiz D, Muftuoglu O, Garcia MJ (2009) Ten years after photorefractive keratectomy (PRK) and laser in situ keratomileusis (LASIK) for moderate to high myopia (control-matched study). Br J Ophthalmol 93:1313–1318
3. Alió JL, Muftuoglu O, Ortiz D, Artola A, Pérez-Santonja JJ, de Luna GC, Abu-Mustafa SK, Garcia MJ (2008) Ten-year follow-up of photorefractive keratectomy for myopia of more than −6 diopters. Am J Ophthalmol 145:37–45
4. Alió JL, Muftuoglu O, Ortiz D, Artola A, Pérez-Santonja JJ, de Luna GC, Abu-Mustafa SK, Garcia MJ (2008) Ten-year follow-up of photorefractive keratectomy for myopia of less than −6 diopters. Am J Ophthalmol 145:29–36

Part VI

Corneal Inlays Complications

Dear reader,

This chapter describes the complications of an innovative surgical procedure.

Intracorneal inlays are used to correct for presbyopia. Intrastromal corneal ring segments are gaining popularity as a surgical alternative for correcting corneal ectatic disorders such as keratoconus and post-LASIK ectasia.

With an increase in use of such techniques, it is important that ophthalmic surgeons understand the complications of this surgical procedure as well as the best way to manage complications.

This chapter covers topics such as inlay displacement, implant reversibility, management of poor vision following INTACS implantation, management of ectasia, the reversibility of intrastromal corneal ring segments and topography changes. Understanding the complications of intracorneal inlays is essential considering the growing popularity of the technique.

For further reading, we suggest two chapters in the first book of this series: J. L. Alio', D. Azar *Management of Complications in Refractive Surgery*, Chapter 16: Complications of Intrastromal Corneal Ring Segments (pp. 297–305) and Chapter 17: Corneal Inlays (pp. 307–312).

Specific topics covered by the cases include a new device to treat presbyopia and the most common complication (Case 74) and reversibility of AcuFocus (Case 75). Other cases will cover preoperative patient selection in INTACS implantation (Case 76), a new way to treat ectasia and postpone corneal transplantation (Case 77). We end with a case focused on why choosing ICRS may not be a good choice for a patient with irregular corneas (Case 78).

Lesson to Learn

Case 74: Complications of corneal inlays, inlay displacement

The inlay displacement is a frequent complication. How to handle it.

Case 75: Kamra AcuFocus® inlay implant reversibility

A reversible surgical procedure to treat presbyopia. The importance to decide the time of explantation to obtain complete reversibility of the topographic changes induced by the inlay.

Case 76: Corneal melting and neovascularization associated with ring segment extrusion 6 months after the surgery

Ring segment migration is one of the most common causes for INTACS explantation if the segment is going to be extruded or the refraction change is too high.

Case 77: Management of poor vision following INTACS implantation for keratoconus

A poor visual acuity related to the high value of aberrometric data after INTACS implantation was resolved by segment substitution.

Case 78: Refractive surprise after PRK in patient with INTACS. Reversibility of intrastromal corneal ring segment refractive and topography changes

ICRS is not a good choice for a patient with irregular cornea. Unstable or artefact refraction may happen as a consequence of the corneal changes induced by the ICRS in a keratoconic cornea.

Complications of Corneal Inlays (Inlay Displacement)

74

Florence Cabot and Damien Gatinel

Contents

F. Cabot, MD
Bascom Palmer Eye Institute, University of Miami, Miller School of Medicine, Miami, FL, USA
e-mail: florence.cabot@gmail.com

D. Gatinel (✉)
Fondation Rothschild,
25 rue Manin, 75019, Paris, France

Why Is This Case Relevant for the Refractive Surgeon?

Corneal inlay repositioning is considered an uncomplicated procedure. However, care should be taken to place the cornea inlay in an appropriate position. In patients with a significant kappa angle, the inlay should be placed halfway between the corneal vertex and the center of the entrance pupil [1, 2].

Case Background

A 56-year-old man was referred to our department for a refractive surgery evaluation. His manifest refraction was +1.50 D in the right eye and +1.00 D in the left eye. The best corrected visual acuity (BCVA) was 20/20 in both eyes and corneal topography performed with Orbscan II (Technolas Perfect Vision GmbH) did not show any anomalies. Laser-assisted in situ keratomileusis (LASIK) was performed in both eyes, and an inlay implantation was associated with the LASIK procedure in the left eye. The right eye was targeted for plano and the left eye was targeted for −0.75D. A 130 μm-thick flap in the right eye and a 200 μm-thick flap in the left eye were created by the IntraLase 60 kHz femtosecond laser. The Bausch and Lomb 217z excimer laser with eye tracking, including cyclorotational tracking, was used for corneal ablation. The right eye surgery was uneventful.

J.L. Alió et al. (eds.), *Difficult and Complicated Cases in Refractive Surgery*,
DOI 10.1007/978-3-642-55238-0_74, © Springer-Verlag Berlin Heidelberg 2015

During the excimer laser ablation in the left eye, the patient had difficulty maintaining fixation on the microscope light. One week postoperatively, the patient complained of monocular diplopia in the left eye. Uncorrected visual acuity was 20/20 Jaeger (J)5 in the right eye and 20/50 J4 in the left eye (BCVA =20/40 with manifest refraction −0.50 in the left eye).

Main Problem to Solve

Monocular diplopia suggested a corneal inlay displacement, prompting the question of in what direction to move and place the inlay. Also of consideration was whether to use corneal vertex or pupil image to recenter the inlay.

Ancillary Tests

The Acutarget Diagnostic Unit (AcuFocus, Inc., Irvine, CA) showed that the center of the inlay was 735 μm nasal and 469 μm inferior to the pupil image center. The center of the inlay was also 250 μm nasal and 112 μm inferior to the corneal vertex (Purkinje image). The Acutarget image obtained after primary surgery is shown in Fig. 74.1. Corneal topography and wavefront analysis were not relevant for this case.

Surgical/Medical Intervention

In order to recenter the inlay, a second surgery was scheduled 2 weeks later and the flap was lifted. According to the Acutarget Diagnostic Unit measurements, the inlay was recentered temporally and superiorly, between the corneal vertex and the pupil image center.

Outcome

One month after recentration, the uncorrected visual acuity was 20/30 J2 in the left eye and the patient had no more complaints of double vision. The Acutarget image (Fig. 74.2) shows the inlay recentration within the pupil area.

What to Learn from This Case

In refractive surgery, the common method for ablation centration is to use the center of the entrance pupil [3, 4]. The inlay manufacturer

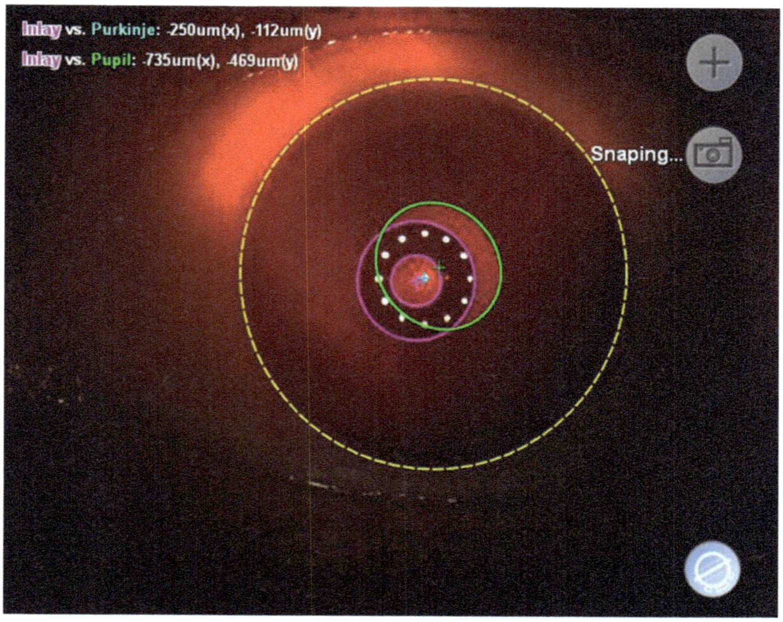

Fig. 74.1 Acutarget photo recorded after the primary surgery. The inlay is decentered nasally and inferiorly

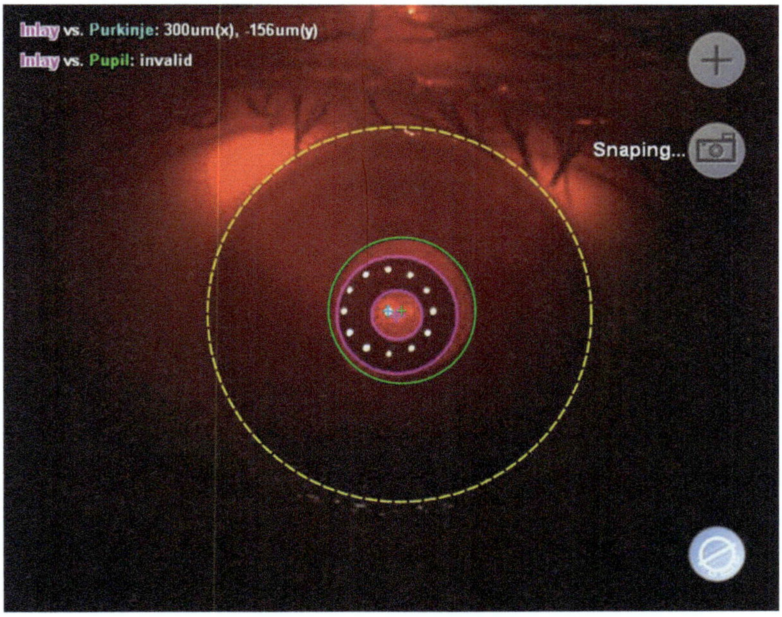

Fig. 74.2 Acutarget image recorded after inlay recentration. The corneal inlay is within the pupil area, placed halfway between the corneal vertex (Purkinje image) and the center of the entrance pupil

recommends centering the inlay on the corneal vertex. However, in patients with a significant kappa angle, the inlay should be placed halfway between the corneal vertex and the center of the entrance pupil. To achieve optimal centration, the surgeon should try to identify the coaxial light reflex and its position versus the center of the entrance pupil. The Acutarget Diagnostic Unit is a useful tool to provide an objective measurement of the distance and direction of the Purkinje image (virtual image behind the cornea resulting from the reflection of a light source by the anterior surface of the cornea) versus the pupil center.

References

1. Seyeddain O, Hohensinn M, Riha W et al (2012) Small-aperture corneal inlay for the correction of presbyopia: 3-year follow-up. J Cataract Refract Surg 38:35–45
2. Gatinel D, El Danasoury A, Rajchles S, Saad A (2012) Recentration of a small-aperture corneal inlay. J Cataract Refract Surg 38(12):2186–2191. doi: 10.1016/j.jcrs.2012.09.009
3. Pande M, Hillman JS (1993) Optical zone centration in keratorefractive surgery: entrance pupil center, visual axis, coaxially sighted corneal reflex or geometric corneal center? Ophthalmology 100:1230–1237
4. Uozato H, Guyton DL (1987) Centering corneal surgical procedures. Am J Ophthalmol 103:264–275

AcuFocus® Inlay Implant Reversibility

75

Emilia M. Mulet, Jorge L. Alió, and Alessandro Abbouda

Contents

E.M. Mulet, MD, PhD (✉)
Department of Refractive Surgery, Vissum Corporacion Oftalmológica, Alicante, Spain
e-mail: memulet@hotmail.com

J.L. Alió, MD, PhD
Department of Refractive Surgery, Vissum Corporación Oftalmológica, Alicante, Spain
e-mail: jlalio@vissum.com

A. Abbouda, MD
Department of Refractive Surgery, Vissum Corporación Oftalmológica, Alicante, Spain

Department of Ophthalmology-Policlinico Umberto I of Rome, University of Rome "Sapienza", Viale del Policlinico, 155, 00186 Roma, Italy

R&D Department, Vissum Corporación Oftalmológica, 03016, Alicante, Spain
e-mail: a.abbouda@gmail.com

Why Is This Case Relevant for the Refractive Surgeon?

Small-aperture intrastromal inlay removal is considered safe, resulting in a good recovery of corneal topography and corneal aberrometry in the months following removal.

Presbyopia is a multifocal physiological aging mechanism that leads to the progressive loss of functional near vision [1]. One method to correct presbyopia is intracorneal inlay implantation which increases the depth of field through the principle of small-aperture optics with the goal of improving intermediate and near vision without markedly affecting distance vision. The disadvantages of inlays are necrosis of corneal tissues and corneal haze [2–4], but the new material and the multiple holes allow water and nutrient permeability which reduces or eliminates these adverse effects [5]. These new materials allow the reversibility of the process if the technique is not effective.

Case Background

A 50-year-old male with near vision problems who does not wear glasses visited our clinic. His preoperative uncorrected distance visual acuity (UCDVA) was 20/20 in the right eye (RE) and 20/25 in the left eye (LE). The preoperative uncorrected near visual acuity (UCNVA) was 20/100 in both eyes. The corrected distance visual acuity

J.L. Alió et al. (eds.), *Difficult and Complicated Cases in Refractive Surgery*,
DOI 10.1007/978-3-642-55238-0_75, © Springer-Verlag Berlin Heidelberg 2015

(CDVA) was 20/20 in both eyes with a refraction of +0.5 −0.5 × 130° in the RE and +0.75 −0.5 × 125° in the LE, and his corrected distance visual acuity (CDVA) was 1 with an addition of +2 diopters (D). The preoperative central keratometry was 45.13 × 153° and 45.74° × 63° in the RE and 44.51 × 138° and 45.23° × 48° in the LE. The RMS was 3.03 µm with an AK (Apical Curvature Gradient) of 46.63 D and the KPI (keratoconus prediction index) was 0 %. The total pachymetry was 580 µ in the corneal center and 610 µ in the periphery. The stromal residual bed measured intraoperatively was 375 µ.

We performed inlay implantation in the patient's nondominant left eye using an AcuFocus inlay KAMRA® (ACI 700, AcuFocus Inc.) with a 5 mm microperforated artificial aperture (3.8 mm outer diameter,1.6 mm inner diameter). The ACI was made of polyvinylidene fluoride (PVDF) and had 8,400 laser-drilled porosity holes (diameter from 5 to 11 mm). The inlay was centered on the line of sight after the creation of a corneal flap using the femtosecond laser (IntraLase FS Laser, 60 kHz; Abbott Medical Optics, Santa Ana, California).

The Main Problem to Solve

One month after implantation, the patient could not read the newspaper or perform other near vision tasks with a postoperative UCNV of 20/70 and a loss of distance visual acuity to 20/32. He needed an addition of +1.75 D.

Ancillary Tests

We evaluated UCNVA, UCDVA, CDVA, slit lamp examination, central keratometry, computerized corneal topography (CSO), and aberrometry before and after inlay implantation and anterior segment optical coherence tomography (Visante OCT (Zeiss)) after implantation (Fig. 75.1).

Surgical/Medical Intervention

The slit lamp exploration showed a nasal inferior inlay decentration (Fig. 75.2). The RMS was 0.80, the AK was 50.50D, and the KPI was 8 %. Visual acuity did not improve and we decided on inlay recentration 4 months after the implant. Following recentration, the patient was dissatisfied with the UCDVA of 20/40 and UCNVA of 20/50. Nine months after the implant, we explanted the AcuFocus inlay.

Outcome

The slit lamp exploration showed a small annular haze that progressively disappeared over 1 month (Fig. 75.3). One week post inlay explantation, the UCDVA was 20/30, the CDVA was 20/20 with +1.25 −0.5 × 150°, and the CNVA was 20/20 with an addition of +2.5 D. Three months after the explantation, the UCDVA was 20/25, the UCDVA was 20/125, and the CNVA was 20/20 with an addition of +2.25. The RMS was 0.79, the AK

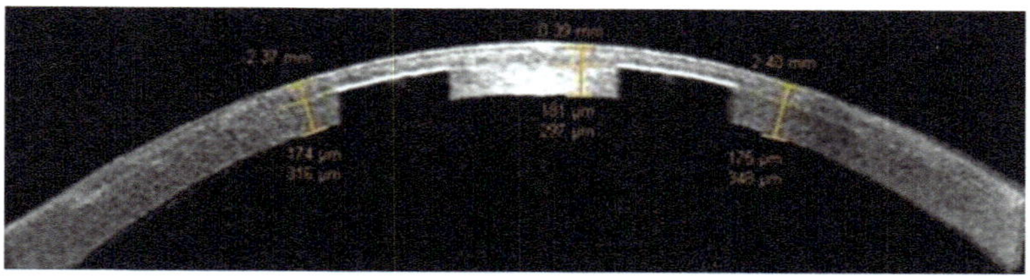

Fig. 75.1 Anterior segment OCT Visante® image of the AcuFocus inlay implantation

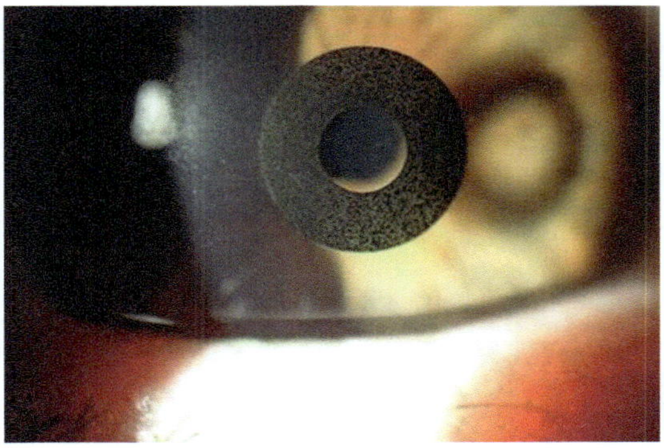

Fig. 75.2 Decentration of the inlay implantation

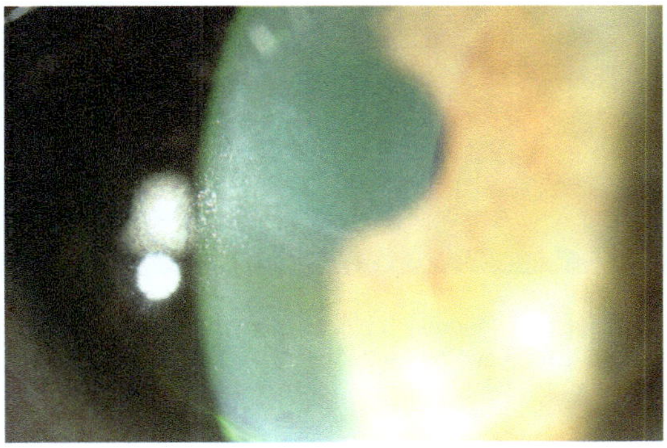

Fig. 75.3 Slit lamp examination revealed small annular haze

was 50.97, and the KPI of 5 % was 1. The inlay postexplantation keratometry was 44.83 × 141° and 45.27 × 51°. The RMS was 0.79, the AK was 50.15, and the KPI was 5 %. Three years after the AcuFocus inlay explantation, we treated the residual defect with an Amaris laser (Schwind, Geneva).

What to Learn from This Case

This case shows the safety and reversibility of the corneal inlay implantation with recovery of the preoperative corneal conditions (Fig. 75.4). AcuFocus KAMRA inlay removal is safe and results in a good recovery of corneal topography and corneal aberrometry in the months following removal. In our study [6], patients who had the corneal inlay removed early tended to have a better result regarding visual acuity, corneal topography, and corneal biomicroscopy compared to patients in whom the corneal inlay removal was performed after a longer time.

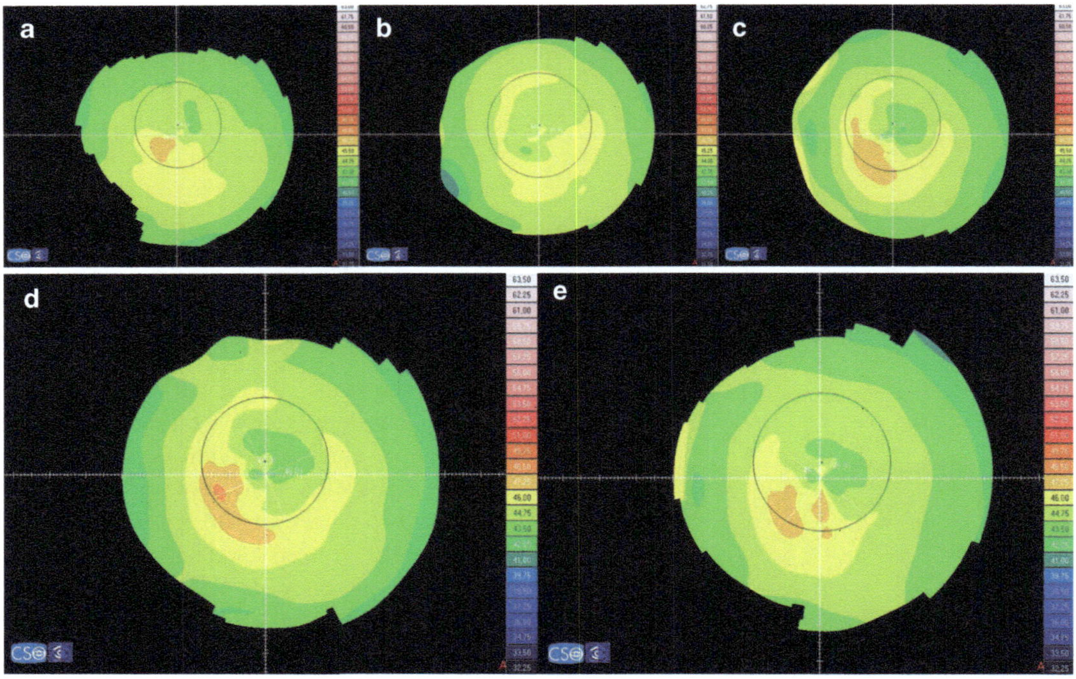

Fig. 75.4 These figures show a topography evolution and axial scan. This case shows a complete reversibility of topography aspect. (**a**) Before the implant. (**b**) After the implant at 3 months. (**c**) After the explants at 1 month. (**d**, **e**) After 3 and 6 months

References

1. Alio JL, Azar D, Kalliopi S, Soria F (2013) Chapter 3.10: Surgical correction of presbyopia. In: Yanoff M, Duker JS (eds) Ophthalmology, 4th edn. Elsevier, Oxford, pp 150–160e1
2. Mulet ME, Alió JL, Knorz MC (2009) Hydrogel intracorneal inlays for the correction of hyperopia: outcomes and complications after 5 years of follow-up. Ophthalmology 116:1145–1160
3. Alió J, Shabayek MH (2006) Hyperopic Lasik following intracorneal hydrogel lens explantation. J Refract Surg 22:205–207
4. Alió JL, Shabayek MH, Montes-Mico R, Mulet ME, Ahmed AG, Merayo J (2005) Intracorneal hydrogel lenses and corneal aberrations. J Refract Surg 21: 247–252
5. Seyeddain O, Hohensinn M, Riha W, Nix G, Ruckl T, Grabner G, Dexl AK (2012) Small-aperture corneal inlay for the correction of presbyopia: 3-year follow-up. J Cataract Refract Surg 38:35–45
6. Alio JL, Abbouda A, Huseynli S, Knorz M, Mulet Homs ME, Durrie D (2013) Removability of a small aperture intracorneal inlay for presbyopia correction. J Refract Surg 29(8):550–6

Corneal Melting and Neovascularization Associated with Ring Segment Extrusion 6 Months After the Surgery

76

Jorge L. Alió, Alessandro Abbouda, and Angelo Rampone

Contents

J.L. Alió, MD, PhD (✉)
Department of Refractive Surgery, Vissum Corporación Oftalmológica, Alicante, Spain
e-mail: jlalio@vissum.com

A. Abbouda, MD
Department of Refractive Surgery, Vissum Corporación Oftalmológica, Alicante, Spain

Department of Ophthalmology-Policlinico Umberto I of Rome, University of Rome "Sapienza", Viale del Policlinico, 155, 00186 Roma, Italy

R&D Department, Vissum Corporación Oftalmológica, 03016, Alicante, Spain
e-mail: a.abbouda@gmail.com

A. Rampone, MD
Department of Ophthalmology, Seconda Università degli Studi di Napoli, Naples, Italy

R&D Department, Vissum Corporacion, 03016, Alicante, Spain
e-mail: angelo.rampone@gmail.com

Why Is This Case Relevant for the Surgeon?

Intracorneal ring segment (ICRS) implantation was initially used for the correction of mild to moderate myopia but recently has been used for the surgical management of keratoconus and iatrogenic postoperative corneal ectasia [1]. ICRS is a safe and reversible alternative to penetrating keratoplasty (PKP) and does not affect the central visual axis of the cornea. Segment implantation is used to delay or avoid corneal grafts and to reduce the progression of keratoconus. Two types of ICRS are used by ophthalmic surgeons: INTACS® and KERARING®. Here, we present a case of INTACS ICRS associated with corneal melting of the manual implant after 4 months.

The refractive surgeon should be able to recognize and manage complications related to ICRS in order to achieve an optimal visual outcome.

Case Background

A 42-year-old woman presented at our clinic with a diagnosis of keratoconus in both eyes and contact lens intolerance and complaining of a gradual loss of vision in both eyes. Her manifest refraction was −12.0, −5.0×5° in the right eye

J.L. Alió et al. (eds.), *Difficult and Complicated Cases in Refractive Surgery*,
DOI 10.1007/978-3-642-55238-0_76, © Springer-Verlag Berlin Heidelberg 2015

(RE) and −6.50, −4.25 × 150° in the left eye (LE). Her best corrected visual acuity (BCVA) was 20/50 in the RE and 20/70 in the LE for distance. The slit lamp examination showed the presence of a peripheral leucoma in the LE. The topography showed a corneal inferior steepening to the corneal vertex in the LE (Fig. 76.1) and a vertical bow tie with rule astigmatism in the RE; the keratometric value in the LE was 45.94/48.93 × 81°. We decided to implant an ICRS following the nomogram type (www.mediphacos.com.br/en/productos_implanteIntraEstromalKeraring.asp).

The postoperative period was uneventful; the slit lamp examination showed no abnormalities. At 4 months, the patient complained of sharp pain in her LE. The slit lamp examination showed an epithelial defect at the incision area. We prescribed topical antibiotics, steroid and cycloplegic drops (tobramycin and dexamethasone four times per day tapering to one drop every week for a total of 4 weeks, ciprofloxacin one drop four times per day and cyclopentolate two times per day for 1 week), and a contact lens was applied. After 2 months, the patient returned with sharp pain and discomfort in her LE. The slit lamp examination showed cornea nasal melting with neovascularization and an extensive ring segment extrusion (Fig. 76.2).

Main Problem to Solve

We were presented with the challenge of managing this case of corneal nasal melting and neovascularization. Ring segment extrusion and dissatisfaction with outcomes are the most

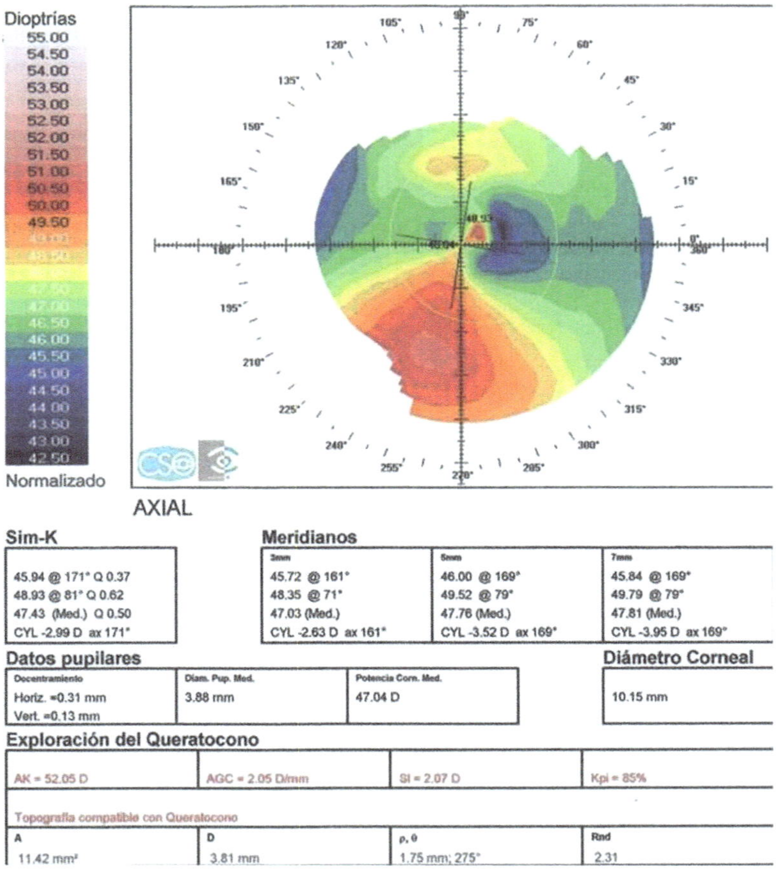

Fig. 76.1 Corneal inferior steepening to corneal vertex and a vertical bow tie

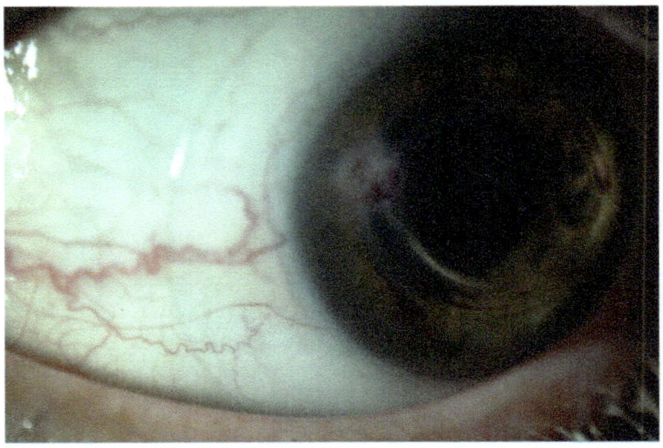

Fig. 76.2 Cornea nasal melting with neovascularization and extensive ring segment extrusion

common causes of explantation. Seven cases of extrusion have been observed in eyes implants using mechanical dissection [2].

Ancillary Tests

Segment migration and decentration (superficial or horizontal displacement) occur most frequently in allergic and atopic patients. High degrees of migration can cause change in the refraction or segment extrusion. Patient education, especially with atopic patients, is important to prevent complications. In addition, a topical antihistamine drops can help relieve allergy symptoms. However, segment explantation is indicated with severe migration with corneal oedema.

Surgical/Medical Intervention

The corneal ring segment was explanted.

Outcome

One month after the INTACS explantation, the patient's manifest refraction was −5.0, −5.0 × 160° in the LE with a BCVA 20/50. Although the quality of the vision was not perfect, the patient did not complain of discomfort. The slit lamp examination showed a stromal opacification in the place of the tunnel with neovascularization inside.

What to Learn from This Case

The use of femtolaser to create a tunnel can help to avoid this complication and to provide a better clinical outcome [3]. Matching the procedure with appropriate patient candidates is also helpful in avoiding postoperative visual complications [4].

References

1. Piñero D, Alio JL (2010) Intracorneal ring segments in ectatic corneal disease – a review. Clin Experiment Ophthalmol 38:154–167
2. Pokroy R, Levinger S (2006) Intacs adjustment surgery for keratoconus. J Cataract Refract Surg 32: 986–992
3. Shabayek M, Alió JL (2008) Chapter 16. Complication of intrastromal corneal ring segment page. In: Alio JL, Azar D (eds) Management of complications in refractive surgery. Springer, Berlin/Heidelberg, pp 297–305
4. Zare MA, Hashemi H, Salari MR (2007) Intracorneal ring segment implantation for the management of keratoconus: safety and efficacy. J Cataract Refract Surg 33:1886–1891

Management of Poor Vision Following INTACS Implantation for Keratoconus

77

Jorge L. Alió and Alessandro Abbouda

Contents

Why Is This Case Relevant for the Refractive Surgeon?

A refractive surgeon should be able to implant an intracorneal ring segment into an appropriate patient before considering a more aggressive procedure.

Corneal ectasia is one of the most serious complications of laser-assisted in situ keratomileusis (LASIK), with an estimated incidence between 0.04 and 0.66 % [1–3]. The main symptoms are progressive myopia, irregular astigmatism, and loss of corrected distance visual acuity (CDVA) [4]. Risk factors for this complication are high myopia, undiagnosed forme fruste keratoconus, low residual stromal bed thickness, a large optical zone, and multiple enhancement procedures.

Case Background

A 38-year-old man arrived at our department complaining of low vision in his left eye (LE) for the past 2 years. He underwent refractive treatment 14 years ago in a different clinic and we had no data about the previous surgery. At the first visit to our clinic, his manifest refraction was $-1 \times 70°$ in the RE and $-4.5 \times 95°$ in the LE. His BCVA was 20/20 in the RE and 20/70 in the LE. Keratometry reading in the LE was $39.5/43.37 \times 11°$. The aberrometric data showed a coma-like RMS of 2.7 μm. The corneal topography showed inferior steepening according to

J.L. Alió, MD, PhD (✉)
Department of Refractive Surgery, Vissum Corporación Oftalmológica, Alicante, Spain
e-mail: jlalio@vissum.com

A. Abbouda, MD
Department of Refractive Surgery, Vissum Corporación Oftalmológica, Alicante, Spain

Department of Ophthalmology-Policlinico Umberto I of Rome, University of Rome "Sapienza", Viale del Policlinico, 155, 00186 Roma, Italy

R&D Department, Vissum Corporación Oftalmológica, 03016, Alicante, Spain
e-mail: a.abbouda@gmail.com

J.L. Alió et al. (eds.), *Difficult and Complicated Cases in Refractive Surgery*,
DOI 10.1007/978-3-642-55238-0_77, © Springer-Verlag Berlin Heidelberg 2015

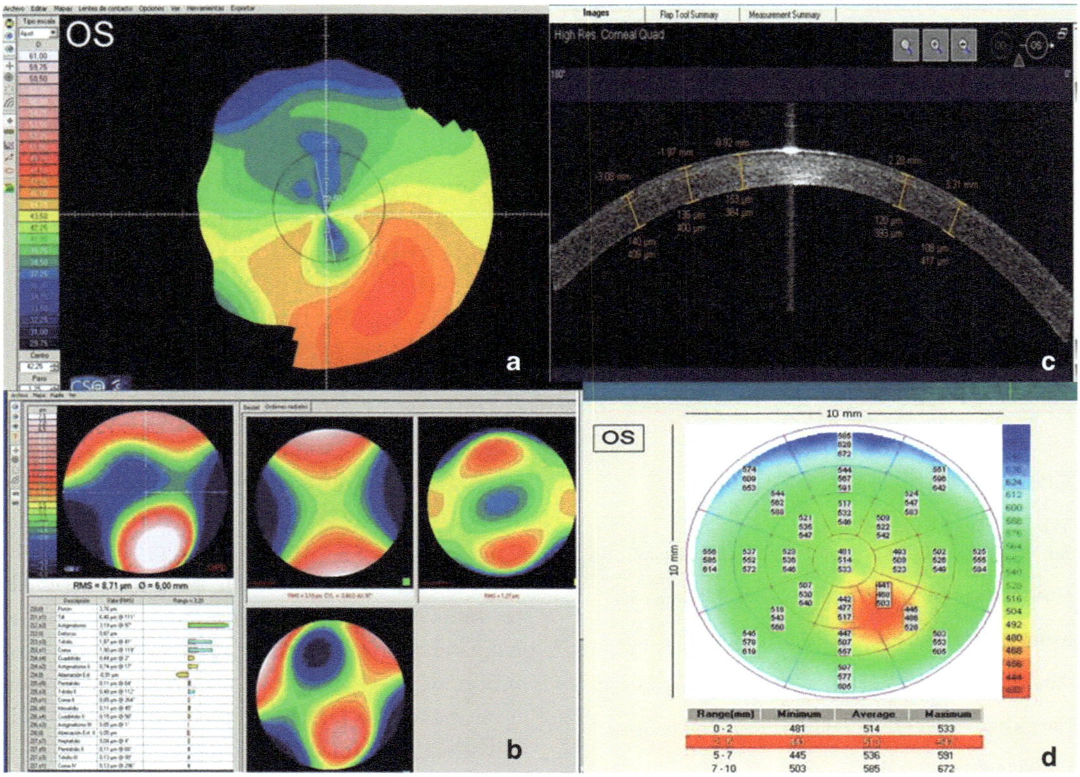

Fig. 77.1 (**a**) Corneal topography showed an ectasia aspect. (**b**) Aberrometric data showed a high value of coma aberration. (**c–d**) OCT Visante. Flap depth and pachymetry

ectatic disorder. The OCT Visante showed a flap depth of 120 μm, residual stroma of 393 μm, and a minimum pachymetry value of 441 μm in the LE (Fig. 77.1a–c). The value of corneal hysteresis (CH) measured by ORA showed a pathological result of 7.8 (Fig. 77.2). The patient was diagnosed with ectasia post LASIK. He did not tolerate rigid gas permeable contact lenses and his cornea was clear. He did not suffer of any form of allergies. We decided to implant an INTACS® segment. A tunnel dissection was performed by femtosecond laser IntraLase at a depth of 310 μm. The tunnel diameter was 5.8 mm × 7.1 mm. According to the ectasia type and the refractive data, we implanted two segments of 120/200 μm. After 6 weeks, the patient's manifest refraction was +1 = −2.25 × 40° and his BCVA was 20/63 (Figs. 77.3 and 77.4).

Main Problem to Solve

Poor visual acuity related to the high value of aberrometric data was noted in patients with grade I and II of keratoconus or in eyes with a preoperative coma <3 μm [5]. Another cause of poor visual acuity is the placement and the thickness of the segment [6].

Ancillary Tests

The keratometry reading in the LE was 39/41.67 × 129°. The topography showed a flattened superior area and a centered cone of ectasia. The aberrometric data showed a significant increase of total corneal aberration of RMS 17.82 μm and a coma-like RMS value of 4.76 μm.

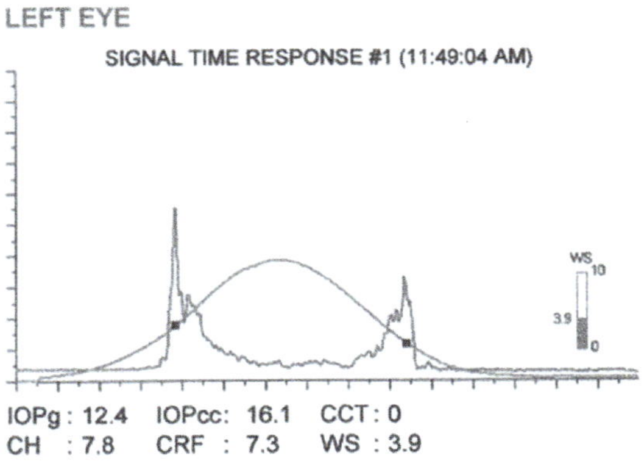

Fig. 77.2 ORA examination showed low value of CH

Surgical/Medical Intervention

Explantation of the superior ring and substitution of the inferior ring with a ring of 120/250 μm were performed.

Outcome

After 1 year, the patient's manifest refraction was +1 −2×45° and his BCVA was 20/25. The keratometry reading was 39/42×110°. The cone of ectasia was centered and the aberrometric data showed a coma-like RMS of 0.7 μm.

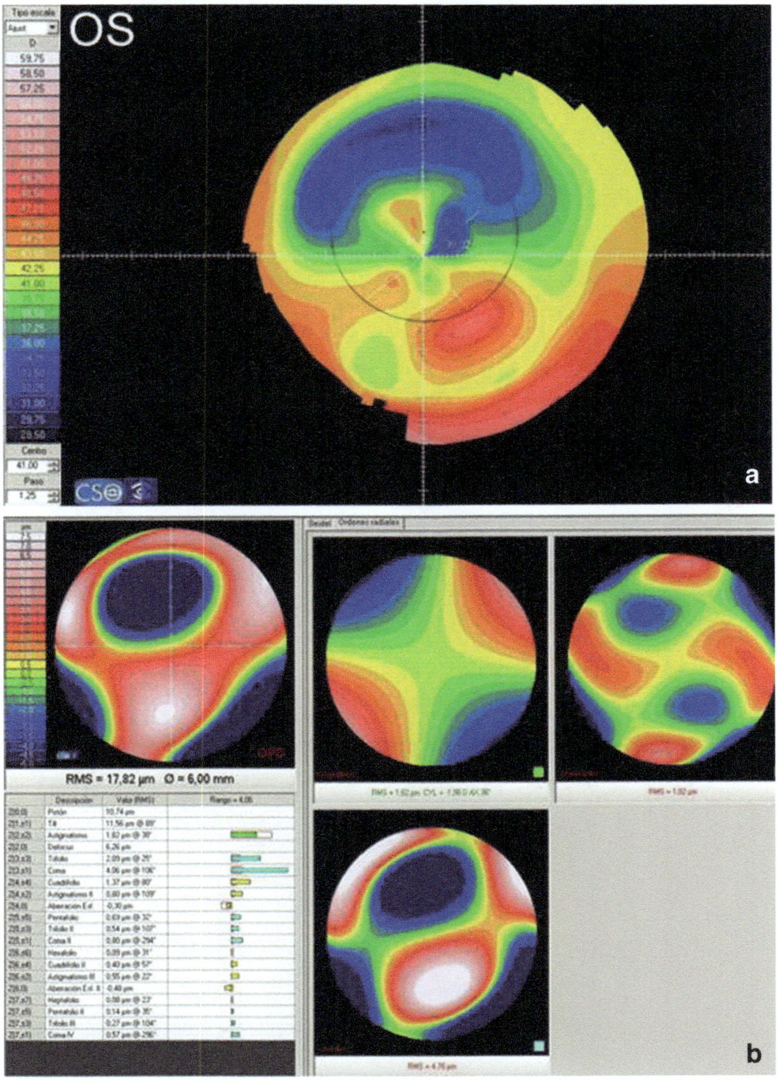

Fig. 77.3 (**a**) Corneal topography after the first implant showed a flattened area and the apex of ectatic centered. (**b**) Aberrometric data showed an increase of aberrometric value

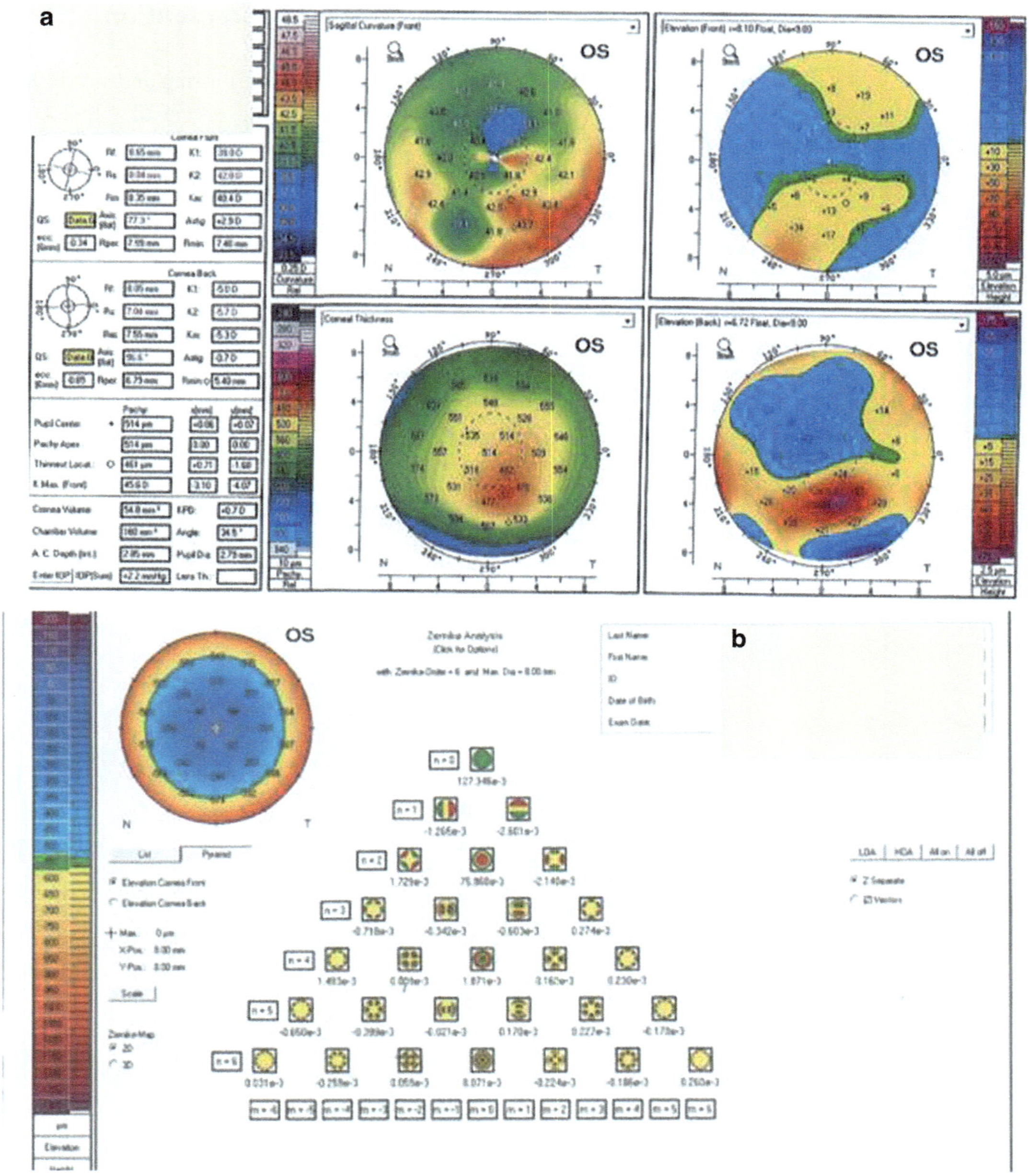

Fig. 77.4 (**a**) Corneal topography 3 months after the second surgery. (**b**) Aberrometric data showed a reduction of coma values

What to Learn from This Case

Intrastromal corneal ring segments are a good treatment option for ectatic corneal disorder. Proper patient selection, appropriate symmetrical or asymmetrical implantation, and segment thickness can promote good visual acuity [7].

References

1. Randleman JB, Russell B, Ward MA, Thompson KP, Stulting RD (2003) Risk factors and prognosis for corneal ectasia after LASIK. Ophthalmology 110: 267–275
2. Lyle WA, Jin GJC (2001) Laser in situ keratomileusis with the VISX Star laser for myopia over −10.0 diopters. J Cataract Refract Surg 27:1812–1822
3. Pallikaris IG, Kymionis GD, Astyrakakis NI (2001) Corneal ectasia induced by laser in situ keratomileusis. J Cataract Refract Surg 27:1796–1802
4. Argento C, Cosentino MJ, Tytiun A, Rapetti G, Zarate J (2001) Corneal ectasia after laser in situ keratomileusis. J Cataract Refract Surg 27:1440–1448
5. Alió JL, Shabayek MH (2006) Corneal higher order aberrations: a method to grade keratoconus. J Refract Surg 22:539–545
6. Alió JL, Shabayek MH (2006) Intracorneal asymmetrical rings for keratoconus: where should the thicker segment be implanted? J Refract Surg 22:307–309
7. Alió JL, Shabayek MH, Belda JI et al (2006) Analysis of results related to good and bad outcome of INTACS implantation for correction of keratoconus. J Cataract Refract Surg 32:756–761

Refractive Surprise After PRK in Patient with INTACS. Reversibility of Intrastromal Corneal Ring Segments. Refractive and Topographic Changes

78

Jorge L. Alió, Dominika Wróbel, and Alessandro Abbouda

Contents

J.L. Alió, MD, PhD (✉)
Department of Refractive Surgery, Vissum Corporación Oftalmológica, Alicante, Spain
e-mail: jlalio@vissum.com

D. Wróbel, MD
Glaucoma Diagnostic and Microsurgery Department, Medical University of Lublin, Lublin, Poland

R&D Department, Vissum Corporacion, Alicante, Spain
e-mail: ddudzinska@interia.pl

A. Abbouda, MD
Department of Refractive Surgery, Vissum Corporación Oftalmológica, Alicante, Spain

Department of Ophthalmology-Policlinico Umberto I of Rome, University of Rome "Sapienza", Viale del Policlinico, 155, 00186 Roma, Italy

R&D Department, Vissum Corporación Oftalmológica, 03016, Alicante, Spain
e-mail: a.abbouda@gmail.com

Why Is This Case Relevant for the Refractive Surgeon?

Intrastromal corneal ring segments (ICRS) were first proposed by Fleming and Reynolds in the late 1970s for the correction of various degrees of myopia [1, 2]. ICRS have gained popularity as a method to correct corneal ectatic diseases such as keratoconus, pellucid marginal corneal degeneration, and post-LASIK ectasia with encouraging results [3].

ICRS insertion may be a good therapeutic option for patients with thin corneas and keratoconus [4], but the procedure is not free from under/overcorrection or regression of the initial refractive error. Insertion may also influence the outcome of later refractive procedures.

Case Background

A 45-year-old woman presented for refractive surgery evaluation. She had worn hard contact lenses for many years. Her manifest refraction was −3.5 in the right eye (RE) and −3.75 in the left eye (LE). Her best corrected visual acuity (BCVA) was 20/20 in both eyes. Intraocular pressure was 12 mmHg in both eyes. Both slit lamp and fundus examinations were normal. The corneal topography was irregular with a steepening area in the center. The keratometric values were 44.1 and 44.37 × 135° in the RE and 43.6 and 44.36 × 94° in the LE. Keratoconus prediction

J.L. Alió et al. (eds.), *Difficult and Complicated Cases in Refractive Surgery*,
DOI 10.1007/978-3-642-55238-0_78, © Springer-Verlag Berlin Heidelberg 2015

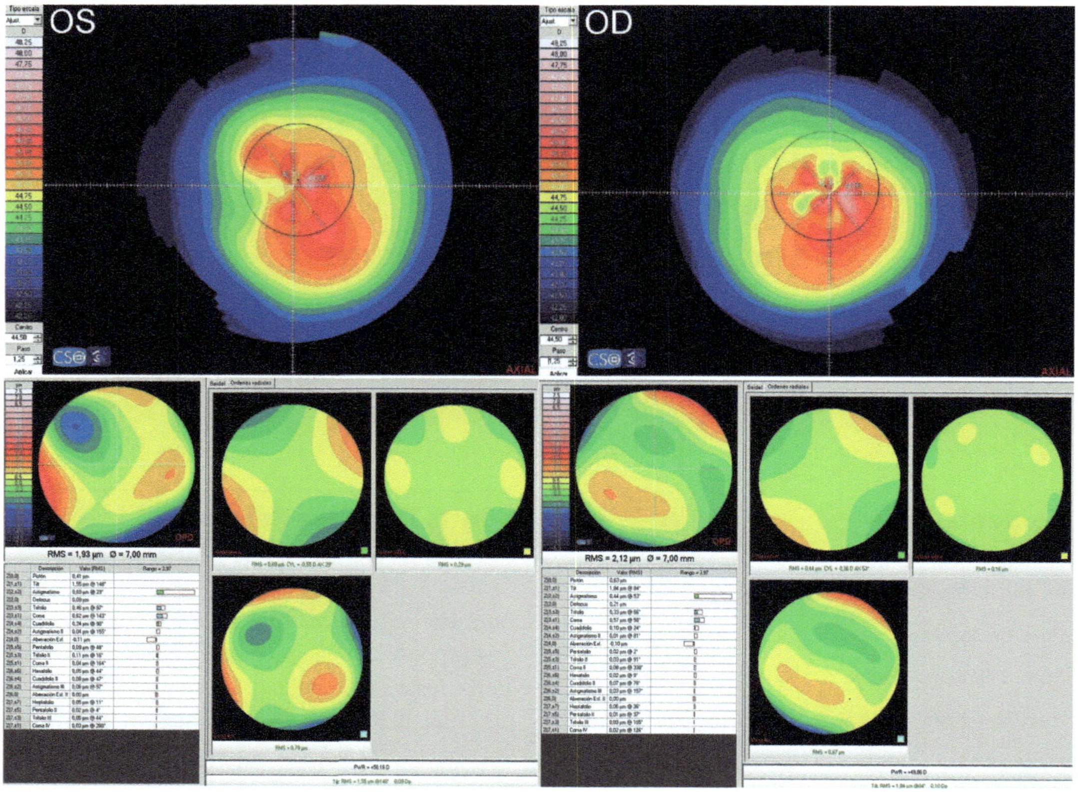

Fig. 78.1 Corneal topography before ICRS implantation

index (KPI) was 31 % in the RE and 32 % in the LE. The surface asymmetry index (SAI) was 0.74 in the RE and 0.59 in the LE. Apical keratometry (AK) was 46.39 in the RE and 46.51 in the LE. The symmetry index (SI) was 1.34 in the RE and 1.25 in the LE. The index of high order of aberration (HOA) had a value of RMS 2.12 μm in the RE and 1.93 μm in the LE. The coma value was 0.57 μm in the RE and 0.62 μm in the LE (Fig. 78.1). Her right eye pachymetry was 430 μm, and her left eye pachymetry was 440 μm. Corneal hysteresis (CH) was 7.6 mmHg in the RE and 7.3 mmHg in the LE. Moreover, the corneal resistance factor (CRF) values were 6.5 mmHg in the RE and 6.1 mmHg in the LE.

Considering all this information, including the patient's thin corneas and risk of keratoconus development, we proposed ICRS implantation to correct the patient's myopia. She underwent ICRS implantation in both eyes with no intraoperative complications. Postoperative medication included tobramycin and dexamethasone (TobraDex; Alcon) one drop four times a day. After 1 month, the UCVA was 20/125 in the RE and 20/200 in the LE. The slit lamp examination showed no anomalies. After 6 months, the patient remained undercorrected with induced astigmatism. UCVA was 20/63 in both eyes. Her manifest refraction was −2.00 −1.50 130° in the RE and −1.50 in the left eye. The BCVA was 20/20 in both eyes. The topography showed that the ICRS created a flattened area in the center of both corneas. The keratometric values were 41.55 and 43.66 × 66° in the RE and 41.7 and 43.73 × 93° in the LE. Keratoconus prediction index (KPI) was 9 % in the RE and 13 % in the LE. The surface asymmetry index (SAI) was 0.25 in the RE and 0.77 in the LE. The apical keratometry (AK) was 71.87 in the RE and 131.10 in the LE. The symmetry index (SI) was 1.48 in the RE and 2.22 in the LE. The index of high order of aberration (HOA) had a value of RMS 3.29 μm in the RE and 4.71 μm in the LE. The coma value was

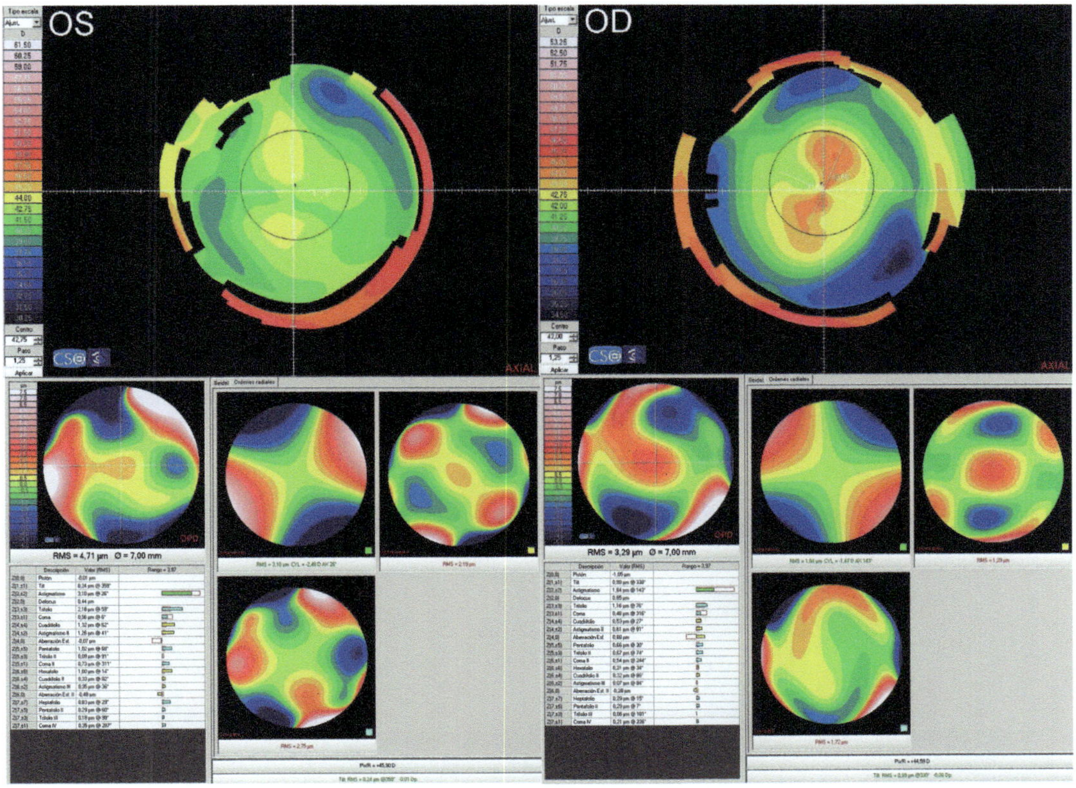

Fig. 78.2 Corneal topography after ICRS implantation

0.48 µm in the RE and 0.56 µm in the LE (Fig. 78.2). The patient was not satisfied with the refractive outcome; thus we proposed ICRS explantation.

Main Problem to Solve

We faced a problem of improving visual acuity given the patient's thin cornea and keratoconus. A refractive shift or an aberrometric rate may cause poor outcomes.

Ancillary Tests

UCVA, BCVA, pachymetry, pupil diameter, topography, CORNEAL ABERROMETRY, corneal hysteresis (CH), corneal resistance factor (CRF), aberrometric data, keratoconus prediction index (KPI), surface asymmetry index (SAI), apical keratometry (AK), symmetry index (SI), and coma value

Surgical/Medical Intervention

The 0.45 mm ICRS were implanted in both eyes using femtosecond laser (IntraLase). The corneal incisions were located on the steep meridian 140° in the RE and 180° in the LE. ICRS explantation was performed in both eyes.

Outcome

Three months after the ICRS explantation, the UCVA was 20/20 in the RE and 20/25 in the LE. The BCVA was 20/20 with −0.50 −1.00 20° in the LE. The IOP was 10 mmHg in both eyes. The keratometry reading was 42.61 and 42.9 × 35° in the RE and 41.73 and 42.08 × 103° in the LE. The topography showed an irregular aspect. The keratoconus prediction index (KPI) was 22 % in the RE and 42 % in the LE. The surface asymmetry index (SAI) was 1.18 in the RE and

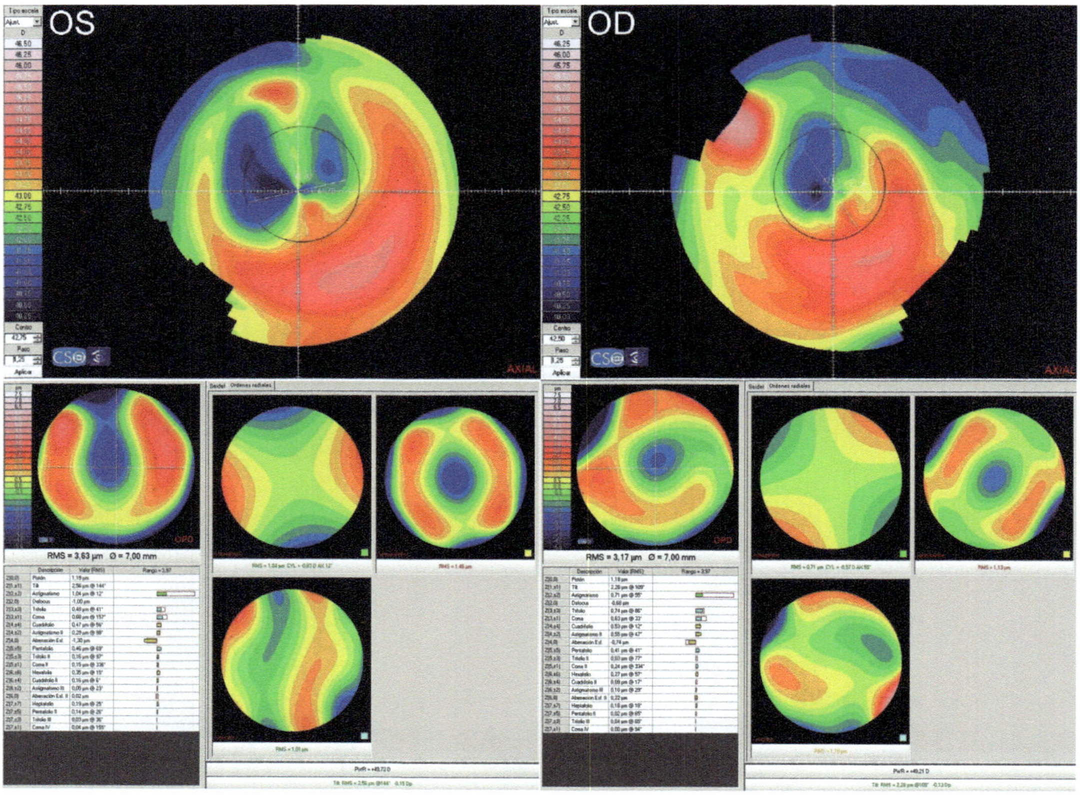

Fig. 78.3 Corneal topography after ICRS explantation

0.91 in the LE. The apical keratometry (AK) was 45.83 in the RE and 48.1 in the LE. The symmetry index (SI) was 1.87 in the RE and 1.95 in the LE. The index of high order of aberration (HOA) was RMS 3.17 μm in the RE and 3.63 μm in the LE. The coma value was 0.63 μm in the RE and 0.68 μm in the LE (Fig. 78.3). The slit lamp examination revealed transparent corneas without fluorescein staining with closed tunnels of previous ICRS. The treatment included dexamethasone (Maxidex® Alcon) four times a day and artificial tears five times a day.

What to Learn from This Case

Intrastromal corneal ring segments, because of their reversibility and exchangeability [5, 6], seem to be a good surgical method to correct myopia in cases of thin cornea and a high risk of keratoconus development. In our case we did not exchange the ICRS because of the thin cornea, which did not permit thicker segments. This case suggested that the ICRS is not a good option for a patient with irregular corneas. Unstable or artifact refraction may occur as a consequence of the corneal changes induced by ICRS in a keratoconic cornea.

References

1. Hofling-Lima AL, Branco BC, Romano AC et al (2004) Corneal infections after implantation of ICRS. Cornea 23:547–549
2. Rau M, Dausch D (2003) Intrastromal corneal ring implantation for the correction of myopia: 12-month follow-up. J Cataract Refract Surg 29:322–328
3. Alio' JL, Shabayek MH (2006) Intracorneal implants. In: Kohen T, Koch D (eds) Essentials in ophthalmology—cataract and refractive surgery II. Springer, Berlin/Heidelberg/New York, pp 159–169

4. Vega-Estrada A, Alio JL, Brenner LF, Javaloy J, Plaza Puche AB, Barraquer RI, Teus MA, Murta J, Henriques J, Uceda-Montanes A (2013) Outcome analysis of intracorneal ring segments for the treatment of keratoconus based on visual, refractive, and aberrometric impairment. Am J Ophthalmol 155: 575–584.e1
5. Chan SM, Khan HN (2002) Reversibility and exchangeability of intrastromal corneal ring segments. J Cataract Refract Surg 28:676–681
6. Shabayek MH, Alió JL (2007) Intrastromal corneal ring segment implantation by femtosecond laser for keratoconus correction. Ophthalmology 114: 1643–1652

Part VII

Phakic Intraocular Lens Complications

Dear reader,

In the last two decades, phakic intraocular lenses (PIOLs) have proved to be a safe and reliable method for correcting high myopia, hyperopia, and astigmatism when they fit patient needs. However, it is important to realize that complications relating to PIOLs can be more severe and disabling than those of keratorefractive surgery.

In this section, we cover cases involving different types and models of PIOLs with varied intraoperative and postoperative complications. For example, cases include artisan lens dislocation, angle-supported phakic IOL migration, ICL and pupillary block, choroidal neovascularization, and retinal detachment. It is essential that ophthalmic surgeons understand the complications of this surgical procedure and are competent in handling complications related to different phakic IOL models.

For further reading, we suggest the first book of this series: J.L. Alio', D. Azar *Management of Complications in Refractive Surgery*, Chapter 13: Phakic Intraocular Lens Complications (pp. 226–262).

Specific topics covered by the cases include how to manage PIOL dislocation (Case 79), what to do with an iatrogenic anterior capsule rupture (Case 80), and how to manage the reduction of safety zone between PIOL and endothelium in light of anterior chamber depth changing with age (Case 81). Other cases cover management of PIOL separation (Case 82), restoring angle-supported phakic IOL (Case 83), the importance of the sulcus anatomy for the ICL (Case 84), and how to manage a bilateral pupillary block associated with ICL (Case 85). We included also a case focused on piggyback IOL to correct residual refractive errors in eyes with previous a history of radial keratotomy (Case 86), a rare case of choroidal neovascularization after PIOL (Case 87), and risk of retinal detachment after PIOL (Case 87).

Lesson to Learn

Case 79: Artisan phakic lens dislocation

The luxation of the iris-supported lens is a possible long-term complication. How to manage this dislocation.

Case 80: Iris and crystalline lens damage during phakic IOL surgery
The less aggressive procedure to follow when an iatrogenic anterior capsule rupture occurs.
Case 81: Angle-supported phakic IOL
Anterior chamber depth changing by age. How to manage the reduction of safety zone between PIOL and endothelium.
Case 82: Phakic IOL optic luxation in a two-piece (Kelman Duet) lens separation
The optic of Kelman Duet PIOL may divide from its haptic following a trauma. If the surgical reposition is done immediately, the corneal endothelium does not seem to be damaged.
Case 83: Angle-supported phakic IOL migration following trauma
The rotation of the angle-supported PIOL is a possible long-term complication. In patients exposed to a frequent risk of blunt trauma, it is advised to avoid the implantation of this lens.
Case 84: Strange case of misaligned STAAR toric implantable collamer lens (ICL)
The importance of the proper axis orientation to achieve the desired visual and optical quality results and the sulcus anatomy for the ICL.
Case 85: ICL implantation and bilateral pupillary block
Pupillary block after phakic ICL implantation may occur if the peripheral iridotomies do not include properly the full thickness of the iris.
Case 86: Complications of phakic intraocular lenses: refractive lens exchange and piggyback
Why piggyback IOL would be the best choice to correct residual refractive errors in eyes with previous history of radial keratotomy.
Case 87: Choroidal neovascularization after phakic intraocular lens implantation
CNV is a possible but infrequent complication in high myopic patients after PIOL implantation.
Case 88: Retinal detachment
In eyes with an axial length of more than 30.24 mm, the high risk of retinal detachment after PIOL implantation must be always remembered.

Artisan Lens Dislocation

79

Jorge L. Alió and Alessandro Abbouda

Contents

J.L. Alió, MD, PhD (✉)
Department of Refractive Surgery,
Vissum Corporación Oftalmológica,
Alicante, Spain
e-mail: jlalio@vissum.com

A. Abbouda, MD
Department of Refractive Surgery,
Vissum Corporación Oftalmológica, Alicante, Spain

Department of Ophthalmology-Policlinico Umberto I of Rome, University of Rome "Sapienza", Viale del Policlinico, 155, 00186 Roma, Italy

R&D Department, Vissum Corporación Oftalmológica, 03016, Alicante, Spain
e-mail: a.abbouda@gmail.com

Why Is This Case Relevant for the Refractive Surgeon?

Luxation of the PIOL is a possible long-term complication of iris-supported PIOL [1]. It is caused either by insufficient iris tissue enclavated in the claw of the lens or by atrophy of the iris grasped at the claw level [2, 3].

Case Background

A 30-year-old man with a history of astigmatism in both eyes had a toric Artisan implanted at the age of 20. Refraction prior to surgery was +6.75 $-3\times5°$ in the right eye (RE) and +6.75 $-3\times175°$ in the left eye (LE). An Artisan lens was implanted in the RE at 5 grades and in the LE at 175 degree. The postoperative was uneventful. Two weeks after surgery, the patient's best corrected visual acuity (BCVA) was 20/20 in both eyes. After 2 years, the patient arrived at our department complaining of foggy vision in the LE. His BCVA was 20/20 in the RE and 20/100 in the LE. The slit lamp examination showed conjunctival hyperemia, corneal edema at the inferior limbus, and dislocation of the lens. The left haptic was completely free, lying down touching the endothelium.

J.L. Alió et al. (eds.), *Difficult and Complicated Cases in Refractive Surgery*,
DOI 10.1007/978-3-642-55238-0_79, © Springer-Verlag Berlin Heidelberg 2015

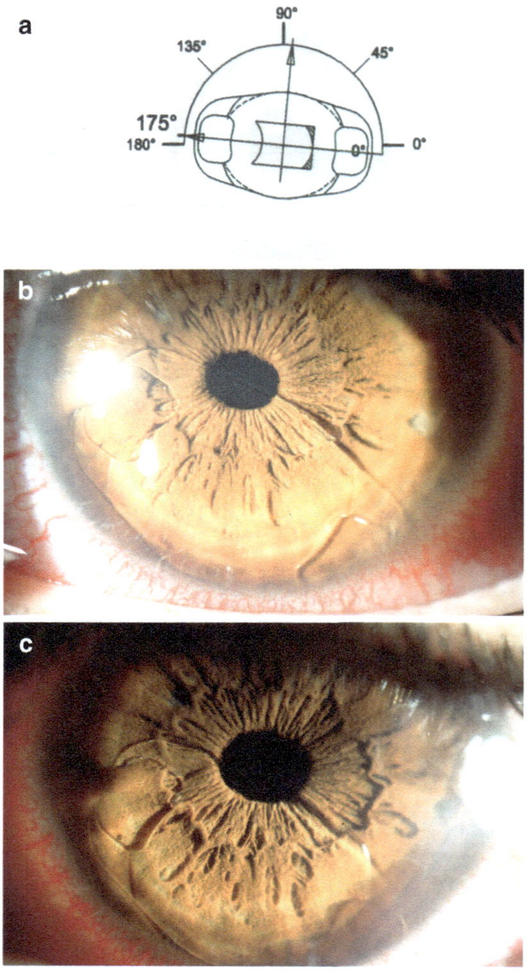

Fig. 79.1 (**a**) Plan of implantation. (**b**, **c**) Aspect of dislocation

Main Problem to Solve

Spontaneous luxation of the lens is very rare. Repositioning must be immediate in order to avoid corneal decompensation.

Ancillary Tests

The Konan 5500 (Konan Camera Research Institute Inc., Hyogo, Japan) was used to analyze the corneal endothelial cell. The endothelial cell count before the first surgery was 3,283 cells/mm^2 in the RE and 3,418 cells/mm^2 in the LE. On the day of dislocation, there were 2,841 cells/mm^2 in the RE and 2,811 cells/mm^2 in the LE.

Surgical/Medical Intervention

The same day the lens was re-centered, enclavation of the nasal and iris bridge was performed with an iris enclavation needle as is typical.

Outcome

At 2 weeks, BCVA was 20/20 in both eyes and the patient was satisfied. The ECC after 10 years was 2,404 cells/mm^2 in the RE and 1,876 cells/mm^2 in the LE. No further loss of ECC was observed.

What to Learn from This Case

An iris claw PIOL can dislocate over time. However, immediate surgical repositioning can prevent damage to the corneal endothelium [1–3], even with a lower cell count in the eye after 10 years.

References

1. Marinho A (2008) Chapter 13.2. Complications of iris supported phakic IOLs. In: Alio JL, Azar D (eds) Management of complications in refractive surgery. Springer, Berlin/Heidelberg, pp 238–244
2. Budo C (2004) Complications. In: Budo C (ed) The ARTISAN lens. Highlights of Ophthalmology International, El Dorado
3. Marinho A, Salgado R (2005) Complications of phakic IOLs. In: Garg A, Alió J, Marinho A et al (eds) Lens-based refractive surgery (phakic IOLs). Jaypee Brothers, New Delhi

Iris and Crystalline Lens Damage During Phakic IOL Surgery

80

Jorge L. Alió and Alessandro Abbouda

Contents

Electronic supplementary material The online version of this chapter (10.1007/978-3-642-55238-0_80) contains supplementary material, which is available to authorized users.

J.L. Alió, MD, PhD (✉)
Department of Refractive Surgery, Vissum Corporación Oftalmológica, Alicante, Spain
e-mail: jlalio@vissum.com

A. Abbouda, MD
Department of Refractive Surgery, Vissum Corporación Oftalmológica, Alicante, Spain

Department of Ophthalmology-Policlinico Umberto I of Rome, University of Rome "Sapienza", Viale del Policlinico, 155, 00186 Roma, Italy

R&D Department, Vissum Corporación Oftalmológica, 03016, Alicante, Spain
e-mail: a.abbouda@gmail.com

Why Is This Case Relevant for the Refractive Surgeon?

A refractive surgeon should be comfortable with handling complications during phakic IOL surgery, including accidental damage to the iris and crystalline lens.

Case Background

A 48-year-old man was evaluated for refractive surgery. His manifest refraction was $-17=-1.25\times 50°$ in the right eye (RE) and $-16=-2\times 70°$ in the left eye (LE). His best corrected visual acuity (BCVA) was 20/20 in the RE and 20/25 in the LE. The preoperative central thickness was 526 μm in the RE and 519 μm in the LE. Keratometry reading was $44.9/46\times 120°$ in the RE and $45/46.4\times 150°$ in the LE. Corneal topography and corneal aberrometry were normal. The endothelial cell count was 3,257 cells/mm^2 in the RE and 2,865 cells/mm^2 in the LE. The anterior chamber depth measured by OCT Visante was 3.12 mm and 3.16 mm. We decided to implant an iris-supported phakic IOL.

Surgical/Medical Intervention

We made a small nasal incision of 6 mm from 12 o'clock. The anterior chamber was filled with viscoelastic. The Artisan was introduced at

J.L. Alió et al. (eds.), *Difficult and Complicated Cases in Refractive Surgery*, DOI 10.1007/978-3-642-55238-0_80, © Springer-Verlag Berlin Heidelberg 2015

12 o'clock with special implantation forceps (forceps of Worst-Fechner or Budo) and centered. The enclavation of the nasal and then the iris bridge was performed using an iris enclavation needle. We removed the viscoelastic and sutured the incision. In the LE, we decided to perform a limbal relaxing incision at 1 mm with 2.4 mm knife. The knife was blunt, and inadvertently, we cut the iris and anterior capsule (see Video 80.1).

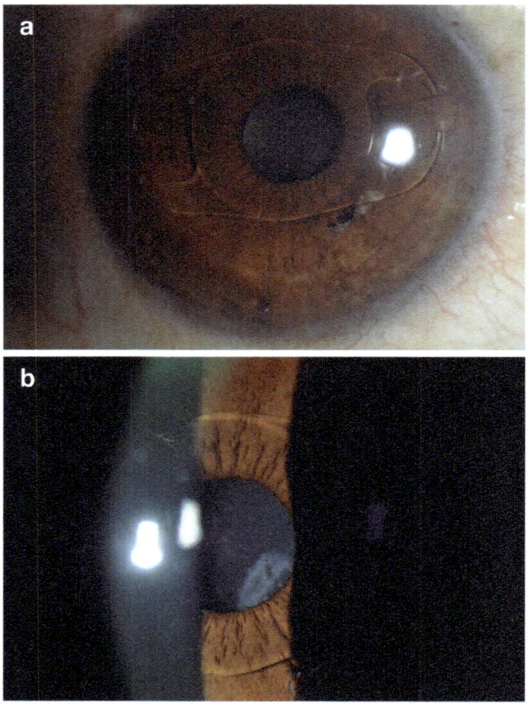

Fig. 80.1 Slit lamp examination at (**a**) 3 months and (**b**) 6 months

Main Problem to Solve

Damage to the iris and anterior capsule is a rare complication of phakic IOL surgery. To manage this complication, one should avoid dilating the pupil in the days following surgery, allowing the iris to repair the capsular wound until the iris posterior synechia is visible. This way, the aqueous cannot penetrate the crystalline lens, preventing development of an intumescent cataract.

Ancillary Tests

Follow-up with a slit lamp biomicroscopy and BCVA examination. Patient explanation and coaching are also very important.

Outcome

After three months, the visual acuity in the LE was 20/20 with a manifest refraction of $+0.75 = -0.75 \times 120°$. The slit lamp examination showed a focal opacity of the crystalline lens (Fig. 80.1). This opacity did not change after 6 months (Fig. 80.2).

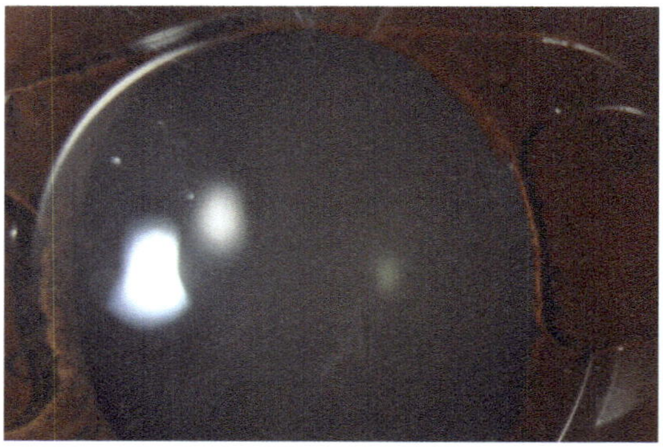

Fig. 80.2 Slit lamp examination at 6 months. The opacity of the crystalline lens was unchanged

What to Learn from This Case

When such a complication occurs during surgery, it is important not to allow anxiety to guide decision-making. In this case, some surgeons would choose a lensectomy surgery to resolve the anterior capsular damage. However, a lensectomy is more aggressive and we must consider the risk of retinal detachment in high myopes following lens removal [1]. Instead, we recommend allowing the iris itself to repair the wound.

Reference

1. Alió JL (2011) Lens surgery (cataract and refractive lens exchange) and retinal detachment risk in myopes: still an issue? Br J Ophthalmol 95:301–303

Angle-Supported Phakic IOL

81

Alessandro Abbouda and Jorge L. Alió

Contents

Electronic supplementary material The online version of this chapter (10.1007/978-3-642-55238-0_81) contains supplementary material, which is available to authorized users.

A. Abbouda, MD (✉)
Department of Refractive Surgery, Vissum Corporación Oftalmológica, Alicante, Spain

Department of Ophthalmology-Policlinico Umberto I of Rome, University of Rome "Sapienza", Viale del Policlinico, 155, 00186 Roma, Italy

R&D Department, Vissum Corporación Oftalmológica, 03016, Alicante, Spain
e-mail: a.abbouda@gmail.com

J.L. Alió, MD, PhD
Department of Refractive Surgery, Vissum Corporación Oftalmológica, Alicante, Spain
e-mail: jlalio@vissum.com

Why Is This Case Relevant for the Refractive Surgeon?

Over the last two decades, phakic intraocular lenses (PIOLs) have been proven as a safe and reliable method for correcting high myopia, hyperopia, and astigmatism with adequate inclusion criteria for implantation [1–3]. Long-term complications for eyes implanted with PIOLs have been reported in several articles [4, 5]. Endothelial cell loss (ECL) was reported [5] to be 1.78 % every year in patients implanted with PIOLs.

Anterior chamber morphology changes with age and the safety distance of Angle Supported PIOL from the endothelium must be respected. This case describes a long-term follow-up and the onset of complication in an older patient. Because PIOLs are common, it is essential that a refractive surgeon be able to respond to complications.

Case Background

A 62-year-old woman with a history of high myopia in both eyes was implanted with a ZB5M0 PIOL when she was 24. She arrived at our department complaining of visual acuity loss in the left eye for 2 weeks. Her manifest refraction was −1 in the right eye (RE) and −4.5 in the left eye (LE). Her best corrected visual acuity (BCVA) was 20/20 in the RE and 20/50 in the LE. Slit lamp examination revealed corneal

J.L. Alió et al. (eds.), *Difficult and Complicated Cases in Refractive Surgery*,
DOI 10.1007/978-3-642-55238-0_81, © Springer-Verlag Berlin Heidelberg 2015

edema in correspondence to the haptic of the lens (Fig. 81.1). The intraocular pressure was 18 mmHg in the RE and 21 mmHg in the LE and a nuclear cataract was diagnosed. The endothelial cell count was 1,289 cells/mm^2 (RE) and 666 cells/mm^2 (LE) (Fig. 81.2a).

Fig. 81.1 Slit lamp examination at the beginning showed corneal edema

Main Problem to Solve

We were faced with proceeding with PIOL explantation (bilensectomy) and cataract surgery while avoiding an increase of ECL.

Ancillary Tests

We found the OCT Visante exam useful. The anterior chamber measurement showed a considerable reduction of the distance between the lens and the endothelium (Fig. 81.3a). The safe value was defined as 1.5 mm. In this case, the temporal and nasal distances between the

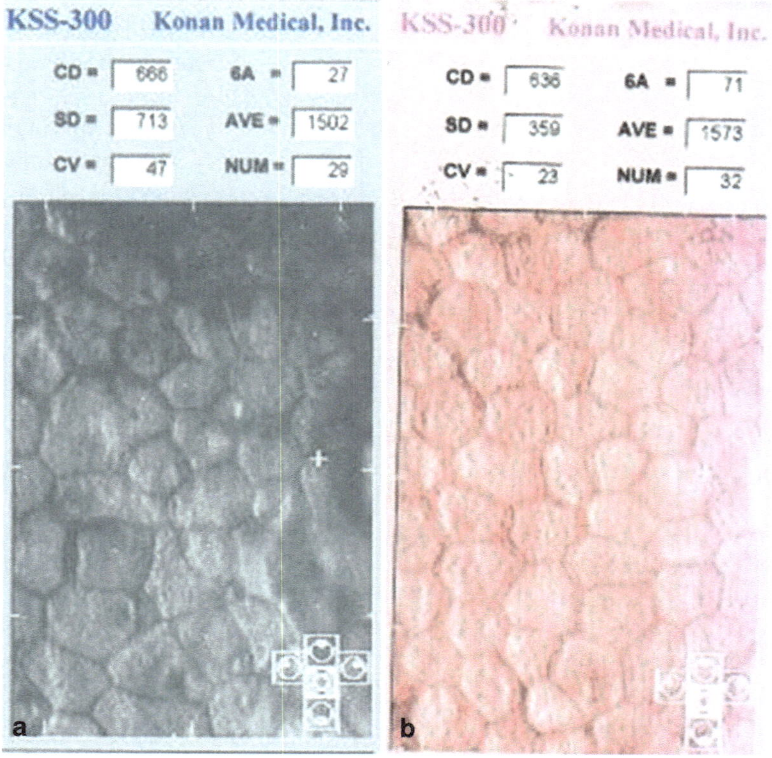

Fig. 81.2 (**a**) Endothelial cell count before and 3 months after the cataract surgery (**b**)

endothelium and the lens were 1.3 mm and 1.4 mm, respectively. The crystalline rise was 1,090 µm.

Surgical/Medical Intervention

Cataract surgery was performed under peribulbar anesthesia, using a 5.5 mm superotemporal scleral tunnel. A dispersive ophthalmic viscosurgical device (OVD) was injected over and below the AS PIOL. We gently grasped the optic with McPherson forceps and removed it from the eye without enlarging the incision. Micro incisional cataract surgery (MICS) was performed with low energy to minimize surgical trauma. The effective phaco time (EPT) was 0.02. The mean ultrasound power was 1 %. A posterior chamber hydrophobic acrylic three-piece lens of 4 diopters (AcrySof MA60, Alcon) was implanted in the capsular bag (Video 81.1).

Outcome

Three months after surgery, visual acuity in the patient's left eye was 20/20 with −0.75/5. The endothelial cell count was 636 cells/mm^2(Fig. 81.2b). The OCT Visante showed an anterior chamber depth of 3.22 mm (Fig. 81.3b).

What to Learn from This Case

Because of age changes related to crystalline size, thorough postoperative examinations are recommended for patients over 40 years. We also realize the importance of analyzing anterior chamber and angle depth modifications and recommending PIOL explantation in cases where the safety zone between the PIOL and endothelium is insufficient. A recent paper [6] recommended explanting ZB5m PIOL before

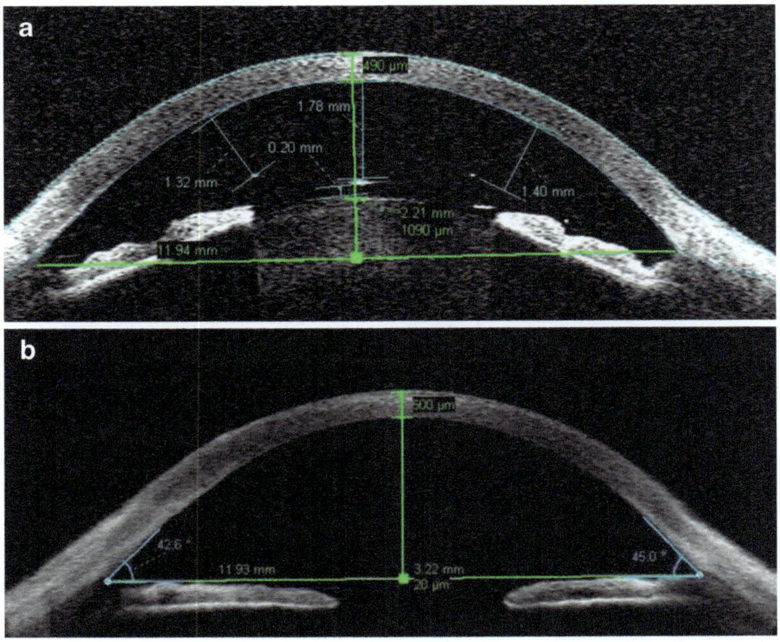

Fig. 81.3 OCT Visante and anterior chamber measurement (**a**) preoperatively and (**b**) postoperatively

30 years of implantation, because the ECC would be less than 600 cells/mm^2 in patients with a preoperative SE of −25D, or before 40 years in patients with SE of −20D. Furthermore, the safety zone of 1.5 mm between the endothelium and the lens will not be respected after 20 years of implantation in patients with a preoperative SE of −20D or after 15 years in patients with an SE of −25D.

References

1. Tahzib NG, Nuijts RM, Wu WY, Budo CJ (2007) Long-term study of Artisan phakic intraocular lens implantation for the correction of moderate to high myopia: 10-year follow-up results. Ophthalmology 114:1133–1142
2. Budo C, Hessloehl JC, Izak M et al (2000) Multicenter study of the Artisan phakic intraocular lens. J Cataract Refract Surg 26:1163–1171
3. Dick HB, Alio J, Bianchetti M et al (2003) Toric phakic intraocular lens: European multicenter study. Ophthalmology 110:150–162
4. Javaloy J, Alió JL, Iradier MT, Abdelrahman AM, Javaloy T, Borrás F (2007) Outcomes of ZB5M angle-supported anterior chamber phakic intraocular lenses at 12 years. J Refract Surg 23:147–158
5. Alio JL, Abbouda A, Huseyinly S, Peña-Garcia P (2013) Follow up study of over 15 years of an angle supported phakic intraocular lens model (ZB5M) for high myopia: outcomes and complications. JAMA Ophthalmol 131(12):1541–1546. doi: 10.1001/jamaophthalmol.2013.5595
6. Alio JL, Abbouda A, Peña-Garcia P (2013) Anterior segment optical coherence tomography of long term phakic angle supported intraocular lenses. Am J Ophthalmol 156(5):894–901.e2 doi: 10.1016/j.ajo.2013.06.018. Epub 2013 Aug 12.

Phakic IOL Optic Luxation in a Two-Pieces (Kelman Duet) Lens Separation

82

Jorge L. Alió and Alessandro Abbouda

Contents

J.L. Alió, MD, PhD (✉)
Department of Refractive Surgery, Vissum Corporación Oftalmológica, Alicante, Spain
e-mail: jlalio@vissum.com

A. Abbouda, MD
Department of Refractive Surgery, Vissum Corporación Oftalmológica, Alicante, Spain

Department of Ophthalmology-Policlinico Umberto I of Rome, University of Rome "Sapienza", Viale del Policlinico, 155, 00186 Roma, Italy

R&D Department, Vissum Corporación Oftalmológica, 03016, Alicante, Spain
e-mail: a.abbouda@gmail.com

Why Is This Case Relevant for the Refractive Surgeon?

This case describes an unusual complication in a patient implanted with a very particular type of angle-supported phakic IOL: Kelman Duet Phakic IOL. The Kelman Duet Implant (Tekia Inc., Irvine, California) is a two-part, angle-supported PIOL that is implantable through a small incision. The main advantage of this kind of lens is the exchangeability of the haptic and optic lens [1, 2]. A refractive surgeon using a Kelman Duet Phakic IOL should be aware of related complications, including division of the haptic and optic lenses.

Case Background

A 40-year-old man with a history of myopia and astigmatism in both eyes was implanted at 35 years of age with the Kelman Duet Implant (Tekia Inc., Irvine, California). Refraction before surgery was $-17=-2\times110°$ in the right eye (RE) and $-13.5=-2\times130°$ in the left eye (LE). The Kelman Duet Implant had a power of −17 in the RE and -14 in the LE. The postoperative was uneventful. Two weeks after surgery, the patient's best corrected visual acuity (BCVA) was 20/32 in the RE and 20/20 in the LE. After 5 years, the patient was referred for accidental trauma from a lollypop. He complained of foggy vision in the RE. His BCVA in the RE was finger

J.L. Alió et al. (eds.), *Difficult and Complicated Cases in Refractive Surgery*,
DOI 10.1007/978-3-642-55238-0_82, © Springer-Verlag Berlin Heidelberg 2015

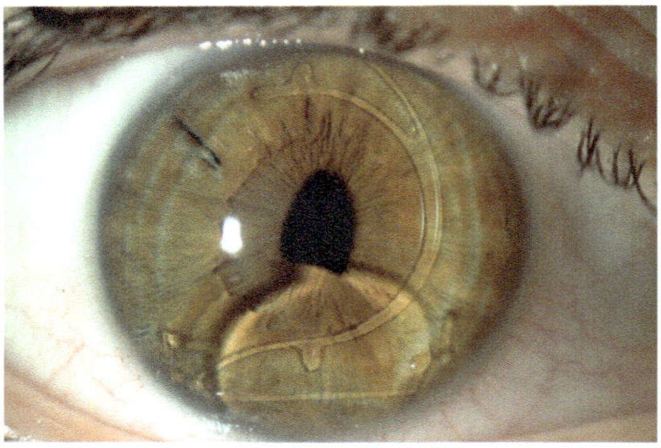

Fig. 82.1 Slit lamp examination showed a complete separation between the optic and the haptic

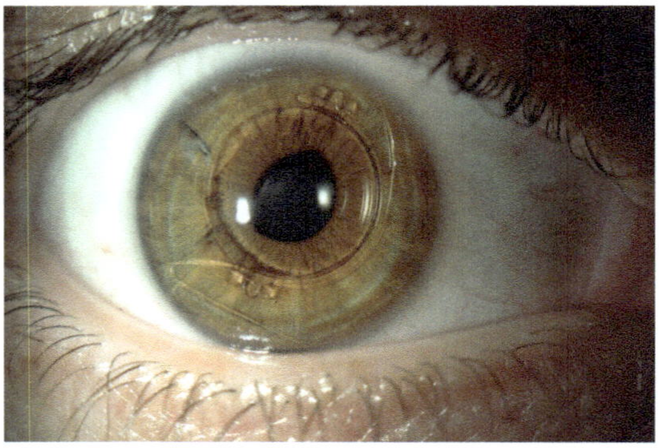

Fig. 82.2 Slit lamp examination at the end of follow-up showed a normal position

count. Slit lamp examination revealed division of the optic from the haptic lens and dislocation at the inferior limbus touching the endothelium (Fig. 82.1).

Main Problem to Solve

Repositioning was necessary in order to avoid corneal decompensation.

Ancillary Tests

We used the Konan 5,500 analyzer (Konan Camera Research Institute Inc., Hyogo, Japan) to analyze the corneal endothelial cells. The endothelial cell count before the first surgery was 2,183 cells/mm^2 in the RE. At the day of dislocation, it was 1,992 cells/mm^2.

Surgical/Medical Intervention

The lens was re-centered on the same day. The first incision was made at 3 o'clock and a hook was used to hold the near tab of the optic, bringing over the bayonet on the haptic. The second hook was introduced at 9 o'clock and was used to place the other haptic over the bayonet.

Outcome

At 2 weeks, the BCVA was 20/20. Slit lamp examination showed normal positions of the lens (Fig. 82.2). The patient was satisfied. The ECC after 5 years was 1,876 cells/mm^2. No further loss of ECC was observed.

What to Learn from This Case

The optic lens of Kelman Duet PIOL may divide from its haptic lens following trauma. Immediate surgical repositioning can prevent damage to the corneal endothelium.

References

1. Alió JL, Piñero D, Bernabeu G, Galal A, Vargas JM, Ismail MM (2007) The Kelman Duet phakic intraocular lens: 1-year results. J Refract Surg 23:868–879
2. Alió JL, Kelman C (2003) The Duet-Kelman lens: a new exchangeable angle-supported phakic intraocular lens. J Refract Surg 19:488–495

Angle-Supported Phakic IOL Migration Following Trauma

83

Jorge L. Alió, Jaime Javaloy, and Alessandro Abbouda

Contents

Electronic supplementary material The online version of this chapter (10.1007/978-3-642-55238-0_83) contains supplementary material, which is available to authorized users.

J.L. Alió, MD, PhD (✉)
Department of Refractive Surgery, Vissum Corporación Oftalmológica, Alicante, Spain
e-mail: jlalio@vissum.com

J. Javaloy, MD, PhD
Department of Anterior Segment and Refractive Surgery, Vissum Corporacion Oftalmológica, Alicante, Spain
e-mail: jjavaloy@coma.es

A. Abbouda, MD
Department of Refractive Surgery, Vissum Corporación Oftalmológica, Alicante, Spain

Department of Ophthalmology-Policlinico Umberto I of Rome, University of Rome "Sapienza", Viale del Policlinico, 155, 00186 Roma, Italy

R&D Department, Vissum Corporación Oftalmológica, 03016, Alicante, Spain
e-mail: a.abbouda@gmail.com

Why Is This Case Relevant for the Refractive Surgeon?

Rotation of the angle-supported PIOL is a potential long-term complication of phakic IOL [1]. Rotation can occur in all models of AS PIOLs, especially following trauma. The Kelman Duet anterior chamber intraocular lens, because of its three-point fixation, can rotate in a counterclockwise direction [2].

Case Background

A 40-year-old woman with a history of myopia and astigmatism in both eyes was implanted at age 32 with a Kelman Duet angle-supported phakic IOL. Refraction before surgery was −14-0.75 × 60° in the right eye (RE) and −14.5-2 × 115° in the left eye (LE). Preoperative data showed a keratometric value 43.2/43.8 × 84° in the RE and 43.5/44.2 × 11° in the LE. Her best corrected visual acuity (BCVA) was 20/20 in both eyes. The preoperative central thickness was 470 μm in both eyes. The endothelial cell count showed 2,283 cell/mm^2 in the RE and 2,045 cell/mm^2 in the LE. Measurement of the anterior chamber was performed with the OCT Visante. In the RE, the anterior chamber depth was 3.13 mm and the angle-to-angle distance was 11.43 mm. In the left eye, these measurements were 2.98 mm and 11.34 mm, respectively. A Kelman Duet was implanted.

J.L. Alió et al. (eds.), *Difficult and Complicated Cases in Refractive Surgery*,
DOI 10.1007/978-3-642-55238-0_83, © Springer-Verlag Berlin Heidelberg 2015

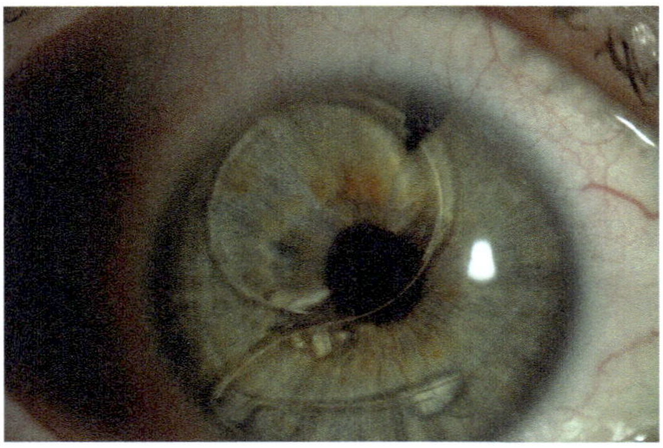

Fig. 83.1 Slit lamp examination 18 months after the first surgery revealed IOL displacement

The lens power was −14 diopters in both eyes with a relaxing incision in the LE. The diameter was 12 mm. The postoperative period was uneventful. After 18 months, the patient presented to our department complaining of foggy vision in the RE after an incidental blunt trauma. Her BCVA was 20/32 in the RE and 20/20 in the LE. The slit lamp examination revealed a lens rotation in a counterclockwise direction and the displacement of the haptic of the lens through the peripheral iridectomy, with the double support dislocated into the anterior chamber (Fig. 83.1). The lens was centered, removing the haptic from the ciliary sulcus and rounding the lens in 2 clockwise directions. The postoperative was uneventful with speedy and satisfactory recovery of visual acuity. After 3 years, the patient returned to our clinic with the same symptoms. She referred a new blunt trauma 3 days before in the RE. The slit lamp examination revealed the same dislocation.

Main Problem to Solve

Decentration of the lens optic due to poor selection of lens size occurs in a low percentage of cases. Decentration produces an imbalance in the forces of angle support [3]. Although the lens size was correct in this case, trauma managed to displace the lens.

Ancillary Tests

The endothelial count was performed excluding damage and endothelial cell loss related to frequent trauma. The cell count was 2,045 cell/mm^2 in the RE. We decided to recenter the lens and not explant it.

Surgical/Medical Intervention

Under topical anesthesia, a paracentesis was performed in the limbus at 10 h. After injecting 0.1 ml of acetylcholine, the anterior chamber was filled with cohesive ophthalmic viscosurgical devices (OVD). Using a Sinskey hook, the lens was rotated in a clockwise direction, removing the haptic from the ciliary sulcus (Video 83.1).

Outcome

Three days after surgery, the patient's manifest refraction was −0.5/70° and her BCVA was 20/20. The slit lamp examination revealed a centered lens and haptics (Fig. 83.2).

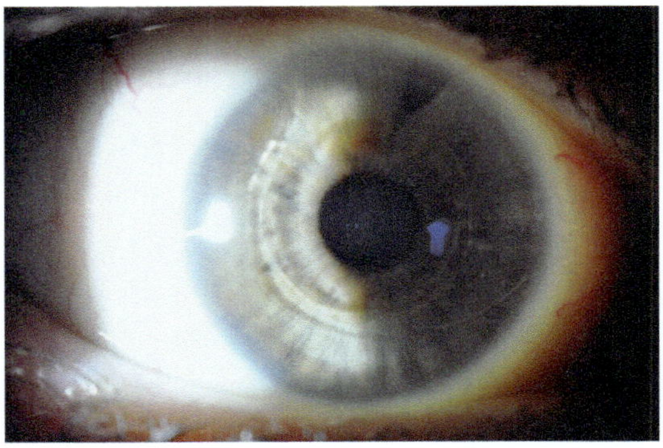

Fig. 83.2 Slit lamp examination after surgery revealed a centered IOL

What to Learn from This Case

In cases of blunt trauma in a patient implanted with an angle-supported phakic IOL, it seems that prompt management can prevent severe complications such as endothelial decompensation. Furthermore, obtaining a patient's detailed history is advised in order to avoid implanting devices in patients exposed to a frequent risk of blunt trauma.

References

1. Mutuologlu O, Alio' JL (2008) Chapter 13.1: Anterior chamber angle supported complications prevention and treatment. In: Alio JL, Azar D (eds) Management of complications in refractive surgery. Springer, Berlin/Heidelberg, pp 226–236
2. Assia EI, Blotnick CA, Powers TP, Legler UF, Apple DJ (1994) Clinicopathologic study of ocular trauma in eyes with intraocular lenses. Am J Ophthalmol 117: 30–36
3. Lovisolo CF, Fabio M, Reinstein DZ, Timothy A (2012) Chapter-04 proper patient assessment, selection and preparation. In: Alio' JL, Perez-Santonja JJ (eds) Refractive surgery with Phakic IOL, Fundamentals and clinical practice. Jaypee, Panama, pp 126–146

Misaligned STAAR Toric Implantable Collamer Lens (ICL)

84

Jaime Javaloy and Alessandro Abbouda

Contents

J. Javaloy, MD, PhD (✉)
Anterior Segment and Refractive Surgery Department, Vissum Corporación Oftalmológica, Alicante, Spain
e-mail: jjavaloy@coma.es

A. Abbouda, MD
Department of Refractive Surgery, Vissum Corporación Oftalmológica, Alicante, Spain

Department of Ophthalmology-Policlinico Umberto I of Rome, University of Rome "Sapienza", Viale del Policlinico, 155, 00186 Roma, Italy

R&D Department, Vissum Corporación Oftalmológica, 03016, Alicante, Spain
e-mail: a.abbouda@gmail.com

Why Is This Case Relevant for the Refractive Surgeon?

The toric implantable collamer lens (TICL; STAAR Surgical Co., Monrovia, Calif) is a posterior chamber, sulcus-supported, phakic IOL used to reduce or eliminate myopia, hyperopia, or astigmatism [1, 2]. The refractive surgeon should use proper axis orientation to achieve the desired optical results.

Case Background

A 26-year-old woman with bilateral myopic astigmatism presented for a refractive surgery evaluation. Her manifest refraction was −5.75 −4 × 10 in the right eye and −6.25 − 4 × 170 in the left eye. Her best corrected visual acuity (BCVA) was 20/20 in both eyes. Her preoperative central thickness was 552 μm in the right eye and 530 μm in the left eye. The keratometry reading was 42.28/44.384 × 93 in the right eye and 42.69/44.86 × 93 in the left eye. Papillary sizes were 6 mm under mesopic light condition. The corneal topography showed asymmetrical bowtie patterns. To avoid the risk of ectasia post-LASIK and to provide the best

J.L. Alió et al. (eds.), *Difficult and Complicated Cases in Refractive Surgery*,
DOI 10.1007/978-3-642-55238-0_84, © Springer-Verlag Berlin Heidelberg 2015

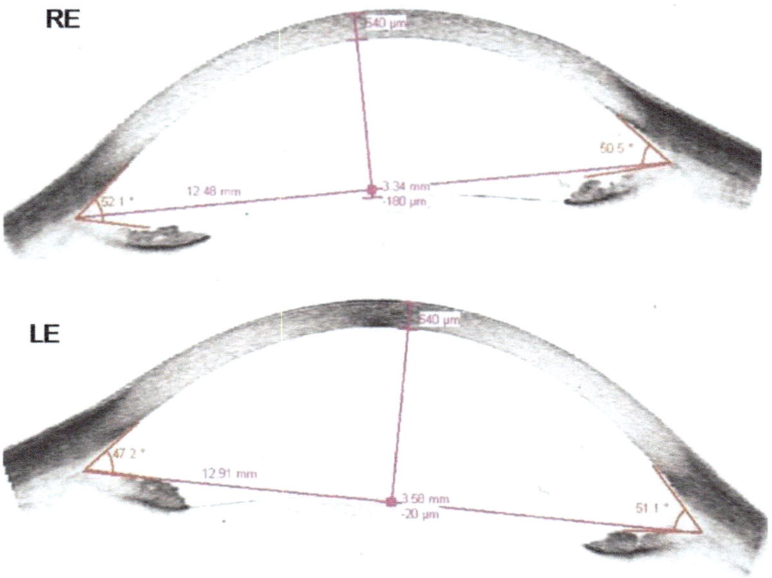

Fig. 84.1 OCT Visante and anterior chamber measurement in the right and left eye

quality vision, we decided to implant a posterior chamber phakic IOL. The endothelial cell count was 3,534 cell/mm^2 in the right eye and 3,344 cell/mm^2 in the left eye. Measurement of the anterior chamber was performed with the OCT Visante (Fig. 84.1). The anterior chamber depth was 3.34 mm and the width was 12.48 mm in the RE; anterior chamber depth was 3.51 mm and width was 12.91 mm in the LE. The TICL calculation software selected a lens power for the right eye of $-11+4\times93$ with a diameter of 13.2 mm and for the left eye a power of $-11.5+4.5\times99$ with a diameter of 13.2 mm. Calculating software guided the plan to implant the lens at 7° clockwise in the right eye and 19° clockwise in the left. Two days after implantation, the patient was not satisfied. She had a manifest refraction of $+1.5-3.5\times10$ in the right eye and $+0.75-2.50\times20$ in left. Her BCVA was 1 in both eyes. A slit lamp examination showed that the lenses were rotated based on the original plan. Both lenses were rotated at 30° clockwise and were replaced. However, at 2 weeks the patient again complained of foggy vision in the left eye. The slit lamp examination showed a new rotation at 30° clockwise. The lens was replaced and on the same day an autorefractometry was performed which showed emmetropia. The day after, the lens was again at 30°.

Main Problem to Solve

We had to determine why the lens implanted in the LE experienced recurrent rotation, even when the size of the IOL had been calculated according to the recommendations of STAAR.

Ancillary Tests

The most helpful tool to calculate the treatment was to repeat the measurement of the anterior chamber width through OCT Visante and IOL master Zeiss. Both instruments showed similar values.

Surgical/Medical Intervention

We decided to replace the lens with one of larger diameter. The TICL calculation software selected a lens power of $-11.5+4\times8$ and a diameter of 13.7 mm with the plan of explantation at 2° clockwise.

Outcome

After 2 months of the last treatment, the uncorrected visual acuity in both eyes was 20/20 and the marks of the lens indicating the axis of the

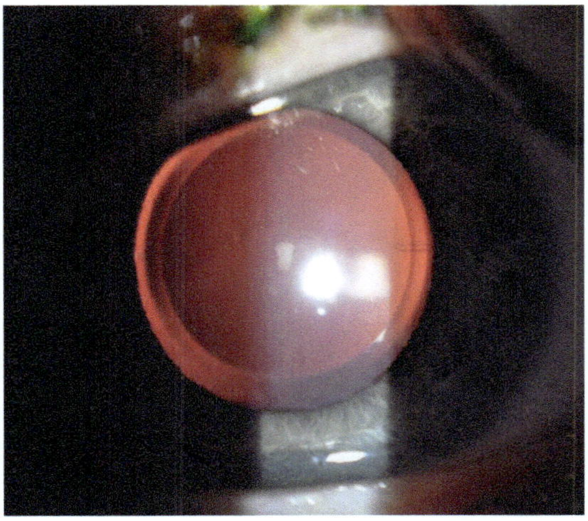

Fig. 84.2 Slit lamp examination showed lens alignment to the axis of astigmatism

astigmatism were aligned according to the desired orientation (Fig. 84.2).

What to Learn from This Case

A recent article [3] suggests that the sulcus diameter is the most important measure to obtain the best predictable postoperative vault height. One of the most difficult things about the phakic IOL implantation in the ciliary sulcus is estimating the correct distance between the sulci. New instruments such as the IOL master and OCT Visante can help size the PIOL implantation. In this case we had to use empirical algorithms to estimate the distance. Reinstein et al. [3] measured the sulcus diameter using Artemis 2 very high-frequency (VHF) digital ultrasound (ArcScan Inc.). Frequent misalignment of the lens is related to an inadequate sulcus diameter, with the only solution to change the lens.

References

1. Sanders DR, Schneider D, Martin R, Brown D, Dulaney D, Vukich J, Slade S, Schallhorn S (2007) Toric Implantable Collamer Lens for moderate to high myopic astigmatism. Ophthalmology 114:54–61
2. Park SC, Kwun YK, Chung ES, Ahn K, Chung TY (2009) Postoperative astigmatism and axis stability after implantation of the STAAR Toric Implantable Collamer Lens. J Refract Surg 25:403–409
3. Reinstein DZ, Lovisolo CF, Archer TJ, Gobbe M (2013) Comparison of postoperative vault height predictability using white-to-white or sulcus diameter-based sizing for the visian implantable collamer lens. J Refract Surg 29:30–35

ICL and Sequential Bilateral Pupillary Block

85

Jaime Javaloy and Alessandro Abbouda

Contents

J. Javaloy, MD, PhD (✉)
Department of Anterior Segment and Refractive Surgery, Vissum Corporacion Alicante, Alacant, Spain
e-mail: jjavaloy@coma.es

A. Abbouda, MD
Department of Refractive Surgery, Vissum Corporación Oftalmológica, Alicante, Spain

Department of Ophthalmology-Policlinico Umberto I of Rome, University of Rome "Sapienza", Viale del Policlinico, 155, 00186 Roma, Italy

R&D Department, Vissum Corporación Oftalmológica, 03016, Alicante, Spain
e-mail: a.abbouda@gmail.com

Why Is This Case Relevant for the Refractive Surgeon?

The refractive surgeon should be aware of the risk of pupillary block after Implantable Collamer Lens (ICL) implantation. If surgery before a neodymium:YAG (Nd:YAG) laser iridotomy is performed, the surgeon must be aware of the complete permeability of these iridotomies. The Visian Implantable Collamer Lens (ICL; STAAR Surgical) is a sulcus-placed, phakic, posterior chamber intraocular lens (PIOL) used to manage myopia, hyperopia, and myopic compound astigmatism in phakic patients [1, 2]. The ICL is designed to vault anteriorly to avoid contact with the crystalline lens. The vault is at risk of causing pupillary block; thus ICL surgery requires prophylactic placement of laser peripheral iridotomies. If the peripheral iridotomies are imperforate, pupillary-block angle closure can develop. Block can be treated with additional laser peripheral iridotomies [3, 4]. The new model of ICL surgery includes a small central hole to ensure adequate aqueous humor circulation, even in the absence of a peripheral iridotomy.

Case Background

A 38-year-old woman with bilateral myopic astigmatism presented for a refractive surgery evaluation. Her manifest refraction was $-8.75-1.25\times95$ in the right eye and $-11-1\times180$ in the left eye. Her

J.L. Alió et al. (eds.), *Difficult and Complicated Cases in Refractive Surgery*,
DOI 10.1007/978-3-642-55238-0_85, © Springer-Verlag Berlin Heidelberg 2015

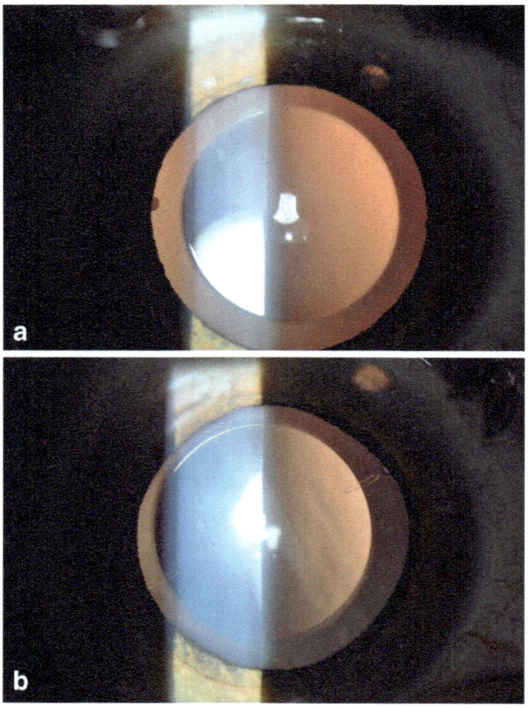

Fig. 85.1 The slit lamp examination at the end showed full iridotomy and normal vault in both eyes (**a**, **b**)

best corrected visual acuity (BCVA) was 20/20 in both eyes. Her preoperative central thickness was 491 μm in the right eye and 509 μm in the left eye. Her keratometry reading was 44.78/45.38 × 13 in the right eye and 45.36/45.36 × 180 in the left eye. Corneal topography showed asymmetric astigmatism with a KPI (keratoconus probability index elevated) pattern in both eyes. To avoid the risk of ectasia post-LASIK, we decided to implant a posterior chamber phakic IOL. The endothelial cell count was 2,646 cell/mm^2 in the right eye and 2,208 cell/mm^2 in the left eye. Measurement of the anterior chamber was performed with the OCT-Visante (Fig. 85.1). The anterior chamber depth was 3.3 mm and the width was 11.6 mm in the right eye; the anterior chamber depth was 3.3 mm and the width was 11.8 mm in the left eye. The TICL calculation software selected a lens power for the right eye of −8.5 − 1.25 × 90 with a diameter of 12.6 mm and for the left eye a power of −10.5 − 1 × 180 with a diameter of 12.6 mm. The model implanted was ICM, STAAR Surgical lens. The implant was uneventful under local anesthesia and a peripheral iridotomy was performed in both eyes at 7 h.

On the first day after surgery, the patient complained of headache, nausea, and low vision in the left eye. The intraocular pressure (IOP) in the LE was 32 mmHg. A slit lamp examination revealed shallow anterior chamber and a partial thickness iridotomy which did not include the pigmentary epithelium. This peak of IOP was successfully treated, as described later. The right eye had a wide pharmacologic mydriasis and IOP of 8 mmHg the first day, but the next day the IOP was 30 mmHg. Slit lamp examination of the RE the second day was comparable to that of the LE the previous day.

Main Problem to Solve

Angle closure in the context of a shallow anterior chamber following the ICL placement has at least three possible etiologies: (1) Malignant glaucoma: the crystalline lens is displaced anteriorly and the space between the ICL and the anterior capsule is diminished or absent. The anterior chamber is shallow. (2) Pupillary block: Result of imperforate peripheral iridotomies. The chamber is shallow and lens vaulting is exaggerated. (3) Angle closure occurs secondary to direct angle compression from oversized and excessively vaulted ICLs.

Ancillary Tests

Slit lamp examination, OCT, and a record of the IOP are used to manage this situation. Pupil dilation and observation over 12–24 h can differentiate these three conditions [4]. If dilation results in immediate deepening of the anterior chamber and a reduction in the IOP, phakic PC IOL pupillary block is present. On the contrary, an oversized phakic PC IOL does not permit anterior chamber deepening after mydriasis. Posterior chamber viscoelastic block resolves over 12–24 h as the viscoelastic material vacates the posterior chamber. Anterior segment OCT helps in diagnosis. Malignant glaucoma is evident if there is no space between the crystalline lens and ICL. Pupillary block is present if there is a large space between the crystalline lens and ICL. High ICL vaulting occurs with marked anterior displacement of the iris.

Surgical/Medical Intervention

Slit lamp examination revealed that the peripheral iridotomy was not appropriately thick; each iridotomy was completed with a neodymium:YAG (Nd:YAG) laser under high power. YAG laser treatment was applied over the pigmentary epithelium. A single burst of 3.0 mJ was enough to perforate the pigmentary epithelium. A flow of aqueous from the posterior to anterior chamber occurred instantly upon penetration of the iris pigment epithelium, with immediate deepening of the peripheral anterior chamber and normalization of the ICL vault. Oral acetazolamide and brimonidine tartrate/timolol maleate drops 2 times a day were prescribed.

Outcome

Three months after surgery, the patient's visual acuity was 20/20 in both eyes. The slit lamp examination revealed a normal anterior segment (Fig. 85.1).

What to Learn from This Case

Pupillary block and cataract formation are potential complications of all phakic IOLs. Pupillary block after phakic PC IOL implantation can occur despite the presence of incomplete peripheral iridotomies if they do not include the full thickness of the iris [4]. In our case, the persistence of a wide mydriasis in the first visit prevented elevation of the IOP in the first 24 h. The key clinical feature of phakic PC IOL pupillary block, which distinguishes it from malignant glaucoma, is the absence of a forward displacement of the crystalline lens.

References

1. Sanders DR, Vukich JA, Doney K, Gaston M, Implantable Contact Lens in Treatment of Myopia Study Group (2003) U.S. Food and Drug Administration clinical trial of the Implantable Contact Lens for moderate to high myopia. Ophthalmology 110:255–266
2. Huang D, Schallhorn SC, Sugar A, Farjo AA, Majmudar PA, Trattler WB, Tanzer DJ (2009) Phakic intraocular lens implantation for the correction of myopia: a report by the American Academy of Ophthalmology. Ophthalmology 116:2244–2258
3. Apel A, Stephensen D (2007) Surgical management of acute angleclosure glaucoma after toric ICL implantation. J Cataract Refract Surg 33:1672
4. Bylsma SS, Zalta AH, Foley E, Osher RH (2002) Phakic posterior chamber intraocular lens pupillary block. J Cataract Refract Surg 28:2222–2228

Complications of Phakic Intraocular Lenses: Refractive Lens Exchange and Piggyback

86

Jorge L. Alió, Dominika Wróbel, and Alessandro Abbouda

Contents

J.L. Alió, MD, PhD (✉)
Department of Refractive Surgery, Vissum Corporación Oftalmológica, Alicante, Spain
e-mail: jlalio@vissum.com

D. Wróbel, MD
Glaucoma Diagnostic and Microsurgery Department, Medical University of Lublin, Lublin, Poland

R&D Department, Vissum Corporacion, Alicante, Spain
e-mail: ddudzinska@interia.pl

A. Abbouda, MD
Department of Refractive Surgery, Vissum Corporación Oftalmológica, Alicante, Spain

Department of Ophthalmology-Policlinico Umberto I of Rome, University of Rome "Sapienza", Viale del Policlinico, 155, 00186 Roma, Italy

R&D Department, Vissum Corporación Oftalmológica, 03016, Alicante, Spain
e-mail: a.abbouda@gmail.com

Why Is This Case Relevant for the Refractive Surgeon?

Radial keratotomy in myopic patients may induce severe hyperopic shift, which can be corrected with hyperopic laser in situ keratomileusis. Moreover, postoperative unexpected hyperopia can occur after cataract surgery in eyes that underwent previous keratorefractive surgery. It is very important to understand the mechanism of hyperopic refractive error after cataract surgery in order to choose a reliable method for accurate IOL power calculation.

The refractive surgeon should be aware of three options to correct residual refractive ametropia. The first option is cornea refractive surgery; however, this was not useful in our case because of coexisting abnormal topography and higher-order aberrations. Another option is IOL exchange, although it has relevant complications. The third possibility is a piggyback IOL placement that seems to be a reliable and relatively easier strategy to correct residual refraction [1–5].

Case Background

A 62-year-old woman presented for refractive and cataract surgeries.

The patient preferred to undergo bilateral radial keratotomy for high myopia, with −8.0 diopters (D) in the right eye and −6.0 D in the left eye, 14 years ago. Hyperopic laser in situ keratomileusis

J.L. Alió et al. (eds.), *Difficult and Complicated Cases in Refractive Surgery*,
DOI 10.1007/978-3-642-55238-0_86,

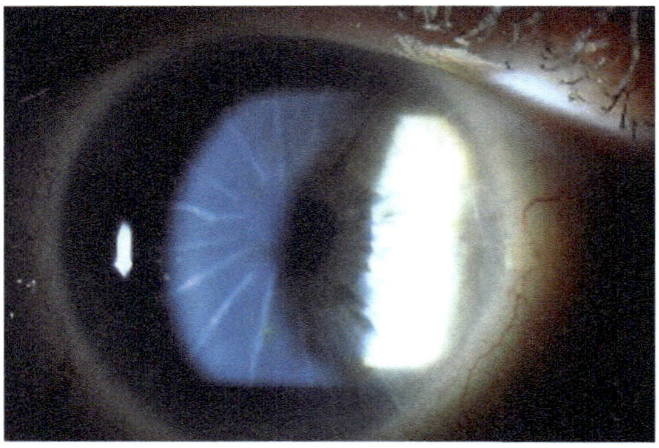

Fig. 86.1 Patient's eye after radial keratotomy and cataract surgery

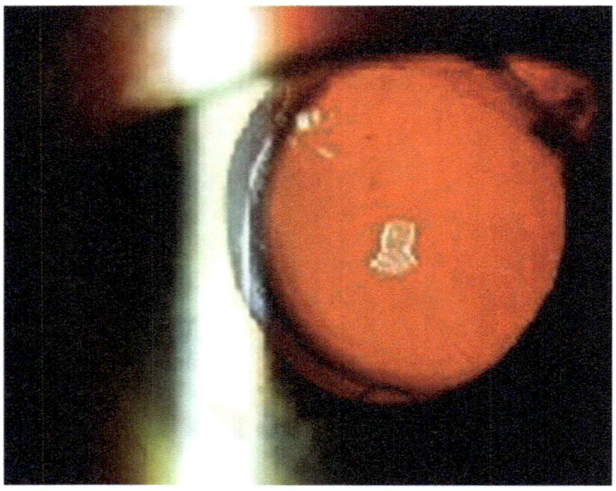

Fig. 86.2 Slit lamp examination showing piggyback lens

(H-LASIK) was then performed for consecutive hyperopia (Fig. 86.1).

Visual acuity improved after the refractive procedures only for a short period of time. In 2009, the woman presented to our department complaining of deteriorating vision.

The patient's manifest refraction was +2.50 in the right eye (RE) and −1.00 160° in the left eye (LE). Her best corrected visual acuity (BCVA) was 20/32 in the right eye and 20/25 in the left eye. Uncorrected visual acuity (UCVA) was 20/63 in the right eye and 20/50 in the left eye. Slit lamp examination revealed 16 deep corneal incisions, no epithelial defects at the flap edge, a clear interface, and a well-positioned flap. Cataracts were diagnosed in both eyes. Fundus examinations were normal. Intraocular pressure (IOP) was 12 mmHg in both eyes.

The topography showed an irregular and flattening cornea surface in the right eye (K1 35.74/36.78 × 22°) and flattening surface in the left eye (K1 35.67/36.25 × 104°). Total cornea aberration was higher, at RMS 5.02 μm. Trefoils and coma aberrations were prevalent in both eyes. The patient's right eye pachymetry was 518 μm and her left eye pachymetry was 508 μm.

After 1 year, the patient underwent uneventful cataract surgeries (with a monthly interval between the right and the left eye) with implantation of Oculentis LS-312MF15 lenses.

Calculation using Aramberri double-K modified formula selected a lens power of +22.0 D for the right eye and +19.0 D for the left eye. Postoperative treatment was ciprofloxacin (Oftacilox® Alcon) one drop three times a day for 7 days and dexamethasone (Maxidex® Alcon) one drop three times a day for 15 days. Postoperative evaluation of the right eye was normal. The slit lamp examination showed no anomalies; the lens was centered and the IOP was normal.

At 3 months, the slit lamp examination showed no anomalies and no changes in cornea, and the lenses were centered. The IOP was 12 mmHg in both eyes. BCVA was 20/25 with +1.0 D in the right eye and 20/20 with +2.00 − 1.25 15° in the left eye.

At 6 months, the refractive surprise was stable. The patient's refraction was +0.75 − 0.50 65° in the right eye and +2.00 − 1.00 15° in the left eye. Uncorrected visual acuity (UCVA) was 20/32 in the right eye and 20/50 in the left eye. The patient's BCVA was 20/32 for distance in the right eye and BCVA 20/20 in the left eye. Slit lamp, IOP, and fundus examinations were normal.

The patient's expectations were not satisfied. Therefore, a wavefront examination and topography were performed. The topography of both eyes did not show any differences in relation to the previous one. ORK wavefront analysis showed a value of total aberration of RMS 1.72 μm, and the index of high order of aberration (HOA) was 1.37 μm.

There were no contraindications to implant a piggyback IOL (no pigment dispersion, no glaucoma, no pseudoexfoliation, and no trauma). The lens calculation software selected a lens power of +2.0 D for the left eye (using Holladay formula). The lens Alcon AcrySof MA60MA was implanted in the ciliary sulcus (Fig. 86.2), which was uneventful. Postoperative treatment was the same as the previous. Postoperative recovery was normal.

Main Problem to Solve

RK treatment is commonly associated with hyperopic shift and is not a stable treatment.

Changes in the cornea occur over time, making a definite solution difficult. The main problem we were presented with was how to manage an unsatisfactory postoperative refraction in a patient who had undergone previous refractive procedures.

Ancillary Tests

Best corrected visual acuity (BCVA), uncorrected visual acuity (UCVA), manifest and cycloplegic refraction, slit lamp biomicroscopy, applanation tonometry fundus examination, corneal topography, pachymetry, IOL biometry, keratometry, and ORK wavefront examination.

Surgical/Medical Intervention

The patient underwent bilateral radial keratotomy in 1999, with the hyperopic shift treated by LASIK. With the appearance of cataracts in both eyes, the patient underwent cataract surgeries with the implantation of Oculentis LS-312MF 15 lenses in the posterior chamber. A historical method was used for the IOL calculation. Six months after previous surgery, residual refractive error in the patient's left eye was corrected by secondary piggyback implantation lens (Alcon AcrySof MA60MA).

Outcome

After 1 year, manifest refraction in the patient's left eye was +0.50 D. Corrected distance visual acuity (CDVA) was 20/20 in the left eye. The postoperative evaluation was normal and the slit lamp examination showed no anomalies.

What to Learn from This Case

It is very challenging to predict the refractive outcome after cataract surgery in patients with prior refractive procedures. The success of radial keratotomy in myopic patients is not guaranteed, with many reports that this method may induce severe unexpected hyperopic shift. H-LASIK can be used to correct RK-induced hyperopia. Piggyback IOL is the best choice to correct residual refractive errors in eyes with a previous history of refractive and cataract surgeries. Piggyback IOL has minimal risk, excellent refractive predictability, and rapid visual rehabilitation.

References

1. Habor-Wilner Z, Sachs D (2005) Refractive results with secondary piggyback implantation to correct pseudophakic refractive errors. J Cataract Refract Surg 31:2101–2103
2. DeMill DL, Hsu M (2011) Evaluation of the American Society of Cataract and Refractive Surgery intraocular lens calculator for eyes with prior radial keratotomy. Clin Ophthalmol 5:1243–1247
3. Francesconi CM, Nosé RAM (2000) Hyperopic laser-assisted in situ keratomileusis for radial keratotomy induced hyperopia the annual meeting of the American Academy of Ophthalmology, Dallas
4. Gayton JL, Sanders V, Van Der Karr M et al (1999) Piggybacking intraocular implants to correct pseudophakic refractive error. Ophthalmology 106:56–59
5. Rubenstein JB (2012) Piggyback IOLs for residual refractive error after cataract surgery. Cataract Refract Surg Today. http://bmctoday.net/crstoday/2012/08/article.asp?f=piggyback-iols-for-residual-refractive-error-after-cataract-surgery

Part VIII

Corneal Cross-Linking Complications

Dear reader,

Corneal cross-linking (CXL) has gained worldwide popularity over the past several years as an effective treatment that strengthens the cornea and reduces the progression of corneal ectatic disorders. CXL's ability to impede keratoconus indicates its relevance for children, although application is controversial.

Although the long-term complications of CXL have not been studied extensively, reports of several short-term complications have been documented, including postoperative infection/ulcer and stromal haze. In addition to keratoconus, corneal cross-linking may be used to correct iatrogenic keratectasia secondary to LASIK, in treating corneal melt, or as an adjunct therapy in intrastromal ring implantation. Some researchers have also proposed an adjunctive role for CXL in the treatment of corneal infection because the procedure enhances corneal resistance against enzymatic degradation.

In this section, we report some of the complications and limitations of CXL, including haze, infection, and Acanthamoeba keratitis, considerations of delayed wounding, and use in pediatrics. Evaluating short and long-term consequences of CXL is important in understanding how best to apply the treatment to patients.

Specific topics covered by the cases include a new and interesting way to manage the haze after CXL (Case 89) and how to manage infection post-CXL (Case 90). Other cases cover how corneal collagen cross-linking may allow surface refractive surgery several years posttreatment (Case 91) and the new use of CXL in infectious keratitis (Case 92). We end with cases focused on what to do when epithelial growth after CXL is delayed (Case 93) and CXL use in the progression of keratoconus in children (Case 94).

Lesson to Learn

Case 89: Treating haze with corneal cross-linking

The accelerated transepithelial cross-linking can be a new tool for corneal haze following cross-linking treatments probably because it is more stromal compared to the classical haze post PRK which is mainly fibrotic.

Case 90: Infection post-corneal collagen cross-linking

This case illustrates the risk for microbial keratitis after CXL with riboflavin–UVA and emphasizes the need for a surgical procedure conducted under sterile techniques.

Haze

87

Roberto Pinelli

Contents

Why Is This Case Relevant for the Refractive Surgeon?

The technique of choice for the treatment of corneal haze following refractive surgery through excimer laser [1] is phototerapeutic keratectomy (PTK) implying the application of mitomycin C. However, in this case we decided to treat haze after epithelium-off corneal cross-linking (CXL) with a transepithelial CXL treatment because of the following considerations:

- PTK's use of epithelium scraping may not be suitable for keratoconus cases due to the natural irregularity of corneal surface and the subsequent risk of irregular epithelium regrowth after surface scraping [2].
- Following epithelium-off CXL, the corneal haze reported in this clinical case was characterized by stromal opacity and a regular epithelial surface, which is not typical in haze cases after refractive surgery.
- The undamaged epithelium appearance was receptive to osmosis [3].

Case Background

One year after having undergone a traditional epithelium-off CXL treatment in another clinic – where an initial diagnosis of keratoconus in the LE was made – a patient arrived at our center complaining of blurred and distorted vision. According to the patient, the visual problems

R. Pinelli, MD
ILMO Istituto Laser Microchirurgia Oculare, Brescia, Italy
e-mail: pinelli@ilmo.it

J.L. Alió et al. (eds.), *Difficult and Complicated Cases in Refractive Surgery*,
DOI 10.1007/978-3-642-55238-0_87, © Springer-Verlag Berlin Heidelberg 2015

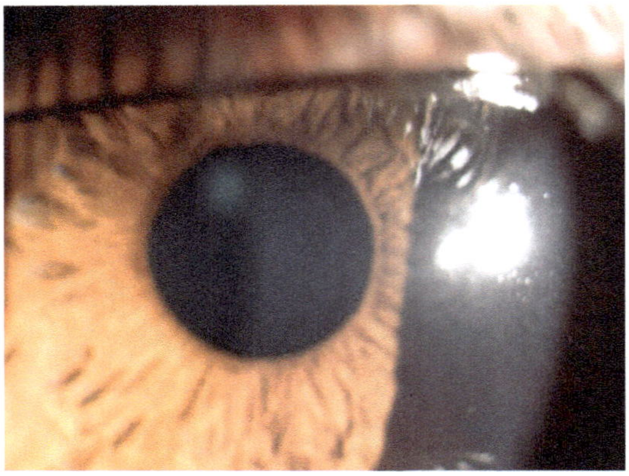

Fig. 87.1 Visible corneal haze at preop slit-lamp examination

started during the postoperative settlement right after the traditional cross-linking treatment.

Main Problem to Solve

During the preoperative assessment, an accurate slit-lamp examination confirmed the presence of corneal haze in the LE (Fig. 87.1). It is our understanding that this unexpected event arose as a postoperative complication following the traditional cross-linking procedure.

Preop Data Were as Follows

LE: UCVA 20/100; BCVA 20/50 corrected sph −1.00 cyl −2.25 ax 165°

Ancillary Tests

Traditional epi-off is a standard treatment for keratoconus cases [4]. However, if we consider that after the initial treatment the LE pachymetry value was 440 μm, traditional haze removal – involving further corneal desepithelisation and mitomycin C treatment (0.01 mg/ml, 60 s) – was not considered the best way to proceed.

In order to reduce halos and improve the overall quality of vision, osmotic accelerated transepithelial cross-linking was offered as the most suitable choice. Its features including quickness, noninvasivity, and absence of pain were particularly attractive to the patient.

No other solutions seemed able to reduce haze, increase BCVA, and improve corneal transparency, like the transepithelial approach (Fig. 87.3).

Surgical/Medical Intervention

The accelerated transepithelial cross-linking was performed by combining ParaCel osmotic riboflavin and high-intensity UVA rays. ParaCel is a transepithelial osmotic riboflavin solution produced by Avedro, Inc. (Waltham, MA), based on the osmotic properties of the corneal epithelium. The KXL system, produced by the same company, produces high-density ultraviolet light rays directed toward the treated cornea.

The transepithelial accelerated CXL application protocol of choice was the following:

- Instillation of 2 preservative-free proparacaine drops
- Application of 2 ParaCel drops
- Soak for 4 min, applying 1 drop of ParaCel every 30 s during soaking
- UVA irradiation with using the KXL device for 2 min 40 s at 45 mW/cm^2, instilling 1 drop of ParaCel every 20 s
- Instillation of 1–2 additional drops of proparacaine during irradiation
- Complete rinsing of the eye with artificial tears

Outcome

The postop visual assessment at 1 month confirmed the following data:

LE: UCVA 20/80; BCVA 20/40 corrected sph −1.00 cyl −2.25 ax 172°

The slit-lamp examination confirmed a decrease of corneal haze (Fig. 87.2), as well as an overall reduction of K values (Fig. 87.3), both of which led to improved BCVA and improved corneal transparency

At 6-month postop, a new assessment delivered the following data:

LE: UCVA 20/80; BCVA 20/32 corrected sph −1.50 cyl −1.50 ax 170°

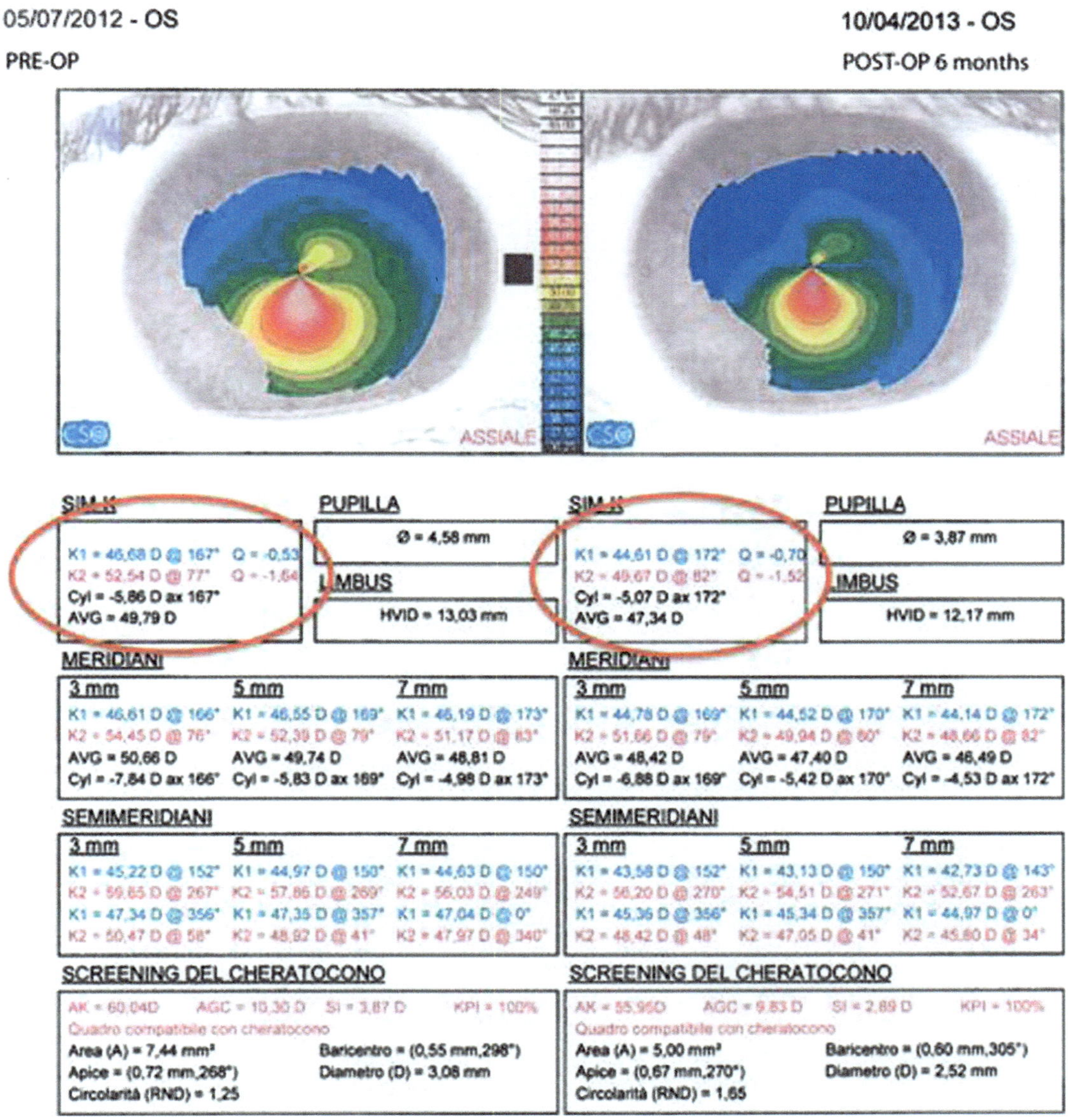

Fig. 87.2 Slit-lamp examination at 1-month postop

A new slit-lamp examination showed further improved corneal transparency (Fig. 87.4) and improved BCVA via reduced K values (Fig. 87.5).

What to Learn from This Case

Results show that accelerated transepithelial cross-linking is an acceptable choice for corneal haze cases following traditional cross-linking treatments [5]. Haze post cross-linking is more stromal compared to classical haze post-PRK which is mainly fibrotic. Transepithelial cross-linking may be effective because it respects the epithelium which is an osmotic membrane; through it, haze reduction may be a reestablishment of collagen parallelism and consequentially corneal transparency. Reduced haze, improved corneal transparency, and improved BCVA and UCVA are all positive outcomes noted; however, more data is needed to support this treatment.

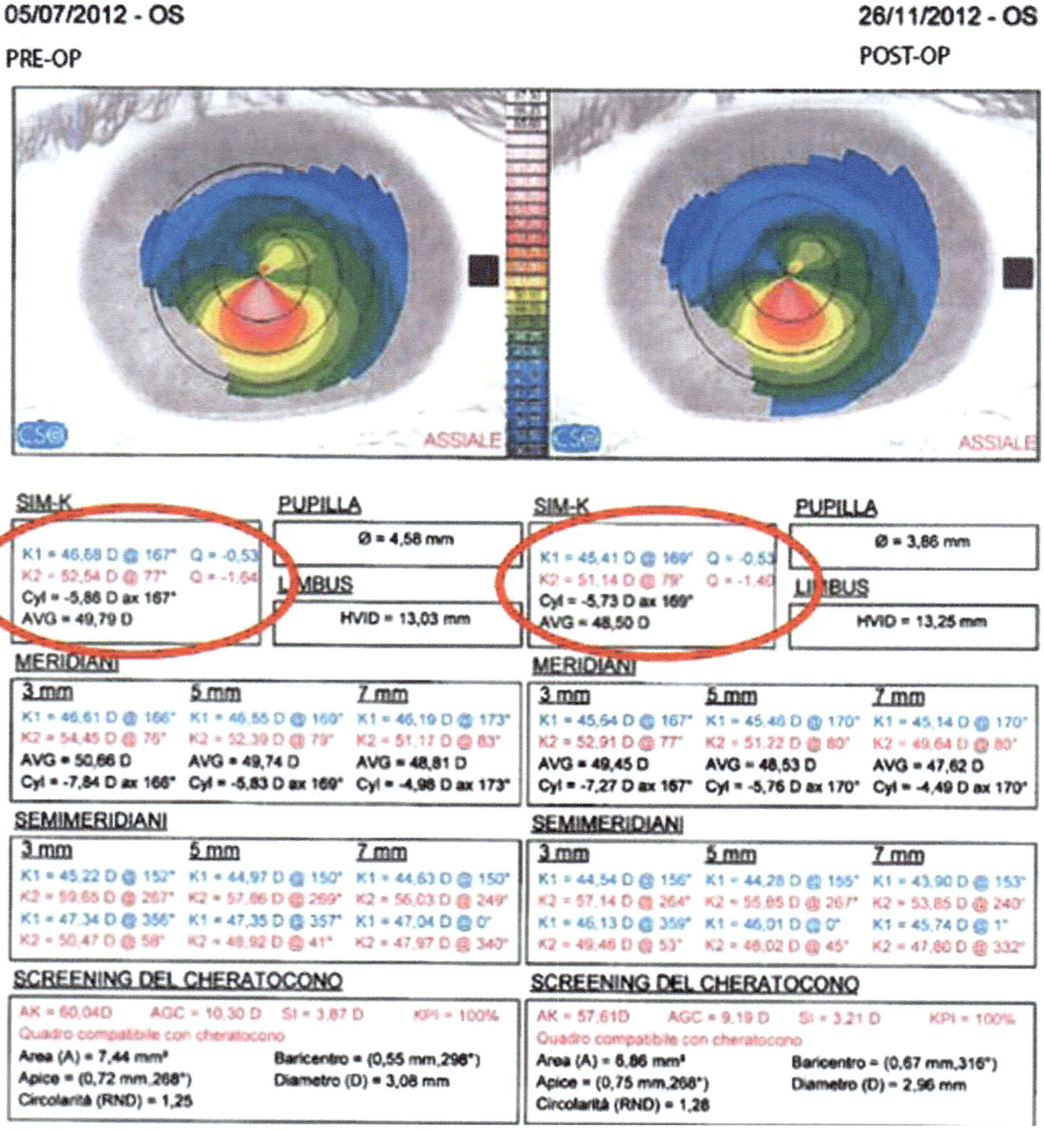

Fig. 87.3 Preop and 1-month postop corneal topography

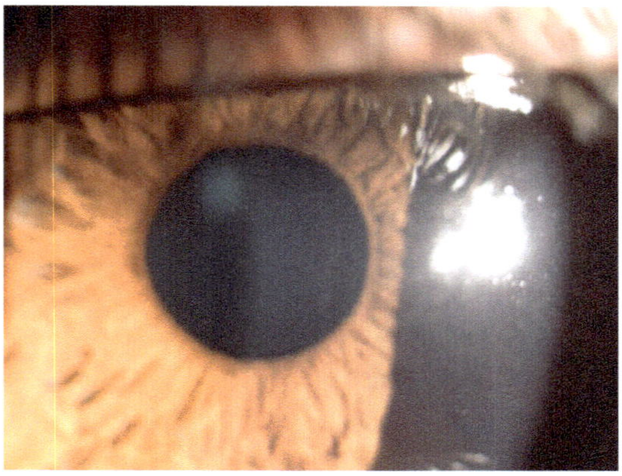

Fig. 87.4 Slit-lamp examination at 6-month postop

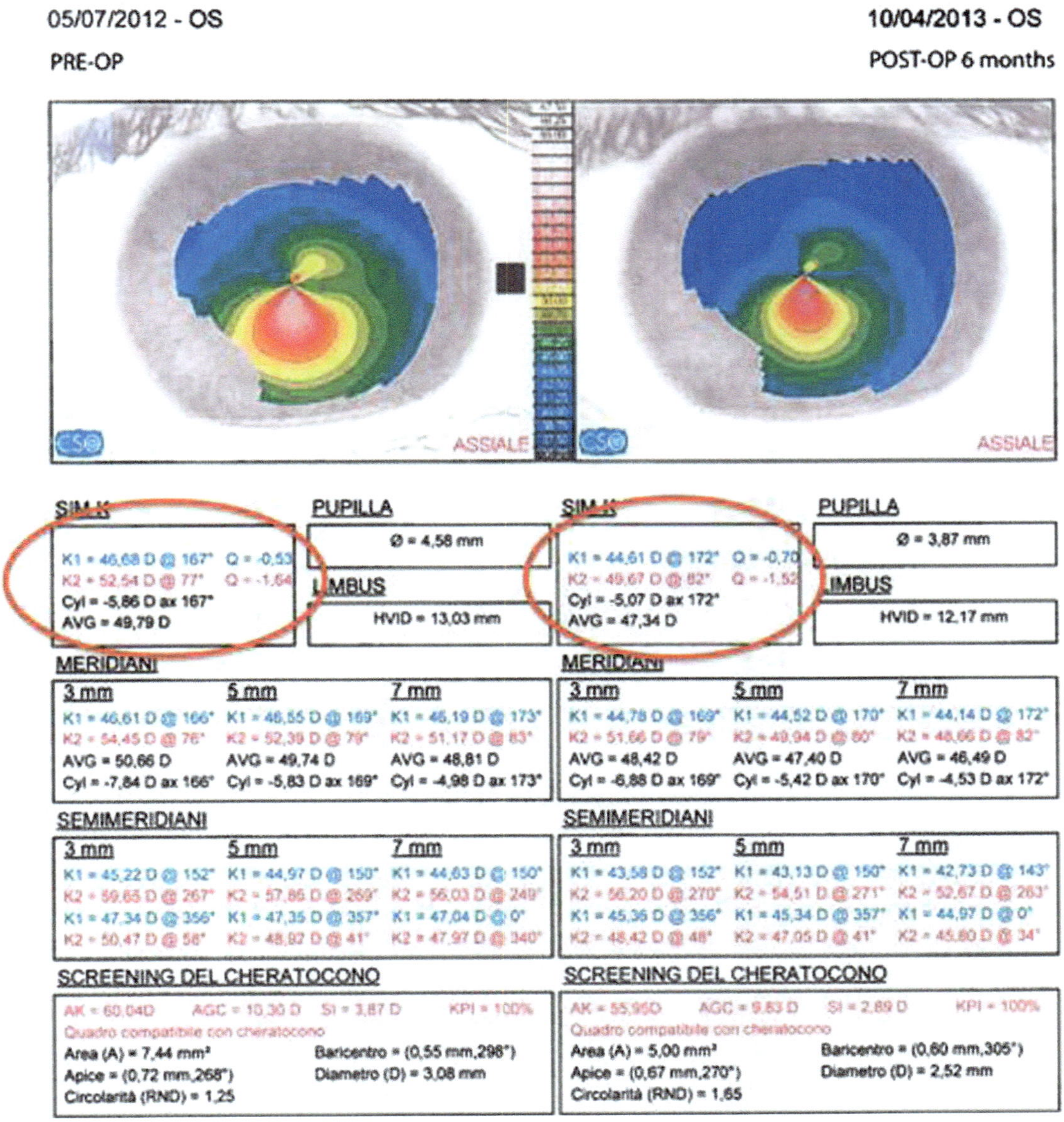

Fig. 87.5 Preop and 6-month postop corneal topography

References

1. Porges Y et al (2003) Phototerapeutic keratectomy with mytomicin C for corneal haze following photorefractive keratectomy for myopia. J Refract Surg 19: 40–43
2. Hersh PS et al (1996) Excimer laser phototerapeutic keratectomy. Ophthalmology 103:1210–1222
3. Raiskup F, Pinelli R, Spoerl H (2012) Riboflavin osmolar modification for transepithelial corneal crosslinking. Curr Eye Res 37:234–238
4. Kanellopoulos AJ (2009) Collagen cross-linking in early keratoconus with riboflavin in a femtosecond laser-created pocket: initial clinical results. J Refract Surg 25:1034–1037
5. Boxer Wachler BS, Pinelli R, Ertan A, Chan CC (2010) Safety and efficacy of transepithelial crosslinking (C3-R/CXL) [letter]. J Cataract Refract Surg 36:186–818; author reply 188–189

Microbial Keratitis After Corneal Collagen Cross-Linking

88

Alberto Artola

Contents

A. Artola, MD, PhD
Department of Surgery, Oftalmar Medimar Hospital Internacional, Universidad Miguel Hernández De Elche, Elche, Spain
e-mail: alberto.artola@umh.es; albertoartola@coma.es

Why Is This Case Relevant for the Refractive Surgeon?

Collagen cross-linking with riboflavin–UVA is a minimally invasive method. However, a refractive surgeon should be aware of its use on epithelial removal, which can be a predisposing factor for bacterial keratitis.

Case Background

A 29-year-old woman was referred to our clinic in February 2008 for correction of progressive keratoconus. She did not have general health problems but was unable to wear contact lenses. Her best spectacle-corrected visual acuity (BSCVA) was 20/25 in the right eye (RE) and 20/32 in the left eye (LE), and her manifest refraction was −0.25 − 0.25 × 125 in the RE and −1.00 × 120 in the LE. Biomicroscopy results of the anterior segment were normal for the right eye; light Vogt striae were observed in the left eye. Intraocular pressure was 12 mmHg in each eye. Ophthalmoscopy revealed normal fundus in both eyes. Corneal thickness, measured with ultrasonic pachymetry (DGH-500 pachymeter, DGH Technology), was 450 and 430 μm in the right eye and left eye, respectively. Videokeratography showed a pattern consistent with keratoconus in both eyes (asymmetric bow-tie with skewing of the radial axis above and below the horizontal meridian and inferonasal

J.L. Alió et al. (eds.), *Difficult and Complicated Cases in Refractive Surgery*,
DOI 10.1007/978-3-642-55238-0_88, © Springer-Verlag Berlin Heidelberg 2015

steepening). The videokeratography-derived indices keratometry (K) (central K-reading) and inferior–superior (I–S) dioptric asymmetry were 47 diopters (D) and 2.3 D, respectively, in the right eye and 51.2 D and the 4.1 D, respectively, in the left eye. Based on these data, Krumeich stage 1 keratoconus was diagnosed in the right eye and Krumeich stage 2 keratoconus was diagnosed in the left eye.

The patient was scheduled for CXL with riboflavin–UVA light in the right eye and intracorneal ring segment implantation in the left eye. The risks of the surgery were fully explained to the patient in accordance with the Declaration of Helsinki. In March 2008, uneventful intracorneal ring segment implantation (Ferrara ring, Mediphacos) was performed in the left eye after a stromal tunnel was created with a femtosecond laser (IntraLaser Corp.). Three months after surgery, the uncorrected visual acuity (UCVA) was 20/20, the manifest refraction was −0.25 × 130, and the cornea was clear and quiet under biomicroscopy.

In April 2008, the patient had CXL with riboflavin–UVA in the right eye. The surgical procedure was conducted under sterile techniques using topical anesthesia of oxybuprocaine 0.4 %, 1 drop every 10 min twice before surgery. After the patient was placed under the operating microscope, an 8.5 mm circle was traced on the epithelium with a corneal marker, and the epithelium within the circle was removed with a blunt spatula. This was followed by instillation of four drops of a solution containing riboflavin 0.1 % and dextran 20 % (Ricrolin) for approximately 10 min. The penetration of the cornea and the presence of riboflavin in the anterior chamber (riboflavin shielding) were monitored by slit lamp examination. After 2–4 additional drops of the riboflavin solution were instilled, the UV lamp was turned on to irradiate an 8.0 mm diameter of the central cornea. Riboflavin 0.1 % solution was applied every 5 min during the irradiation. The UV (wavelength 370 nm) source was a solid-state device consisting of 1 UV diode (Vega X linker, Compagnia Strumenti Oftalmici). The source was focused on the apex of the cornea at a distance of 50 mm to obtain a radiant energy of 3 mW/cm^2. The cornea was irradiated with the UVA diode for 30 min.

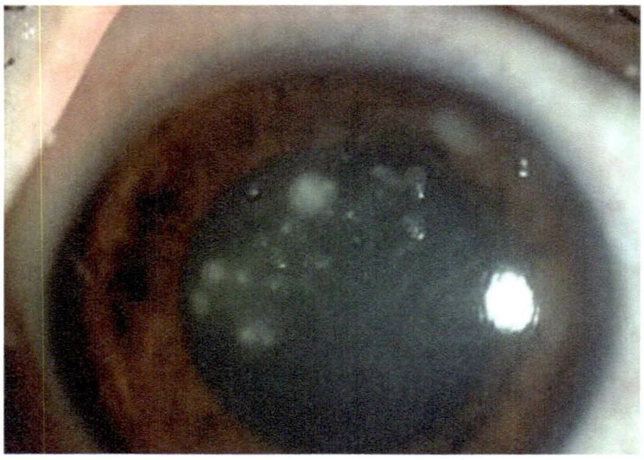

Fig. 88.1 Right eye slit lamp photograph showing four well-defined, gray-white stromal infiltrates surrounded by small satellite lesions in the upper midperipheral cornea 4 days after CXL with riboflavin (Fig. 88.2)

After treatment, the eye surface was washed with 20 mL balanced salt solution, medicated with two drops of ciprofloxacin (Oftacilox) and two drops of cyclopentolate (Ciclopléjico), and dressed with a soft contact lens (Focus NIGHT & DAY, CIBA VISION). After the procedure, the patient was given paracetamol–codeine (500/30 mg) every 8 h for 2 days, cyclopentolate eyedrops three times a day for 2 days, and ciprofloxacin eyedrops four times a day for 5 days. At the first follow-up visit 2 days after surgery, the patient complained of photophobia and blurriness in the right eye. Slit lamp examination revealed ciliary injection and four well-defined white nodules surrounded by small satellite lesions and hazy stromal infiltrate in the upper midperipheral cornea (Fig. 88.1). Epithelial defects were present overlying the corneal infiltrates and in the central cornea due to epithelial repair. The anterior chamber reaction was mild.

Main Problem to Solve

The problem we faced was early diagnosis and treatment of microbial keratitis after CXL.

Ancillary Tests

The corneal samples were placed on a microscope slide for Gram staining; on blood, chocolate, and MacConkey agar and thioglycolate broth for bacterial culture; and on Sabouraud agar for fungal culture.

Surgical/Medical Intervention

The smears revealed no microorganisms, but hourly topical fortified cefazolin (50 mg/mL) and topical fortified tobramycin (15 mg/mL) were started on the same day. Cultures were subsequently (after 48 h of incubation) positive for *Staphylococcus epidermidis*. The organisms were identified based on their morphology, stain features, ability to produce catalase, inability to produce coagulase, and antibiotic susceptibility to novobiocin. Twenty-four hours after organism identification, an antibiotic-sensitivity test (Kirby-Bauer disk-diffusion method) showed that the isolated organism was sensitive to tobramycin/gentamicin, fluoroquinolones, and vancomycin but resistant to cefazolin. The treatment regimen was then changed to topical ofloxacin 0.3 % (Exocin) and topical fortified tobramycin (15 mg/mL), which were given at 1 h intervals around the clock for 2 days and decreased to 2 h intervals for 5 days.

Outcome

The patient's condition improved rapidly, with regression of the ocular inflammation and corneal infiltrates, and topical antibiotic agents were reduced to four times a day for two more weeks. One week after the antibiotic-sensitivity test, topical fluorometholone 0.10 % (FML) three times a day was added to the antibiotic regimen. One month after CXL, an eye examination revealed moderate leucomas surrounded by stromal haze in the upper midperipheral cornea. Topical fluorometholone was continued twice a day for an additional month. Five months after the treatment, the UCVA in the right eye was 20/32 and the BSCVA was 20/22. The postoperative refraction was +1.00−2.50×40. Slit lamp examination disclosed a mild haze in the upper midperipheral area (Fig. 88.2), and the central corneal thickness was 405 μm.

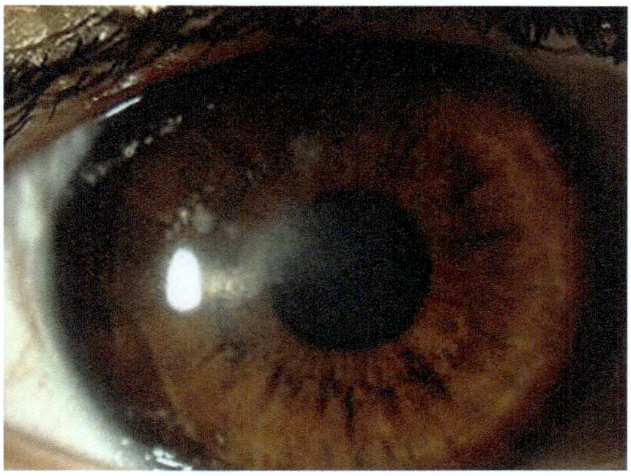

Fig. 88.2 Slit lamp view of the right eye showing mild haze in the upper midperipheral cornea 5 months after treatment

What to Learn from This Case

This case illustrates the risk of microbial keratitis after CXL that employs riboflavin–UVA for the treatment of keratoconus. The case also emphasizes the need for surgical procedure conducted under sterile techniques. Infections are a risk especially considering postoperative contamination, contact lens use, a long recovery time, and the teratogenic effects of UV that weaken local host defenses. Postoperative surveillance and postoperative topical antibiotic agents are important in providing the best results for patients who elect for this keratoconus treatment.

References

1. Perez-Santonja JJ, Artola A, Javaloy J, Alio JL, Abad JL (2009) Microbial keratitis after corneal collagen crosslinking. J Cataract Refract Surg 35:1138–1140

2. Colin J, Velou S (2003) Current surgical options for keratoconus. J Cataract Refract Surg 29:379–386
3. Wollensak G, Spoerl E, Seiler T (2003) Riboflavin/ultraviolet-A-induced collagen crosslinking for the treatment of keratoconus. Am J Ophthalmol 135:620–627
4. Caporossi A, Baiocchi S, Mazzotta C, Traversi C, Caporossi T (2006) Parasurgical therapy for keratoconus by riboflavin-ultraviolet type A rays induced cross-linking of corneal collagen; preliminary refractive results in an Italian study. J Cataract Refract Surg 32:837–845
5. Raiskup-Wolf F, Hoyer A, Spoerl E, Pillunat LE (2008) Collagen crosslinking with riboflavin and ultraviolet-A light in keratoconus: long-term results. J Cataract Refract Surg 34:796–801

Limitations of PRK After ICRS and Corneal Collagen Cross-Linking for Keratoconus

89

Kaitlyn Wallace and Dimitri Azar

Contents

K. Wallace (✉)
UIC Department of Ophthalmology and Visual Sciences, Illinois Eye and Ear Infirmary, Chicago, IL, USA
e-mail: kaitlyn.m.wallace@gmail.com

D. Azar, MD, MBA
Department of Ophthalmology, Pharmacology and Bioengineering, College of Medicine, University of Illinois at Chicago, Chicago, IL, USA
e-mail: dazar@uic.edu

Why Is This Case Relevant for the Refractive Surgeon?

Corneal collagen cross-linking (CXL) is an emerging treatment in slowing the progression of keratectasia in patients with keratoconus (KCN) [1]. Today, there are over 40 clinical trials under way that involve CXL and KCN. With current estimates that 10–15 % of KCN patients will need penetrating keratoplasty (PKP) in their lifetime [2], many patients hope that treatments such as CXL will reduce the likelihood of requiring future PKP. It is postulated that CXL may allow surface photorefractive keratectomy (PRK) to correct the refractive error following CXL.

Here we present the complicated clinical course of a woman with KCN who previously underwent intracorneal ring segment (ICRS) and collagen cross-linking (CXL). The patient underwent PRK OS, but the postoperative refraction was not stable. It is essential for the refractive surgeon to be aware that corneal collagen cross-linking may not preclude the possibility of surface refractive surgery several years posttreatment.

As demonstrated in this case, CXL for KCN did not sufficiently stabilize the corneal shape after PRK.

Case Background

A 37-year-old female school teacher presented at our clinic complaining of contact lens discomfort and blurry vision. She had been diagnosed with

J.L. Alió et al. (eds.), *Difficult and Complicated Cases in Refractive Surgery*,
DOI 10.1007/978-3-642-55238-0_89, © Springer-Verlag Berlin Heidelberg 2015

keratoconus at age 31. Nine months previously, she had intracorneal ring segments placed in both eyes and underwent CXL at another location. Her manifest refraction was −6.25 diopters (D) + 6.75 D × 005 in the right eye and −3.25 D + 5.50 D × 170 in the left eye. Her corresponding spectacle-corrected Snellen visual acuity was 20/40 in both eyes. Despite previous collagen cross-linking, the patient experienced worsening discomfort and significant astigmatism. As shown in Fig. 89.1, her right eye had a significant amount of irregular astigmatism. Thus, she underwent PKP in her right eye. Her postoperative Snellen visual acuity was 20/20 in her right eye with successful contact lens fitting. Eighteen months following PKP surgery OD, the patient complained of left eye discomfort with a multitude of unsuccessful contact lens trials.

Main Problem to Solve

Given the patient's history of keratoconus OS, intracorneal ring segment insertion OS, and CXL OS, we had to determine the best treatment option. Possibilities included intracorneal ring segment or photorefractive keratectomy (PRK).

Ancillary Tests

The patient's corneal topography OS (Fig. 89.2), with contact lenses removed for 2 weeks, showed the thinnest corneal thickness to be 361 mm, whereas it was 464 mm according to ultrasound pachymetry. Her wavefront analysis OS showed a large astigmatic error of −9.24 D + 4.23 D × 055. Considering her history of cross-linking and ICRS OS, it was possible that her cornea was sufficiently stable to withstand surface treatment. Furthermore, if the cornea proved unstable, the patient knew that PKP would be performed after PRK. After weighing the risks and benefits, the patient decided to undergo PRK.

Surgical/Medical Intervention

A PRK treatment plan (of −4.79 + 3.13 × 026) aimed at undercorrection of the patient's myopic error was performed OS. She tolerated the procedure well, and Fig. 89.3 shows her topography 1 month postoperatively. Two months later, her manifest refraction OS was −2.00 D + 2.00 D × 066. She was still unhappy with her contact lenses and chose to undergo a second PRK treatment OS. Her wavefront-guided retreatment plan, performed 4 months after original treatment, was −1.52 D + 1.98 D × 056 (Fig. 89.4).

Outcome

The topography of the patient's left eye at the 1-month postoperative visit showed a healing pattern including an astigmatism with an axis at 90° (Fig. 89.5). Manifest refraction at this time was −1.25 D + 0.75 D × 095. The patient still had discomfort in her LE and was not content with her quality of vision (despite reduced refractive error measurements). Ultimately, the patient has ICRS removal and 2 months later underwent PKP in the left eye.

What to Learn from This Case

It was postulated that in this patient with progressive keratoconus OS, who had undergone ICRS and collagen cross-linking, her cornea had theoretically been strengthened by the CXL sufficiently enough to withstand PRK. However, the CXL was unsuccessful in stabilizing her cornea prior to PRK OS, requiring a retreatment OS. Although the patient's visual acuity and refractive error improved, her decreased quality necessitated PKP OS. It is possible that repeat CXL OS prior to PRK may have improved the likelihood of successful PRK.

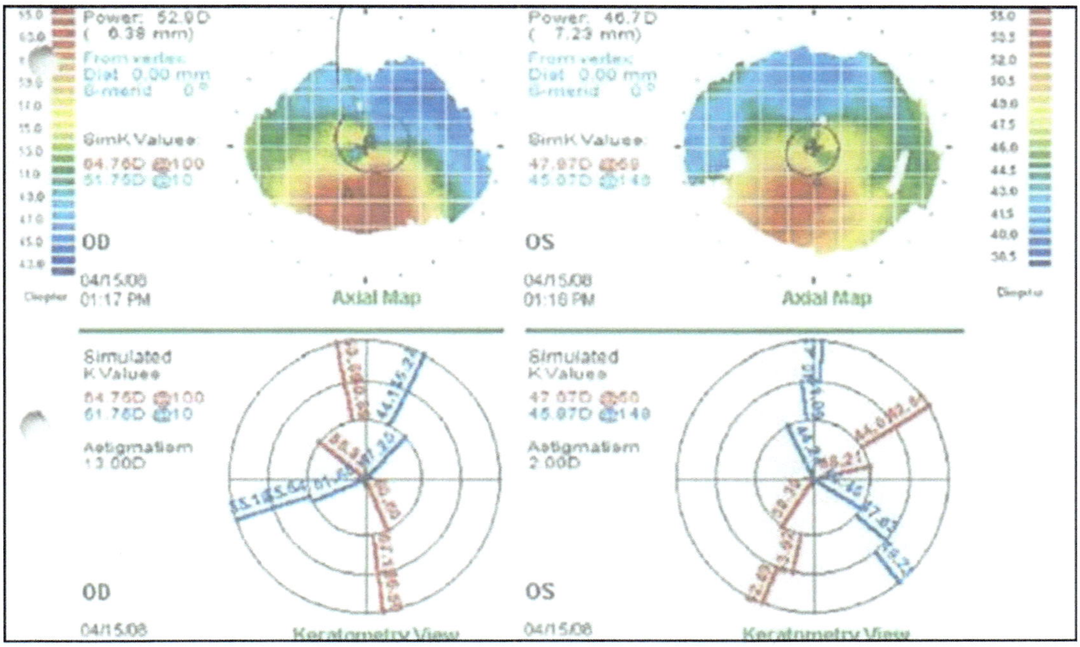

Fig. 89.1 Corneal topographical maps following ICRS and CXL for KC OU

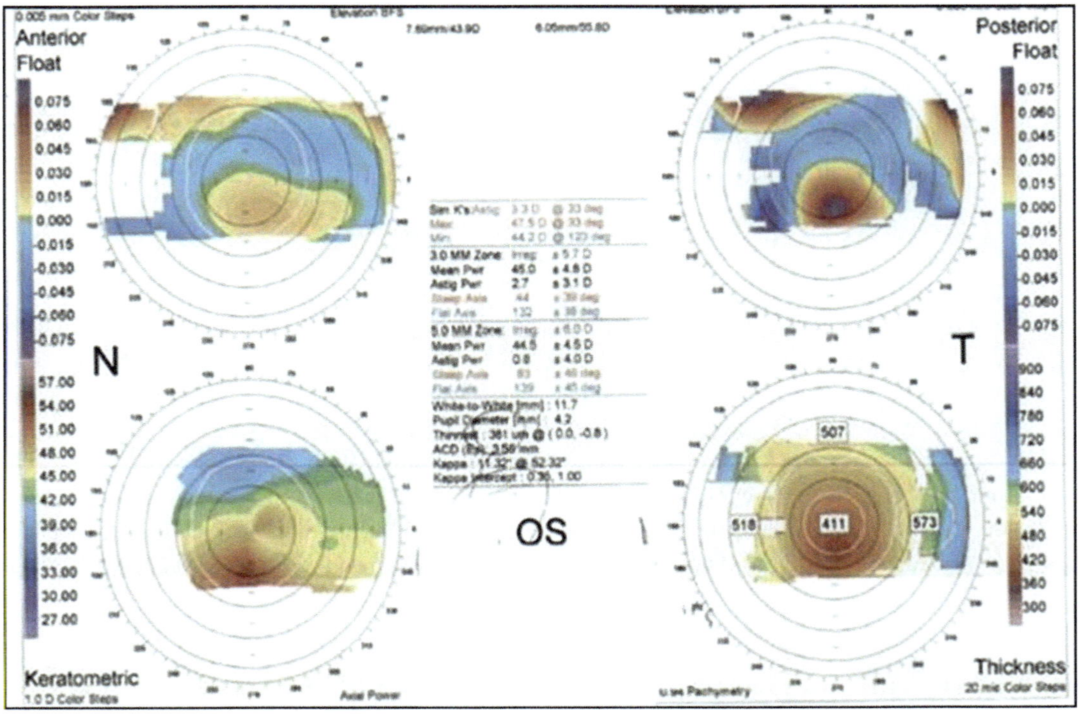

Fig. 89.2 Corneal topography OS prior to PRK

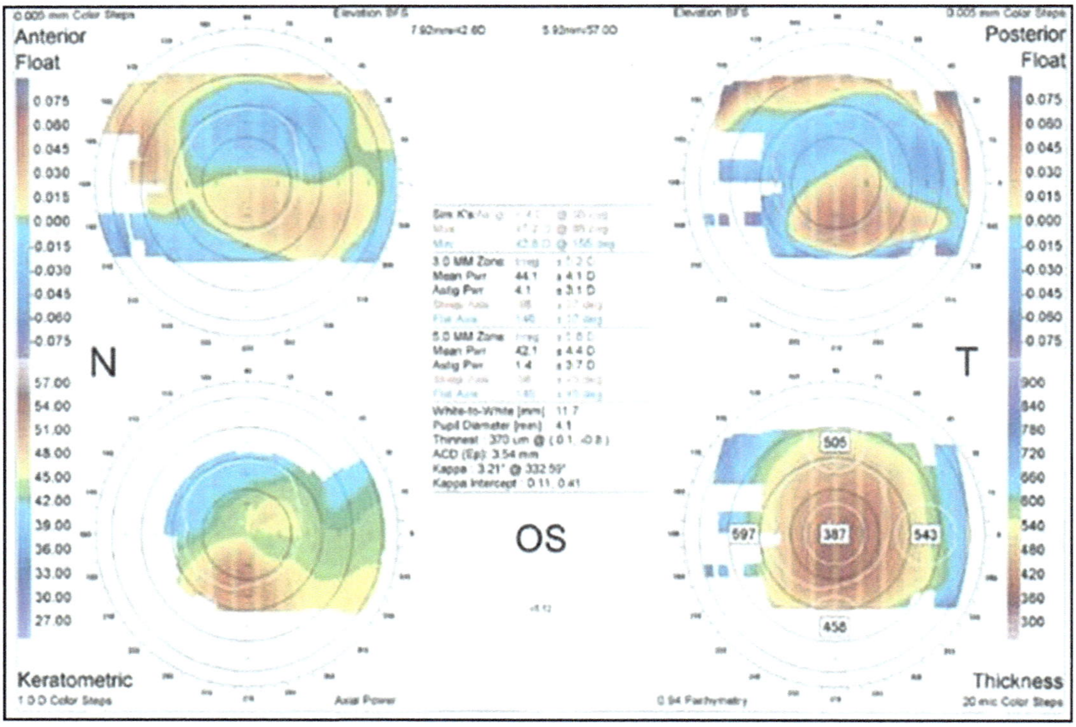

Fig. 89.3 Corneal topography 1 month after PRK OS

Some longitudinal case series show outcomes of corneal collagen cross-linking for keratoconus. Viswanathan and Males found that, at a mean follow-up of 14.38=9.36 months, cross-linking was statistically significant in flattening of maximum keratometry (0.96+2.33 D, $p=0.005$) and in improving visual acuity (0.05=0.13 logMAR, $p=0.04$) compared to control eyes [3]. Asri et al. described a case series from two referral centers in France. At 12 months, keratoconus progression had stopped in 42 eyes (68.8 %) and the maximum K value had decreased by more than 2.0 D in 13 eyes (21.3 %) [4]. Brooks et al. found that patients who completed a subjective questionnaire regarding their symptoms both before and 1 year after CXL noted improvement in various visual symptoms and foreign body sensation [5].

Most reports have follow-up periods of 18 months or less and are in retrospective case-series format. Among the exceptions, the Sienna eye cross study reported outcomes of CXL for 44 eyes with keratoconus with a minimum follow-up of 48 months in an open, non-randomized phase II clinical trial. The mean *K* value was reduced by a mean of 2 D, and coma aberration reduction with corneal symmetry improvement was observed in more than 85 % of cases. The mean BCVA improved by 1.9 lines on the Snellen chart. Fellow eyes, prior to joining the treatment arm at 24 months, showed a mean progression of 1.5 D in more than 65 % [6].

Despite these promising long-term results, there is still need for more data over an extended period. The case presented here is unique in that the patient underwent cross-linking several years prior to photorefractive keratectomy and ultimately PKP. Although cross-linking has less severe side effects than PKP for keratoconus treatment, CXL use may not preclude the need for future treatment.

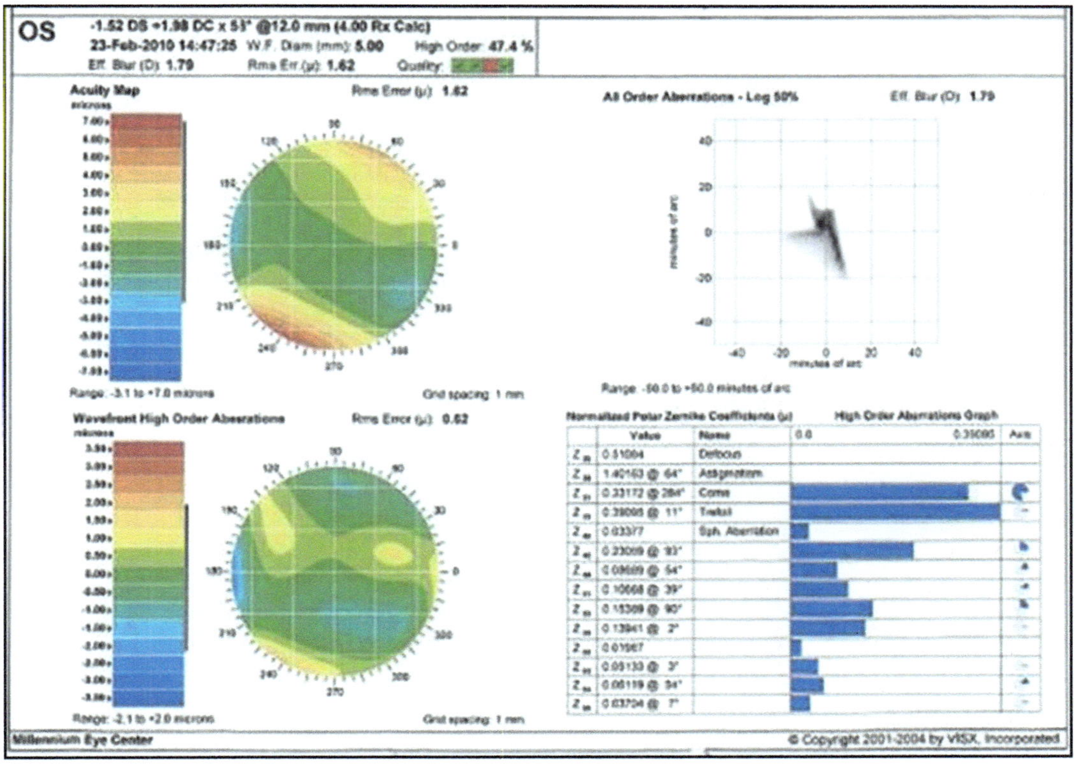

Fig. 89.4 Wavefront error OS prior to PRK retreatment OS

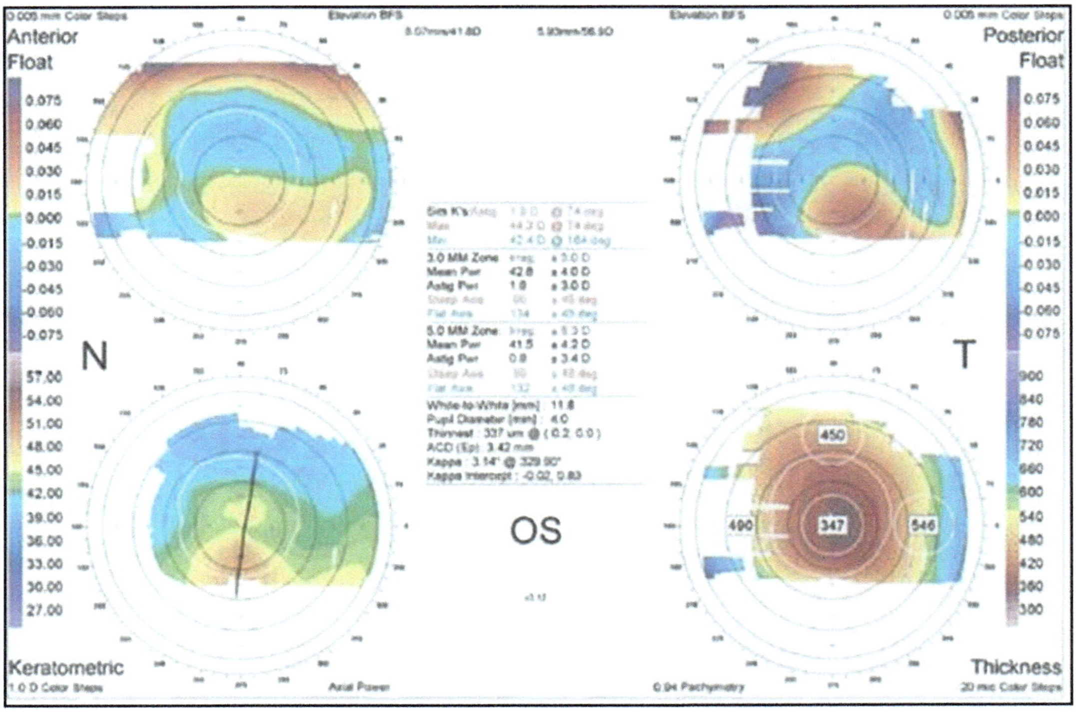

Fig. 89.5 Corneal topography 1 month after PRK retreatment OS

References

1. A service of the U.S. National Institutes of Health ClinicalTrials.gov. 17 Nov 2012. http://www.clinicaltrials.gov/. Search: "keratoconus" AND "crosslinking"
2. Richoz O, Schultz JS, Pajic B, Coskunseven E, Hafezi F (2012) Crosslinking for recurrent keratoconus. Ophthalmology 119:878–878.e2
3. Viswanathan D, Males J (2013) Prospective longitudinal study of corneal collagen crosslinking in progressive keratoconus. Clin Experiment Ophthalmol 41(6): 531–536
4. Asri D, Touboul D, Fournie P, Malet F, Garra C, Gallois A, Malecaze F, Colin J (2011) Corneal collagen crosslinking in progressive keratoconus: multicenter results from the French National Reference Center for Keratoconus. J Cataract Refract Surg 37:2137–2143
5. Brooks NO, Greenstein S, Fry K, Hersh PS (2012) Patient subjective visual function after corneal collagen crosslinking for keratoconus and corneal ectasia. J Cataract Refract Surg 38:615–619
6. Caporossi A, Mazzotta C, Baiocchi S, Caporossi T (2010) Long-term results of riboflavin ultraviolet a corneal collagen cross-linking for keratoconus in Italy: the Siena eye cross study. Am J Ophthalmol 149:585–593

PACK-CXL Treatment of Acanthamoeba Keratitis Following PRK

90

Alessandro Abbouda and Jorge L. Alió

Contents

A. Abbouda, MD (✉)
Department of Refractive Surgery, Vissum Corporación Oftalmológica, Alicante, Spain

Department of Ophthalmology-Policlinico Umberto I of Rome, University of Rome "Sapienza", Viale del Policlinico, 155, 00186 Roma, Italy

R&D Department, Vissum Corporación Oftalmológica, 03016, Alicante, Spain
e-mail: a.abbouda@gmail.com

J.L. Alió, MD, PhD
Department of Refractive Surgery, Vissum Corporación Oftalmológica, Alicante, Spain
e-mail: jlalio@vissum.com

Why Is This Case Relevant for the Refractive Surgeon?

Keratitis has a very poor prognosis and can lead to severe reducion of visual acuity. This is a case of a patient who developed Acanthamoeba keratitis (AK) after PRK in which we employed Collagen Cross-Linking with Photoactivated Riboflavin (PACK-CXL) treatment with good results. The refractive surgeon should be aware of the potentials of CXL.

Case Background

A 19-year-old man underwent PRK treatment 2 months prior, with a manifest refraction before the surgery of −4 diopters (D). He reported frequent use of contact lenses in the past. He arrived at our department complaining of photophobia and pain in the right eye (RE) for 3 days. His best corrected visual acuity (BCVA) was 20/80 in the RE. Slit lamp examination revealed conjunctival injection, multiple white stromal infiltrates in the central cornea, and a moderate anterior chamber reaction (Fig. 90.1). The appearance was suspect for AK. An epithelial scraping was performed and sent to the ocular pathology laboratory. The patient started chlorhexidine (CHX) 0.02 % drops every hour while awake and polyhexamethylene biguanide (PHMB) 0.02 % drops four times a day. Over follow-up appointments, the cornea opacified further, with white opacities

J.L. Alió et al. (eds.), *Difficult and Complicated Cases in Refractive Surgery*,
DOI 10.1007/978-3-642-55238-0_90, © Springer-Verlag Berlin Heidelberg 2015

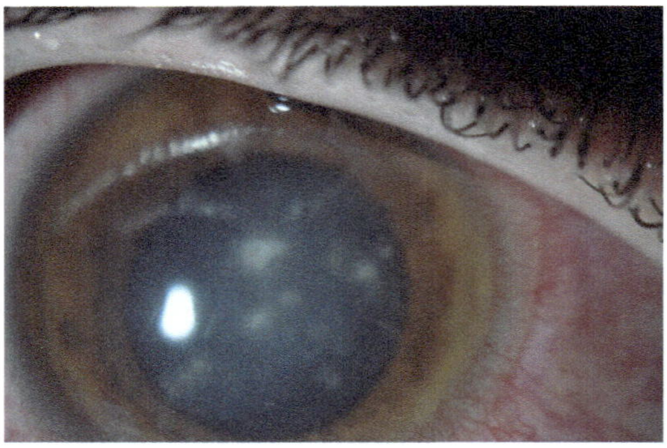

Fig. 90.1 Slit lamp examination at the presentation revealed white stromal infiltrates

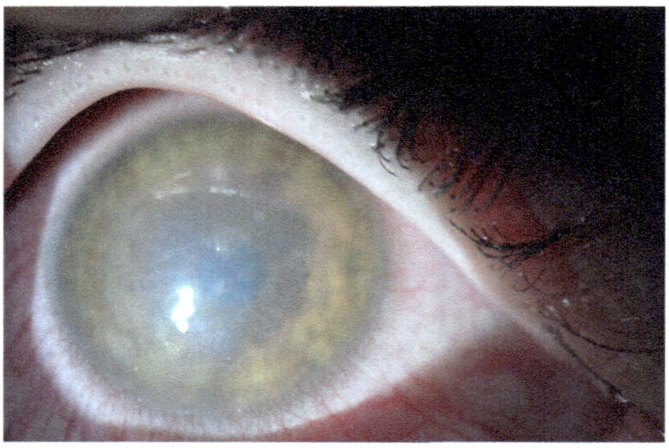

Fig. 90.2 Slit lamp examination 1 week after topic treatment revealed a worsening of stromal infiltrate appearance and corneal edema

forming around the peri-limbal cornea. Visual acuity was reduced to 20/100 secondary to persistent dense stromal infiltrates and corneal edema (Fig. 90.2). Epithelial scraping results confirmed an AK infection.

Main Problem to Solve

The spreading of AK in stroma topical treatment can be prolonged and unsatisfactory. We had to consider whether a more conservative treatment was appropriate for this young patient.

Ancillary Tests

We decided to treat this patient with PACK-CXL. In Acanthamoeba, the free radicals generated by irradiating UVA and riboflavin combined with

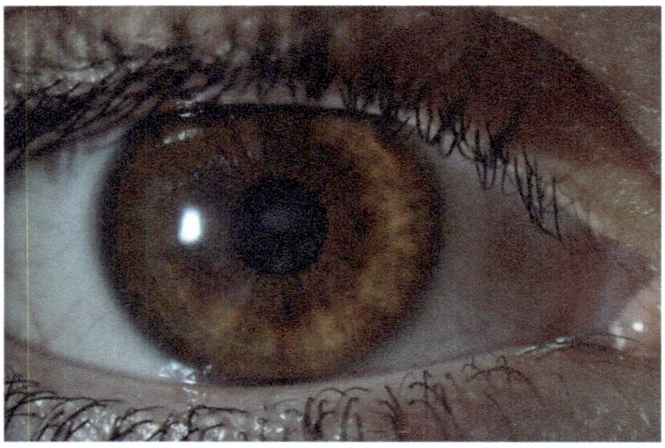

Fig. 90.3 Slit lamp examination 6 months after CXL revealed a complete resolution of edema and the presence of stromal scars

hydrogen peroxide-based oxidation seem to successfully neutralize the Acanthamoeba cyst [2].

Before the procedure, it is essential to check the corneal pachymetry. Ultrasound pachymetry confirmed a value of 435 μm, indicating that it was safe to proceed.

Surgical/Medical Intervention

After topical anesthesia of the cornea, the corneal epithelium within a 9 mm diameter zone including all microbial infiltrates was removed. After inserting a lid speculum, 0.1 % riboflavin drops were administered every 2 min for 30 min. Successful penetration of riboflavin through the cornea was assured by visualizing the riboflavin in the anterior chamber by slit lamp biomicroscopy (using blue light). Then, the eye was irradiated at 3 mW/cm^2 for 30 min with UVA. During that time, the cornea was moistened every 2 min with 0.1 % riboflavin drops. At the end of the procedure, a contact lens bandage was applied. CHX 0.02 % drops every hour for 1 week, followed by one drop every 2 h for 4 weeks and finally one drop four times a day for 4 months, were prescribed.

Outcome

After 6 months, the patient appeared in good condition. His visual acuity was 20/20 in the RE. The slit lamp examination revealed tender stromal opacity in the central cornea (Fig. 90.3).

What to Learn from This Case

According to recent studies [1–6], CXL is an emerging treatment option for infectious keratitis. In order to establish CXL as a therapy against bacterial or infectious keratitis, the procedure has to be more extensively studied to determine whether it is sufficient for effective eradication of microorganisms. CXL should be considered before undertaking emergency keratoplasty.

References

1. Alio JL, Abbouda A, Valle DD, Del Castillo JM, Fernandez JAL (2013) Corneal cross linking and infectious keratitis: a systematic review with a meta-analysis of reported cases. J Ophthalmic Inflamm Infect 3:47
2. Khan YA, Kashiwabuchi RT, Martins SA, Castro-Combs JM, Kalyani S, Stanley P, Flikier D, Behrens A (2011) Riboflavin and ultraviolet light a therapy as an adjuvant treatment for medically refractive acanthamoeba keratitis: report of 3 cases. Ophthalmology 118:324–331
3. Anwar HM, El-Danasoury AM, Hashem AN (2011) Corneal collagen crosslinking in the treatment of infectious keratitis. Clin Ophthalmol 5:1277–1280
4. Makdoumi K, Mortensen J, Sorkhabi O, Malmvall BE, Crafoord S (2012) UVA-riboflavin photochemical therapy of bacterial keratitis: a pilot study. Graefes Arch Clin Exp Ophthalmol 50:95
5. Price MO, Tenkman LR, Schrier A, Fairchild KM, Trokel SL, Price FW Jr (2012) Photoactivated riboflavin treatment of infectious keratitis using collagen cross-linking technology. J Refract Surg 28: 706–713
6. Said DG, Elalfy MS, Gatzioufas Z, El-Zakzouk ES, Hassan MA, Saif MY, Zaki AA, Dua HS, Hafezi F (2014) Collagen cross-linking with photoactivated riboflavin (PACK-CXL) for the treatment of advanced infectious keratitis with corneal melting. Ophthalmology.;121(7):1377–82. doi: 10.1016/j.ophtha.2014.01.011. Epub 2014 Feb 25

CXL and Delayed Wound Healing

91

Alfredo Vega Estrada

Contents

A. Vega Estrada, MD, MSc
Department of Keratoconus,
Vissum Corporacion Oftalmológica,
Alicante, Spain

Universidad Miguel Hernandez,
Alicante, Spain
e-mail: alfredovega@vissum.com

Why Is This Case Relevant for the Refractive Surgeon?

Although delayed wound healing after corneal collagen cross-linking is not a common complication, when present it can deteriorate the visual function of the patient and cause complications such as infectious keratitis and corneal scarring. Due to its harmful complications, ophthalmic surgeons should be aware of how to identify and treat this pathological condition.

Case Background

A 22-year-old male patient had a history of intracorneal ring segment implantation (ICRS) due to keratoconus. One year after ICRS implantation, keratoconus progression was confirmed by an increase of more than 1 diopter in the corneal topography in the steepest keratometric reading and a reduction of 1 line in the corrected distance visual acuity. We decided to perform an Epi-off UVA/riboflavin corneal cross-linking procedure in order to halt keratoconus progression. The surgical procedure was uneventful. Treatment with topical ciprofloxacin, preservative-free dexamethasone and artificial tears commenced, and a bandage contact lens was placed on the affected eye. The ophthalmological examination at 24 h was normal. The ophthalmological evaluation 5 days after the procedure revealed a 2 mm central area of the cornea that was absent of epithelium (Fig. 91.1). We decided to increase the artificial

J.L. Alió et al. (eds.), *Difficult and Complicated Cases in Refractive Surgery*,
DOI 10.1007/978-3-642-55238-0_91, © Springer-Verlag Berlin Heidelberg 2015

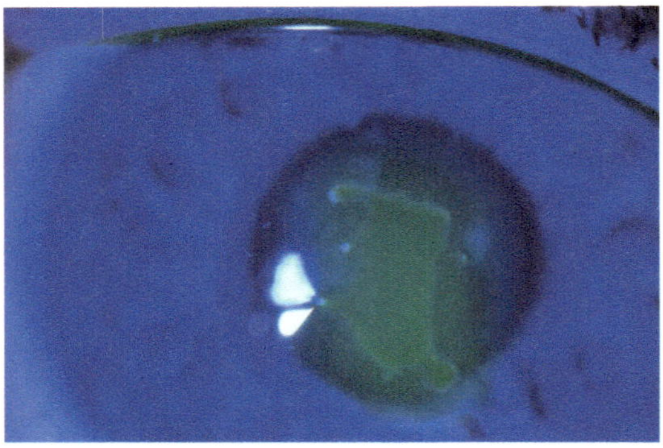

Fig. 91.1 Slit lamp photograph with fluorescein staining 5 days after the corneal cross-linking procedure showing the epithelial defect

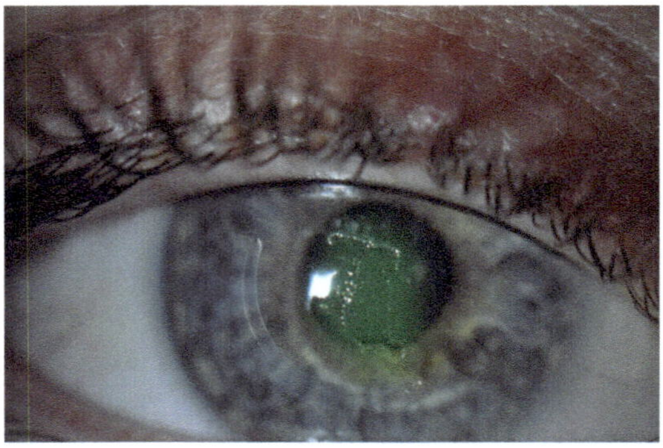

Fig. 91.2 Slit lamp photograph of the patient 5 days after mechanical debridement of the ulcer's edge, showing minimal improvement of the corneal epithelial defect

tear dosage to 6–8 times a day and evaluate the patient after 48 h. Two days later (1 week after the procedure), the patient complained of a foreign body sensation. The slit lamp evaluation revealed that the epithelial defect was still present and without significant change.

Main Problem to Solve

Delayed closure of the epithelial defect after the Epi-off UVA/riboflavin corneal cross-linking procedure presented a problem. Appropriate management was necessary in order to promote a successful refractive outcome and to prevent complications such as infectious keratitis and corneal scarring.

Ancillary Tests

Refraction, BCVA, corneal topography and slit lamp photo with fluorescein during the follow-up.

Surgical/Medical Intervention

One week after the corneal cross-linking procedure, we performed a mechanical debridement of the edge of the ulcer to promote the wound healing and asked the patient to stop the preservative-free dexamethasone. The patient was examined 5 days after the epithelial debridement, and the epithelial defect, although slightly smaller (approx. 1.5 mm), was still present (Fig. 91.2). We then decided to use a treatment-based topical platelet-rich plasma (PRP) six times a day.

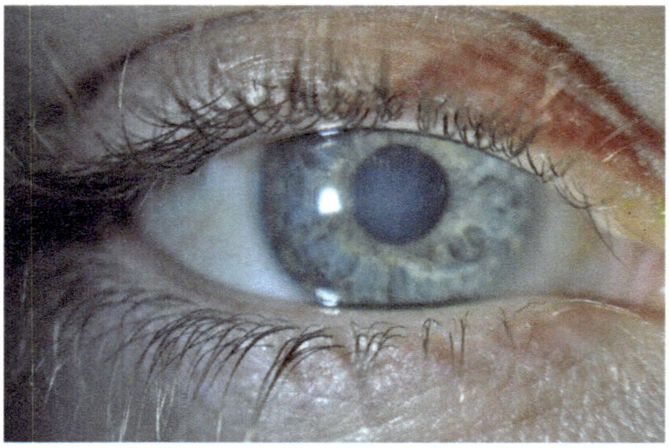

Fig. 91.3 Slit lamp photograph of the patient 1 week after treatment with topical platelet-rich plasma. The epithelial defect is completely healed

Outcome

One week after the PRP regimen began, the patient had no symptoms and the corneal epithelial defect had completely healed (Fig. 91.3). We recommended the patient continue the PRP topical treatment for only five additional days. One month after the initial surgical intervention, the patient had a refraction of sphere −0.50 cylinder −1.00 at 30 and the corrected visual acuity was 20/25. The slit lamp examination showed no signs of epithelial defect or corneal scarring.

What to Learn from This Case

We learned three main things in handling this case. First, it is important to ensure close follow-up in a patient who has undergone new surgical alternatives such as an Epi-off UVA/riboflavin corneal cross-linking procedure. Second, identifying clinical signs of complications is essential in order to start adequate treatment immediately to avoid compromise of visual function and eye integrity. Third, we realized the importance of modern and effective therapies for the treatment of corneal epithelial defects such as platelet-rich plasma [1].

References

1. Alio JL, Abad M, Artola A, Rodriguez-Prats JL, Pastor S, Ruiz-Colecha J (2007) Use of autologous platelet-rich plasma in the treatment of dormant corneal ulcers. Ophthalmology 114:1286–1293.e1

Bibliography

Touboul D, Efron N, Smadja D, Praud D, Malet F, Colin J (2012) Corneal confocal microscopy following conventional, transepithelial, and accelerated corneal collagen cross-linking procedures for keratoconus. J Refract Surg 28:769–776

Koppen C, Vryghem JC, Gobin L, Tassignon MJ (2009) Keratitis and corneal scarring after UVA/riboflavin cross-linking for keratoconus. J Refract Surg 25:S819–S823

Alio JL, Arnalich-Montiel F, Rodriguez AE (2012) The role of "Eye Platelet Rich Plasma" (E-PRP) for wound healing in ophthalmology. Curr Pharm Biotechnol 13:1257–1265

CXL in Pediatric Age

92

Alessandro Abbouda and Alfredo Vega Estrada

Contents

A. Abbouda, MD (✉)
Department of Refractive Surgery,
Vissum Corporación Oftalmológica, Alicante, Spain

Department of Ophthalmology-Policlinico Umberto I of Rome, University of Rome "Sapienza", Viale del Policlinico, 155, 00186 Roma, Italy

R&D Department, Vissum Corporación Oftalmológica, 03016, Alicante, Spain
e-mail: a.abbouda@gmail.com

A. Vega Estrada, MD, MSc
Department of Keratoconus, Vissum Corporacion Oftalmologica, Alicante, Spain

Universidad Miguel Hernandez, Alicante, Spain
e-mail: alfredovega@vissum.com

Why Is This Case Relevant for the Refractive Surgeon?

Keratoconus is often diagnosed after adolescence by modern corneal topography; however, the corneal ectasia process begins much earlier, with the disease underdiagnosed in children. Reports [1–6] demonstrating the efficacy and safety of CXL in children call for the refractive surgeon to consider the utility of the procedure in pediatric patients.

Case Background

A 7-year-old child came to our clinic complaining of visual difficulties during daily activities at school. His manifest refraction was +3.5 − 5 × 180° in the right eye (RE) and +4 − 5 × 170° in the left eye (LE).His best corrected visual acuity (BCVA) was 20/25 in both eyes. The keratometry reading in the RE was 42.18/47 × 94°. He had an AK of 47.5 and KPI of 25 %. In the LE, the keratometric index was 42.5/47.2 × 79°, the AK 47.8 and the KPI 28 %. The topography aspect showed an irregular astigmatism with inferosuperior asymmetry and skewing of the main topographic axis (Fig. 92.1a, b). A diagnosis of keratoconus was made. After 1 year, the manifest refraction was +3.5 − 5.5 × 5° in the RE and +3.5 − 5.5 × 170° in the LE. His best corrected visual acuity (BCVA) was 20/32 in both eyes. Keratometry

J.L. Alió et al. (eds.), *Difficult and Complicated Cases in Refractive Surgery*,
DOI 10.1007/978-3-642-55238-0_92, © Springer-Verlag Berlin Heidelberg 2015

reading in the RE was 42.9/47.7 × 98°, the AK 48 and the KPI 26 %. In the LE, the keratometric index was 42.5/47.1 × 82°, the AK 47.9 and the KPI 31 %. The topography aspect was comparable to the previous examination (Fig. 92.1c, d). At 2-years follow-up, the child's refraction was +3.5 − 5 × 180° in the RE and +4 − 5 × 170° in the LE. His best corrected visual acuity (BCVA) was 20/30 in the RE and 20/50 in the LE. The keratometry reading of the RE was 43.5/48.2 × 100°, AK 48 and KPI 25 %. In the LE, the keratometric index was 43.1/48.3 × 80°, AK 48 and KPI 39 %. The topography aspect showed asymmetrical astigmatism with rule (Fig. 92.2a, b). The corneal aberrometry showed a coma-like value in both eyes of 0.66 μm. We decided to perform CXL in the LE.

Main Problem to Solve

Considering the progression of keratoconus, when is it appropriate to perform CXL in a child?

Ancillary Tests

Refraction, BCVA, corneal topography, and aberrometry.

Surgical/Medical Intervention

Topical anesthesia of the cornea was performed, and the corneal epithelium within a 9 mm diameter zone was removed. After inserting a lid speculum, 0.1 % riboflavin drops were administered

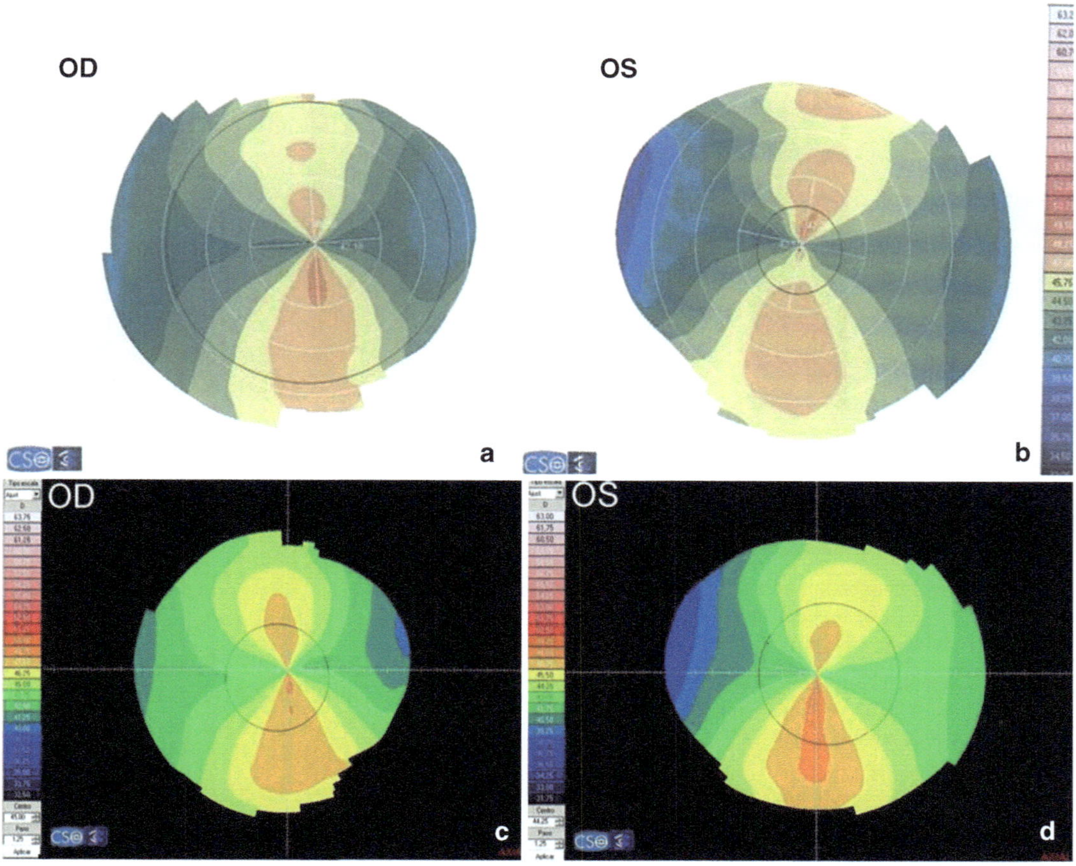

Fig. 92.1 Corneal topography at the first visit (**a**, **b**) and then after 1 year (**c**, **d**)

every 2 min for 30 min. Successful penetration of riboflavin through the cornea was assured by visualizing the riboflavin in the anterior chamber by slit lamp biomicroscopy (using blue light). Thereafter, the eye was irradiated for 30 min with UVA (UVA) with an irradiance of 3 mW/cm^2. During that time, the cornea was moistened every 2 min with 0.1 % riboflavin drops. At the end, a contact lens was applied. Topical ofloxacin and dexamethasone were prescribed.

Outcome

Three years after the procedure, the patient's manifest refraction was $+1.25-2.5\times15°$ in the LE. His best corrected visual acuity (BCVA) was 20/25. The keratometry reading was $42.4/47.6\times80$. AK was 48 and KPI was 38 %. The topography aspect was substantially similar to the previous examination (Fig. 92.3). The corneal aberrometry showed a coma-like value of 0.4 μm.

What to Learn from This Case

Although traditionally CXL is performed only after the documentation of the progression of keratoconus in children and adolescents, recent studies [1–6] suggest that CXL should be performed as soon as the diagnosis has been made. Some authors [3] suggested CXL for children with advanced disease in their fellow eyes, without waiting for keratoconus progression. Early treatment could potentially prevent loss of visual acuity at an amblyogenic age and reduce the need for an early corneal graft. However, the arrest of disease progression may not be as long lasting as in adults; therefore, a longer follow-up is needed to verify this trend. However, the good visual outcome demonstrated in this case suggests the positive outcomes of pediatric CXL.

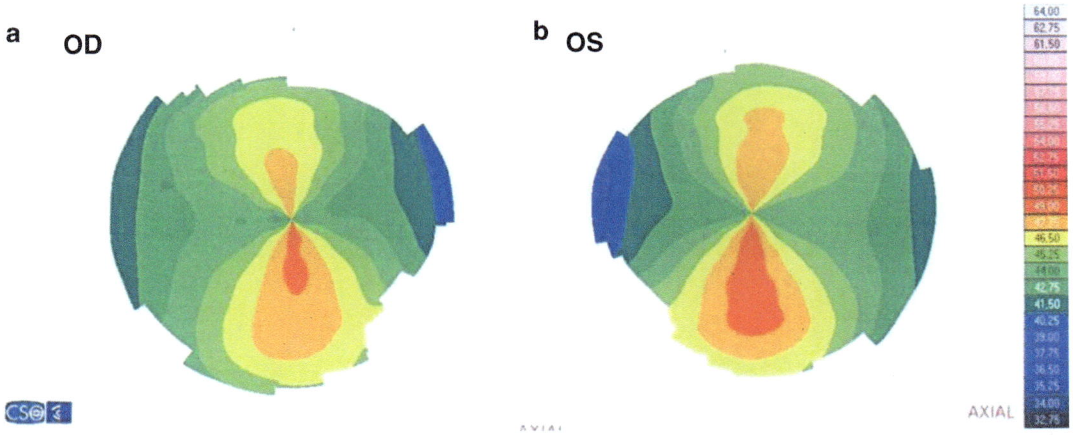

Fig. 92.2 Corneal topography at 2 years (**a**, **b**)

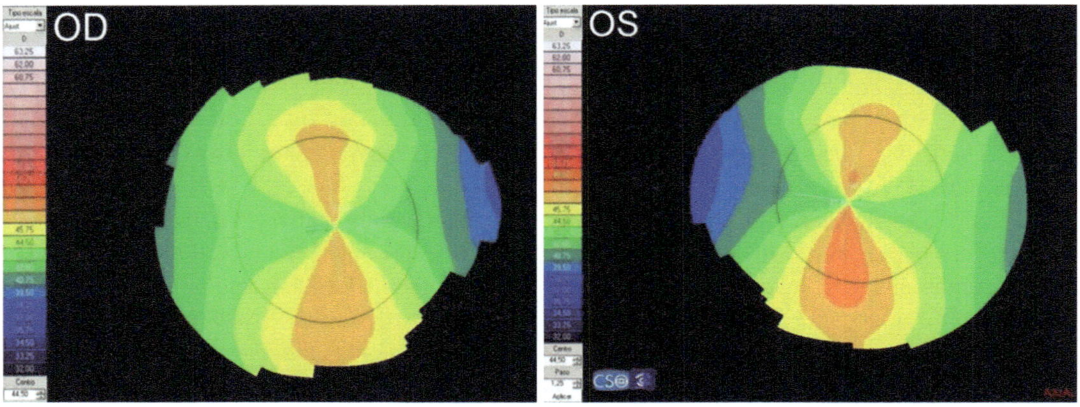

Fig. 92.3 Corneal topography at the last follow-up. Three years after CXL treatment

References

1. Zotta PG, Moschou KA, Diakonis VF, Kymionis GD, Almaliotis DD, Karamitsos AP, Karampatakis VE (2012) Corneal collagen cross-linking for progressive keratoconus in pediatric patients: a feasibility study. J Refract Surg 28:793–799
2. Buzzonetti L, Petrocelli G (2012) Transepithelial corneal cross-linking in pediatric patients: early results. J Refract Surg 28:763–767
3. Arora R, Gupta D, Goyal JL, Jain P (2012) Results of corneal collagen cross-linking in pediatric patients. J Refract Surg 28:759–762
4. Chatzis N, Hafezi F (2012) Progression of keratoconus and efficacy of pediatric corneal collagen cross-linking in children and adolescents. J Refract Surg 28(11):753–758
5. Magli A, Forte R, Tortori A, Capasso L, Marsico G, Piozzi E (2013) Epithelium-off corneal collagen cross-linking versus transepithelial cross-linking for pediatric keratoconus. Cornea 32:597–601
6. Caporossi A, Mazzotta C, Baiocchi S, Caporossi T, Denaro R, Balestrazzi A (2012) Riboflavin-UVA-induced corneal collagen cross-linking in pediatric patients. Cornea 31:227–231

Part IX

Refractive Keratotomy Complications

Dear reader,

Post-refractive keratotomy patients present a significant challenge for cataract surgeons because of the risks they pose, including complications and hyperopic results in the early postoperative period.

Accurate IOL power calculations are more difficult and require accurate refractive measurements of the corneal power. Moreover, previous corneal refractive procedures may present complications such as RK incision rupture, a frequent complication especially during phaco surgery or LASIK re-treatment.

In this section, we describe some refractive complications following RK, variations among RK cases, and concerns with cataract surgery. Our hope is to promote understanding of some of the serious risks associated with RK.

To further clarify this subject, we suggest the first book in this series: J. L. Alio', D. Azar *Management of Complications in Refractive Surgery*, Chapter 15: Complications of Radial Keratotomy (pp. 285–289).

Specific topics covered by the cases include how to solve hyperopic shift after RK (Case 95), remarkable irregular astigmatism after RK and its management (Case 96), understanding cataract surgery in the development of hyperopic shift in eyes with RK (Case 97), and how to perform a LASIK procedure after arcuate lamellar keratotomy (Case 98).

Lesson

Case 95: Solving refractive complications after RK correction of a hyperopic shift

How transepithelial PRK with Mitomycin C 0.02 % was used in hyperopic shift after RK.

Case 96: Variability of astigmatic keratotomy and approaches to solve the problems

Remarkable irregular astigmatism after an intraoperative mistake was solved using a transepithelial PRK. This treatment results effective for the presence of an epithelium with different thicknesses.

Solving Refractive Complications after RK Correction of Hyperopic Shift

93

Massimo Camellin, Diego Ponzin, and Samuel Arba-Mosquera

Contents

Why Is This Case Relevant for the Refractive Surgeon?

IOL calculation in eyes that have previously undergone RK is difficult. In these cases, we face two main challenges: a change in the fictitious refractive index and a difficult determination of the basal ray of the cornea, because of the high asphericity of the optical zone. The refractive surgeon needs to be able to handle complications following RK correction of hyperopic shift [1–3].

Case Background

A 47-year-old female underwent incisional surgery 20 years prior (6 cuts, radial keratotomy, RK) in her right eye. Previous myopia in the right eye was −6.5 D (the left eye presented a −3.5 D and underwent a 4 cut-RK). When the patient presented at our clinic, she had a refraction and visual acuity of +3 sph/+0.25 cyl@170 (8/10, 20/25) in the right eye and +1.75 sph (8/10, 20/25) in the left eye. The patient complained of progressive worsening of near vision, due to increasing presbyopia associated with hyperopia, and haloes in night vision due to a small optical zone. The patient also presented an initial cataract which would likely require future operation.

In our experience, hyperopic shift can reach a spherical equivalent of +3/+4 D and then, with the exception of rare cases of dehiscence, flatten-

M. Camellin, MD (✉)
SEKAL Rovigo Microsurgery, Rovigo, Italy
e-mail: cammas@tin.it

D. Ponzin
The Veneto Eye Bank Foundation, Venice, Italy
e-mail: diego.ponzin@fbov.it

S. Arba-Mosquera
SCHWIND Eye-Tech-Solutions, Kleinostheim, Germany
e-mail: samuel.arba.mosquera@eye-tech.net

J.L. Alió et al. (eds.), *Difficult and Complicated Cases in Refractive Surgery*,
DOI 10.1007/978-3-642-55238-0_93, © Springer-Verlag Berlin Heidelberg 2015

ing stops. Therefore, there is a rationale to operate in such cases.

Main Problem to Solve

We proposed to reduce the hyperopia to improve near and far vision and moreover to enlarge the optical zone (OZ), thus reducing the haloes and enabling a more precise IOL calculation.

Ancillary Tests

Corneal wavefront showed a high spherical aberration. The functional OZ zone, or the area in which the diameter of spherical aberration was less than 0.25 D, had a value of 3.75 mm (Figs. 93.1, 93.2, and 93.3).

Surgical/Medical Intervention

The programmed surgery was a topo–aberrometric link procedure in which the topography was converted into corneal wavefronts, and these data were linked to the laser. The platform was the excimer laser SCHWIND AMARIS with a particular eye tracker (6 axes) that allowed a perfect matching of the topography with the eye.

The procedure was a transepithelial link in which the laser took into account the elimination of epithelium during treatment. Its great advantage is that it is a non-touch procedure able to perfectly match the analyzed cornea with the laser program and the optimized epithelial ablation, which is determined by the diameter of the treatment.

Mitomycin C (MMC) 0.02 % was applied for 2 min with a Merocel sponge (as is typical in all re-treatments). A contact lens was then applied for 4 days. The topical post-op treatment was gentamicin for 7 days and steroid (clobetasone) for 1 month, twice a day (Figs. 93.4 and 93.5).

Outcome

The postoperative result was excellent, and the spherical aberration was strongly reduced. The post-op visual acuity was +0.75 sph/−0 75 cyl@15 (8/10, 20/25) for the right eye. There was no haze, and the OZ measured on the cornea was now 8.6 mm.

The same simulation with a pupil of 5 mm shows little difference. However, in high-order aberrations besides coma and spherical, there is typically a huge reduction from pre-op to post-op.

What to Learn from This Case

An eye that has undergone RK has a high risk for developing hyperopia. Problems in night vision related to the small optical zone (high spherical aberration) can now be solved with a simple customized procedure. A topo–aberrometric link is based on the analysis of the surface and, therefore, it is better to operate on the surface for a better correspondence of measured shape and ideal final profile. A LASIK procedure, particularly following RK, can compromise the flap's integrity with the presence of radial cuts and therefore induce errors.

MMC is fundamental to reducing the risk of haze in surface treatments following RK.

Trans-PRK procedure reduces all small irregularities detected with a high-order analysis (Fig. 93.6).

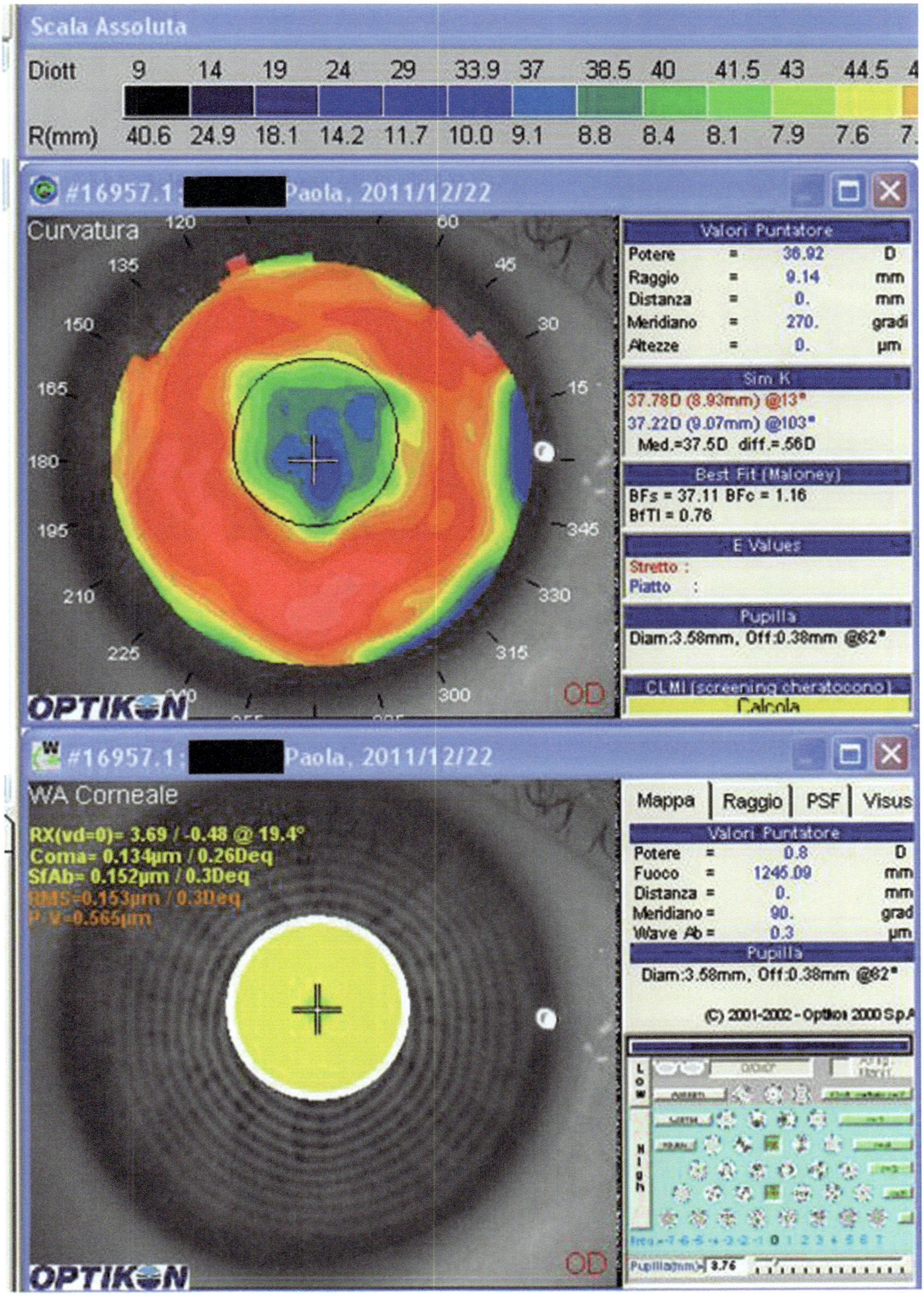

Fig. 93.1 Topography and corneal wavefront following RK. The diameter of the OZ is determined by the spherical aberration which value must be less than 0.25 D. In this case, the OZ is 3.75 mm. A Scheimpflug camera analysis is important in detecting the pachymetry, the position and aspect of the incisions

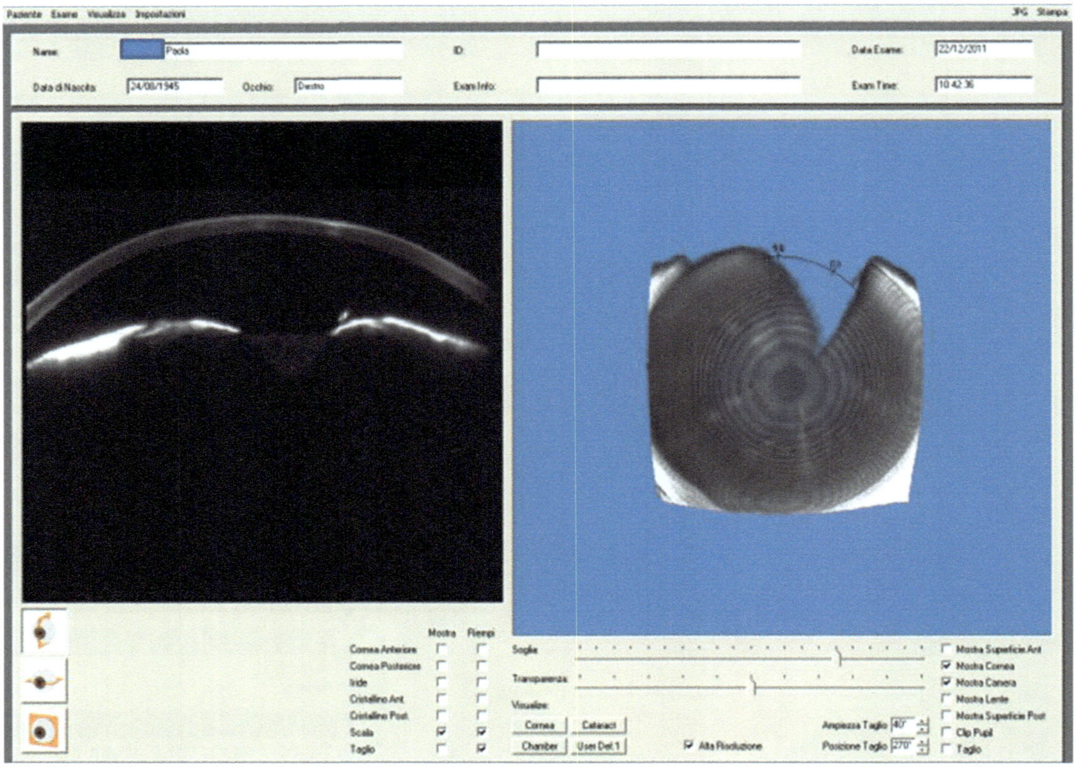

Fig. 93.2 Scheimpflug tomography with Pentacam shows 6 scars on the surface

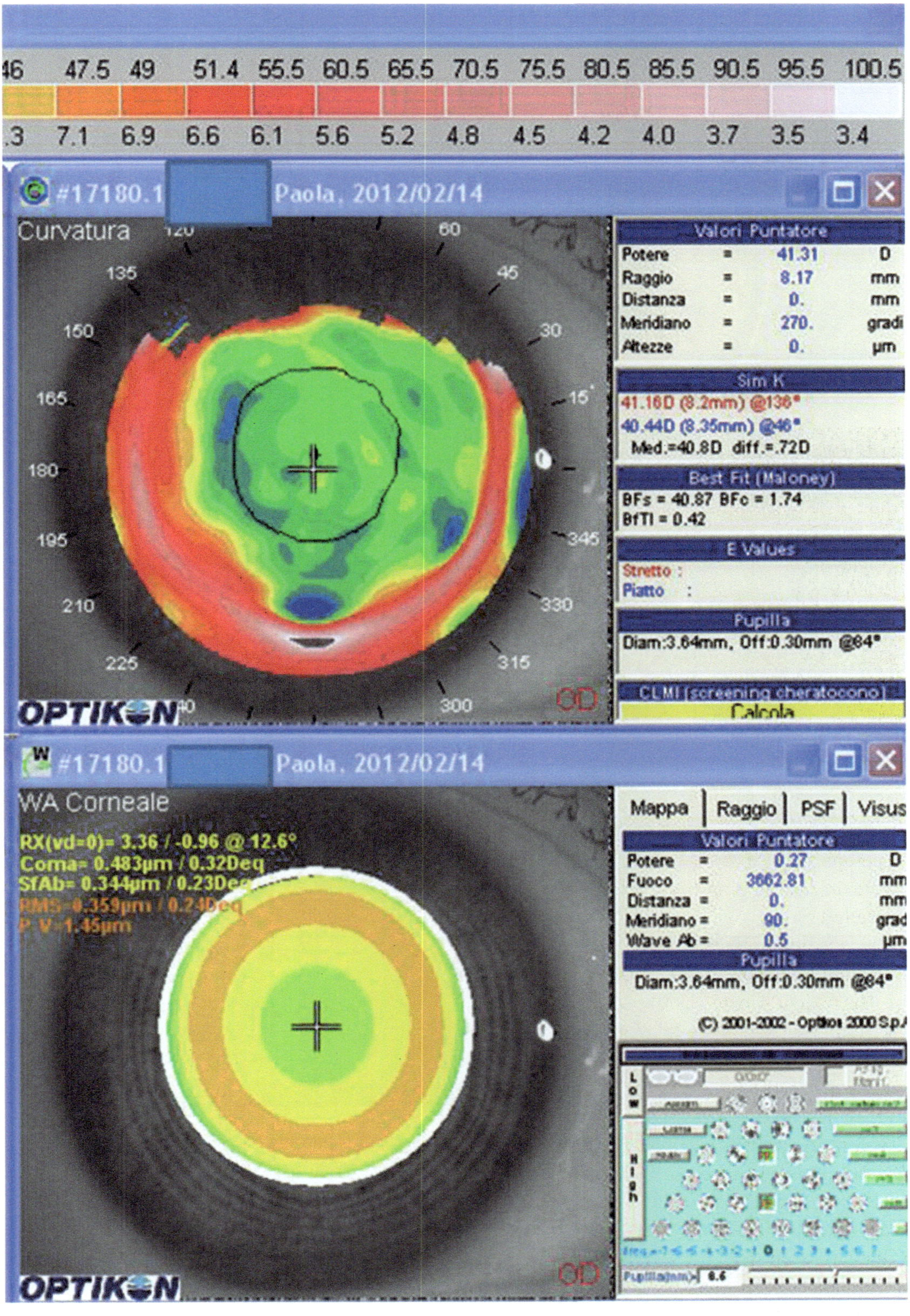

Fig. 93.3 Topography and corneal wavefront following transepithelial link. The OZ with a spherical aberration less than 0.25 D is 8.6 mm. We can simulate the BCVA through the corneal wavefront analysis, and we can see that there is a great difference between the pre-op and the post-op corneal wavefront in 7 mm

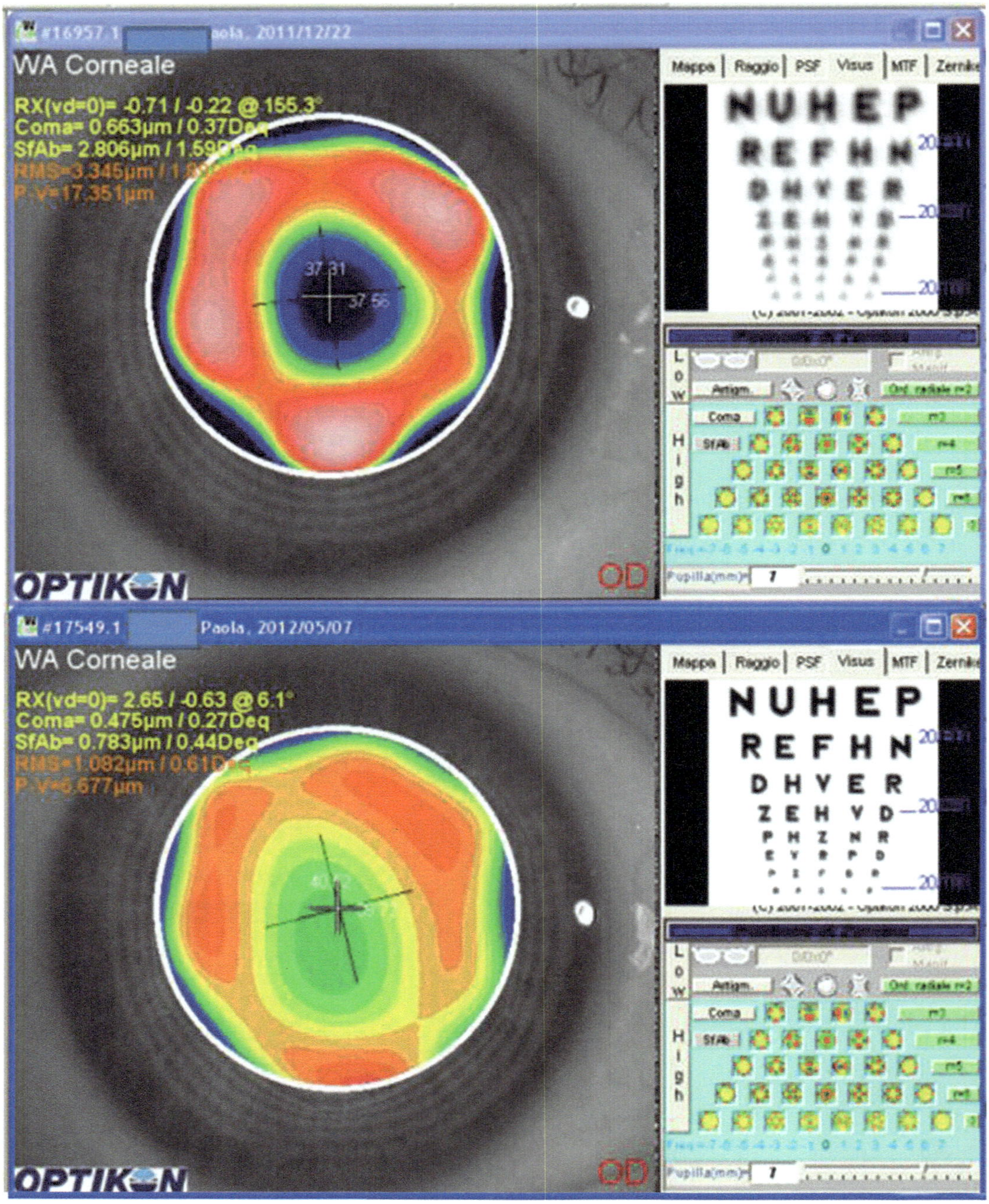

Fig. 93.4 The corneal wavefront in scotopic condition with a 7 mm pupil shows a great difference in pre-op and post-op

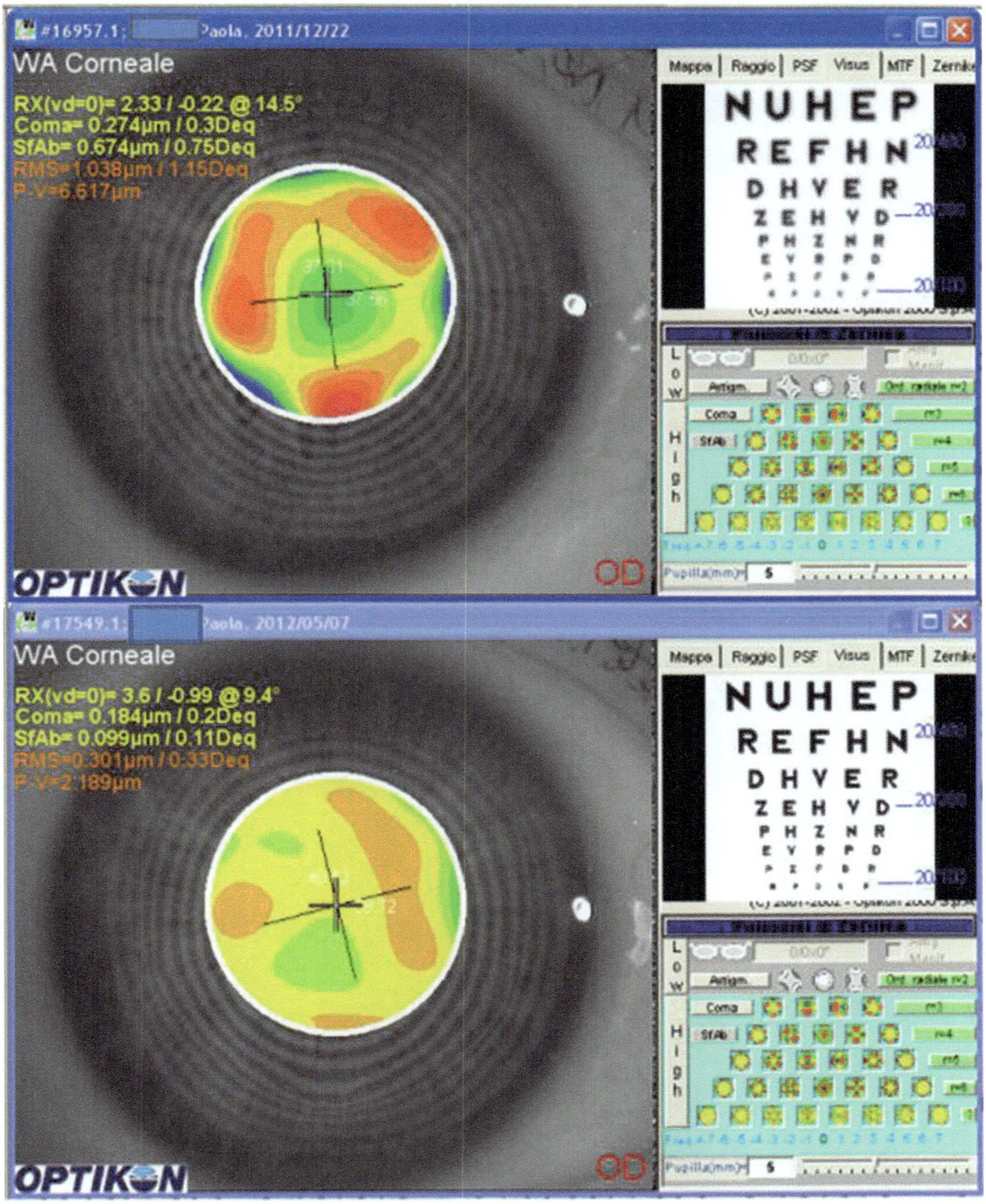

Fig. 93.5 Corneal wavefront in mesopic condition (5 mm pupil). The pre-op visual acuity is quite good

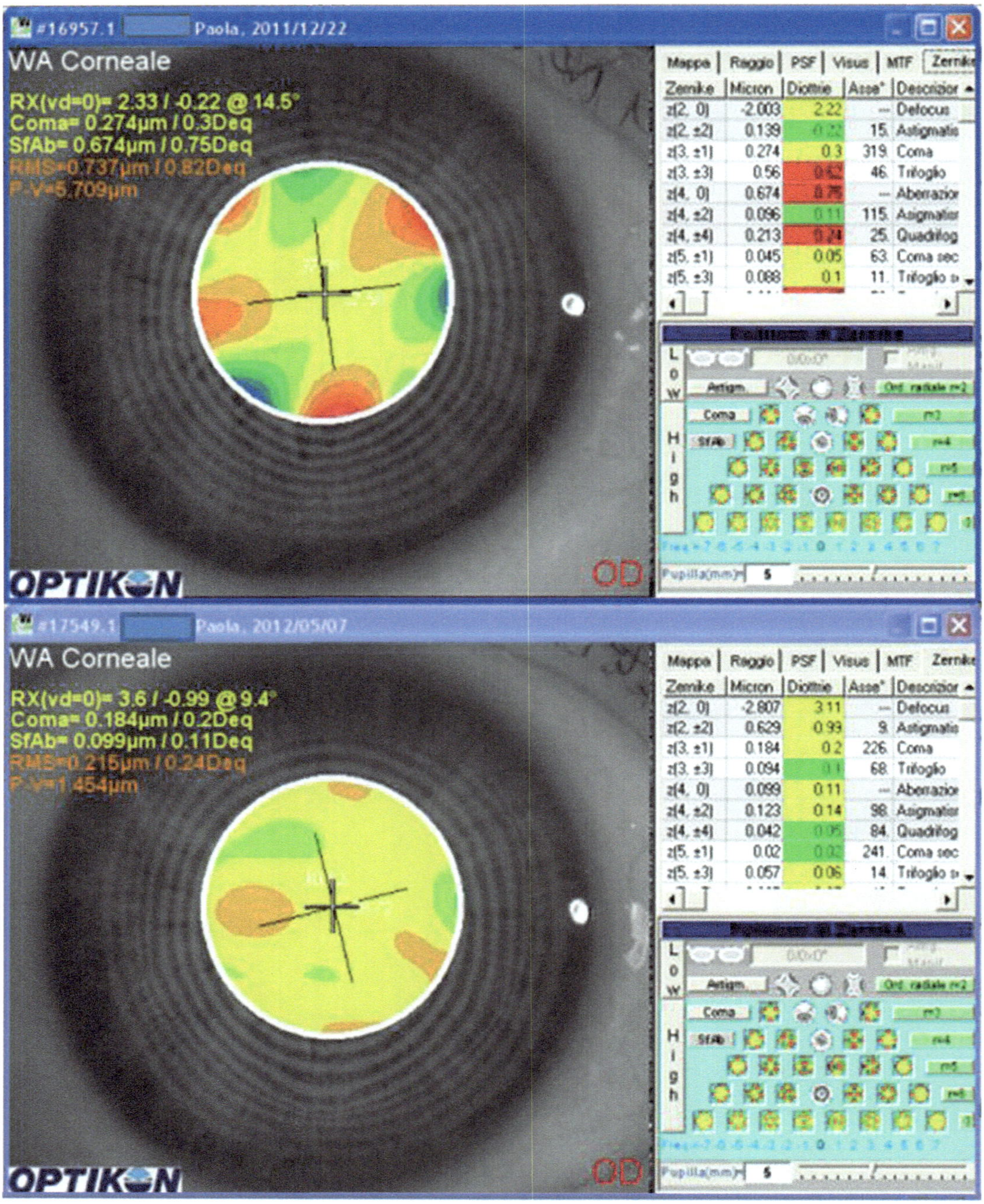

Fig. 93.6 Reduction of high-order aberrations following customized trans-PRK. In cases of impending cataracts, it is valuable to perform a customized ablation to improve the precision of the IOL calculation

References

1. Camellin M, Calossi A (2006) A new formula for intraocular lens power calculation after refractive corneal surgery. J Refract Surg 22:187–199
2. Camellin M, Savini G, Hoffer KJ, Carbonelli M, Barboni P (2012) Scheimpflug camera measurement of anterior and posterior corneal curvature in eyes with previous radial keratotomy. J Refract Surg 28:275–279
3. Camellin M, Mosquera SA (2011) Aspheric optical zones: the effective optical zone with the Schwind Amaris. J Refract Surg 27:135–146

Variability of Astigmatic Keratotomy

94

Massimo Camellin, Diego Ponzin,
and Samuel Arba-Mosquera

Contents

M. Camellin, MD (✉)
SEKAL Rovigo Microsurgery, Rovigo, Italy
e-mail: cammas@tin.it

D. Ponzin
The Veneto Eye Bank Foundation, Venice, Italy
e-mail: diego.ponzin@fbov.it

S. Arba-Mosquera
SCHWIND Eye-Tech-Solutions, Kleinostheim, Germany

Why Is This Case Relevant for the Refractive Surgeon?

This is a case of remarkable irregular astigmatism post-radial keratotomy (RK). In the patient's right eye, four radial and two arcuate incisions were made to correct myopic astigmatism. In the left eye, four radial and four arcuate incisions were present. The reason for this peculiar surgical protocol was related to intraoperative error. The surgeon realized the error in the axis just after performing the two arcuate incisions and intended to fix the problem by performing two additional arcuate incisions on the correct axis.

This led to different complications. The right eye developed a typical astigmatic overcorrection (hyperopic shift-like effect) with a prevalent coma aberration due to the excessive ectasia of the inferior incisions. The left eye showed instead a residual astigmatism, worse than pre-RK but with the same axis, and a tetrafoil aberration. The new incisions neutralized the incorrect ones. A topo–aberrometric laser link on the surface of the cornea allows a refractive surgeon to solve various irregularities caused by previous incisional surgery. Responding to errors and irregular astigmatisms is essential for the refractive surgeon (Figs. 94.1 and 94.2).

J.L. Alió et al. (eds.), *Difficult and Complicated Cases in Refractive Surgery*,
DOI 10.1007/978-3-642-55238-0_94, © Springer-Verlag Berlin Heidelberg 2015

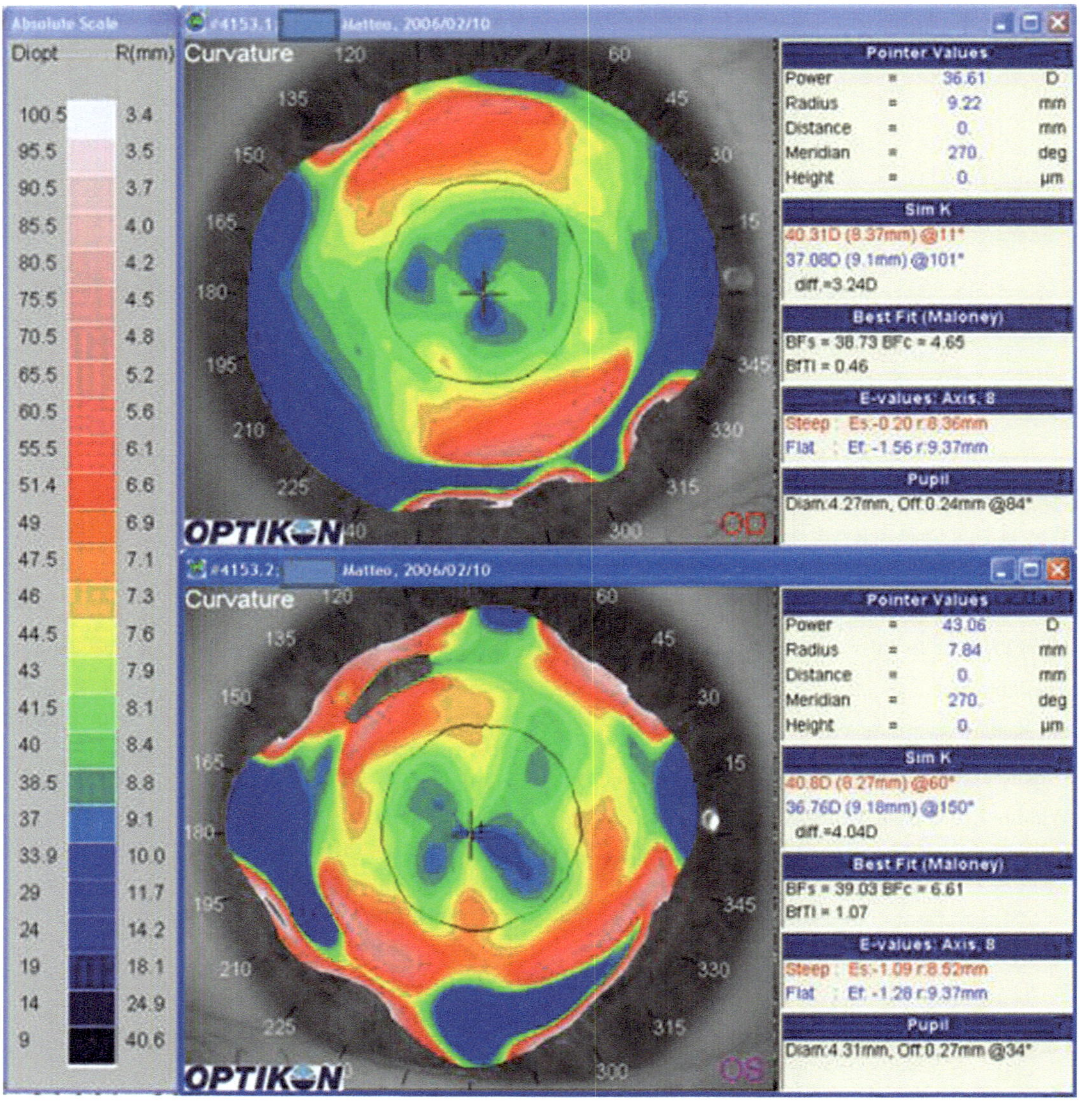

Fig. 94.1 Topographic analysis (instantaneous algorithm) of the right and left eye. The overcorrection produced by the arcuate incisions in the right eye and the tetrafoil aspect of the optical zone in the left eye are both evident

Case Background

A 20-year-old male underwent incisional surgery 9 years prior. In the right eye, he endured 4 cuts radial keratotomy (RK), plus 2 cuts arcuate keratotomies (AK). In the left eye, he had 4 cuts RK and 4 cuts AK. His pre-RK refraction and visual acuity was −3.75 sph/−4 cyl@5 (10/10, 20/20) in the right eye and −2.75 sph/−4 cyl@160 (10/10, 20/20) in the left eye. When he presented at our clinic 9 years after surgery, his post-RK refraction and visual acuity was −3 sph/−4 cyl@95 (8/10, 20/25) in the right eye and −1 sph/−7 cyl@170 (6–7/10, 20/30) in the left eye.

We supposed that, because of his young age, the patient's myopia could not be completely stabilized, as it had a negative refraction despite previous incisional operations.

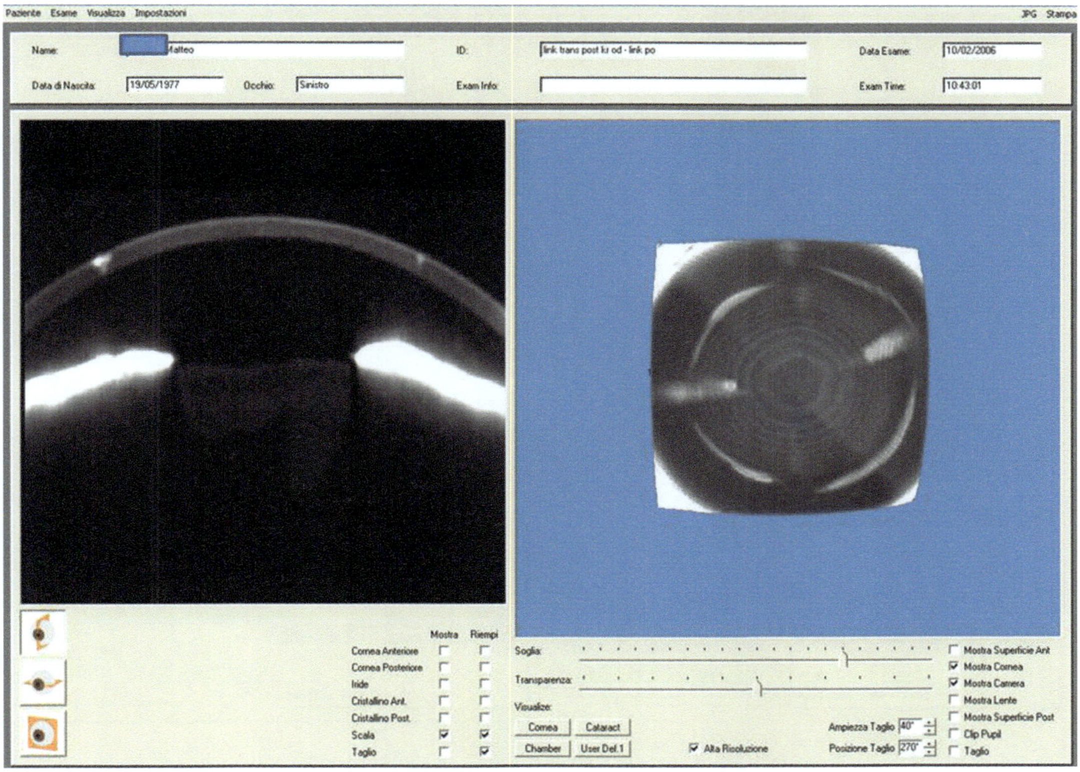

Fig. 94.2 Tomography with Pentacam shows the position of the incisions in the left eye (four radial plus four arcuate)

Main Problem to Solve

Both eyes presented with myopic irregular astigmatism. There was a component of coma in the right eye and a tetrafoil aberration in the left eye. Reoperation was intended to eliminate both low-order and high-order aberrations.

Ancillary Tests

Photokeratoscopy is the most appropriate exam to analyze the shape of the cornea. We chose a short-distance analysis instrument, the Keratron Scout (Optikon 2000, Rome, Italy), that could project the rings in the extreme periphery of the cornea.

Routine protocol included the slit lamp evaluation. Pentacam analysis (Oculus, Germany) was particularly useful to highlight the scars with the tomography option.

Cornea wavefront analysis was performed to determine which aberration was prevalent, enabling us to analyze the coma in the right eye and tetrafoil aberration in the left eye.

Surgical/Medical Intervention

The programmed surgery was a topo–aberrometric link procedure in which the topography was converted in corneal wavefront and these data linked to the laser. The platform was the excimer laser SCHWIND ESIRIS. The procedure consisted of two steps. In the first, the customized ablation was performed over the epithelium, and later a PTK procedure with a 50 μm depth completed the ablation (Figs. 94.3 and 94.4).

The procedure was a non-touch PRK procedure able to perfectly match the analyzed cornea with the laser program and perform the optimized epithelial ablation determined by the diameter of the

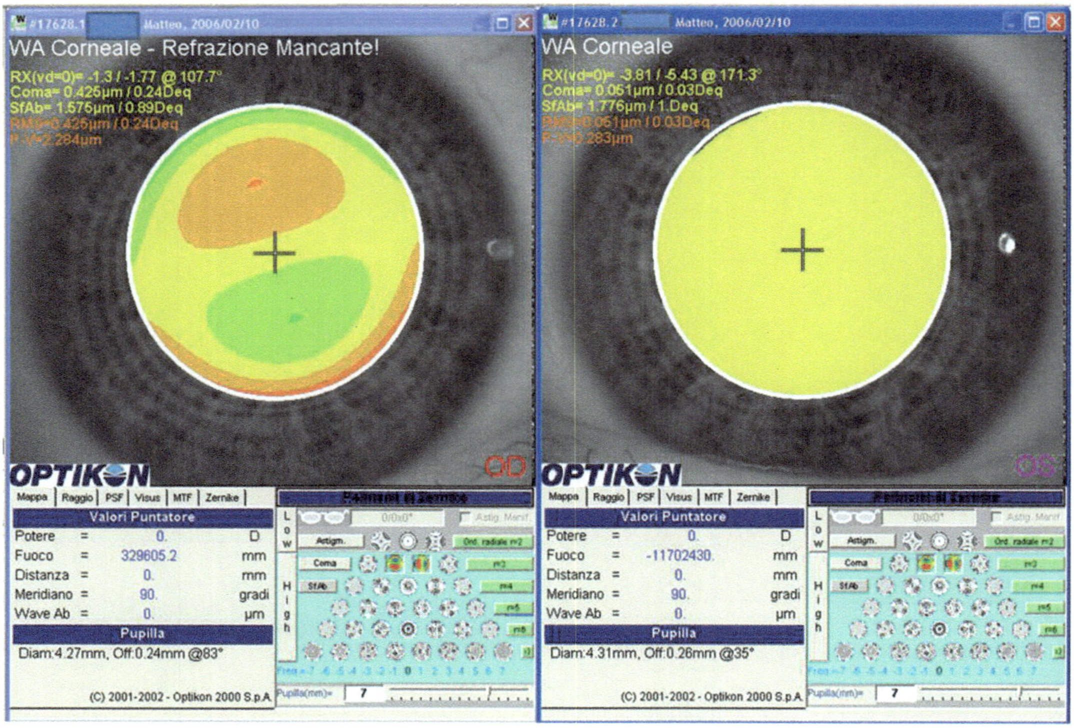

Fig. 94.3 Corneal wavefront analysis of coma in both eyes shows an abnormal coma only in the right eye

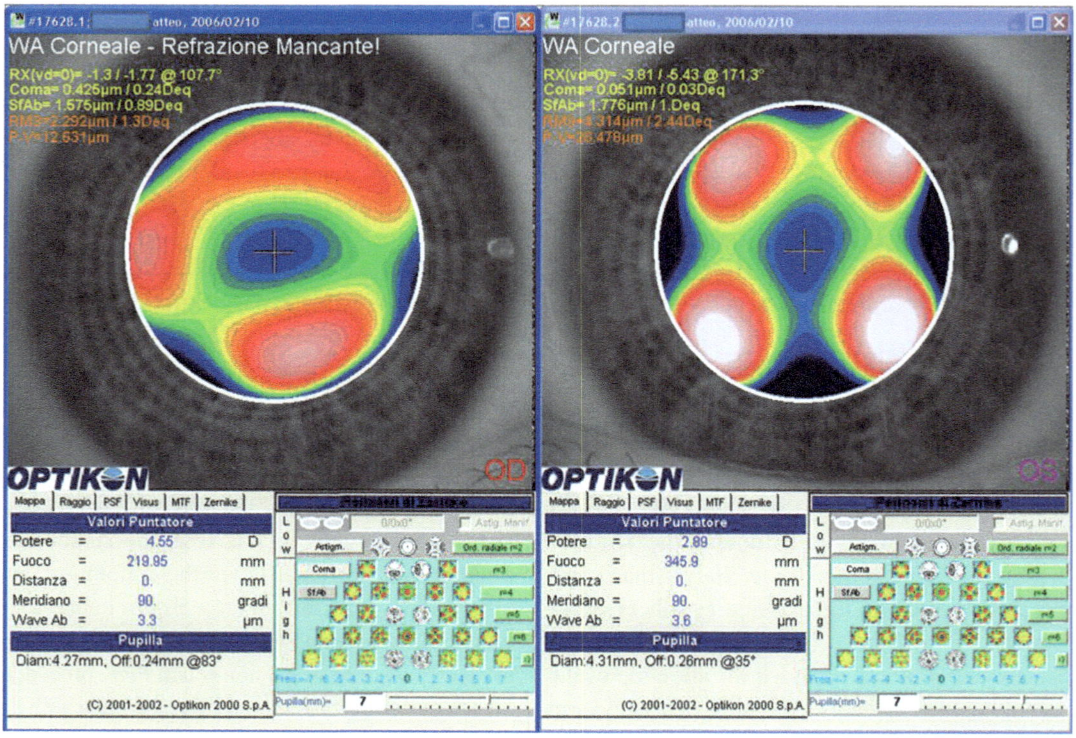

Fig. 94.4 Corneal wavefront analysis of high-order aberrations without coma and spherical aberration. Tetrafoil is evident in the left eye

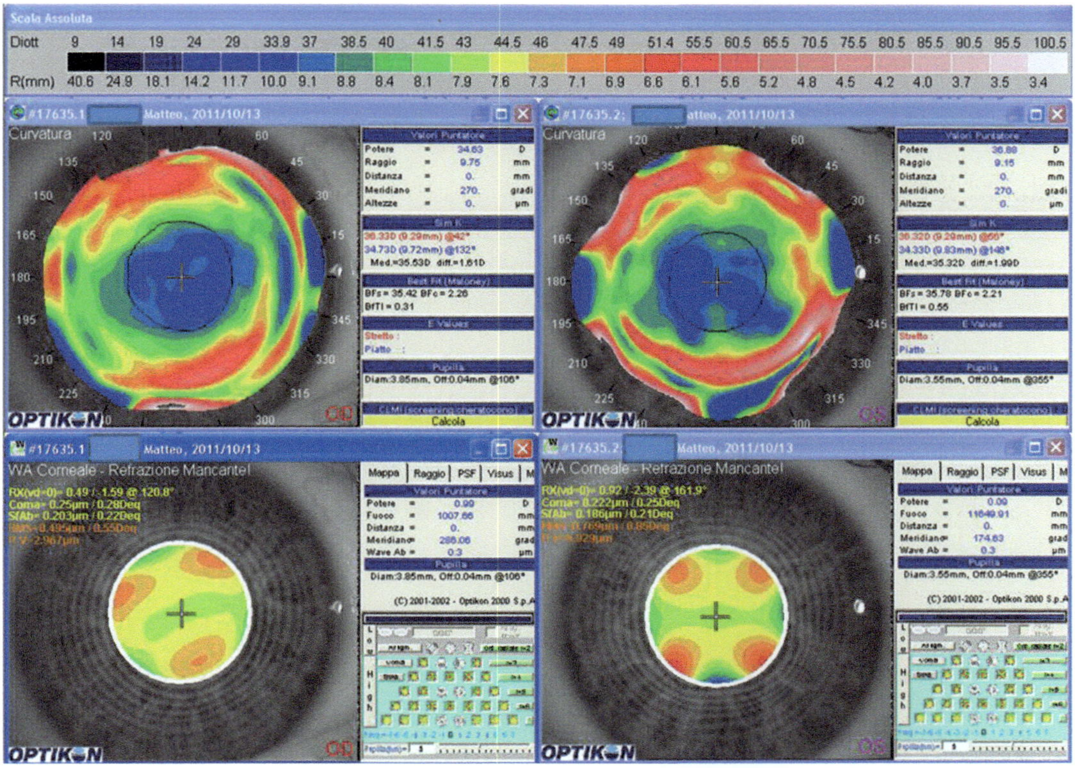

Fig. 94.5 The topography shows a wide optical zone in both eyes and a great reduction of all aberrations

treatment. 0.02 % MMC was applied for 2 min with a Merocel sponge, as is typical in re-treatments. A contact lens was applied for 4 days. Topical treatment with gentamicin (7 days) and a steroid (clobetasone bid for 1 month) was suggested.

Outcome

Postoperative care was uneventful and haze was 0 in both eyes. The refraction and visual acuity were the following: −1.25/−1@125 (8/10, 20/25) in the right eye and −0.5/−1.75@170 (9/10, 20/25) in the left eye. Stability remains excellent 6 years after the laser surgery (Fig. 94.5).

What to Learn from This Case

RK with AK often creates astigmatic overcorrection. Thanks to the topo–aberrometric link, it is possible to correct the "hyperopic-like" shift. In our case, the stability of the result was excellent over a 6-year follow-up. MMC can prevent the development of haze in eyes with previous RK.

The transepithelial PRK procedure is effective in irregular corneas, where we suspect the presence of an epithelium with different thicknesses due to scars or other irregularities [1, 2].

References

1. Camellin M, Mattioli R, Tripoli NK (2012) Topo-aberrometry with keratron onda. Corneal topography. Slack Incorporated, Thorofare, pp 184–190
2. Camellin M, Mosquera SA (2010) Simultaneous aspheric wavefront-guided transepithelial photorefractive keratectomy and phototherapeutic keratectomy to correct aberrations and refractive errors after corneal surgery. J Cataract Refract Surg 36:1173–1180

Cataract Surgery Complications of Radial Keratotomy

95

Massimo Camellin, Diego Ponzin, and Samuel Arba-Mosquera

Contents

M. Camellin, MD (✉)
SEKAL Rovigo Microsurgery, Rovigo, Italy
e-mail: cammas@tin.it

D. Ponzin
The Veneto Eye Bank Foundation, Venice, Italy
e-mail: diego.ponzin@fbov.it

S. Arba-Mosquera
SCHWIND Eye-Tech-Solutions, Kleinostheim, Germany

Why Is This Case Relevant for the Refractive Surgeon?

Curved keratotomies were common in the past and today have a new use in the femtosecond growing technique. Unfortunately, they can be unstable and overcorrect the original astigmatism. In case of a reached stability of overcorrection, it is possible to use customized laser ablation.

Incisional surgery creates unstable curvature of the cornea. Corneas treated with both RK and AK can increase in curvature in the case of ocular hypertension. Furthermore, even many years after the first surgery, mild trauma can open cuts.

In the case of cataract operations, there may be remarkable changes in intraocular pressure, and it is common to observe a hyperopic shift that generally declines after one month. Unfortunately, AK are more sensitive to high pressure, and this case shows an increased, stable astigmatism following the cataract operation [1].

Case Background

A 44-year-old male underwent a right eye 2 arcuate keratotomies (AK) in 1992 for congenital astigmatism. In 2004 he underwent a cataract operation OD, with pre-RK refraction and visual acuity pre-AK right eye of −2.5 sph/+5 cyl@135 (6/10, 20/30). Post-AK refraction and visual acuity in the right eye was −0.25 sph/+0.5 cyl@135 (6/10, 20/30).

J.L. Alió et al. (eds.), *Difficult and Complicated Cases in Refractive Surgery*,
DOI 10.1007/978-3-642-55238-0_95, © Springer-Verlag Berlin Heidelberg 2015

Post-cataract surgery, refraction and visual acuity in the right eye was −1 sph/−3 cyl@115 (6–7/10, 20/30). After cataract surgery, the incisions had an increased effect, and the refraction resulted in myopic astigmatism. The patient complained of poor near and far visual acuity and refused to wear spectacles.

Main Problem to Solve

The shape of an astigmatism following AK is typically irregular, with a dehiscence of the previous incisions. The atypical shape prevents a standard astigmatic ablation.

Although it is possible also to suture the incisions, healing with a stable scar requires several months. Moreover, some astigmatism can remain.

Ancillary Tests

Topography and corneal wavefront analysis are both necessary. A Scheimpflug camera has been used to study the features of the incisions (Figs. 95.1 and 95.2).

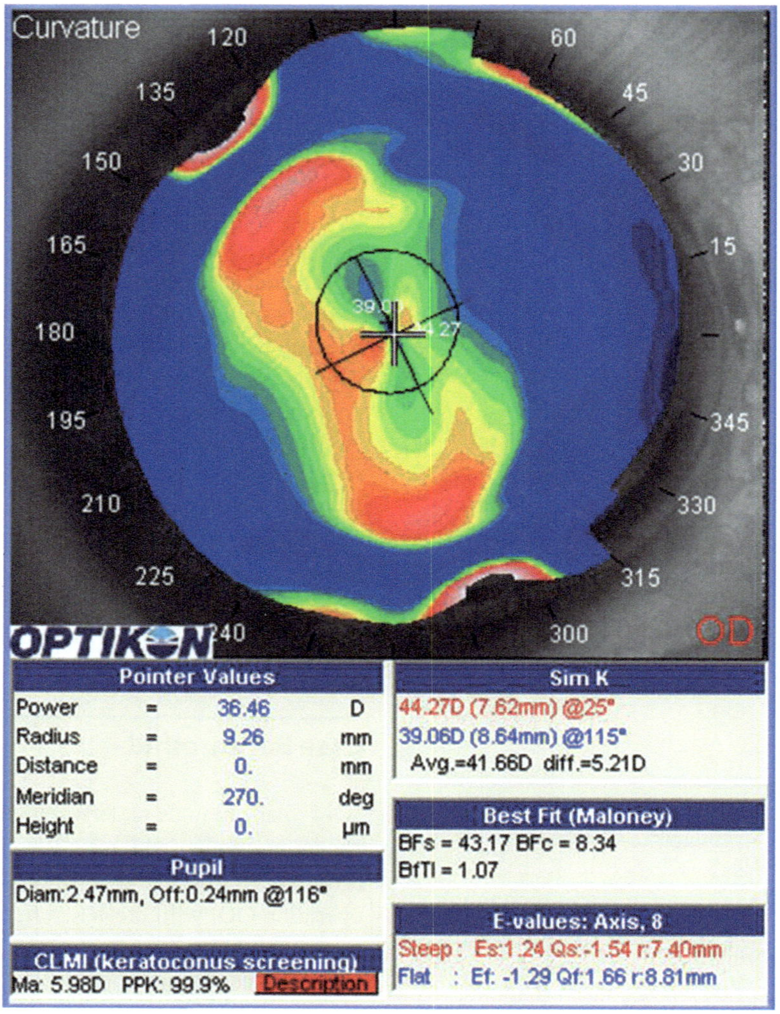

Fig. 95.1 Topography in tangential analysis shows the two arcuate keratotomies that are over dilated

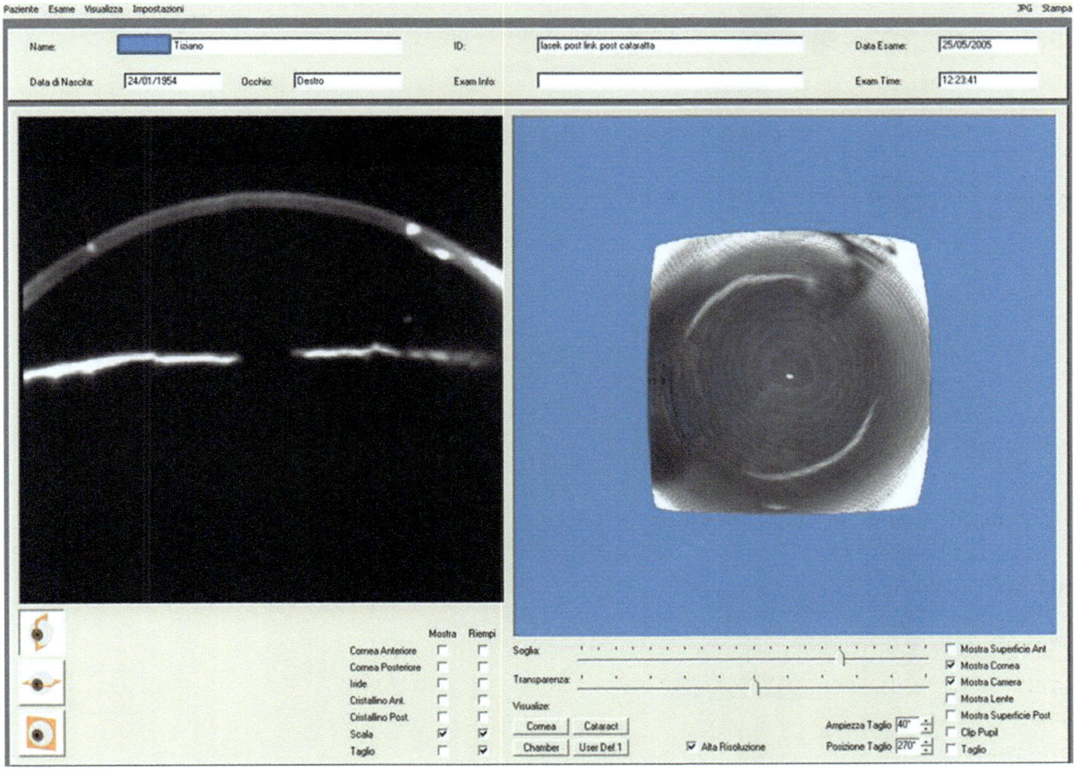

Fig. 95.2 Tomography with Scheimpflug camera

Surgical/Medical Intervention

The programmed surgery was a topo–aberrometric link procedure in which the topography was converted in corneal wavefront, and these data linked to the laser [2].

The platform used was the excimer laser SCHWIND AMARIS with a particular eye tracker (6 axes) that allows a perfect matching of the topography with the eye (Fig. 95.3).

The procedure used was a transepithelial link in which the laser takes into account the elimination of epithelium during the treatment. It is a non-touch procedure that is able to perfectly match the analyzed cornea with the laser program and the optimized epithelial ablation, determined from the diameter of the treatment.

0.02 % MMC was applied for 2 min with a Merocel sponge, as is typical in re-treatments. A contact lens was applied for 4 days. A topical treatment with gentamicin (7 days) and a steroid (clobetasone bid for 1 month) was suggested.

Outcome

The postoperative course was uneventful, haze was 0, and the stability was excellent three years following surgery. The right eye refraction and visual acuity was −0.25 sph/−0.5 cyl@180 (6–7/10, 20/30) (Figs. 95.4, 95.5, and 95.6).

What to Learn from This Case

It is important to be cautious in operating on cataracts in post-AK patients, as the pressure can have an increased effect of the incisions. A topo–aberrometric link is useful because it is relatively quick and has extreme precision.

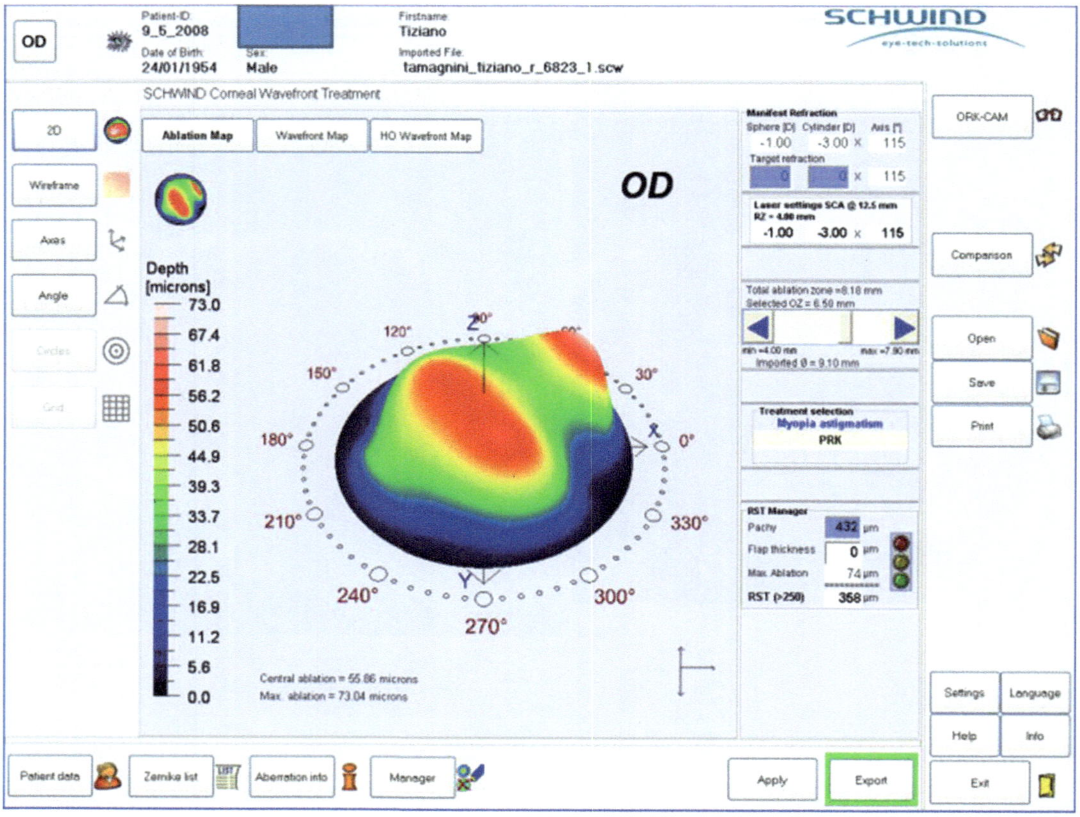

Fig. 95.3 File shot of the SCHWIND AMARIS. The ablations corresponding with the arcuate incisions are not of the same amplitude. The inferior one is deeper

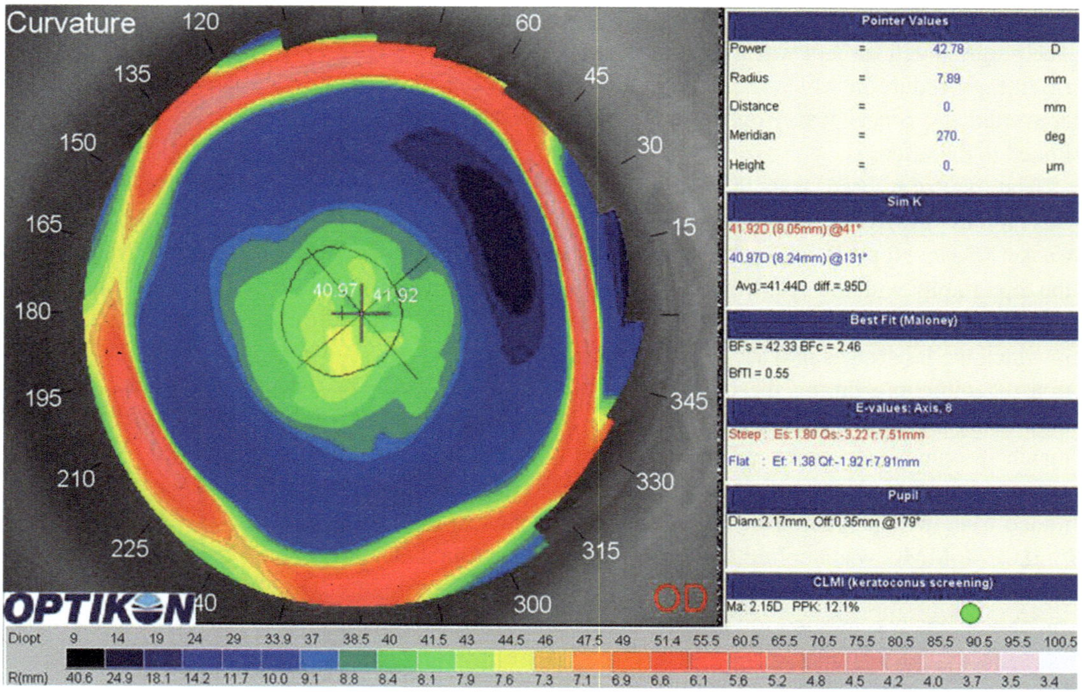

Fig. 95.4 Post-link topography. The aspect is that of a typical hyperopic pattern. There are no traces of the previous incisions

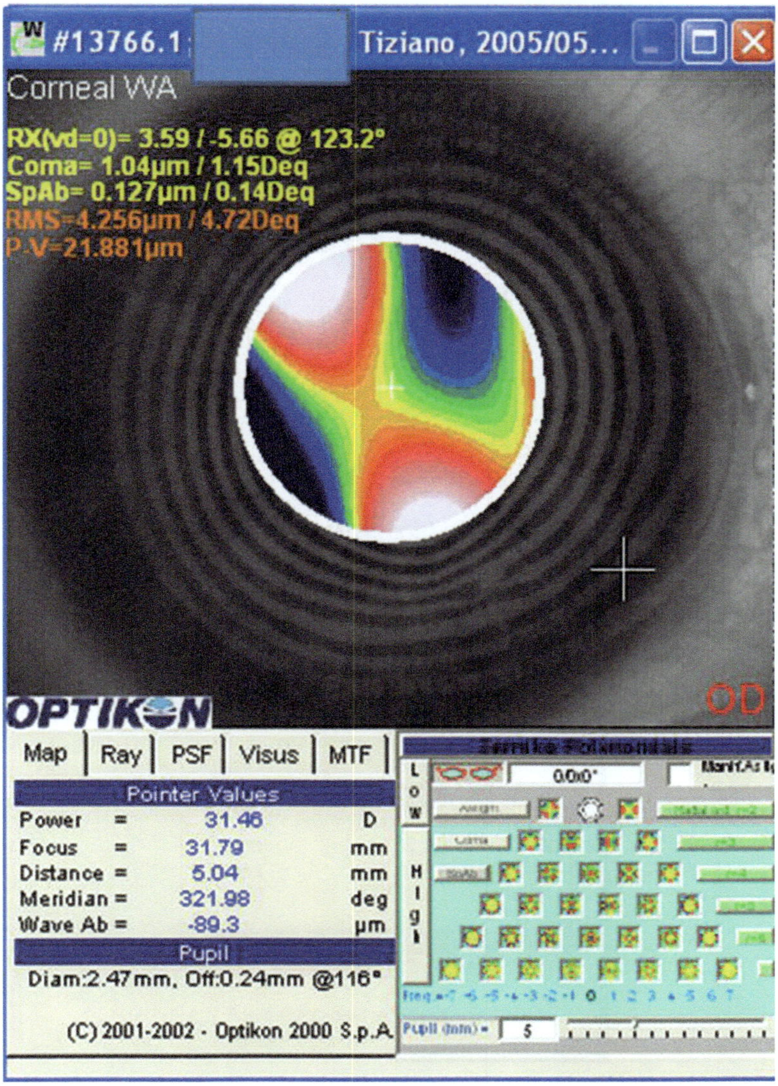

Fig. 95.5 Pre-link corneal wavefront. RMS value within 5 mm is 4.25 u

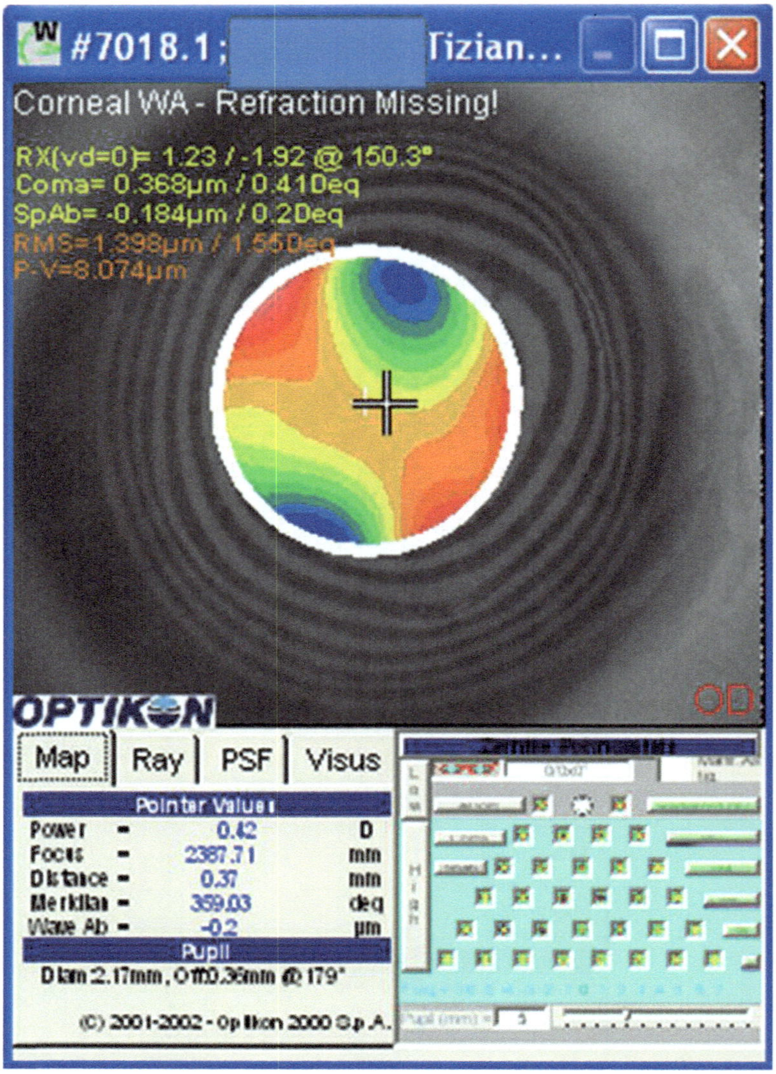

Fig. 95.6 Post-link corneal wavefront. RMS value within 5 mm is now reduced to 1.39 u

References

1. Camellin M, Mosquera SA (2012) Aspheric refractive correction of irregular astigmatism. In: Astigmatism optics, physiology and management. In Tech, Croatia, pp 103–124
2. Camellin M, Mosquera SA (2010) Simultaneous aspheric wavefront-guided transepithelial photorefractive keratectomy and phototherapeutic keratectomy to correct aberrations and refractive errors after corneal surgery. J Cataract Refract Surg 36:1173–1180

96 Lasik Surgery After Arcuate Lamellar Keratotomy

Jorge L. Alió and Alessandro Abbouda

Contents

J.L. Alió, MD, PhD (✉)
Department of Refractive Surgery, Vissum Corporación Oftalmológica, Alicante, Spain
e-mail: jlalio@vissum.com

A. Abbouda, MD
Department of Refractive Surgery, Vissum Corporación Oftalmológica, Alicante, Spain

Department of Ophthalmology-Policlinico Umberto I of Rome, University of Rome "Sapienza", Viale del Policlinico, 155, 00186 Roma, Italy

R&D Department, Vissum Corporación Oftalmológica, 03016, Alicante, Spain
e-mail: a.abbouda@gmail.com

Why Is This Case Relevant for the Refractive Surgeon?

When surgeons have to perform a second surgical procedure in an eye previously treated by radial keratotomy (RK) or, as in this case, arcuate lamellar keratotomy (ALK), they should be aware of the potential risk of flap adhesions and the possibility of tearing and damaging the flap.

Case Background

A 48-year-old man came to our department complaining of blurred vision in both eyes. Some years before, he underwent another ocular surgery, although he was not able to specify which one. His manifest refraction was +2 in the RE and $+0.25 = -0.25 \times 40°$ in the LE. His BCVA was 20/20 in both eyes. The corneal topography showed an astigmatic profile ablation (Fig. 96.1a). The keratometric index was $44.10/44.60 \times 98°$ in the RE and $44.88/44.91 \times 73°$ in the LE. The ultrasound pachymetry showed a value of 450 and 423 μm. The slit lamp examination revealed a centered corneal flap and ALK in both eyes. The patient had a strong motivation to be free from glasses.

J.L. Alió et al. (eds.), *Difficult and Complicated Cases in Refractive Surgery*,
DOI 10.1007/978-3-642-55238-0_96, © Springer-Verlag Berlin Heidelberg 2015

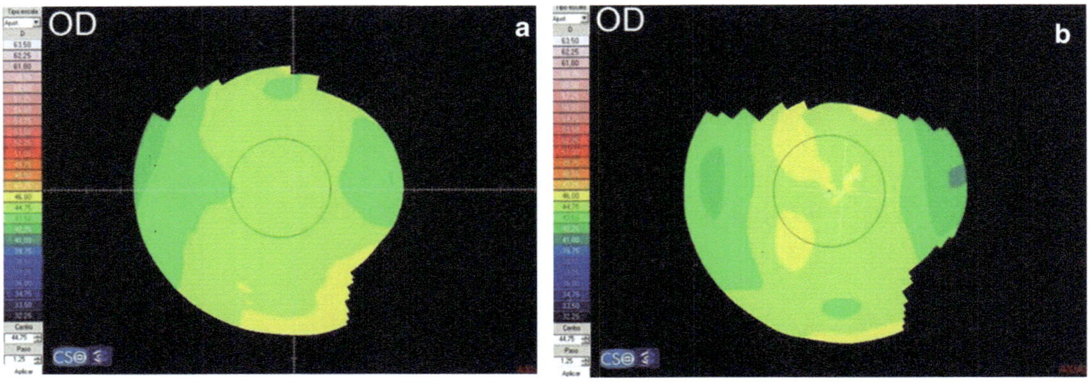

Fig. 96.1 Corneal topography at (**a**) the beginning and (**b**) the end of follow-up

Main Problem to Solve

We needed to determine whether PRK or ALK was more suitable for the patient. On the one hand, PRK seemed safer than ALK; on the other hand, PRK was associated with a five- to tenfold increase in haze formation and at least 20 % reduction in refractive predictability in RK-/ALK-treated eyes [1, 2]. We could not confirm whether the flap was created by a microkeratome or femtosecond laser, although its appearance suggested it was made by an FM. According to the amount of the defect to treat, the perfect condition of the flap, and the residual stroma bed, we decided to create a new deeper flap and then perform a hyperopic ablation.

Ancillary Tests

Manifest refraction, BCVA, corneal topography and aberrometry, and ultrasound pachymetry.

Surgical/Medical Intervention

The flap was created at 180 μm with double raster parameter at high energy. The tip of the Sinskey hook was used to open the flap margin for 1 clock hour at this location. The edge of the flap was grasped gently with a sponge and retracted across the superior conjunctiva. When the hook arrived at the side of the ALK, we found a very strong adhesion. The hook was moved up and down very gently until all the adhesions broke. The excimer laser ablation was applied, and the remainder of the procedure and postoperative care were identical to that of a normal LASIK procedure.

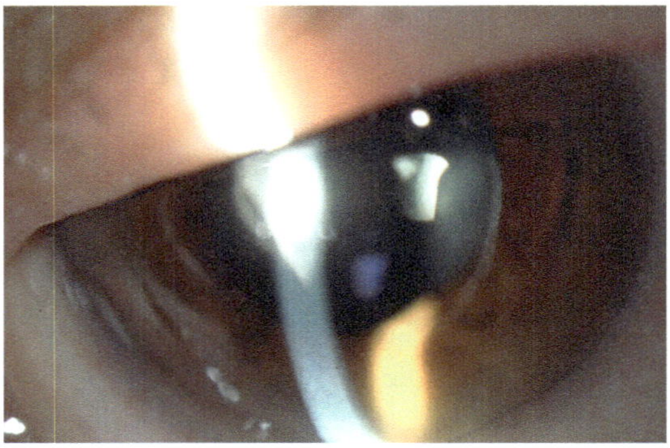

Fig. 96.2 Slit lamp examination following LASIK procedure showed ALK and the large LASIK flap. The flap margin is visible in the temporal side

Outcome

After 15 days, the manifest refraction in the patient's RE was plano and BCVA was 20/20. The corneal topography showed an increasing steepening in the central area. The keratometric index was 44.71/44.91 × 86° (Fig. 96.1b). The slit lamp examination revealed a normal flap with previous arcuate lamellar keratotomy (Fig. 96.2).

What to Learn from This Case

A careful preoperative evaluation may help avoid complications such as reopening of incisions during surgery or postoperative ingrowths of epithelium beneath the corneal flap. The patient must first be informed of any possible alternative treatments. In this case, a new deeper femtosecond flap resulted in effective correction of refractive error following AKT, even when the surgical procedure was somewhat difficult [3].

References

1. Azar T, Tuli S, Benson RA, Hardten DR (1998) Photorefractive keratectomy for residual myopia after radial keratotomy. J Cataract Refract Surg 24:303–311
2. Gimbel HV, Sun R, Chin PK, van Westenbrugge J (1997) Excimer laser photorefractive keratectomy for residual myopia after radial keratotomy. Can J Ophthalmol 32:25–30
3. Forseto AS, Nosé RA, Francesconi CM, Nosé W (1999) Laser in situ keratomileusis for undercorrection after radial keratotomy. J Refract Surg 15:424–428

Part X

Optical Neuropathy and Retinal Complications After Refractive Surgery

Dear reader,

In the final chapter of this book, we emphasize severe complications that may be associated with refractive surgical procedures. Although incidence is low, complications can lead to issues of clinical misunderstandings and medicolegal litigation.

We include some topics such as: choroidal neovascularization, flap displacement, NIAON, macular hole, and retinal detachment occured post-LASIK. It is very important to inform patients, especially those with severe myopia, about the risks of vitreoretinal stress and macular disease associated with some refractive surgical procedures. We report cases associated with these complications and how to manage them.

For further reading, we suggest the first book of this series: J. L. Alio', D. Azar *Management of Complications in Refractive Surgery*, Chapter 8: Optical Neuropathy and Retinal Complications After Refractive Surgery (pp. 155–165).

Specific topics covered by the cases include choroidal neovascularization after LASIK (Cases 99), lacquer cracks after LASIK (Case 100), and unusual and interesting case of intraoperative complication related to flap displacement (Case 101). We end with cases focused on NIAON after LASIK (Case 102), macular lesion after LASIK and the role of vitreous traction (Case 103), and risk factors of retinal detachment following LASIK (Case 104).

Lesson to Learn

Case 99: Choroidal neovascularization following after LASIK

In high myopic eyes with lacquer cracks, does inflammatory reaction induced by LASIK, increasing VEGF levels and induce CNV development?

Case 100: Lacquer cracks after LASIK

The increase in intraocular pressure during suction and the excimer laser shock wave that is transmitted to the eye may open the gap in Bruch's membrane and generate lacquer cracks.

Case 101: LASIK flap displacement during vitrectomy

Unusual and interesting case of intraoperative complication related to the flap displacement after corneal epithelial debridement during a scleral buckling procedure.

Case 102: NIAON after LASIK

Intraocular pressure elevation during LASIK may cause deterioration in perfusion of the optic nerve head or a compression of the ganglion cells/nerve fiber layer leading a posterior cupping of the optic nerve and damage to the nerve fibers, with resultant visual defect.

Case 103: Macular hole after LASIK

A mechanism for development of peripheral retinal tears or macular disease could be anterior-posterior compression and expansion during the suction.

Case 104: Retinal detachment after LASIK

Refractive surgeons should ask their patients to assess the condition of the peripheral retina before and after the LASIK procedure in order to prevent or treat risky lesions that could predispose to retinal detachment.

CNV After LASIK

97

J. Fernando Arevalo

Contents

J.F. Arevalo, MD, FACS
Vitreoretinal Division, The King Khaled Eye Specialist Hospital, Riyadh, Saudi Arabia

Department of Ophthalmology,
Wilmer Eye Institute, The Johns Hopkins University, Baltimore, MD, USA
e-mail: arevalojf@jhmi.edu

Why Is This Case Relevant for the Refractive Surgeon?

The risk of developing lacquer cracks in highly myopic patients corrected by LASIK, though uncommon, must be kept in mind. This is true especially in highly myopic patients with myopic retinopathy in whom LASIK could be used to correct residual defects after posterior chamber or phakic intraocular lens implantation [1].

Case Background

A 52-year-old female patient underwent LASIK to correct bilateral myopia (SE −8.00 D RE and −13.00 D LE) in January 1999. Twenty-four months later, she complained of decreased visual acuity in her LE. At that time, best-corrected visual acuity (BCVA) in her RE was 20/40 (SE −2.75 D) and 10/200 (SE −5.75 D) in her LE. A CNV was diagnosed with fluorescein angiography (Fig. 97.1a).

Main Problem to Solve

Lacquer cracks are often underdiagnosed because of their small size and the difficulty of detecting them in myopic fundi. Lacquer cracks often lead to poor visual outcomes because of choroidal neovascularization and macular atrophy in pathologic myopia. When Bruch's membrane ruptures, it allows the progression of

J.L. Alió et al. (eds.), *Difficult and Complicated Cases in Refractive Surgery*,
DOI 10.1007/978-3-642-55238-0_97, © Springer-Verlag Berlin Heidelberg 2015

CNV. Due to early treatment will allow better success, the surgeons must be aware of this condition.

Ancillary Tests

Fluorescein angiography (FA) and optic coherence tomography (OCT) are the best tests to be done in order to diagnose and follow the treatment of the CNV. At the time we reported this case, the only feasible diagnostic test available was the FA.

Surgical/Medical Intervention

Our patient underwent Lasik procedure in 1999. At that time the CNV was treated with two sessions of photodynamic therapy (PDT) with verteporfin 6 months apart (current CNV treatment has evolved to anti-VEGF therapy).

Outcome

After the second PDT treatment, the CNV was totally closed with subretinal fibrosis, and a final BCVA of 20/200 was observed 6 months later (Fig. 97.1b).

What to Learn from This Case

Choroidal neovascularization is related to myopia itself, and its incidence varies from 4 to 11 % in patients with high myopia. In addition, lacquer cracks have been found to be associated with CNV in up to 82 % of cases with myopia [2]. Theoretically, when a break in Bruch's membrane occurs, it allows the progression of the neovascular complex under the retina. The increase in intraocular pressure (IOP) to levels over 60 mmHg during suction with the microkeratome suction ring up to 4 mm posterior to the limbus may exert traction and compression posteriorly. In addition, we have to consider that the excimer laser is responsible for a shock wave that is transmitted to the eye. These mechanisms may open the gap in Bruch's membrane even more [1]. Because this condition may lead to an irreversible visual lost, it is extremely important to adopt preventive measures. Patients with high myopia and lacquer cracks in the macula are at high risk to develop macular hemorrhage or CNV after the IOP is raised with the suction ring during the procedure. Patients with angioid streaks and traumatic choroidal ruptures are in the same category of risk [3]. We believe that in patients with high myopia and lacquer cracks, LASIK should be considered

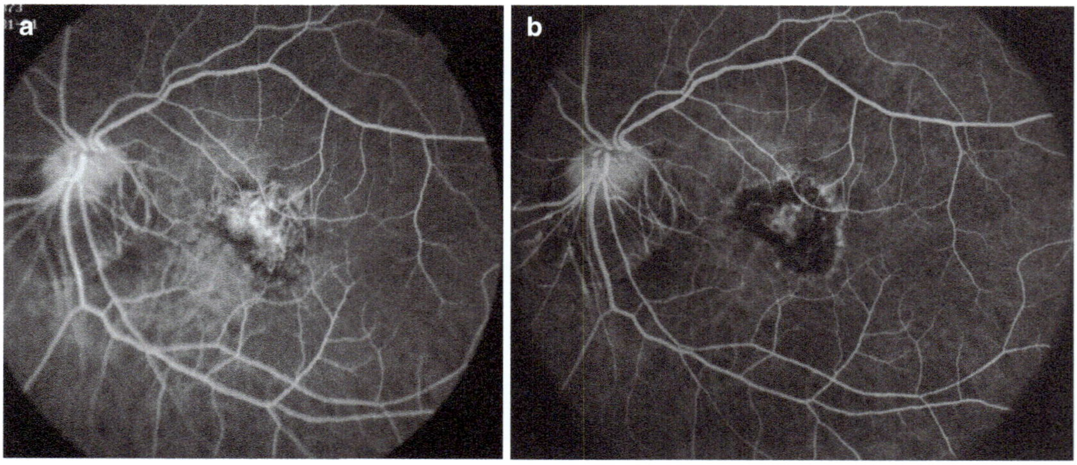

Fig. 97.1 (**a**) A CNV was diagnosed with fluorescein angiography. (**b**) After the second PDT treatment, the CNV was totally closed with subretinal fibrosis and a final BCVA of 20/200 6 months later

contraindicated and some other methods of refractive surgery offered.

Nowadays, myopic CNVs are treated with antiangiogenic agents (bevacizumab [Avastin®] or ranibizumab [Lucentis®]; Genentech, San Francisco, CA, USA or aflibercept [EYLEA], Regeneron, Tarrytown, NY, USA and Bayer HealthCare, Berlin, Germany). Intravitreal anti-VEGF therapy resulted in long-term visual improvement in myopic CNV in recent studies [4, 5]. Patients would be given an initial injection and re-treatment based on BCVA and OCT. The treatment efficacy in terms of visual gain and number of re-treatments appears to be similar between bevacizumab and ranibizumab. The mean number of injections was 3.8 for both bevacizumab and ranibizumab groups at 2 years in a recent study [4].

References

1. Ruiz-Moreno JM, Montero J, Alio JL (2003) Lacquer crack formation after LASIK. Ophthalmology 110:1669–1671
2. Amat-Peral P, Lugo F, Montero JA, de la Vega C, Arévalo JF, Alió Y, Sanz JL (2008) Photodynamic therapy with verteporfin in choroidal neovascularization after refractive surgery. Arch Soc Esp Oftalmol 83:539–544
3. Arevalo JF (2008) Posterior segment complications after laser-assisted in situ keratomileusis. Curr Opin Ophthalmol 19:177–184
4. Lai TY, Luk FO, Lee GK, Lam DS (2012) Long-term outcome of intravitreal anti-vascular endothelial growth factor therapy with bevacizumab or ranibizumab as primary treatment for subfoveal myopic choroidal neovascularization. Eye (Lond) 26: 1004–1011
5. Neo HY, Neelam K, Yip CC, Quah HM, Au Eong KG (2013) Choroidal neovascularization following laser in situ keratomileusis for high myopia: a case series. Int Ophthalmol 33:27–34

LASIK Flap Displacement During Vitrectomy

98

J. Fernando Arevalo

Contents

J.F. Arevalo, MD, FACS
Vitreoretinal Division, The King Khaled Eye Specialist Hospital, Riyadh, Saudi Arabia

Department of Ophthalmology, Wilmer Eye Institute, The Johns Hopkins University, Baltimore, MD, USA
e-mail: arevalojf@jhmi.edu

Why Is This Case Relevant for the Refractive Surgeon?

Displacement of a corneal flap after LASIK is a serious complication which has been identified after corneal epithelial debridement during a scleral buckling procedure and vitrectomy. It is extremely important for the refractive surgeon to detect and treat certain conditions before LASIK, including misdiagnosed posterior pole diseases such as epiretinal membranes, vitreomacular traction syndrome, and others. In addition, diabetic retinopathy is a relative contraindication to LASIK as these patients may require vitreoretinal surgery in their future. If a posterior pole complication develops after LASIK, the refractive surgeon should consult with the vitreous surgeon about the past ocular history.

Background

In this case, a dislocated corneal flap (Fig. 98.1) occurred from corneal epithelial debridement during vitrectomy 69 months after LASIK. Similar cases have been reported [1–3], in which patients underwent vitreous surgery between 4 and 12 months after LASIK.

J.L. Alió et al. (eds.), *Difficult and Complicated Cases in Refractive Surgery*,
DOI 10.1007/978-3-642-55238-0_98, © Springer-Verlag Berlin Heidelberg 2015

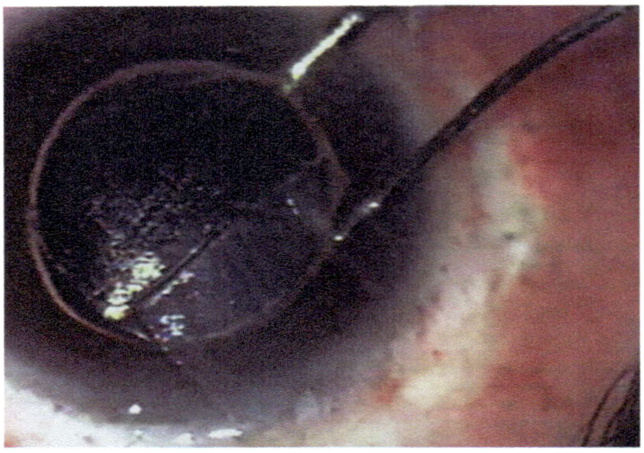

Fig. 98.1 A dislocated corneal flap occurred from corneal epithelial debridement during vitrectomy 69 months after LASIK

The Problem

Possible problems include losing the cap, epithelial ingrowth, interface particles, and striae in the flap. Trauma to the flap may affect the final refractive status.

Ancillary Tests

This condition should be diagnosed clinically. However, ancillary tests can document complications such as anterior segment optical coherence tomography, ultrabiomicroscopy, Orbscan, or Pentacam [4].

Surgical/Medical Intervention

Management of a displaced corneal flap includes repositioning the flap, patching, and topical steroids. Refractory cases may require suture fixation. A bandage contact lens may be useful if striae develop. Striae that persist are an indication to elevate and reposition the flap.

Outcome

Our patient's case was successfully managed with repositioning of the flap, a bandage contact lens at the end of the vitreous surgery, and topical steroids.

What We Learned

When vitreoretinal surgeons treat an eye with a history of LASIK, they are cautioned to avoid debridement of the corneal epithelium. In cases when corneal debridement is necessary, it is recommended to start the procedure nasally and advance temporally (most cases have a nasal hinge). Refractive surgeons should avoid LASIK in patients who face the potential of vitreoretinal surgery in their future, including cases of diabetic retinopathy or vitreomacular traction syndrome. A preoperative OCT of the posterior pole is important to rule out vitreomacular adhesions. If a posterior pole complication develops, the refractive surgeon should alert the vitreous surgeon to the past ocular history (LASIK).

References

1. Chaudhry NA, Smiddy WE (1998) Displacement of corneal cap during vitrectomy in a post-LASIK eye. Retina 18:554–555
2. Tosi GM, Tilanus MA, Eggink C, Mittica V (2005) Flap displacement during vitrectomy 24 months after in situ keratomileusis. Retina 25:1101–1103
3. López-Guajardo L, Drake-Rodríguez P, Paz-Moreno J, Teus-Guezala M, Pareja-Esteban J (2007) Possibility of flap displacement during retinal surgery. Retina 27:393–394
4. Mannino G, Perdicchi A, Medori EM, Recupero SM (2007) Ultrabiomicroscopy (UBM) in flap dislocation following LASIK: a case report. Eur J Ophthalmol 17:259–261

NIAON After LASIK

99

J. Fernando Arevalo

Contents

J.F. Arevalo, MD, FACS
Vitreoretinal Division, The King Khaled Eye Specialist Hospital, Riyadh, Saudi Arabia

Department of Ophthalmology, Wilmer Eye Institute, The Johns Hopkins University, Baltimore, MD, USA
e-mail: arevalojf@jhmi.edu

Why Is This Case Relevant for the Refractive Surgeon?

Although this complication is extremely rare, optic neuropathy after LASIK surgery is a significant vision-threatening complication. During LASIK, an uncontrolled and unpredictable rise in intraocular pressure occurs. The rise may lead to the development of optic neuropathy, which can cause irreversible and untreatable visual loss, even legal blindness. Although controversial, the use of systemic corticosteroids may help improve visual function in some patients and should be given during the very early stages of the disease. In cases where the physician is not aware of this complication, delaying treatment is of no benefit. Finally, a proper diagnosis can allow the surgeon to take preventative measures to avoid optic nerve damage.

Case Background

A 39-year-old man had loss of vision 1 day after bilateral LASIK. He described a hazy quality of vision in both eyes immediately after LASIK. His medical history showed no other risk factors for optic neuropathy. Examination revealed a visual acuity of 20/20 in both eyes, normal color vision, increased cupping of the optic nerve, and a relative afferent pupillary defect in the right eye (RE) (Fig. 99.1).

J.L. Alió et al. (eds.), *Difficult and Complicated Cases in Refractive Surgery*,
DOI 10.1007/978-3-642-55238-0_99, © Springer-Verlag Berlin Heidelberg 2015

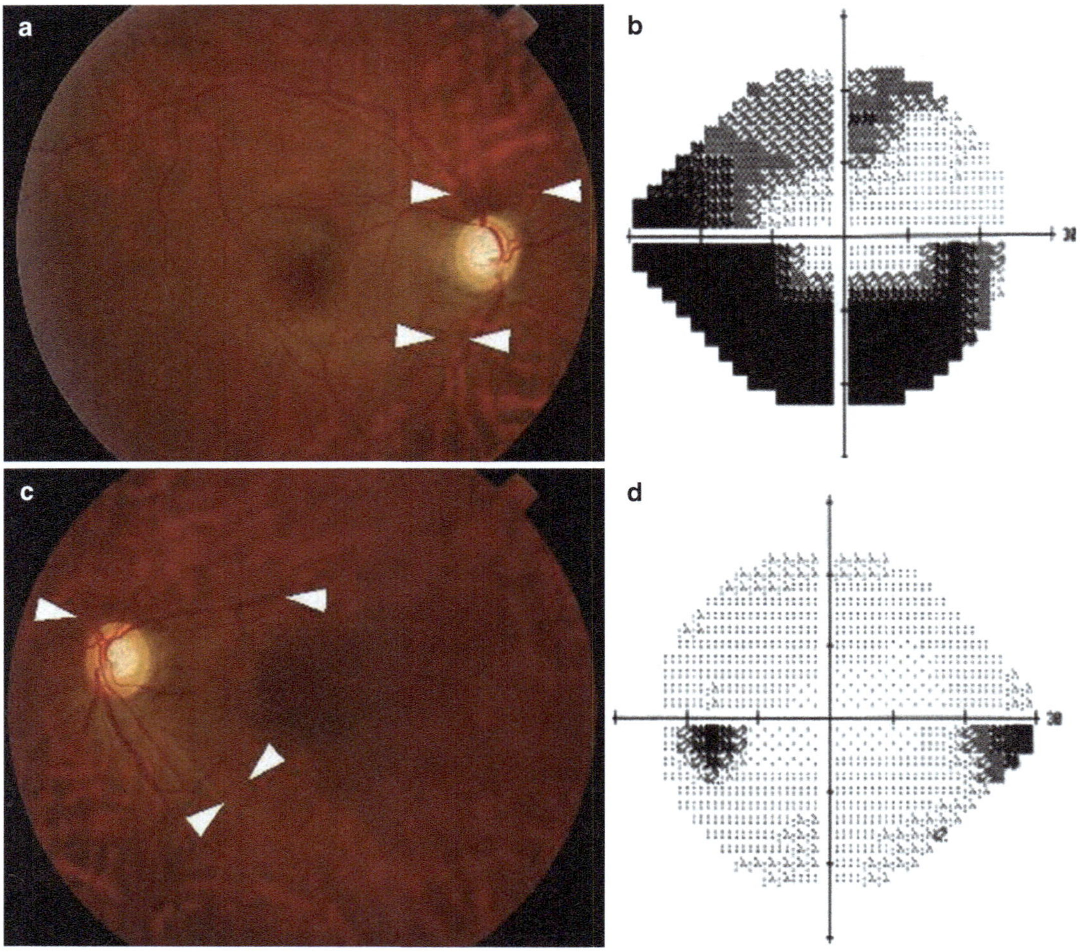

Fig. 99.1 (**a**) A fifty-degree fundus photo of the RE shows diffuse loss of retinal nerve fiber layer (RNFL) at the superior pole of the disc and early wedge defects in the RNFL at the inferior pole of the disc (*arrowheads*). (**b**) The visual field shows a dense inferior nerve fiber bundle-type scotoma and a moderate superior nerve fiber bundle-type scotoma corresponding to the disc and RNFL defects in the RE. (**c**) Fifty-degree fundus photo of the left eye (LE) shows diffuse loss of RNFL at the superior pole of the disc and a wedge defect in the inferotemporal RNFL corresponding to the notch in the inferior neuroretinal rim (*arrows*). (**d**) Visual field shows an early inferior nerve fiber bundle-type scotoma corresponding to the loss of superior RNFL in the LE (Modified and reprinted from Cameron et al. [1], with permission from the American Academy of Ophthalmology)

Main Problem to Solve

Visual field defects and loss of vision are the main problems; however, because no real treatment exists for this condition, it is extremely important to adopt preventive measures.

Ancillary Tests

At the onset of optic neuropathy after LASIK, the patient can present postoperative visual acuity and color vision deterioration, relative afferent pupillary defect, variable swelling of the disc, and optic nerve-related visual field defects. Deep cupping of the optic nerve, focal changes in the neuroretinal rim, and decreased thickness of the retinal nerve fiber layer can be seen 2 or 3 months after the onset of AION and sometimes as soon as 6 weeks [1, 2].

Surgical/Medical Intervention

Treatment options for AION are controversial. Some advocate for steroid treatment for the non-arteritic type of AION. A number of reports suggest that systemic corticosteroids given during the very early stages of the disease may help improve visual function in some patients. Hayreh found definite evidence of significant visual improvement with steroids in a small group of patients, particularly those with incipient non-arteritic AION, treated early [3].

Surgical treatment including optic nerve fenestration was advocated for AION until the completion of the Ischemic Optic Neuropathy Decompression Trial (IONDT). This study showed no conclusive effect of the surgical procedure [4].

Because there is no real treatment for this condition, prevention is extremely important. Prevention should include (1) avoiding any sudden fall in systemic arterial blood pressure (hypotensive anesthesia, congestive heart failure), (2) improving systemic circulatory hemodynamics by medical therapy, (3) preventing any sudden rise in intraocular pressure (angle closure and intraocular surgery such as cataract extraction), and (4) keeping intraocular pressure as low as possible by medical means [3, 5].

Patients with personal or family histories of coagulopathies, hereditary neuropathies, or AION; optic nerves at risk such as a small crowded optic nerve; tilted disc; glaucoma; a family history of glaucoma; or glaucoma suspects should be cautioned of LASIK-associated visual field loss prior to the procedure. Most neuropathies after LASIK occur in patients over 35 years old, so age is another consideration. For many patients, photorefractive keratectomy, intrastromal corneal ring segments, or continued use of contact lens or eyeglasses may offer satisfactory vision without subjecting the optic nerve to the small but real risk of pressure-associated visual field loss.

Outcome

The functional and structural changes that occur in neuropathies after LASIK procedures are typically permanent.

What to Learn from This Case

Intraocular pressure elevation during LASIK may cause deterioration in perfusion of the retina and optic nerve head, posterior displacement of the lamina cribrosa, and a decline in ocular perfusion pressure of the posterior ciliary arteries. Although IOP elevation is temporary, the potential for ischemic or pressure-induced damage to the optic nerve head and the retinal nerve fiber layer exists. Others believe that LASIK-related optic neuropathy could be due to barotrauma, with compression of the ganglion cells, nerve fiber layer, and lamina cribrosa. This leads to posterior cupping of the optic nerve and damage to the nerve fibers, with a resultant visual defect. Optic neuritis may occur in predisposed LASIK cases with vascular ischemic risk factors.

References

1. Cameron BD, Saffra NA, Strominger MB (2001) Laser in situ keratomileusis-induced optic neuropathy. Ophthalmology 108:660–665
2. Lee AG, Kohnen T, Ebner R et al (2000) Optic neuropathy associated with laser in situ keratomileusis. J Cataract Refract Surg 26:1581–1584
3. Hayreh SS (1996) Acute ischemic disorders of the optic nerve: pathogenesis, clinical manifestations and management. Ophthalmol Clin North Am 9:407–442
4. Optic Neuropathy Decompression group. Ischemic Optic Neuropathy Decompression Trial: twenty-four-month update (2000) Arch Ophthalmol 118:793–798
5. Shaikh NM, Shaikh S, Singh K, Manche E (2002) Progression to end-stage glaucoma after laser in situ keratomileusis. J Cataract Refract Surg 28:356–359

Macular Hole After LASIK

100

J. Fernando Arevalo

Contents

J.F. Arevalo, MD, FACS
Vitreoretinal Division, The King Khaled
Eye Specialist Hospital, Riyadh, Saudi Arabia

Department of Ophthalmology, Wilmer Eye Institute,
The Johns Hopkins University, Baltimore, MD, USA
e-mail: arevalojf@jhmi.edu

Why Is This Case Relevant for the Refractive Surgeon?

Posterior pole complications after LASIK tend to occur months to years after the procedure. The surgeon must maintain a close observation of his patients over a long period of time in order to diagnose and treat these complications promptly. In the largest reported series of macular hole, the hole formed between 1 and 83 months after the procedure (mean: 12.1 months). All eyes were myopic. Posterior vitreous detachment was not present before but was documented after LASIK on 55 % of the eyes; a vitrectomy closed the macular hole on all 20 eyes that underwent surgical management. These 20 eyes reflect an incidence of 0.02 % (20/83,938 eyes) [1–3]. Although very rare, the occurrence of a macular hole after LASIK may definitively compromise the central visual function of a patient.

Case Background

A 30-year-old woman with −13.00 D of myopia in the right (RE) and −10.00 D in the left eye (LE) underwent bilateral laser in situ keratomileusis in June 2001. Six months after surgery, she noted the onset of blurred vision in her LE. Retinal examination revealed a stage 4 macular hole in the LE (Fig. 100.1a) associated with a posterior pole retinal detachment and a best-corrected visual acuity (BCVA) of counting fingers.

J.L. Alió et al. (eds.), *Difficult and Complicated Cases in Refractive Surgery*,
DOI 10.1007/978-3-642-55238-0_100,

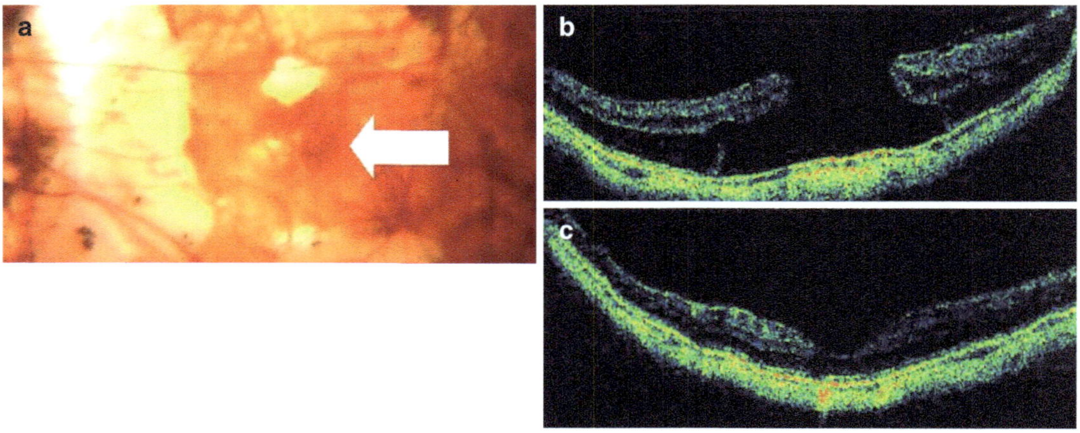

Fig. 100.1 (**a**) Retinal examination revealed a stage 4 macular hole (*arrow*) in the LE associated with a posterior pole retinal detachment and a BCVA of counting fingers. (**b**) The optical coherence tomography (OCT) image showed features of both foveal retinal detachment and retinoschisis. (**c**) Best-corrected visual acuity recovered to 20/150 with macular hole closure 4 months after a successful vitrectomy

Main Problem to Solve

Noting the development and treating a macular hole early promote better surgical results.

Ancillary Tests

Optical coherence tomography (OCT) is the premier test that allows a surgeon to diagnose macular holes soon after LASIK. In some circumstances, the atrophic myopic macular changes do not allow the surgeon to diagnose the condition. In our case, the OCT image showed features of both foveal retinal detachment and retinoschisis (Fig. 100.1b).

Surgical/Medical Intervention

Pars plana vitrectomy with internal limiting membrane peeling and a fluid-gas exchange.

Outcome

BCVA recovered to 20/150 with macular hole closure 4 months after a successful vitrectomy (Fig. 100.1c).

What to Learn from This Case

When the suction ring induces an increase in IOP and is suddenly released, the anterior segment is rapidly drawn into a vacuum chamber with a rapid change in shape, and all structures posterior to the suction ring are compressed and decompressed in sequence. A mechanism for the development of peripheral retinal tears or macular disease could be anterior-posterior compression and expansion. The eye elongates along the anterior-posterior axis, and the diameter of the globe may increase. At the same time, because the eye is a closed system, the eye is constricted in the equatorial plane (Fig. 100.2a). As the anterior segment is drawn into a vacuum, the lens may be displaced forward along with the anterior hyaloid. This can accelerate vitreous detachment or cause traction at the vitreous base. When the suction is suddenly released, decompression leads to a dynamic overshooting with equatorial expansion and shortening in the anterior-posterior dimension (Fig. 100.2b). These events may cause acute vitreoretinal traction at the vitreous base and posterior pole. In addition, when the excimer laser light ablates tissue, energy is released anteriorly as a plume of ablated tissue and is thrown into the air in front of the cornea.

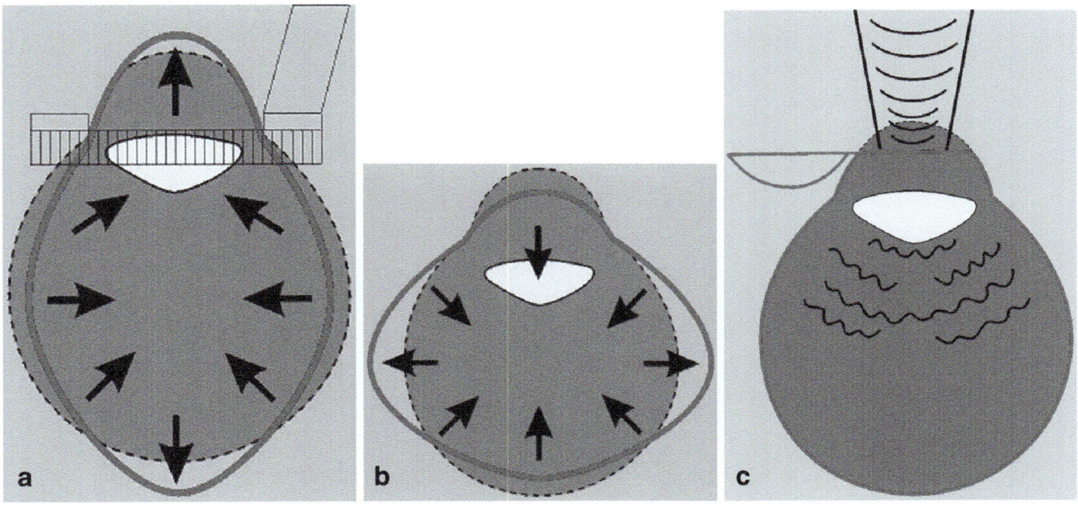

Fig. 100.2 (**a**) When the suction ring induces an increase in IOP, the eye is constricted in the equatorial plane. (**b**) When the suction is suddenly released, decompression leads to a dynamic overshooting with equatorial expansion and shortening in the anterior-posterior dimension. (**c**) In addition, when the excimer laser light ablates tissue posteriorly, energy is transmitted in the form of a shockwave

Such a powerful force might also be associated with backward force into the vitreous. Posteriorly, energy is transmitted in the form of a shockwave (Fig. 100.2c). The effect of shockwaves and posteriorly radiated energy on the vitreous integrity is unknown [4].

References

1. Arevalo JF, Mendoza AJ, Velez-Vazquez W, Rodriguez FJ, Rodriguez A, Rosales-Meneses JL, Yepez JB, Ramirez E, Dessouki A, Chan CK, Mittra RA, Ramsay RC, Garcia RA, Ruiz-Moreno JM (2005) Full-thickness macular hole after LASIK for the correction of myopia. Ophthalmology 112:1207–1212
2. Arevalo JF (2008) Posterior segment complications after laser-assisted in situ keratomileusis. Curr Opin Ophthalmol 19:177–178
3. Arevalo JF, Rodriguez FJ, Rosales-Meneses JL, Dessouki A, Chan CK, Mittra RA, Ruiz-Moreno JM (2005) Vitreoretinal surgery for macular hole after laser assisted in situ keratomileusis for the correction of myopia. Br J Ophthalmol 89:1423–1426
4. Arevalo JF, Ramirez E, Suarez E, Cortez R, Antzoulatos G, Morales-Stopello J, Ramirez G, Torres F, Gonzalez-Vivas R (2001) Rhegmatogenous retinal detachment in myopic eyes after laser in situ keratomileusis. Frequency, characteristics, and mechanism. J Cataract Refract Surg 27:674–680

Retinal Detachment After LASIK

101

J. Fernando Arevalo

Contents

J.F. Arevalo, MD, FACS
Vitreoretinal Division, The King Khaled Eye Specialist Hospital, Riyadh, Saudi Arabia

Department of Ophthalmology, Wilmer Eye Institute, The Johns Hopkins University, Baltimore, MD, USA
e-mail: arevalojf@jhmi.edu

Why Is This Case Relevant for the Refractive Surgeon?

In some patients with retinal detachments, a delay in referral to the vitreoretinal specialist is due to a belief that the visual symptoms were related to a refractive or corneal problem after LASIK. A refractive surgeon must be aware of complications related to retinal detachment post-LASIK and refer patients to a retinal specialist appropriately, to promote the best visual outcome.

Case Background

A 60-year-old man with myopia (−6.50 D OD and −6.75 D OS) complained of visual loss OS 1 month after a LASIK procedure. His visual acuity was 20/80, and his biomicroscopy showed a nuclear sclerosis of 2+. A dilated fundoscopy showed a subtotal retinal detachment (macula off) from 10:00 to 5:00 o'clock, posterior vitreous detachment, and round and horseshoe retinal tears at 5:30 o'clock (Figs. 101.1 and 101.2).

Main Problem to Solve

Factors related to high myopia (including myopic degeneration and amblyopia) can detract from the final functional results, despite a high anatomic success rate of myopic cases. Chan and

J.L. Alió et al. (eds.), *Difficult and Complicated Cases in Refractive Surgery*,
DOI 10.1007/978-3-642-55238-0_101, © Springer-Verlag Berlin Heidelberg 2015

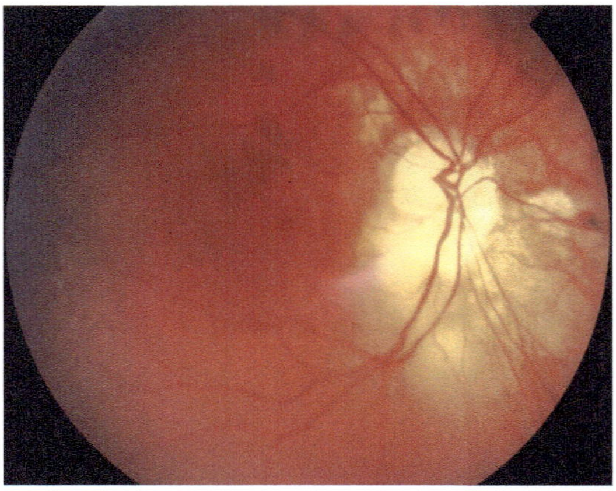

Fig. 101.1 Fundus photograph of a subtotal inferotemporal retinal detachment (macula off) after laser in situ keratomileusis

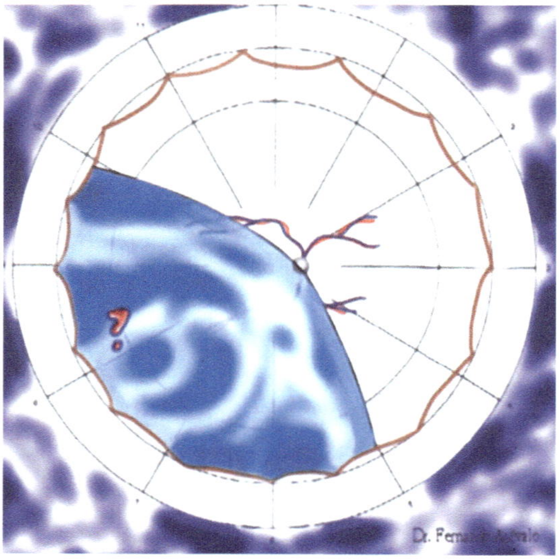

Fig. 101.2 Retinal drawing of the same case with partial posterior vitreous detachment, a horseshoe retinal tear at 8 o'clock and a retinal hole at the same location

coworkers [1] describe the characteristics of a large number of eyes (60) with substantial myopia (mean myopia −9.5 ± 5.8 D) with pre-LASIK retinal examinations (14 eyes had documented lattice degeneration or small retinal breaks) and characteristics of post-LASIK retinal breaks and rhegmatogenous retinal detachments. Many of these eyes developed complex vitreoretinal complications (53.3 % with 2 or more breaks, 26.7 % eyes with 3 or more breaks, 30 % with bilateral conditions, 8.3 % with total RD, 8.3 % with PVR, 6.7 % with giant tears, and 5.0 % with extensive retinal dialysis). Forty percent developed vitreoretinal complications within 6 months of LASIK.

Ancillary Tests

Retinal detachment should be diagnosed clinically. However, a B-scan ultrasound can be performed when the posterior segment view is difficult due to anterior segment opacities.

Surgical/Medical Intervention

A scleral buckling procedure was performed with cryotherapy, with 0.5 cc of 100 % SF6 in the vitreous cavity. Topical steroids and cycloplegics were prescribed.

Outcome

One month later, the patient's LE visual acuity was 20/40 with a completely attached retina.

What to Learn from This Case

Refractive surgeons should recommend that their patients see for a retina specialist before and after the LASIK procedure in order to prevent or treat lesions that could develop retinal detachments such as tears or lattice-risk areas. The referring refractive surgeon should be aware of retinal detachment symptoms (floaters, flashes of light, a shadow or curtain effect across part of the visual field, new or sudden vision loss) to prevent missing an unexpected retinal complication. Due to delay in referral to a vitreoretinal specialist or the particular myopic conditions of the post-LASIK eyes, detachments tend to be more complicated to solve than those occurring in regular conditions [1–4].

References

1. Chan CK, Arevalo JF, Akbatur HH et al (2004) Characteristic of sixty myopic eyes with pre-laser in situ keratomileusis retinal examination and post-laser in situ keratomileusis retinal lesions. Retina 24:706–713
2. Arevalo JF, Ramirez E, Suarez E et al (2000) Retinal detachments after laser-assisted in situ keratomileusis (LASIK) for the correction of myopia. Retina 20:338–341
3. Arevalo JF, Ramirez E, Suarez E et al (2001) Rhegmatogenous retinal detachment in myopic eyes after laser in situ keratomileusis. Frequency, characteristics, and mechanism. J Cataract Refract Surg 27:674–680
4. Arevalo JF, Ramirez E, Suarez E et al (2002) Retinal detachment in myopic eyes after laser in situ keratomileusis. J Refract Surg 18:708–714

Erratum

Difficult and Complicated Cases in Refractive Surgery

Jorge L. Alió • Dimitri T. Azar • Alessandro Abbouda • Amr El Aswad

ISBN 978-3-642-55237-3
ISBN 978-3-642-55238-0 (eBook)
DOI 10.1007/978-3-642-55238-0

Author "Rosario Cobo-Soriano" name is incorrectly captured in chapters 19 and 21 as "Rosario Soriano".

The online version of the original chapters can be found at:
http://dx.doi.org/10.1007/978-3-642-55238-0_19
http://dx.doi.org/10.1007/978-3-642-55238-0_21

J.L. Alió et al. (eds.), *Difficult and Complicated Cases in Refractive Surgery*,
DOI 10.1007/978-3-642-55238-0_102, © Springer-Verlag Berlin Heidelberg 2015

Appendix: Step-By-Step Approach for Planning Refractive Correction of Highly Aberrated Eyes in Excimer Laser Refractive Corneal Surgery

Samuel Arba Mosquera, Tobias Ewering, Jerry Tan, and Por Yong Ming

The controlled change of the corneal curvature to compensate for refractive errors [1] is more accurate than ever. To avoid the induction of aberrations [2] and to try to eliminate already existing aberrations, so-called customized treatments were developed [3]. Customization of the ablation is possible, either using wavefront measurements of the whole eye (obtained, e.g., by Hartmann-Shack wavefront sensors) or by using corneal topography-derived wavefront analyses [4, 5]. Considerations such as duration of treatment, removal [6] and remodeling of tissue, and, in general, the surgical outcomes have made it difficult to establish a universal optimum profile.

Customized laser corneal refractive surgery on aberrated eyes may yield better results than the standard procedure [7–9], but generally results in higher ablation depth, volume, and time. The idea to optimize the customized treatment to reduce the ablated thickness while retaining the positive aspects is therefore pertinent [10].

Samuel Arba Mosquera, Msc
SCHWIND Eye-Tech-Solutions, Mainparkstr. 6-10, D-63801 Kleinostheim, Germany

Grupo de Investigación de Cirugía Refractiva y Calidad de Visión, Instituto de Oftalmobiología Aplicada, University of Valladolid, Valladolid, Spain
samuel.arba.mosquera@eye-tech.net

Tobias Ewering, Dipl.-Ing. (FH),
SCHWIND Eye-Tech-Solutions, Mainparkstr. 6-10, D-63801 Kleinostheim, Germany

Jerry Tan, • Por, Yong Ming, MD,
Jerry Tan Eye Surgery Pte Ltd, Singapore, Singapore

Step-By-Step Approach

Step 1: Decision Tree Analysis

Use first the Decision Tree procedure [11] for determining manifest refraction and for selecting Ocular Wavefront (OW) or Corneal Wavefront (CW) as basis.

Step 2: Refraction

We continue assessing refraction values in order to determine the best starting point for planning the refractive component of the treatment, considering:

(a) Manifest refraction
(b) Aberrometric refraction @ 4 mm
(c) Topographic astigmatism (Maloney @ 3 mm)
(d) WAb astigmatism (without MR input) @ 4 mm
(e) WAb astigmatism (without MR input) @ 6 mm

We select the most representative value for the astigmatism [12].

Step 3: Input Refraction

We load the diagnostic file into the planning software and select the treatment technique [13] as well as the desired optical zone [14] (OZ), planning:

(a) Selected sphere and astigmatism
(b) Selected sphere (consider testing in both negative and positive cylinder conventions, as well as spherical equivalent)
(c) No sphere but selected astigmatism (consider testing in both negative and positive directions, as well as a mixed astigmatism with zero spherical equivalent)

J.L. Alió et al. (eds.), *Difficult and Complicated Cases in Refractive Surgery*,
DOI 10.1007/978-3-642-55238-0, © Springer-Verlag Berlin Heidelberg 2015

For all ablation profiles, we check whether it corresponds to an ablation to regularize the topographic or the wavefront map (plausibility check: if yes, we consider it; otherwise, we discard this possibility), and we note down central and maximum depth (and ablation volume). At this step, we select the refraction resulting in minimum tissue removal.

Step 4: Comparison to Aspheric Treatments

We compare the result of stage 3 (central depth and maximum depth) with the values of an aspheric treatment planned with the same treatment technique as well as OZ, based only on full manifest refraction. We accept the differences in central or maximum ablation of 8–14 µm for 5.25–5.75 mm OZ, 14–16 µm for 5.75–6.25 mm OZ, 16–19 µm for 6.25–6.75 mm OZ, 19–21 µm for 6.75–7.25 mm OZ, and 21–24 µm for >7.25 mm OZ. If the differences are larger than those, we modify the spherical component (iteratively) until the difference for central or maximum ablation depth is within range for the selected OZ.

Step 5: Minimize Tissue Removal

We select Minimize Depth or Minimize Volume [10, 15, 16] (depending on the tissue consumption, in general Minimize Depth for myopic spherical equivalent and Minimize Volume otherwise).

At this point, if we are satisfied with the global savings and the proposed ablation map, we proceed with the plan as is, otherwise, we select Minimize Depth+ or Minimize Volume+ [10, 15, 16].

If we are satisfied with the global savings and the proposed ablation map, we proceed with the plan as is, otherwise, we proceed with the results of the previous stage (comparison to aspheric treatments).

Step 6: Residual Risks

We estimate the refractive risk by comparing the planned refractive correction with the full manifest refraction. We estimate the tissue removal risk by adding the planned customized treatment plus an aspheric treatment planned with the refractive risk and the same treatment technique as well as OZ compared to a full customized treatment using directly the manifest refraction.

Clinical Cases

Case 1

A female patient, who had PRK done in 1993, complained of symptoms of lights smearing inferiorly vertical coma. She refracted to −0.25 DS − 0.75 DC × 167° achieving 6/6 in OD. The Decision Tree procedure [11] recommended CW as a basis for treatment planning (Fig. 1b). We have selected −2.25 DC × 168° as the most representative astigmatism for this eye (Table 1). The spherical component is adjusted to maintain the spherical equivalent, so refraction is rewritten as +0.50 DS − 2.25 DC × 168°.

Manifest sphere input refraction: +0.50 DS has been selected as minimum tissue removal (Table 2, Fig. 1c)

We compared this result with the values of a non-wavefront-guided aspheric treatment planned with the same treatment technique as well as OZ, based only on full manifest refraction (−0.25 DC − 0.75 DC × 167°) (Fig. 1a).

The selected OZ was 6.74, so a difference of up to 19 µm would be acceptable. The actual differences are 15 µm for maximum depth, 7 µm for central depth, and 402 nl for total volume. So we modify the manifest refraction to +0.50 DS − 0.75 DC × 168° (Fig. 1d).

We selected Minimize Volume (Fig. 2):

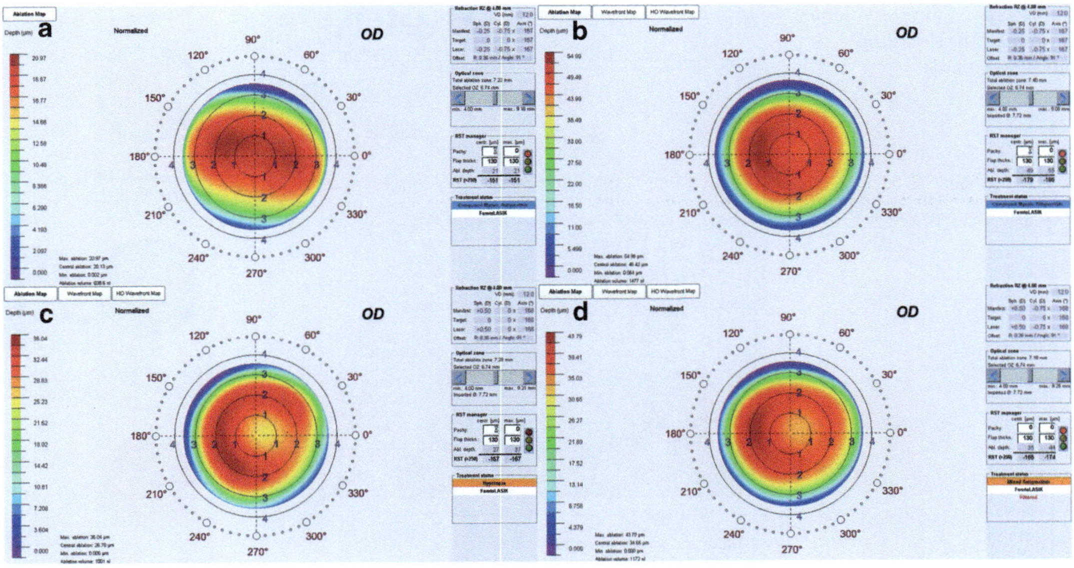

Fig. 1 (**a**) Non-wavefront-guided aspheric treatment planned with the same treatment technique as well as OZ, based only on full manifest refraction (–0.25 DS – 0.75 1DC × 167°). (**b**) Full-wavefront-guided aspheric treatment. (**c**) Input refraction +0.50 DS has been selected as minimum tissue removal. (**d**) Modify the input refraction to +0.50 DS – 0.75 DC × 168° to be closer to the non-wavefront-guided aspheric treatment tissue depth

Table 1 OD refractions for Case 1

Refraction mode	Sphere (D)	Cylinder (D)	Axis (deg)	Spherical equivalent (D)
Manifest refraction	–0.25	–0.75	167	–0.62
Aberrometric refraction at 4 mm	–0.93	–1.54	158	–1.70
Topographic astigmatism (Maloney ai 3 mm)	–	–3.55	166	–
WAb astigmatism (without MR input) at 4 mm	–	–2.38	173	–
WAb astigmatism (without MR input) at 6 mm	–	–2.54	175	–

Table 2 Depth and volume for the different input refractions in combination with the selected wavefront map for Case 1

Refraction mode	Refraction values	Max depth (μm)	Central depth (μm)	Volume (nl)
Selected sphere and astigmatism	+0.50 DS – 2.25 DC × 168°	71	61	2,074
Selected sphere	**+0.50 DS**	**36**	**27**	**1,001**
Selected sphere	–0.63 DS	53	47	1,386
Selected sphere	–1.75 DS	71	67	1,830
Selected astigmatism	0.00 DS – 2.25 DC × 168°	79	71	2,338
Selected astigmatism	+1.13 DS – 2.25 DC × 168°	62	49	1,764
Selected astigmatism	+2.25 DS – 2.25 DC × 168°	50	30	1,482

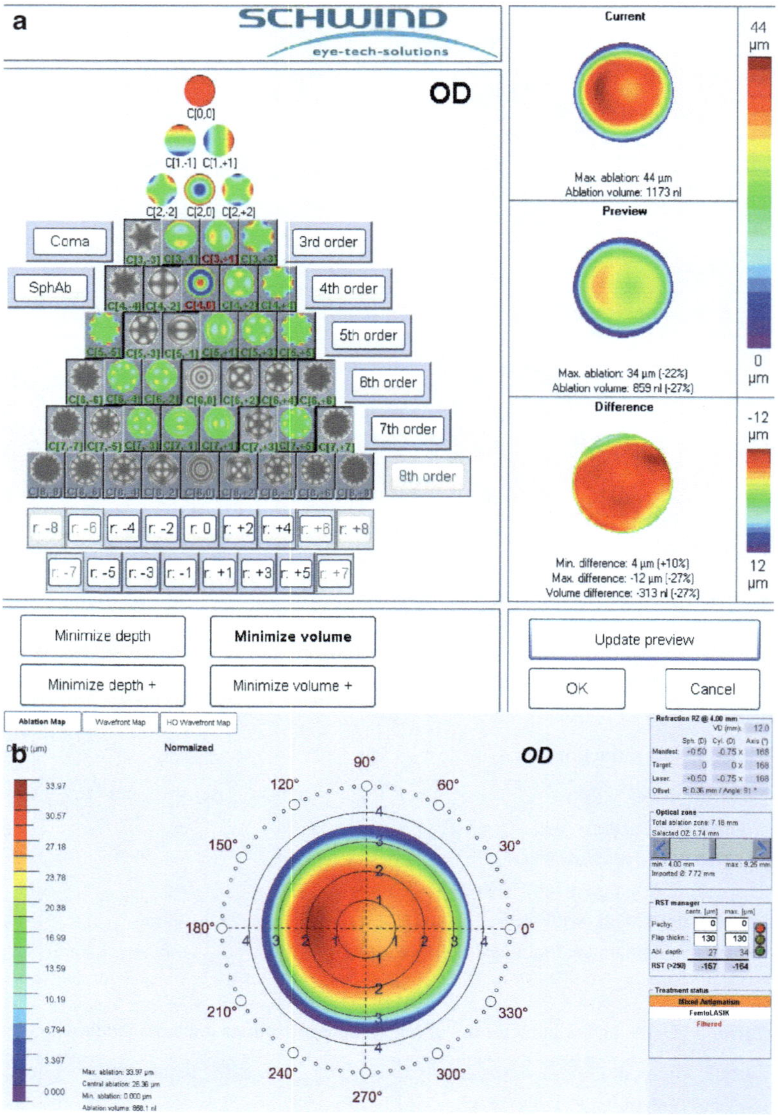

Fig. 2 (**a**) Minimize Volume selection. (**b**) Resulting ablation volume

At this point, the actual differences with the non-wavefront-guided aspheric treatment as reference are 13 µm for maximum depth, 6 µm for central depth, and 259 nl for total volume, whereas the actual differences with the full-wavefront-guided aspheric treatment as reference are −21 µm for maximum depth, −22 µm for central depth, and −619 nl for total volume.

The refractive risk is in this case −0.75 DS, and the tissue removal risk is zero, since the actual differences of adding the planned customized treatment plus an aspheric treatment planned with the refractive risk and the same treatment technique as well as OZ with the full-wavefront-guided aspheric treatment as reference are −5 µm for maximum depth, −7 µm for central depth, and −245 nl for total volume.

Case 2

A male patient, who had bilateral LASIK elsewhere for preoperative myopia of about −5 D in 2010, and postoperatively has been having persistent halos and poor visual quality. He refracted to −0.25 DS − 0.25 DC × 86° achieving 6/4.5 in

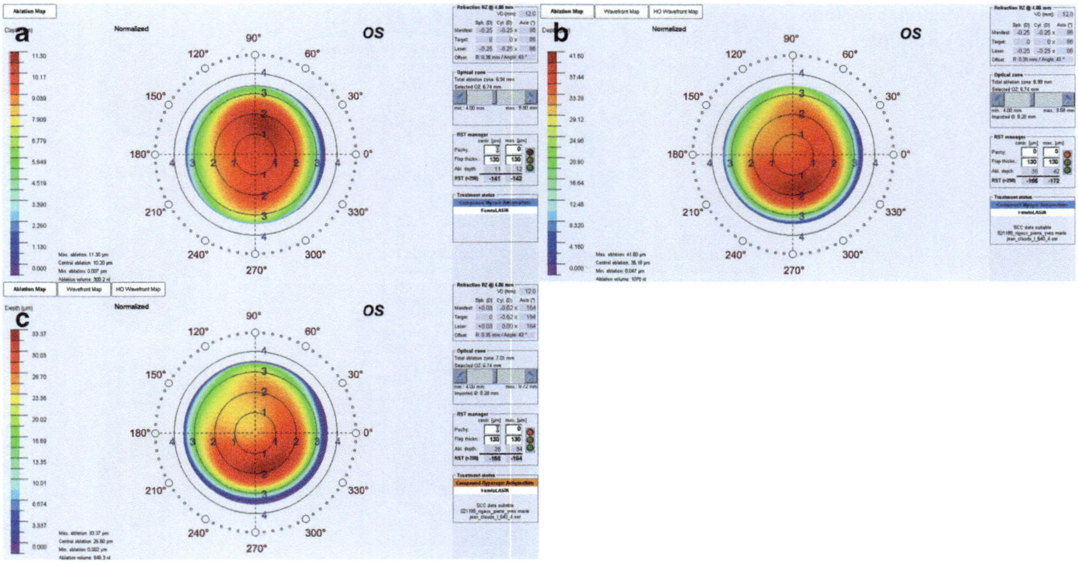

Fig. 3 (**a**) Non-wavefront-guided aspheric treatment planned with the same treatment technique as well as OZ, based only on full manifest refraction (−0.25 DS − 0.25 DC × 86°). (**b**) Full-wavefront-guided aspheric treatment. (**c**) Input refraction +0.03 DS selected as minimum tissue removal

Table 3 OS refractions for Case 2

Refraction mode	Sphere (D)	Cylinder (D)	Axis (deg)	Spherical equivalent (D)
Manifest refraction	−0.25	−0.25	86	−0.38
Aberrometric refraction at 4 mm	−0.17	−0.23	101	−0.28
Topographic astigmatism (Maloney at 3 mm)	–	−1.44	166	–
WAb astigmatism (without MR input) at 4 mm	–	−0.77	171	–
WAb astigmatism (without MR input) at 6 mm	–	−0.97	173	–

Table 4 Depth and volume for the different input refractions in combination with the selected wavefront map for Case 2

Refraction mode	Refraction values	Max depth (μm)	Central depth (μm)	Volume (nl)
Selected sphere and astigmatism	+0.03 DS − 0.62 DC × 164°	43	36	1,149
Selected sphere	**+0.03 DS**	**33**	**26**	**848**
Selected sphere	−0.28 DS	38	31	955
Selected sphere	−0.59 DS	42	37	1,073
Selected astigmatism	0.00 DS − 0.62 DC × 164°	43	36	1,161
Selected astigmatism	+0.62 DS − 0.62 DC × 164°	35	26	959
Selected astigmatism	+0.31 DS − 0.62 DC × 164°	39	31	1,041

OS but he complains of poor visual quality. The Decision Tree procedure [11] recommended CW as a basis for treatment planning (Fig. 3b).

We have selected −0.62 DC × 164° as the most representative astigmatism for this eye (Table 3). The spherical component is adjusted to maintain the spherical equivalent, so refraction is rewritten as +0.03 DS − 0.62 DC × 164°.

Input refraction +0.03 DS has been selected as minimum tissue removal (Table 4, Fig. 3c).

We compared this result with the values of a non-wavefront-guided aspheric treatment planned

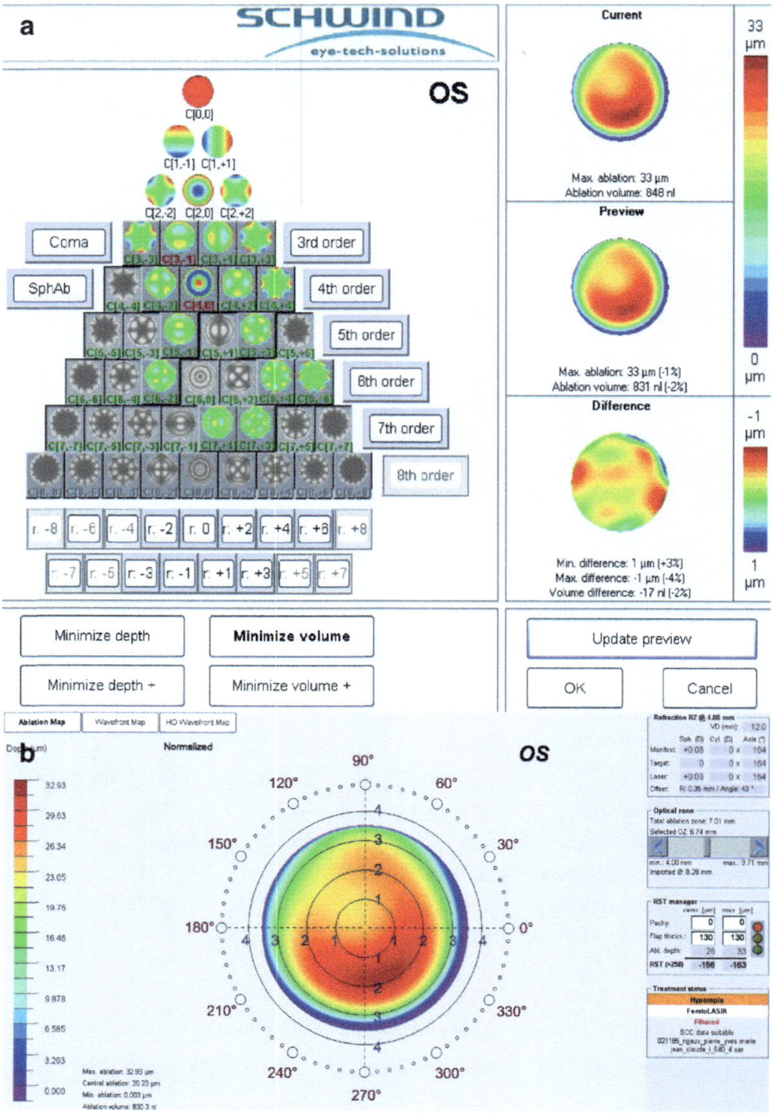

Fig. 4 (**a**) Minimize Volume selection. (**b**) Resulting ablation volume

with the same treatment technique as well as OZ, based only on full manifest refraction (–0.25 DS – 0.25 DC × 86°) (Fig. 3a).

The selected OZ was 6.74, so a difference of up to 19 μm would be acceptable. The actual differences are 22 μm for maximum depth, 16 μm for central depth, and 549 nl for total volume.

We selected Minimize Volume (Fig. 4):

At this point, the actual differences with the non-wavefront-guided aspheric treatment as reference are 22 μm for maximum depth, 15 μm for central depth, and 531 nl for total volume, whereas the actual differences with the full-wavefront-guided aspheric treatment as reference are –9 μm for maximum depth, –10 μm for central depth, and –240 nl for total volume.

The refractive risk is in this case –0.25 DS – 0.25 DC × 86°, and the tissue removal risk is 2 μm for maximum depth, 0 μm for central depth, and 59 nl for total volume.

Case 3

A female patient, who had bilateral LASIK for preoperative myopia of about –10 D back on 2001. Her 3 months post op refraction was +0.75 DS – 0.25 DC × 105° and complained of

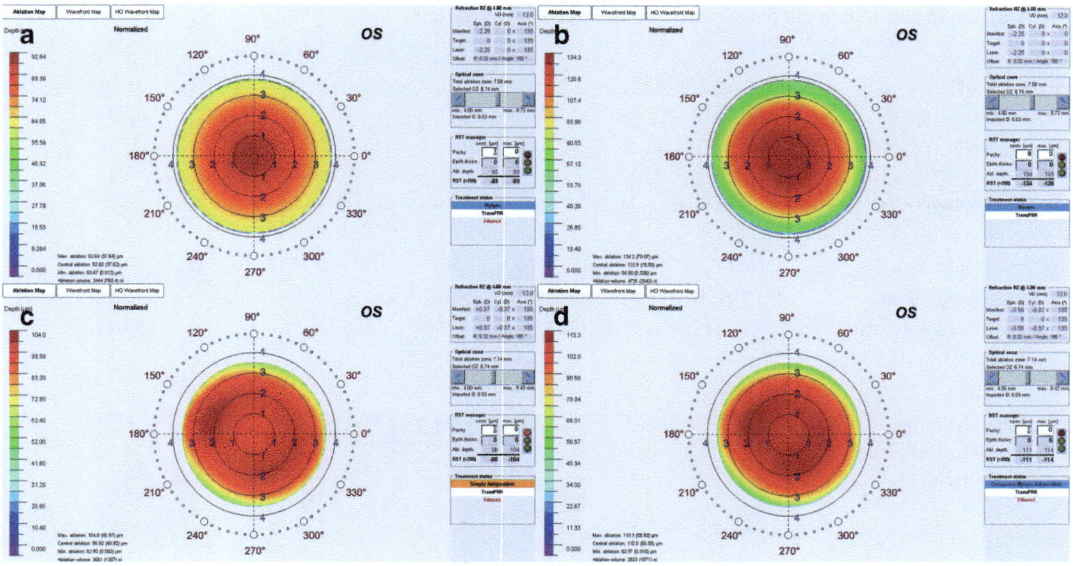

Fig. 5 (**a**) Non-wavefront-guided aspheric treatment planned with the same treatment technique as well as OZ, based only on full manifest refraction (–2.25 DS). (**b**) Full-wavefront-guided aspheric treatment. (**c**) Input refraction (+0.37 DS – 0.37 DC × 135°) selected as minimum tissue removal. (**d**) Modify input refraction to –0.50 DS – 0.37 DC × 135° to be closer to the non-wavefront-guided aspheric treatment tissue depth

Table 5 OS refractions for Case 3

Refraction mode	Sphere (D)	Cylinder (D)	Axis (deg)	Spherical equivalent (D)
Manifest refraction	–2.25	0	0	–2.25
Aberrometric refraction at 4 mm	–2.25	–0.13	150	–2.31
Topographic astigmatism (Maloney at 3 mm)	–	–0.65	32	–
WAb astigmatism (without MR input) at 4 mm	–	–0.35	178	–
WAb astigmatism (without MR input) at 6 mm	–	–0.57	171	–

glare and halos, refraction regressed to –2.25 DS in 10 years. She refracted to –2.25 DS achieving 6/6 in OS but she complained of poor visual quality. The Decision Tree procedure [11] recommended CW as a basis for treatment planning (Fig. 5b).

We have selected –0.37 DC × 135° as the most representative astigmatism for this eye (Table 5). The spherical component is adjusted to maintain the spherical equivalent, so refraction is rewritten as –2.06 DS – 0.37 DC × 135°.

Selected astigmatism as input refraction (+0.37 DS – 0.37 DC × 135°) has been selected as minimum tissue removal (Table 6, Fig. 5c).

We compared this result with the values of a non-wavefront-guided aspheric treatment planned with the same treatment technique as well as OZ, based only on full manifest refraction (–2.25 DS) (Fig. 5a).

The selected OZ was 6.74, so a difference of up to 19 μm would be acceptable. The actual differences are 11 μm for maximum depth, 3 μm for central depth, and 217 nl for total volume. So we modify the input refraction to –0.50 DS – 0.37 DC × 135° (Fig. 5d).

We selected Minimize Depth (Fig. 6):

At this point, the actual differences with the non-wavefront-guided aspheric treatment as

Table 6 Depth and volume for the different input refractions for Case 3

Refraction mode	Refraction values	Maximum depth (µm)	Central depth (µm)	Ablation volume (nl)
Selected sphere and astigmatism	−2.06 DS − 0.37 DC × 135°	137	137	4,833
Selected sphere	−2.06 DS	131	131	4,615
Selected sphere	−2.25 DS	134	134	4,725
Selected sphere	−2.43 DS	137	137	4,839
Selected astigmatism	0.00 DS − 0.37 DC × 135°	108	102	3,774
Selected astigmatism	+0.19 DS − 0.37 DC × 135°	106	99	3,650
Selected astigmatism	**+0.37 DS − 0.37 DC × 135°**	**104**	**96**	**3,661**

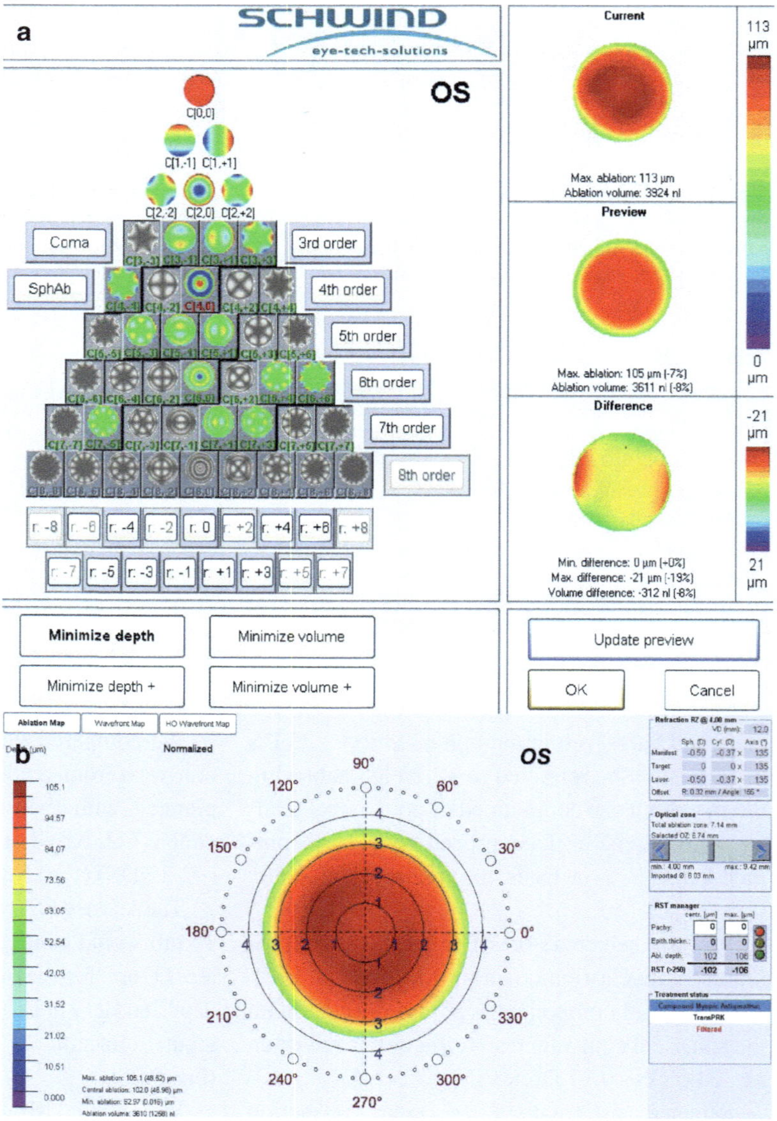

Fig. 6 (**a**) Minimize Depth selection. (**b**) Resulting ablation volume

reference are 12 μm for maximum depth, 9 μm for central depth, and 166 nl for total volume, whereas the actual differences with the full-wavefront-guided aspheric treatment as reference are −29 μm for maximum depth, −32 μm for central depth, and −1,115 nl for total volume.

The refractive risk is in this case −1.35 DS − 0.38 DC × 45°, and the tissue removal risk is zero, since the actual differences of adding the planned customized treatment plus an aspheric treatment planned with the refractive risk and the same treatment technique as well as OZ with the full-wavefront-guided aspheric treatment as reference are 0 μm for maximum depth, −3 μm for central depth, and −489 nl for total volume.

Discussion

Wavefront-guided treatments have a higher risk of overcorrections. CW treatments have a risk for overcorrections higher than OW treatments (especially because CW treatments cannot determine defocus or in general manifest refraction values). The risk for overcorrections in wavefront-guided (WFG) treatments increases for higher wavefront errors. Reasons for these extra risks for overcorrections in generally speaking WFG treatments are:

- They attempt to correct HOA + refraction.
  - In particular they attempt to correct coma + high-order astigmatism (HOAst) + astigmatism (Ast), but manifest Ast is influenced by coma and by HOAst, so they may be correcting manifest Ast "twice" and inducing overcorrections.
  - More often, they attempt to correct SphAb + defocus, but manifest Sph is influenced by SphAb, so they may be correcting manifest defocus "twice" and inducing overcorrections.
- Modern software planning platforms for laser corneal refractive surgery claim to compensate for the refraction of HOAb, but they can only compensate this from an optical basis, whereas manifest refraction has a visual basis. Further the (optical) compensation for this is usually made for a static virtual pupil of given size which is concentric to and within the measured aberrations disk, whereas the actual pupil may be different in size and center. This compensation and the wavefront refraction are based on the optical properties of the wavefront referenced to the pupil center, but the visual axis is the reference for manifest refraction.
- Even if this compensation is optically perfect, at the moment of the ablation due to their simplicity, the parabolic terms (low orders) may be more efficiently corrected than HO terms, so parabolic terms are corrected in full (including optical compensations), but HO terms are corrected in part (undercorrecting the WF part of the treatment), and as a sum it also ends up in refractive overcorrections (you overcompensate parabolic terms to anticipate refractive changes from HO terms. But these refractive changes from HO terms only occur partly due to undercorrection of the HO components).

We have two levels for judging the ablations which we recommend:

1. Compare ablation depth to a non-wavefront-guided aspheric treatment planned with the same treatment technique as well as OZ, based only on full manifest refraction. We do recommend to accept differences in central or maximum ablation compatible with no more than 1D of refractive deviation. If the differences are larger than those, we would recommend to adjust the sphere until the difference is within range for the selected OZ.
2. Use minimize functions [10, 15, 16]. "Minimize Depth" or "Minimize Volume" combines low-order and high-order aberrations out of the pyramid to receive the least amount of depth or volume. Minor coefficient values will be taken out only if they contribute to minimized tissue removal. With the addition "+," moderate coefficients that contribute to tissue sparing can be disabled, as well. Observe always, with the help of the preview, similarities between full HOA correction profile and current selection.

Coupling effects between different high-order aberration terms and between HOAs and manifest refraction have been found [17–19]. These interactions may provide some relative visual benefits [20], but may as well contribute as sources of uncertainty in the conversion of wavefront aberration maps to refractive prescriptions [21, 22].

Since we may manipulate to some extent Sph and Cyl components to accommodate to less tissue removal, we have a risk of under/overcorrections. But consider that those under/overcorrections even when occurring had saved tissue, so the spared tissue is still available for further re-treatments, for which a more regular less aberrated optical system is expected with an easier and more trustable refraction.

Our experience suggests that wavefront-customized treatments can only be successful if pre-existing aberrations are greater than repeatability (e.g., repeatability of diagnostic [23] and treatment devices) and biological noise (e.g., day-to-day variabilities in visual acuity, refraction, or aberration in the same subject). Recently published studies by Stonecipher et al. [24] and by Venter [25] illustrated similar findings.

There are different proposed approaches for minimizing tissue ablation in refractive surgery:

In the multizonal treatments and treatments planned with smaller OZ combined with bigger transition zones, the minimization is based on the concept of progressive decreasing corrections in different OZs. The problem comes from the induced aberrations (especially spherical aberration).

In the treatments planned with smaller OZ for the cylindrical component (in general for the most powerful correction axis), the minimization is based upon the concept of the maximal depth being based on the lowest meridional refraction and the selected OZ, and the effective OZ of the highest meridional refraction is reduced to match the same maximal depth. The problem comes from the induced aberrations (especially high-order astigmatism).

In the Z-shift and Z-clip methods, minimization consists of defining either a "threshold value" or a "saturation depth" for the ablated volume, no points planned to ablate less than the threshold value are ablated, and the rest of the points are ablated by an amount equal to the original planned ablation minus the threshold value, whereas all points planned to ablate deeper than the saturation value are ablated only by an amount equal to the saturation value. The problem comes from the fact that these "threshold value" and "saturation limit" may occur anywhere in the ablation volume, compromising the refraction when they occur close to the ablation center, and the functional OZ when occurring at the periphery, and affecting the induction of aberrations in a complicated way.

The present report could be useful to better understand that not the full refraction and not all aberrations need to be corrected to improve vision in customized treatments in the eyes with previous large amount of aberrations.

References

1. Munnerlyn CR, Koons SJ, Marshall J (1998) Photorefractive keratectomy: a technique for laser refractive surgery. J Cataract Refract Surg 14: 46–52
2. Hersh PS, Fry K, Blaker JW (2003) Spherical aberration after laser in situ keratomileusis and photorefractive keratectomy. Clinical results and theoretical models of etiology. J Cataract Refract Surg 29:2096–2104
3. Mrochen M, Kaemmerer M, Seiler T (2001) Clinical results of wavefront-guided laser in situ keratomileusis 3 months after surgery. J Cataract Refract Surg 27:201–207
4. Salmon TO (1999) Corneal contribution to the Wavefront aberration of the eye. PhD dissertation, p 70
5. Mrochen M, Jankov M, Bueeler M, Seiler T (2003) Correlation between corneal and total wavefront aberrations in myopic eyes. J Refract Surg 19:104–112
6. Gatinel D, Malet J, Hoang-Xuan T, Azar DT (2002) Analysis of customized corneal ablations: theoretical limitations of increasing negative asphericity. Invest Ophthalmol Vis Sci 43:941–948
7. Arbelaez MC, Arba Mosquera S (2009) The SCHWIND AMARIS total-tech laser as an all-rounder in refractive surgery. Middle East Afr J Ophthalmol 16:46–53
8. Arbelaez MC, Vidal C, Arba Mosquera S (2009) Clinical outcomes of corneal wavefront customized ablation strategies with SCHWIND CAM in LASIK treatments. Ophthalmic Physiol Opt 29:487–496

9. Arbelaez MC, Vidal C, Arba Mosquera S (2009) Clinical outcomes of LASIK for myopia using the SCHWIND platform with ocular wavefront customized ablation. J Refract Surg 25:1083–1090
10. Arba Mosquera S, de Ortueta D, Merayo-Lloves J (2009) Tissue-saving zernike terms selection in customized treatments for refractive surgery. J Optom 2:182–196
11. Arbelaez MC, Ewering T, Arba Mosquera S (2010) Decision assistant wizard to standardize optimal outcomes in excimer laser refractive corneal surgery. J Refract Surg 26:980–990
12. Arbelaez MC, Vidal C, Arba Mosquera S (2009) Excimer laser correction of moderate to high astigmatism with a non-wavefront-guided aberration-free ablation profile: six-month results. J Cataract Refract Surg 35:1789–1798
13. Arbelaez MC, Vidal C, Arba Mosquera S (2011) Comparison of LASEK and LASIK with thin and ultrathin flaps after excimer laser ablation with the SCHWIND Aspheric ablation profile. J Refract Surg 27:38–48
14. Camellin M, Arba Mosquera S (2011) Aspheric optical zones: the effective optical zone with the SCHWIND AMARIS. J Refract Surg 27(2):135–46
15. Arba Mosquera S, de Ortueta D (2011) Optimized zernike terms selection in customized treatments for laser corneal refractive surgery: a case report. J Refract Surg 27:148–152
16. Arba-Mosquera S, Arbelaez MC, Merayo-Llovés J (2011) Six-month clinical outcomes of customised treatments minimized for depth and time in laser corneal refractive surgery. Cornea 30:876–888
17. Bará S, Arines J, Ares J, Prado P (2006) Direct transformation of Zernike eye aberration coefficients between scaled, rotated, and/or displaced pupils. J Opt Soc Am A 23:2061–2066
18. MacRae S (2007) Aberration interaction in aberration interaction in wavefront guided custom wavefront guided custom ablation. Wavefront Congress, Santa Fe
19. Bühren J, Yoon GY, Kenner S, Artrip S, MacRae S, Huxlin K (2007) The effect of decentration on lower- and higher-order aberrations after myopic photorefractive keratectomy (PRK) in a cat model. Wavefront Congress, Santa Fe
20. McLellan JS, Prieto PM, Marcos S, Burns SA (2006) Effects of interactions among wave aberrations on optical image quality. Vision Res 46:3009–3016
21. Thibos LN (2004) Unresolved issues in the prediction of subjective refraction from wavefront aberration maps. J Refract Surg 20:S533–536
22. Cheng X, Bradley A, Thibos LN (2004) Predicting subjective judgment of best focus with objective image quality metrics. J Vis 4:310–321
23. Holzer MP, Sassenroth M, Auffarth GU (2006) Reliability of corneal and total wavefront aberration measurements with the SCHWIND Corneal and Ocular Wavefront Analyzers. J Refract Surg 22:917–920
24. Stonecipher KG, Kezirian GM (2008) Wavefront-optimized versus wavefront-guided LASIK for myopic astigmatism with the ALLEGRETTO WAVE: three-month results of a prospective FDA trial. J Refract Surg. 24:S424–S430
25. Venter J (2008) Wavefront-guided custom ablation for myopia using the NIDEK NAVEX laser system. J Refract Surg 24:487–493

GPSR Compliance

The European Union's (EU) General Product Safety Regulation (GPSR) is a set of rules that requires consumer products to be safe and our obligations to ensure this.

If you have any concerns about our products, you can contact us on ProductSafety@springernature.com

In case Publisher is established outside the EU, the EU authorized representative is:

Springer Nature Customer Service Center GmbH
Europaplatz 3
69115 Heidelberg, Germany

Batch number: 10731361

Printed by Printforce, the Netherlands